PRINCIPLES OF
PULMONARY MEDICINE

FIFTH EDITION

PRINCIPLES OF
PULMONARY MEDICINE

Steven E. Weinberger, MD, FACP
Senior Vice President for Medical Education and Publishing
Adjunct Professor of Medicine
University of Pennsylvania School of Medicine
American College of Physicians
Philadelphia, Pennsylvania
Senior Lecturer on Medicine
Harvard Medical School
Boston, Massachusetts

Barbara A. Cockrill, MD
Clinical Director
Pulmonary Vascular Disease Program
Pulmonary and Critical Care Unit
Massachusetts General Hospital
Assistant Professor of Medicine
Harvard Medical School
Boston, Massachusetts

Jess Mandel, MD, FACP
Associate Professor of Medicine
Associate Dean, Division of Medical Education
University of California San Diego School of Medicine
San Diego, California

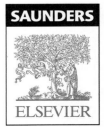

SAUNDERS

ELSEVIER

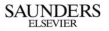

SAUNDERS
ELSEVIER

1600 John F. Kennedy Blvd.
Ste 1800
Philadelphia, PA 19103-2899

PRINCIPLES OF PULMONARY MEDICINE, FIFTH EDITION   ISBN: 978-1-4160-5034-6

Library of Congress Cataloging-in-Publication Data
Weinberger, Steven E.
Principles of pulmonary medicine / Steven E. Weinberger, Barbara A. Cockrill, Jess Mandel. – 5th ed.
   p. ; cm.
Includes bibliographical references and index.
ISBN 978-1-4160-5034-6 (alk. paper)
1. Lungs–Diseases. I. Cockrill, Barbara A. II. Mandel, Jess. III. Title.
[DNLM: 1. Lung Diseases. WF 600 W423p 2008]

RC756.W45 2008
616.2'4–dc22   2007050196

Acquisitions Editor: Dolores Meloni
Developmental Editor: Kimberly DePaul
Project Manager: Bryan Hayward
Design Direction: Steven Stave
Marketing Manager: Bill Veltre

Printed in the United States of America

Working together to grow libraries in developing countries

www.elsevier.com | www.bookaid.org | www.sabre.org

ELSEVIER   BOOK AID International   Sabre Foundation

Last digit is the print number: 9 8 7 6 5 4 3 2 1

To Janet, Eric, and Mark.
Steven Weinberger

To my parents, Fred and Shirley Cockrill.
Barbara Cockrill

To my parents, who first inspired me and who inspire me still.
Jess Mandel

Introduction
to the Fifth Edition

Now in its Fifth Edition, *Principles of Pulmonary Medicine* has remained true to its original goal—serving as a readable introductory text that provides a pathophysiologic approach to disorders affecting the respiratory system. Originally (and still primarily) intended as a text that could be read in its entirety by medical students during their preclinical respiratory pathophysiology course, it has additionally been used by a much wider audience, including medical students during their clinical experiences, house staff and fellows who are particularly interested in an approach that links clinical medicine with its scientific and pathophysiologic foundations, and other health professionals who care for patients with pulmonary disease. The text is based on an integrative approach, correlating diseases with their physiologic effects, the patterns they produce on imaging studies, and their histopathologic appearances. Although the content and the references have been substantially updated from the Fourth Edition, the basic structure of the text is unchanged, with margin notes summarizing some of the key points covered in the text and serving as a valuable review.

There are two particularly important changes in the Fifth Edition. First, two new authors (BC and JM) have joined the single author of the first four editions (SW). All three of us have taught the subject matter of this book to medical students and trainees at all levels and at several different institutions (Harvard University, University of Pennsylvania, University of Iowa, and University of California, San Diego). We have updated this edition based on many years of experience conveying the concepts and information to individuals in the formative stages of learning about pulmonary medicine. Second, we have added a Web-based component that provides the reader with multiple choice self-assessment questions, a more extensive collection of images, and audio files of auscultatory findings in patients with lung disease.

It continues to be a pleasure to work with the editorial staff at Elsevier, and we are particularly grateful to Dolores Meloni and Kim DePaul for their invaluable assistance in preparation of the book. We also wish to thank Elsevier for providing us with material from their extensive library of publications that we could use for the additional Web-based resources that we are providing with this edition. Finally, we are most grateful to our spouses and children, who were most understanding, patient, and supportive to us while we sacrificed a significant amount of our precious time with them in order to develop the new edition of this book.

Steven E. Weinberger, MD, FACP
Barbara A. Cockrill, MD
Jess Mandel, MD, FACP

CONTENTS

CHAPTER 1

Pulmonary Anatomy and Physiology— The Basics

ANATOMY	Oxygen Transport
PHYSIOLOGY	Carbon Dioxide Transport
Mechanical Aspects of the Lungs and Chest Wall	Ventilation-Perfusion Relationships
Ventilation	**ABNORMALITIES IN GAS EXCHANGE**
Circulation	Hypoxemia
Diffusion	Hypercapnia

To be effective at gas exchange, the lungs cannot act in isolation. The lungs must inter-act with the central nervous system (which provides the rhythmic drive to breathe); the diaphragm and muscular apparatus of the chest wall (which respond to signals from the central nervous system and act as a bellows for movement of air); and the circulatory system (which provides blood flow and, therefore, gas transport between the tissues and the lungs). The processes of oxygen uptake and carbon dioxide elimi-nation by the lungs depend on the functioning of all these systems, and a disturbance in any of them can result in clinically important abnormalities in gas transport and thus arterial blood gases. This chapter begins with an initial overview of pulmonary anatomy, followed by a discussion of mechanical properties of the lungs and chest wall and a consideration of some aspects of the contribution of the lungs and the circula-tory system to gas exchange. Additional discussion of pulmonary and circulatory physiology is presented in Chapters 4, 8, and 12; neural, muscular, and chest wall in-teractions with the lungs are discussed further in Chapter 17.

ANATOMY

It is appropriate when discussing the anatomy of the respiratory system to include the entire pathway for airflow from the mouth or nose down to the alveolar sacs. En route to the alveoli, gas flows through the oropharynx or nasopharynx, the larynx, the trachea, and finally a progressively arborizing system of bronchi and bronchioles (Fig. 1-1). The trachea divides at the carina into right and left mainstem bronchi, which branch into lobar bronchi (three on the right, two on the left), segmental bron-chi, and an extensive system of subsegmental and smaller bronchi. These conducting airways divide approximately 15 to 20 times down to the level of terminal bronchioles, which are the smallest units that do not actually participate in gas exchange.

Conducting airways include all airways down to the level of the terminal bronchioles.

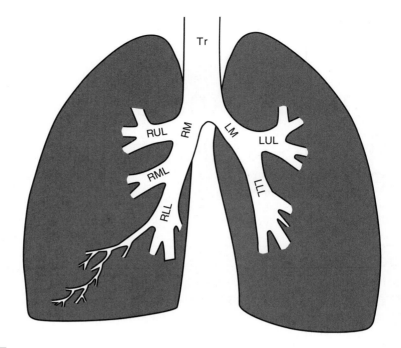

Figure 1-1. Schematic diagram of airway branching. LLL = Left lower lobe bronchus; LM = left mainstem bronchus; LUL = left upper lobe bronchus; RLL = right lower lobe bronchus; RM = right mainstem bronchus; RML = right middle lobe bronchus; RUL = right upper lobe bronchus; Tr = trachea.

The acinus includes structures distal to a terminal bronchiole: respiratory bronchioles, alveolar ducts, and alveoli (alveolar sacs).

Beyond the terminal bronchioles, further divisions include the respiratory bronchioles, the alveolar ducts, and the alveoli. From the respiratory bronchioles on, these divisions form the portion of the lung involved in gas exchange and constitute the terminal respiratory unit or *acinus*. At this level, inhaled gas comes into contact with alveolar walls (septa), and pulmonary capillary blood loads O_2 and unloads CO_2 as it courses through the septa.

The surface area for gas exchange provided by the alveoli is enormous. It is estimated that the adult human lung has on the order of 300 million alveoli, with a total surface area approximately the size of a tennis court. This vast surface area of gas in contact with alveolar walls is a highly efficient mechanism for O_2 and CO_2 transfer between alveolar spaces and pulmonary capillary blood.

The pulmonary capillary network and the blood within provide the other crucial requirement for gas exchange: a transportation system for O_2 and CO_2 to and from other body tissues and organs. After blood arrives at the lungs via the pulmonary artery, it courses through a widely branching system of smaller pulmonary arteries and arterioles to the major locale for gas exchange, the pulmonary capillary network. The capillaries generally allow red blood cells to flow through in single file only so that gas exchange between each cell and alveolar gas is facilitated. On completion of gas exchange and travel through the pulmonary capillary bed, the oxygenated blood flows through pulmonary venules and veins and arrives at the left side of the heart for pumping to the systemic circulation and distribution to the tissues.

Further details about the anatomy of airways, alveoli, and the pulmonary vasculature, particularly with regard to structure-function relationships and cellular anatomy, are given in Chapters 4, 8, and 12.

PHYSIOLOGY

MECHANICAL ASPECTS OF THE LUNGS AND CHEST WALL

The discussion of pulmonary physiology begins with an introduction to a few concepts about the mechanical properties of the respiratory system, which have important implications for assessment of pulmonary function and its derangement in disease states.

The lungs and the chest wall have elastic properties. They have a particular resting size (or volume) that they would assume if no internal or external pressure were exerted on them, and any deviation from this volume requires some additional influencing force. If the lungs were removed from the chest and no longer had the external influences of the chest wall and the pleural space acting on them, they would collapse to the point of being almost airless; they would have a much lower volume than they have within the thoracic cage. To expand these lungs, positive pressure would have to be exerted on the air spaces, as could be done by putting positive pressure through the airway. (Similarly, a balloon is essentially airless unless positive pressure is exerted on the opening to distend the elastic wall and fill it with air.)

Alternatively, instead of positive pressure exerted on alveoli through the airways, negative pressure could be applied outside the lungs to cause their expansion. Thus, what increases the volume of the isolated lungs from the resting, essentially airless, state is the application of a positive *transpulmonary pressure*—the pressure inside the lungs relative to the pressure outside. Internal pressure can be made positive, or external pressure can be made negative; the net effect is the same. With the lungs inside the chest wall, the internal pressure is alveolar pressure, whereas external pressure is the pressure within the pleural space (Fig. 1-2). Therefore, transpulmonary pressure is defined as alveolar pressure (P_{alv}) minus pleural pressure (P_{pl}). For air to be present in the lungs, pleural pressure must be relatively negative compared with alveolar pressure.

> Transpulmonary pressure = $P_{alv} - P_{pl}$.

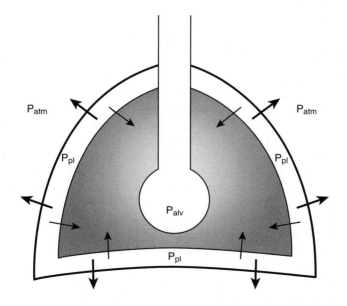

Figure 1-2. Simplified diagram showing the pressures on both sides of the chest wall *(heavy line)* and the lung *(shaded area)*. Thin arrows show the direction of elastic recoil of the lung (at the resting end-expiratory position). Thick arrows show the direction of elastic recoil of the chest wall. P_{alv} = Alveolar pressure; P_{atm} = atmospheric pressure; P_{pl} = pleural pressure.

The relationship between transpulmonary pressure and lung volume can be described for a range of transpulmonary pressures. The plot of this relationship is the *compliance curve* of the lung (Fig. 1-3, *A*). As transpulmonary pressure increases, lung volume naturally increases. However, the relationship is not linear but curvilinear. At relatively high volumes, the lungs reach their limit of distensibility, and even rather large increases in transpulmonary pressure do not result in significant increases in lung volume.

Switching from the lungs to the chest wall, if the lungs were removed from the chest, the chest wall would expand to a larger size when no external or internal pressures were exerted on it. Thus the chest wall has a springlike character. The resting volume is relatively high, and distortion to either a smaller or larger volume requires alteration of either the external or internal pressures acting on it. The pressure across the chest wall is akin to the transpulmonary pressure. Again, with the lungs back inside the chest wall, the pressure across the chest wall is the pleural pressure (internal pressure) minus the external pressure surrounding the chest wall (atmospheric pressure).

The compliance curve of the chest wall relates the volume enclosed by the chest wall to the pressure across the chest wall (Fig. 1-3, *B*). The curve becomes relatively flat at low lung volumes, at which the chest wall becomes stiff. Further changes in the pressure across the chest wall cause little further decrement in volume.

> At FRC, the inward elastic recoil of the lung is balanced by the outward elastic recoil of the chest wall.

In order to examine how the lungs and chest wall behave in situ, remember that the elastic properties of each are acting in opposite directions. At the normal resting end-expiratory position of the respiratory system (*functional residual capacity* [FRC]), the lung is expanded to a volume greater than the resting volume it would have in isolation, whereas the chest wall is contracted to a volume smaller than it would have in isolation. However, at FRC the tendency of the lung to become smaller (the inward or elastic recoil of the lung) is exactly balanced by the tendency of the chest wall to expand (the outward recoil of the chest wall). The transpulmonary pressure at FRC is equal in magnitude to the pressure across the chest wall but acts in an opposite direction (Fig. 1-3, *C*). Therefore pleural pressure is negative, a consequence of the inward recoil of the lungs and the outward recoil of the chest wall.

The chest wall and the lungs can be considered as a unit, the *respiratory system*. The respiratory system has its own compliance curve, which is essentially a combination of the individual compliance curves of the lungs and chest wall (see Fig. 1-3, *C*). The transrespiratory system pressure, again defined as internal pressure minus external pressure, is airway pressure minus atmospheric pressure. At a transrespiratory system pressure of 0, the respiratory system is at its normal resting end-expiratory position, and the volume within the lungs is FRC.

> At TLC, the expanding action of the inspiratory musculature is limited primarily by the inward elastic recoil of the lung.

Two additional lung volumes can be defined, as can the factors that determine each of them. *Total lung capacity* (TLC) is the volume of gas within the lungs at the end of a maximal inhalation. At this point the lungs are stretched well above their resting position, and even the chest wall is stretched beyond its resting position. We are able to distort both the lungs and the chest wall so far from FRC by using our inspiratory muscles, which exert an outward force to counterbalance the inward elastic recoil of the lung and, at TLC, the chest wall. However, at TLC it is primarily the extreme stiffness of the lungs that prevents even further expansion by inspiratory muscle action. Therefore, the primary determinants of TLC are the expanding action of the inspiratory musculature balanced by the inward elastic recoil of the lung.

> At RV, either outward recoil of the chest wall or closure of airways prevents further expiration.

At the other extreme, when we exhale as much as possible, we reach *residual volume* (RV). At this point a significant amount of gas still is present within the lungs; that is, we can never exhale enough to empty the lungs entirely of gas. Again, the reason can be seen by looking at the compliance curves in Figure 1-3, *C*. The chest wall becomes so stiff at low volumes that additional effort by the expiratory muscles is unable to decrease the volume any further. Therefore, RV is determined primarily by the balance of the outward recoil of the chest wall and the contracting action of the

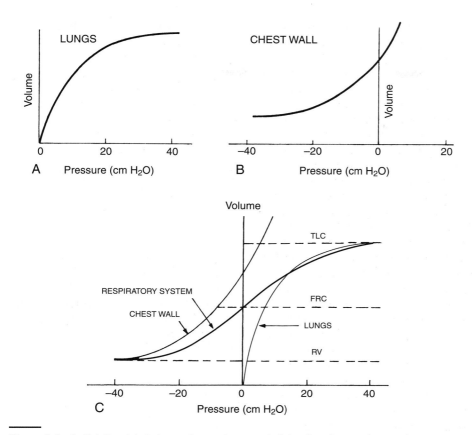

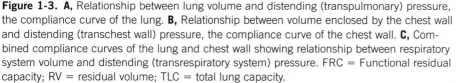

Figure 1-3. A, Relationship between lung volume and distending (transpulmonary) pressure, the compliance curve of the lung. **B,** Relationship between volume enclosed by the chest wall and distending (transchest wall) pressure, the compliance curve of the chest wall. **C,** Combined compliance curves of the lung and chest wall showing relationship between respiratory system volume and distending (transrespiratory system) pressure. FRC = Functional residual capacity; RV = residual volume; TLC = total lung capacity.

expiratory musculature. However, this simple model for RV applies only to the young individual with normal lungs and airways. With age or with disease of the airways, further expulsion of gas during expiration is limited not only by the outward recoil of the chest wall but also by the tendency for airways to close during expiration and for gas to be trapped behind the closed airways.

VENTILATION

To maintain normal gas exchange to the tissues, an adequate volume of air must pass through the lungs for provision of O_2 to and removal of CO_2 from the blood. A normal person at rest typically breathes approximately 500 mL of air per breath at a frequency of 12 to 16 times per minute, resulting in a ventilation of 6 to 8 L/min (*minute ventilation* [$\dot{V}E$]).* The volume of each breath (*tidal volume* [V_T]) is not used entirely for gas exchange; a portion stays in the conducting airways and does not reach the distal part of the lung capable of gas exchange. The portion of the tidal volume that is "wasted"

The volume of each breath (tidal volume [V_T]) is divided into dead space volume (V_D) and alveolar volume (V_A).

*By convention, a dot over a letter adds a time dimension. Hence, $\dot{V}E$ stands for volume of expired gas per minute, that is, minute ventilation. Similar abbreviations used in this chapter are $\dot{V}CO_2$ (volume of CO_2 produced per minute) and $\dot{Q}$ (blood flow per minute).

(in the sense of gas exchange) is termed the *volume of dead space* (V_D), and the volume that reaches the gas-exchanging portion of the lung is the *alveolar volume* (V_A). The *anatomic dead space,* which includes the larynx, trachea, and bronchi down to the level of the terminal bronchioles, is approximately 150 mL in a normal person; thus, 30% of a tidal volume of 500 mL is wasted.

As for CO_2 elimination by the lung, alveolar ventilation ($\dot{V}_A$), which is equal to the breathing frequency (f) multiplied by V_A, bears a direct relationship to the amount of CO_2 removed from the body. In fact, the partial pressure of CO_2 in arterial blood (Pa_{CO_2}) is inversely proportional to $\dot{V}_A$; as $\dot{V}_A$ increases, Pa_{CO_2} decreases. Additionally, Pa_{CO_2} is affected by the body's rate of CO_2 production ($\dot{V}_{CO_2}$); if $\dot{V}_{CO_2}$ increases without any change in $\dot{V}_A$, Pa_{CO_2} shows a proportional increase. Thus, it is easy to understand the relationship given in Equation 1-1:

$$Pa_{CO_2} \propto \dot{V}_{CO_2}/\dot{V}_A \qquad (1\text{-}1)$$

Arterial PCO_2 (Pa_{CO_2}) is inversely proportional to alveolar ventilation ($\dot{V}_A$) and directly proportional to CO_2 production ($\dot{V}_{CO_2}$).	This defines the major factors determining Pa_{CO_2}. When a normal individual exercises, $\dot{V}_{CO_2}$ increases, but $\dot{V}_A$ increases proportionately so that Pa_{CO_2} remains relatively constant.

This defines the major factors determining Pa_{CO_2}. When a normal individual exercises, $\dot{V}_{CO_2}$ increases, but $\dot{V}_A$ increases proportionately so that Pa_{CO_2} remains relatively constant.

As mentioned earlier, the dead space comprises that amount of each breath going to parts of the tracheobronchial tree not involved in gas exchange. The anatomic dead space consists of the conducting airways. In disease states, however, areas of lung that normally participate in gas exchange (parts of the terminal respiratory unit) may not receive normal blood flow, even though they continue to be ventilated. In these areas, some of the ventilation is wasted; such regions contribute additional volume to the dead space.

Hence, a more useful clinical concept than anatomic dead space is *physiologic dead space,* which takes into account the volume of each breath not involved in gas exchange, whether at the level of the conducting airways or the terminal respiratory units. Primarily in certain disease states, in which there may be areas with normal ventilation but decreased or no perfusion, the physiologic dead space is larger than the anatomic dead space.

Quantitation of the physiologic dead space or, more precisely, the fraction of the tidal volume represented by the dead space (V_D/V_T), can be made by measuring PCO_2 in arterial blood (Pa_{CO_2}) and expired gas (PE_{CO_2}) and by using Equation 1-2, known as the *Bohr equation* for physiologic dead space:

The Bohr equation can be used to quantify the fraction of each breath that is wasted, the dead space to tidal volume ratio (V_D/V_T).

$$V_D/V_T = (Pa_{CO_2} - PE_{CO_2})/Pa_{CO_2} \qquad (1\text{-}2)$$

For gas coming directly from alveoli that have participated in gas exchange, PCO_2 approximates that of arterial blood. For gas coming from the dead space, PCO_2 is 0 because the gas never came into contact with pulmonary capillary blood.

Consider the two extremes. If the expired gas came entirely from perfused alveoli, PE_{CO_2} would equal Pa_{CO_2}, and, according to the equation, V_D/V_T would equal 0. On the other hand, if expired gas came totally from the dead space, it would contain no CO_2, PE_{CO_2} would equal 0, and V_D/V_T would equal 1. In practice, this equation is used in situations between these two extremes, and it quantifies the proportion of expired gas coming from alveolar gas ($PCO_2 = Pa_{CO_2}$) versus dead space gas ($PCO_2 = 0$).

In summary, each normal or tidal volume breath can be divided into alveolar volume and dead space, just as the total minute ventilation can be divided into alveolar ventilation and wasted (or dead space) ventilation. Elimination of CO_2 by the lungs is proportional to alveolar ventilation; therefore, Pa_{CO_2} is inversely proportional to alveolar ventilation and not to minute ventilation. The wasted ventilation can be quantified by the Bohr equation, with use of the principle that increasing amounts of dead space ventilation augment the difference between PCO_2 in arterial blood and expired gas.

CIRCULATION

Because the entire cardiac output flows from the right ventricle to the lungs and back to the left side of the heart, the pulmonary circulation handles a blood flow of approximately 5 L/min. If the pulmonary vasculature were similar in structure to the systemic vasculature, large pressures would need to be generated because of the thick walls and high resistance offered by systemic-type arteries. However, pulmonary arteries are quite different in structure from systemic arteries, with thin walls that provide much less resistance to flow. Thus, despite equal right and left ventricular outputs, the normal mean pulmonary artery pressure of 15 mm Hg is much lower than the normal mean aortic pressure of approximately 95 mm Hg.

One important feature of blood flow in the pulmonary capillary bed is the distribution of flow in different areas of the lung. The pattern of flow is explained to a large degree by the effect of gravity and the need for blood to be pumped "uphill" to reach the apices of the lungs. In the upright person, the apex of each lung is approximately 25 cm higher than the base, so the pressure in pulmonary vessels at the apex is 25 cm H$_2$O (19 mm Hg) lower than in pulmonary vessels at the bases. Because flow through these vessels depends on the perfusion pressure, the capillary network at the bases receives much more flow than do capillaries at the apices. In fact, flow at the lung apices falls to 0 during the part of the cardiac cycle when pulmonary artery pressure is insufficient to pump blood up to the apices.

West developed a model of pulmonary blood flow that divides the lung into zones, based on the relationships among pulmonary arterial, venous, and alveolar pressures (Fig. 1-4). As stated earlier, the vascular pressures, that is, pulmonary arterial and venous, depend in part on the vertical location of the vessels in the lung because of the hydrostatic effect. Apical vessels have much lower pressure than do basilar vessels, the difference being the vertical distance between them (divided by a correction factor of 1.3 to convert from cm H$_2$O to mm Hg).

> As a result of gravity, there is more blood flow to dependent regions of the lung.

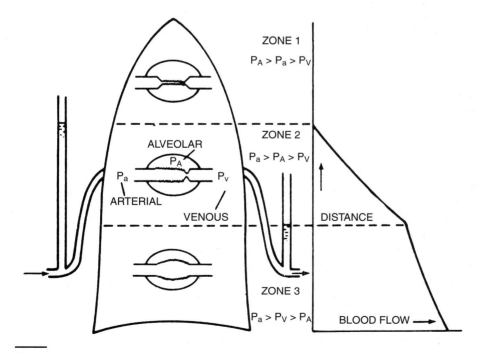

Figure 1-4. Three-zone model of pulmonary blood flow showing relationships among alveolar pressure (PA), arterial pressure (P$_a$), and venous pressure (P$_v$) in each zone. Blood flow (per unit volume of lung) is shown as function of vertical distance on the right. (From West JB, Dollery CT, Naimark A: *J Appl Physiol* 19:713–724, 1964.)

At the apex of the lung (zone 1 in Fig. 1-4), alveolar pressure exceeds arterial and venous pressures, and no flow results. Normally, such a condition does not arise unless pulmonary arterial pressure is decreased or alveolar pressure is increased (by exogenous pressure applied to the airways and alveoli). In zone 2, arterial but not venous pressure exceeds alveolar pressure, and the driving force for flow is determined by the difference between arterial and alveolar pressures. In zone 3, arterial and venous pressures exceed alveolar pressure, and the driving force is the difference between arterial and venous pressures, as is the case in the systemic vasculature.

When cardiac output is increased (e.g., on exercise) the normal pulmonary vasculature is able to handle the increase in flow by recruiting previously unperfused vessels and by distending previously perfused vessels. The ability to expand the pulmonary vascular bed and thus decrease vascular resistance allows major increases in cardiac output with exercise to be accompanied by only small increments in mean pulmonary artery pressure. In disease states that affect the pulmonary vascular bed, however, the ability to recruit additional vessels with increased flow may not exist, and significant increases in pulmonary artery pressure may result.

DIFFUSION

> Normally, equilibration of O_2 and CO_2 between alveolar gas and pulmonary capillary blood is complete in one third the time spent by blood in the pulmonary capillary bed.

For O_2 and CO_2 to be transferred between the alveolar space and blood in the pulmonary capillary, diffusion must take place through several compartments: alveolar gas, alveolar and capillary walls, plasma, and membrane and cytoplasm of the red blood cell. In normal circumstances, the process of diffusion of both gases is relatively rapid, and full equilibration occurs during the transit time of blood flowing through the pulmonary capillary bed. In fact, the Po_2 in capillary blood rises from the mixed venous level of 40 mm Hg* to the end-capillary level of 100 mm Hg in approximately 0.25 second, or one third the total transit time (0.75 second) that an erythrocyte normally spends within the pulmonary capillaries. Similarly, CO_2 transfer is complete within approximately the same amount of time.

Diffusion of O_2 is normally a rapid process, but it is not instantaneous. Resistance to diffusion is provided primarily by the alveolar-capillary membrane and by the reaction that forms oxygenated hemoglobin within the erythrocyte. Each factor provides approximately equal resistance to the transfer of O_2, and each can be disturbed in various disease states. However, as discussed later in this chapter, even when diffusion is measurably impaired, it rarely is a cause of impaired gas exchange. Sufficient time still exists for full equilibration of O_2 or CO_2 unless transit time is significantly shortened, as with exercise.

Even though diffusion limitation rarely contributes to hypoxemia, an abnormality in diffusion may be a useful marker for diseases of the pulmonary parenchyma that affect the alveolar-capillary membrane, the volume of blood in the pulmonary capillaries, or both. Rather than using O_2 to measure diffusion within the lung, clinicians generally use carbon monoxide, which also combines with hemoglobin and is a technically easier test to perform and interpret. The usefulness and meaning of the measurement of diffusing capacity are discussed in Chapter 3.

OXYGEN TRANSPORT

Because the eventual goal of tissue oxygenation requires transport of O_2 from the lungs to the peripheral tissues and organs, any discussion of oxygenation is incomplete without consideration of transport mechanisms.

---

*The units torr and mm Hg can be used interchangeably: 1 torr = 1 mm Hg.

In preparation for this discussion, an understanding of the concepts of *partial pressure, gas content,* and *percent saturation* is essential. The partial pressure of any gas is the product of the ambient total gas pressure and the proportion of total gas composition made up by the specific gas of interest. For example, air is composed of approximately 21% O_2. Assuming a total pressure of 760 mm Hg at sea level and no water vapor pressure, the partial pressure of O_2 (P_{O_2}) is 0.21 × 760, or 160 mm Hg. If the gas is saturated with water vapor at body temperature (37°C), the water vapor has a partial pressure of 47 mm Hg. The partial pressure of O_2 is then calculated on the basis of the remaining pressure, 760 − 47 = 713 mm Hg. Therefore, when room air is saturated at body temperature, P_{O_2} is 0.21 × 713 = 150 mm Hg. Because inspired gas is normally humidified by the upper airway, it becomes fully saturated by the time it reaches the trachea and bronchi, where inspired P_{O_2} is approximately 150 mm Hg.

In clinical situations, we also must consider the concept of partial pressure of a gas within a body fluid, primarily blood. When a liquid is in contact with a gas mixture, the partial pressure of a particular gas in the liquid is the same as its partial pressure in the gas mixture, assuming full equilibration has taken place. Therefore, the partial pressure of the gas acts as the "driving force" for the gas to be carried by the liquid phase.

However, the quantity of a gas that can be carried by the liquid medium depends on the "capacity" of the liquid for that particular gas. If a specific gas is quite soluble within a liquid, more of that gas is carried for a given partial pressure than is a less soluble gas. In addition, if a component of the liquid is able to bind the gas, more of the gas is transported at a particular partial pressure. This is true, for example, of the interaction of hemoglobin and O_2, as more detailed discussion will show.

The content of a gas in a liquid, such as blood, is the actual amount of the gas contained within the liquid. For O_2 in blood, the content is expressed as milliliters of O_2 per 100 mL blood. The percent saturation of a gas is the ratio of the actual content of the gas to the maximal possible content if there is a limit or plateau in the amount that can be carried.

Oxygen is transported in blood in two ways, either dissolved in the blood or bound to the heme portion of hemoglobin. Oxygen is not very soluble in plasma, and only a small amount of O_2 is carried this way under normal conditions. The amount dissolved is proportional to the partial pressure of O_2, with 0.0031 mL dissolved for each millimeter of mercury of partial pressure. The amount bound to hemoglobin is a function of the *oxyhemoglobin dissociation curve,* which relates the driving pressure (P_{O_2}) to the quantity of O_2 bound. This curve reaches a plateau, indicating that hemoglobin can hold only so much O_2 before it becomes fully saturated (Fig. 1-5). At P_{O_2} = 60 mm Hg, hemoglobin is approximately 90% saturated, so only relatively small amounts of additional O_2 are transported at a P_{O_2} above this level.

> Almost all O_2 transported in the blood is bound to hemoglobin; a small fraction is dissolved in plasma.

> Hemoglobin is 90% saturated with O_2 at an arterial P_{O_2} of 60 mm Hg.

This curve can shift to the right or left, depending on a variety of conditions. Thus, the relationships between arterial P_{O_2} and saturation are not fixed. For instance, a decrease in pH or an increase in P_{CO_2} (largely by a pH effect), temperature, or 2,3-diphosphoglycerate (2,3-DPG) levels shifts the oxyhemoglobin dissociation curve to the right, making it easier to unload (or harder to bind) O_2 for any given P_{O_2} (see Fig. 1-5). The opposite changes in pH, P_{CO_2}, temperature, or 2,3-DPG shift the curve to the left and make it harder to unload (or easier to bind) O_2 for any given P_{O_2}. These properties help ensure that oxygen is released preferentially to tissues that are more metabolically active because intense anaerobic metabolism results in decreased pH and elevations in 2,3-DPG, whereas increased heat and CO_2 are generated by intense aerobic metabolism.

Perhaps the easiest way to understand O_2 transport is to follow O_2 and hemoglobin as they course through the circulation in a normal person. When blood leaves the pulmonary capillaries, it has already been oxygenated by equilibration with alveolar

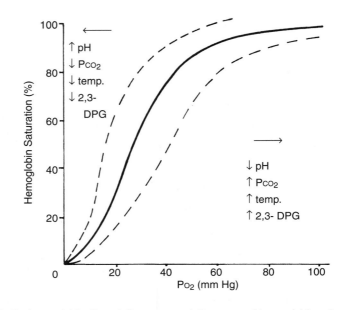

Figure 1-5. Oxyhemoglobin dissociation curve, relating percent hemoglobin saturation and partial pressure of oxygen (Po_2). Oxygen content can be determined on the basis of hemoglobin concentration and percent hemoglobin saturation (see text). Normal curve is depicted with solid line. Curves shifted to right or left (and conditions leading to them) are shown with broken lines. 2,3-DPG = 2,3-Diphosphoglycerate; Pco_2 = partial pressure of carbon dioxide.

gas, and the Po_2 should be identical to that in the alveoli. Because of O_2 uptake and CO_2 excretion at the level of the alveolar-capillary interface, alveolar Po_2 is less than the 150 mm Hg that was calculated for inspired gas within the airways (see discussion on Hypoxemia and Equation 1-7). Alveolar Po_2 in a normal individual (breathing air at sea level) is approximately 100 mm Hg. However, the Po_2 measured in arterial blood actually is slightly lower than this value for alveolar Po_2, partly because of the presence of small amounts of "shunted" blood that do not participate in gas exchange at the alveolar level, e.g., (1) desaturated blood from the bronchial circulation draining into pulmonary veins and (2) venous blood from the coronary circulation draining into the left ventricle via thebesian veins.

Assuming Po_2 = 95 mm Hg in arterial blood, the total O_2 content is the sum of the quantity of O_2 bound to hemoglobin plus the amount dissolved. To calculate the quantity bound to hemoglobin, the patient's hemoglobin level and the percent saturation of the hemoglobin with O_2 must be known. Because each gram of hemoglobin can carry 1.34 mL O_2 when fully saturated, the O_2 content is calculated by Equation 1-3:

$$O_2 \text{ content bound to hemoglobin} = 1.34 \times \text{Hemoglobin} \times \text{Saturation} \tag{1-3}$$

Assume that hemoglobin is 97% saturated at Po_2 = 95 mm Hg and that the individual has a hemoglobin level of 15 g/100 mL blood.

$$
\begin{aligned}
O_2 \text{ content bound to hemoglobin} &= 1.34 \times 15 \times 0.97 \\
&= 19.5 \text{ mL } O_2/100 \text{ mL blood} \tag{1-4}
\end{aligned}
$$

In contrast, the amount of dissolved O_2 is much smaller and is proportional to Po_2, with 0.0031 mL O_2 dissolved per 100 mL blood per mm Hg Po_2. Therefore, at an arterial Po_2 of 95 mm Hg (Equation 1-5):

$$\text{Dissolved } O_2 \text{ content} = 0.0031 \times 95 = 0.3 \text{ mL } O_2/100 \text{ mL blood} \qquad (1\text{-}5)$$

The total O_2 content is the sum of the hemoglobin-bound O_2 plus the dissolved O_2, or $19.5 + 0.3 = 19.8$ mL $O_2/100$ mL blood.

Arterial Po_2 is not the sole determinant of O_2 content; the hemoglobin level is also crucial. With anemia (a reduced hemoglobin level), fewer binding sites are available for O_2, and the O_2 content falls even though Po_2 remains unchanged. In addition, the O_2 content of blood is a static measurement of the quantity of O_2 per 100 mL blood. The actual delivery of oxygen to tissues is dynamic and depends on blood flow (determined primarily by cardiac output but also influenced by regulation at the microvascular level) as well as O_2 content. Thus, three main factors determine tissue O_2 delivery: arterial Po_2, hemoglobin level, and cardiac output. Disturbances in any one of these factors can result in decreased or insufficient O_2 delivery.

Oxygen content in arterial blood depends on arterial Po_2 and the hemoglobin level; tissue oxygen delivery depends on these two factors and cardiac output.

When blood reaches the systemic capillaries, O_2 is unloaded to the tissues, and Po_2 falls. The extent to which Po_2 falls depends on the balance of O_2 supply and demand: The local venous Po_2 of blood leaving a tissue falls to a greater degree if more O_2 is extracted per volume of blood because of increased tissue requirements or decreased supply (e.g., as a result of decreased cardiac output).

On average, in a resting individual Po_2 falls to approximately 40 mm Hg after O_2 extraction occurs at the tissue-capillary level. Because $Po_2 = 40$ mm Hg is associated with 75% saturation of hemoglobin, the total O_2 content in venous blood is calculated by Equation 1-6:

$$\text{Venous } O_2 \text{ content} = (1.34 \times 15 \times 0.75) + (0.0031 \times 40) \qquad (1\text{-}6)$$
$$= 15.2 \text{ mL } O_2/100 \text{ mL blood}$$

The quantity of O_2 consumed at the tissue level is the difference between the arterial and venous O_2 contents, or $19.8 - 15.2 = 4.6$ mL O_2 per 100 mL blood. The total O_2 consumption ($\dot{V}o_2$) is the product of cardiac output and the difference noted previously in arterial-venous O_2 content. Because (1) normal resting cardiac output for a young individual is approximately 5 to 6 L/min and (2) 46 mL O_2 is extracted per liter of blood flow (note difference in units), the resting O_2 consumption is approximately 250 mL/min.

When venous blood returns to the lungs, oxygenation of this desaturated blood occurs at the level of the pulmonary capillaries, and the entire cycle can repeat.

CARBON DIOXIDE TRANSPORT

Carbon dioxide is transported through the circulation in three different forms: (1) as bicarbonate (HCO_3^-), quantitatively the largest component; (2) as CO_2 dissolved in plasma; and (3) as carbaminohemoglobin, bound to terminal amino groups on hemoglobin. The first form, bicarbonate, results from the combination of CO_2 with H_2 to form carbonic acid (H_2CO_3), catalyzed by the enzyme carbonic anhydrase, and subsequent dissociation to H^+ and HCO_3^-. This reaction takes place primarily within the red blood cell, but HCO_3^- within the erythrocyte then is exchanged for Cl^- within plasma.

Carbon dioxide is carried in blood as (1) bicarbonate, (2) dissolved CO_2, and (3) carbaminohemoglobin.

Although dissolved CO_2, the second transport mechanism, constitutes only a small portion of the total CO_2 transported, it is quantitatively more important for CO_2 transport than dissolved O_2 is for O_2 transport, because CO_2 is approximately 20 times more soluble in plasma than is O_2. Carbaminohemoglobin, formed by the combination of CO_2 with hemoglobin, is the third transport mechanism. The oxygenation status of hemoglobin is important in determining the quantity of CO_2 that can be bound, with deoxygenated hemoglobin having a greater affinity for CO_2 than oxygenated hemoglobin (known as the Haldane effect). Therefore, oxygenation of hemoglobin in the pulmonary capillaries decreases its ability to bind CO_2 and facilitates the elimination of CO_2 by the lungs.

In the same way that the oxyhemoglobin dissociation curve depicts the relationship between the Po_2 and O_2 content of blood, a curve can be constructed relating the total CO_2 content to the Pco_2 of blood. However, within the range of gas tensions encountered under physiologic circumstances, the Pco_2–CO_2 content relationship is almost linear compared with the curvilinear relationship of Po_2 and O_2 content (Fig. 1-6).

Pco_2 in mixed venous blood is approximately 46 mm Hg, whereas normal arterial Pco_2 is approximately 40 mm Hg. The 6 mm Hg decrease when going from mixed venous to arterial blood, combined with the effect of oxygenation of hemoglobin on release of CO_2, corresponds to a change in CO_2 content of approximately 3.6 mL per 100 mL blood. Assuming a cardiac output of 5 to 6 L/min, CO_2 production can be calculated as the product of the cardiac output and arteriovenous CO_2 content difference, or approximately 200 mL/min.

VENTILATION-PERFUSION RELATIONSHIPS

Ventilation, blood flow, diffusion, and their relationship to gas exchange (O_2 uptake and CO_2 elimination) are more complicated than initially presented because the distribution of ventilation and blood flow within the lung was not considered. Effective gas exchange depends critically on the relationship between ventilation and perfusion in individual gas-exchanging units. A disturbance in this relationship, even if the total amounts of ventilation and blood flow are normal, is frequently responsible for markedly abnormal gas exchange in disease states.

The optimal efficiency for gas exchange would be provided by an even distribution of ventilation and perfusion throughout the lung so that a matching of ventilation and perfusion is always present. In reality, such a circumstance does not exist, even in normal lungs. Because blood flow is determined to a large extent by hydrostatic and gravitational forces, the dependent regions of the lung receive a disproportionately larger share of the total perfusion, whereas the uppermost regions are relatively underperfused. Similarly, there is a gradient of ventilation throughout the lung, with greater amounts also going to the dependent areas. However, even though ventilation and

From top to bottom of the lung, the gradient is more marked for perfusion ($\dot{Q}$) than for ventilation ($\dot{V}$); thus, the $\dot{V}/\dot{Q}$ ratio is lower in the dependent regions of the lung.

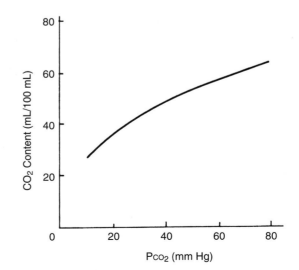

Figure 1-6. Relationship between partial pressure of carbon dioxide (Pco_2) and CO_2 content. Curve shifts slightly to left as O_2 saturation of blood decreases. Curve shown is for blood completely saturated with O_2.

perfusion both are greater in the gravity-dependent regions of the lung, this gradient is more marked for perfusion than for ventilation. Consequently, the ratio of ventilation ($\dot{V}$) to perfusion ($\dot{Q}$) is higher in apical regions of the lung than in basal regions. As a result, gas exchange throughout the lung is not uniform but varies depending on the $\dot{V}/\dot{Q}$ ratio of each region.

To understand the effects on gas exchange of altering the $\dot{V}/\dot{Q}$ ratio, first consider the individual alveolus and then the more complex model with multiple alveoli and variable $\dot{V}/\dot{Q}$ ratios. In a single alveolus, a continuous spectrum exists for the possible relationships between $\dot{V}$ and $\dot{Q}$ (Fig. 1-7). At one extreme, where $\dot{V}$ is maintained and $\dot{Q}$ approaches 0, the $\dot{V}/\dot{Q}$ ratio approaches ∞. When there is actually no perfusion ($\dot{Q} = 0$), ventilation is wasted insofar as gas exchange is concerned, and the alveolus is part of the dead space. At the other extreme, $\dot{V}$ approaches 0 and $\dot{Q}$ is preserved, and the $\dot{V}/\dot{Q}$ ratio approaches 0. When there is no ventilation ($\dot{V} = 0$), a "shunt" exists, oxygenation does not occur during transit through the pulmonary circulation, and the hemoglobin still is desaturated when it leaves the pulmonary capillary.

Again dealing with the extremes, for an alveolar-capillary unit acting as dead space ($\dot{V}/\dot{Q} = \infty$), Po_2 in the alveolus is equal to that in air, that is, 150 mm Hg (taking into account the fact that air in the alveolus is saturated with water vapor), whereas Pco_2 is 0 because no blood and therefore no CO_2 is in contact with alveolar gas. With a region of true dead space, there is no blood flow, so no gas tensions in blood are leaving the alveolus. If there were a minute amount of blood flow, that is, if the $\dot{V}/\dot{Q}$ ratio approached but did not reach ∞, then the blood also would have a Po_2 approaching (but slightly less than) 150 mm Hg and a Pco_2 approaching (but slightly more than) 0 mm Hg. At the other extreme, for an alveolar-capillary unit acting as a shunt ($\dot{V}/\dot{Q} = 0$), blood leaving the capillary has gas tensions identical to those in mixed venous blood, that is, $Po_2 = 40$ mm Hg and $Pco_2 = 46$ mm Hg, assuming the rest of the lung functioned well enough to maintain normal arterial and mixed venous gas tensions.

In reality, alveolar-capillary units fall anywhere along this continuum of $\dot{V}/\dot{Q}$ ratios. The higher the $\dot{V}/\dot{Q}$ ratio in an alveolar-capillary unit, the closer the unit comes to behaving like an area of dead space and the more Po_2 approaches 150 mm Hg and Pco_2 approaches 0 mm Hg. The lower the $\dot{V}/\dot{Q}$ ratio, the closer the unit comes to

Ventilation-perfusion ratios within each alveolar-capillary unit range from $\dot{V}/\dot{Q} = \infty$ (dead space) to $\dot{V}/\dot{Q} = 0$ (shunt).

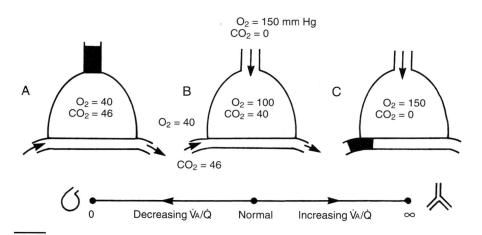

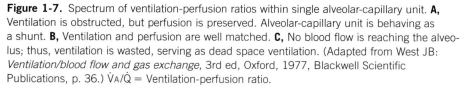

Figure 1-7. Spectrum of ventilation-perfusion ratios within single alveolar-capillary unit. **A,** Ventilation is obstructed, but perfusion is preserved. Alveolar-capillary unit is behaving as a shunt. **B,** Ventilation and perfusion are well matched. **C,** No blood flow is reaching the alveolus; thus, ventilation is wasted, serving as dead space ventilation. (Adapted from West JB: *Ventilation/blood flow and gas exchange,* 3rd ed, Oxford, 1977, Blackwell Scientific Publications, p. 36.) $\dot{V}_A/\dot{Q}$ = Ventilation-perfusion ratio.

behaving like a shunt, and the more the Po_2 and Pco_2 of blood leaving the capillary approach the gas tensions in mixed venous blood (40 and 46 mm Hg, respectively). This continuum is depicted in Figure 1-8, in which moving to the left signifies decreasing the $\dot{V}/\dot{Q}$ ratio and moving to the right means increasing the $\dot{V}/\dot{Q}$ ratio. The ideal circumstance lies between these extremes, in which $Po_2 = 100$ mm Hg and $Pco_2 = 40$ mm Hg.

When multiple alveolar-capillary units are considered, the net Po_2 and Pco_2 of the resulting pulmonary venous blood depend on the total O_2 or CO_2 content and the total volume of blood collected from each of the contributing units. Considering Pco_2 first, areas with relatively high $\dot{V}/\dot{Q}$ ratios contribute blood with a lower Pco_2 than do areas with low $\dot{V}/\dot{Q}$ ratios. However, inasmuch as the relationship between CO_2 content and Pco_2 is nearly linear over the range of concern, if blood having a higher Pco_2 and CO_2 content mixes with an equal volume of blood having a lower Pco_2 and CO_2 content, an intermediate PCO_2 and CO_2 content (approximately halfway between) results.

> Regions of the lung with a high $\dot{V}/\dot{Q}$ ratio and a high PO_2 cannot compensate for regions with a low $\dot{V}/\dot{Q}$ ratio and low PO_2.

In marked contrast, a high Po_2 in blood coming from a region with a high $\dot{V}/\dot{Q}$ ratio cannot compensate for blood with a low Po_2 from a region with a low $\dot{V}/\dot{Q}$ ratio. The difference stems from the shape of the oxyhemoglobin dissociation curve, which is curvilinear (rather than linear) and becomes nearly flat at the top. Therefore, after hemoglobin is nearly saturated with O_2 (on the relatively flat part of the oxyhemoglobin dissociation curve), increasing Po_2 does not significantly boost the O_2 content. Therefore, blood with a higher than normal Po_2 does not have a correspondingly higher O_2 content and cannot compensate for blood with a low Po_2 and low O_2 content.

In the normal lung, regional differences in the $\dot{V}/\dot{Q}$ ratio affect gas tensions in blood coming from specific regions as well as gas tensions in the resulting arterial blood. At the apices, where the $\dot{V}/\dot{Q}$ ratio is approximately 3.3, $Po_2 = 132$ mm Hg and $Pco_2 = 28$ mm Hg. At the bases, where the $\dot{V}/\dot{Q}$ ratio is approximately 0.63, $Po_2 = 89$ mm Hg and $Pco_2 = 42$ mm Hg. As discussed, the net Po_2 and Pco_2 of the combined blood coming from the apices, the bases, and the areas between are a function of the relative amounts of blood from each of these areas and the gas contents of each.

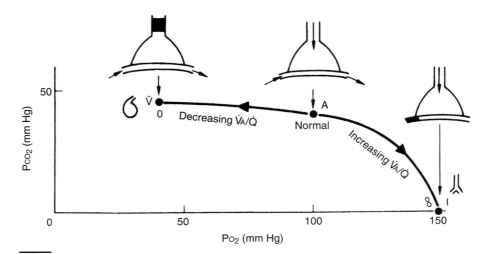

Figure 1-8. Continuum of alveolar gas composition at different ventilation-perfusion ratios within a single alveolar-capillary unit. Line is the "ventilation-perfusion ratio line." At the extreme left side of the line, $\dot{V}/\dot{Q} = 0$ (shunt). At the extreme right side of the line, $\dot{V}/\dot{Q} = \infty$ (dead space). Pco_2 = Partial pressure of carbon dioxide; Po_2 = partial pressure of oxygen. (Adapted from West JB: *Ventilation/blood flow and gas exchange*, 3rd ed. Oxford, 1977, Blackwell Scientific Publications, p. 37.)

In disease states, ventilation-perfusion mismatch frequently is much more extreme, resulting in clinically significant gas-exchange abnormalities. When an area of lung behaves as a shunt or even as a region having a very low $\dot{V}/\dot{Q}$ ratio, blood coming from this area has a low O_2 content and saturation, which cannot be compensated for by blood from relatively preserved regions of lung. $\dot{V}/\dot{Q}$ mismatch that is severe, particularly with areas of a high $\dot{V}/\dot{Q}$ ratio, can effectively produce dead space and therefore decrease the alveolar ventilation to other areas of the lung carrying a disproportionate share of the perfusion. Because CO_2 excretion depends on alveolar ventilation, P_{CO_2} may rise unless an overall increase in the minute ventilation restores the effective alveolar ventilation.

ABNORMALITIES IN GAS EXCHANGE

The net effect of disturbances in the normal pattern of gas exchange can be assessed by measurement of the gas tensions (P_{O_2} and P_{CO_2}) in arterial blood. The information that can be obtained from arterial blood gas measurement is discussed further in Chapter 3, but the mechanisms of hypoxemia (decreased arterial P_{O_2}) and hypercapnia (increased P_{CO_2}) are considered here because they relate to the physiologic principles just discussed.

HYPOXEMIA

Blood that has traversed pulmonary capillaries leaves with a P_{O_2} that should be in equilibrium with and almost identical to the P_{O_2} in companion alveoli. Although it is difficult to measure the O_2 tension in alveolar gas, it can be conveniently calculated by a formula known as the *alveolar gas equation*. A simplified version of this formula is relatively easy to use and can be extremely useful in the clinical setting, particularly when trying to deduce why a patient is hypoxemic. The alveolar O_2 tension (P_{AO_2})* can be calculated by Equation 1-7:

$$P_{AO_2} = F_{IO_2}(P_B - P_{H_2O}) - P_{ACO_2}/R \qquad (1\text{-}7)$$

where F_{IO_2} = fractional content of inspired O_2 (F_{IO_2} of air = 0.21), P_B = barometric pressure (approximately 760 mm Hg at sea level), P_{H_2O} = vapor pressure of water in the alveoli (at full saturation at 37° C, P_{H_2O} = 47 mm Hg), P_{ACO_2} = alveolar CO_2 tension (which can be assumed to be identical to arterial CO_2 tension, P_{aCO_2}), and R = respiratory quotient (CO_2 production divided by O_2 consumption, usually approximately 0.8). In practice, for the patient breathing room air (F_{IO_2} = 0.21), the equation often is simplified. When numbers are substituted for F_{IO_2}, P_B, and P_{H_2O} and when P_{aCO_2} is used instead of P_{ACO_2}, the resulting equation (at sea level) is Equation 1-8:

$$P_{AO_2} = 150 - 1.25 \times P_{aCO_2} \qquad (1\text{-}8)$$

The simplified alveolar gas equation (Equation 1-8) can be used to calculate alveolar P_{O_2} (P_{AO_2}) for the patient breathing room air.

By calculating P_{AO_2}, the expected P_{aO_2} can be determined. Even in a normal person, P_{AO_2} is greater than P_{aO_2} by an amount called the *alveolar-arterial oxygen difference* or *gradient* (AaD_{O_2}). A gradient exists even in normal individuals for two main reasons: (1) A small amount of cardiac output behaves as a shunt, without ever going through the pulmonary capillary bed. This includes venous blood from the bronchial circulation, a portion of which drains into the pulmonary veins, and coronary venous blood draining via thebesian veins directly into the left ventricle. Desaturated blood from these sources lowers O_2 tension in the resulting arterial blood. (2) Ventilation-perfusion

*By convention, "A" refers to alveolar and "a" to arterial.

gradients from the top to the bottom of the lung result in somewhat less-oxygenated blood from the bases combining with better-oxygenated blood from the apices.

$AaDo_2$ normally is less than 15 mm Hg, but it increases with age. $AaDo_2$ may be elevated in disease for several reasons. First, a shunt may be present so that some desaturated blood combines with fully saturated blood and lowers Po_2 in the resulting arterial blood. Common causes of a shunt are as follows:

1. Intracardiac lesions, with a right-to-left shunt at the atrial or ventricular level, for example, in an atrial or ventricular septal defect. Note that although a left-to-right shunt can produce severe long-term cardiac consequences, it does not affect either $AaDo_2$ or arterial Po_2 because its net effect is to recycle already oxygenated blood through the pulmonary vasculature, not to dilute oxygenated blood with desaturated blood.
2. Structural abnormalities of the pulmonary vasculature that result in direct communication between pulmonary arterial and venous systems, for example, pulmonary arteriovenous malformations.
3. Pulmonary diseases that result in filling of the alveolar spaces with fluid (e.g., pulmonary edema) or complete alveolar collapse. Either process can result in complete loss of ventilation to the affected alveoli, although some perfusion through the associated capillaries may continue.

Another cause of elevated $AaDo_2$ is ventilation-perfusion mismatch. Even when total ventilation and total perfusion to both lungs are normal, if some areas receive less ventilation and more perfusion (low $\dot{V}/\dot{Q}$ ratio) while others receive more ventilation and less perfusion (high $\dot{V}/\dot{Q}$ ratio), then $AaDo_2$ increases and hypoxemia results. As just mentioned, the reason for this phenomenon is that areas having a low $\dot{V}/\dot{Q}$ ratio provide relatively desaturated blood with a low O_2 content. Blood coming from regions with a high $\dot{V}/\dot{Q}$ ratio cannot compensate for this problem, inasmuch as the hemoglobin is already fully saturated and cannot increase its O_2 content further by increased ventilation (Fig. 1-9).

In practice, true shunt ($\dot{V}/\dot{Q} = 0$) and $\dot{V}/\dot{Q}$ mismatch (with areas of $\dot{V}/\dot{Q}$ that are low but not 0) can be distinguished by having the patient inhale 100% O_2. In the former case, increasing inspired Po_2 does not add more O_2 to the shunted blood, and O_2 content does not increase significantly. In the latter case, alveolar and capillary Po_2 rise considerably with additional O_2, fully saturating blood coming even from regions with a low $\dot{V}/\dot{Q}$ ratio, and arterial Po_2 rises substantially.

A third cause of elevated $AaDo_2$ occurs primarily in specialized circumstances. This cause is a "diffusion block" in which Po_2 in pulmonary capillary blood does not reach equilibrium with alveolar gas. If the interface (i.e., the tissue within the alveolar wall) between the capillary and the alveolar lumen is thickened, one can hypothesize that O_2 does not diffuse as readily and that the Po_2 in pulmonary capillary blood never reaches the Po_2 of alveolar gas. Even with a thickened alveolar wall, however, there is still sufficient time for this equilibrium. Unless the transit time of erythrocytes through the lung is significantly shortened, failure to equilibrate does not appear to be a problem. A specialized circumstance in which a diffusion block plus more rapid transit of erythrocytes together contribute to hypoxemia occurs during exercise in a patient with interstitial lung disease, as will be discussed later. However, for most practical purposes in the nonexercising patient, a diffusion block should be considered only a hypothetical rather than a real mechanism for increasing $AaDo_2$ and causing hypoxemia.

Increasing the difference between alveolar and arterial Po_2 is not the only mechanism that results in hypoxemia. Alveolar Po_2 can be decreased, which must necessarily lower arterial Po_2 if $AaDo_2$ remains constant. Referring back to the alveolar gas equation, it is relatively easy to see that alveolar Po_2 drops if barometric pressure falls (e.g., with altitude) or if alveolar Pco_2 rises (e.g., with hypoventilation). In the latter

Ventilation-perfusion mismatch and shunting are the two important mechanisms for elevation of the alveolar-arterial O_2 difference ($AaDo_2$).

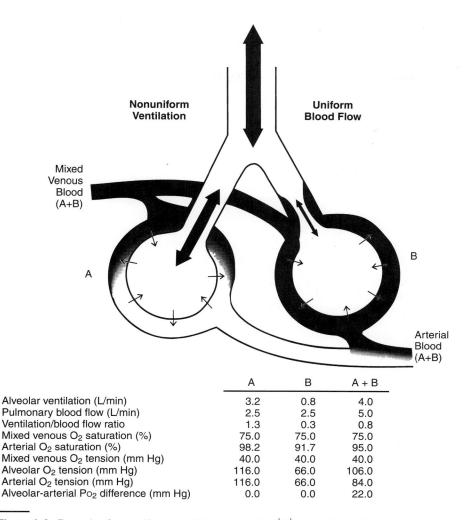

	A	B	A + B
Alveolar ventilation (L/min)	3.2	0.8	4.0
Pulmonary blood flow (L/min)	2.5	2.5	5.0
Ventilation/blood flow ratio	1.3	0.3	0.8
Mixed venous O_2 saturation (%)	75.0	75.0	75.0
Arterial O_2 saturation (%)	98.2	91.7	95.0
Mixed venous O_2 tension (mm Hg)	40.0	40.0	40.0
Alveolar O_2 tension (mm Hg)	116.0	66.0	106.0
Arterial O_2 tension (mm Hg)	116.0	66.0	84.0
Alveolar-arterial P_{O_2} difference (mm Hg)	0.0	0.0	22.0

Figure 1-9. Example of nonuniform ventilation producing $\dot{V}/\dot{Q}$ mismatch in two-alveolus model. In this instance, perfusion is equally distributed between the two alveoli. The calculations demonstrate how $\dot{V}/\dot{Q}$ mismatch lowers arterial P_{O_2} and causes elevated alveolar-arterial oxygen difference. (Adapted from Comroe JH: *The lung,* 2nd ed. Chicago, 1962, Year Book Medical Publishers, p. 94.)

circumstance, when total alveolar ventilation falls, P_{CO_2} in alveolar gas rises at the same time that alveolar P_{O_2} falls. Hypoventilation is relatively common in lung disease and can easily be identified by the presence of a high P_{CO_2} accompanying the hypoxemia. If P_{CO_2} is elevated and AaD_{O_2} is normal, then hypoventilation is the exclusive cause of low P_{O_2}. If AaD_{O_2} is elevated, then either $\dot{V}/\dot{Q}$ mismatch or shunting also contributes to the hypoxemia.

In summary, lung disease can result in hypoxemia for multiple reasons. Shunting and ventilation-perfusion mismatch are associated with elevated AaD_{O_2}. They often can be distinguished, if necessary, by inhalation of 100% O_2, which markedly increases Pa_{O_2} with $\dot{V}/\dot{Q}$ mismatch but not with true shunting. In contrast, hypoventilation (identified by high Pa_{CO_2}) and low inspired P_{O_2} lower alveolar P_{O_2} and cause hypoxemia, although AaD_{O_2} remains normal. Because many of the disease processes examined in this text cause several pathophysiologic abnormalities, it is not at all uncommon to see more than one of the aforementioned mechanisms producing hypoxemia in a particular patient.

When hypoventilation is the sole cause of hypoxemia, AaD_{O_2} is normal.

Mechanisms of hypoxemia:
1. Shunt
2. $\dot{V}/\dot{Q}$ mismatch
3. Hypoventilation
4. Low inspired P_{O_2}

HYPERCAPNIA

As discussed earlier in the section on ventilation, alveolar ventilation is the prime determinant of arterial P_{CO_2}, assuming that CO_2 production remains constant. It is clear that alveolar ventilation is compromised either by decreasing the total minute ventilation (without changing the relative proportion of dead space and alveolar ventilation) or by keeping the total minute ventilation constant and increasing the relative proportion of dead space to alveolar ventilation. A simple way to produce the latter circumstance is to change the pattern of breathing, that is, by decreasing the tidal volume and increasing the frequency of breathing. With a lower tidal volume, a larger proportion of each breath ventilates the anatomic dead space, and the proportion of alveolar ventilation to total ventilation must decrease.

In addition, if significant ventilation-perfusion mismatching is present, well-perfused areas may be underventilated, whereas underperfused areas receive a disproportionate amount of ventilation. The net effect of having a large proportion of ventilation go to poorly perfused areas is similar to that of increasing the dead space. By wasting this ventilation, the remainder of the lung with the large share of the perfusion is underventilated, and the net effect is to decrease the effective alveolar ventilation. In many disease conditions, when such significant $\dot{V}/\dot{Q}$ mismatch exists, any increase in P_{CO_2} stimulates breathing, increases total minute ventilation, and compensates for the effectively wasted ventilation.

> Decrease in alveolar ventilation is the primary mechanism that causes hypercapnia.

Therefore, several causes of hypercapnia can be defined, all of which have in common a decrease in effective alveolar ventilation. The causes include a decrease in minute ventilation, an increase in the proportion of wasted ventilation, and significant ventilation-perfusion mismatch. By increasing the total minute ventilation, however, a patient often is capable of compensating for the latter two situations so that CO_2 retention does not result.

Increasing CO_2 production necessitates an increase in alveolar ventilation to avoid CO_2 retention. Thus, if alveolar ventilation does not rise to compensate for additional CO_2 production, hypercapnia also will result.

As is the case with hypoxemia, pathophysiologic explanations for hypercapnia do not necessarily follow such simple rules so that each case can be fully explained by one mechanism. In reality, several of these mechanisms may be operative, even in a single patient.

REFERENCES

Cotes JE, Chinn DJ, Miller MR: *Lung function: physiology, measurement and application in medicine,* 6th ed, Malden, MA, 2006, Blackwell.

Lumb A, Nunn JF: *Nunn's applied respiratory physiology,* 6th ed. Oxford, 2005, Butterworth Heinemann.

Schwartzstein RM, Parker MJ: *Respiratory physiology: a clinical approach,* Philadelphia, 2006, Lippincott Williams & Wilkins.

Wagner PD, West JB: Ventilation, blood flow, and gas exchange. In Mason RJ, Murray JF, Broaddus VC, et al, editors: *Textbook of respiratory medicine,* 4th ed. Philadelphia, 2005, WB Saunders, pp. 51–86.

Weibel ER: *The pathway for oxygen: structure and function in the mammalian respiratory system,* Cambridge, 1984, Harvard University Press.

Weinberger SE, Schwartzstein RM, Weiss JW: Hypercapnia, *N Engl J Med* 321:1223–1231, 1989.

West JB: *Respiratory physiology—The essentials,* 7th ed. Philadelphia, 2005, Lippincott Williams & Wilkins.

West JB: *Ventilation/blood flow and gas-exchange,* 5th ed. Oxford, 1990, Blackwell Scientific.

2

Presentation of the Patient with Pulmonary Disease

Dyspnea	Hemoptysis
Cough	Chest Pain

The patient with a pulmonary problem generally comes to the attention of the clinician for one of two reasons: (1) complaint of a symptom that can be traced to a respiratory cause, or (2) incidental finding of an abnormality on chest radiograph. Although the former presentation is more common, the latter is not uncommon when a radiograph is obtained either as part of a routine examination or for evaluation of a seemingly unrelated problem. This chapter focuses on the first case, the patient who comes to the physician with a respiratory-related complaint. In the next and subsequent chapters, frequent references are made to abnormal radiographic findings as the clue to the presence of a pulmonary disorder.

Four particularly common and a number of less common symptoms bring the patient with lung disease to the physician: dyspnea (and its variants), cough (with or without sputum production), hemoptysis, and chest pain. Each of these symptoms, to a greater or lesser extent, may result from a nonpulmonary disorder, especially primary cardiac disease. For each symptom, a discussion of some of the important clinical features is followed by the pathophysiologic features and the differential diagnosis.

DYSPNEA

Dyspnea, or shortness of breath, is frequently a difficult symptom for the physician to evaluate because it is such a subjective feeling experienced by the patient. It is perhaps best defined as an uncomfortable sensation (or awareness) of one's own breathing, to which little attention normally is paid. However, the term *dyspnea* probably subsumes several sensations that are qualitatively distinct. As a result, when patients are asked to describe in more detail their sensation of breathlessness, their descriptions tend to fall into three primary categories: (1) air hunger or suffocation, (2) increased effort or work of breathing, and (3) chest tightness.

Not only is the symptom of dyspnea highly subjective and describable in different ways, but the patient's appreciation of it and its importance to the physician depend heavily on the stimulus or amount of activity required to precipitate it. The physician must take into account how the stimulus, when quantified, compares with the patient's usual level of activity. For example, a patient who is limited in exertion by a nonpulmonary problem may not experience any shortness of breath even in the presence of additional and significant lung disease. If the person were more active, however, dyspnea would become readily apparent. A marathon runner who experiences a new symptom of shortness of breath after running 5 miles may warrant more concern than would an elderly man who for many years has had a stable symptom of shortness of breath after walking 3 blocks.

Dyspnea should be distinguished from several other signs or symptoms that may have an entirely different significance. *Tachypnea* is a rapid respiratory rate (greater than the usual value of 12–20/min). Tachypnea may be present with or without dyspnea, just as dyspnea does not necessarily entail the finding of tachypnea on physical examination. *Hyperventilation* is ventilation that is greater than the amount required to maintain normal CO_2 elimination. Hence, the criterion that defines hyperventilation is a decrease in the P_{CO_2} of arterial blood. Finally, the symptom of *exertional fatigue* must be distinguished from dyspnea. Fatigue may be due to cardiovascular, neuromuscular, or other nonpulmonary diseases, and the implication of this symptom is quite different from that of true shortness of breath.

There are some variations on the theme of dyspnea. *Orthopnea,* or shortness of breath on assuming the recumbent position, often is quantitated by the number of pillows or angle of elevation necessary to relieve or prevent the sensation. One of the main causes of orthopnea is an increase in venous return and central intravascular volume on assuming the recumbent position. In patients with cardiac decompensation and either overt or subclinical congestive heart failure, the increment in left atrial and left ventricular filling may result in pulmonary vascular congestion and pulmonary interstitial or alveolar edema. Thus, orthopnea frequently suggests cardiac disease and some element of congestive heart failure. However, some patients with primary pulmonary disease experience orthopnea, such as individuals with a significant amount of secretions who have more difficulty handling their secretions when they are recumbent.

Paroxysmal nocturnal dyspnea is waking from sleep with dyspnea. As with orthopnea the recumbent position is important, but this symptom differs from orthopnea in that it does not occur soon after lying down. Although the implication with regard to underlying cardiac decompensation still applies, the increase in central intravascular volume is due more to a slow mobilization of tissue fluid, such as peripheral edema, than to a rapid redistribution of intravascular volume from peripheral to central vessels.

Variants that are much more uncommon are only mentioned here. *Platypnea* is shortness of breath when the patient is in the upright position; it is the opposite of orthopnea. *Trepopnea* is shortness of breath when the patient lies on his or her side. Patients with this symptom report dyspnea on either the right or the left side. The symptom can be relieved by moving to the opposite lateral position.

Returning to the more general symptom of dyspnea, a number of sources or mechanisms are proposed rather than a single common thread linking the diverse responsible conditions. In particular, neural output reflecting central nervous system respiratory drive appears to be integrated with input from a variety of mechanical receptors in the chest wall, respiratory muscles, airways, and pulmonary vasculature. Presumably, the relative contributions of each source differ from disease to disease and from patient to patient, and they are responsible for the qualitatively different sensations all subsumed under the term *dyspnea*.

In an attempt to link dyspnea with underlying pathophysiologic mechanisms, we can return to the three qualitatively distinct sensations of breathlessness mentioned at the beginning of this section. Patients who describe their breathlessness as a sense of air hunger or suffocation often have increased respiratory drive, which can be related in part to either a high P_{CO_2} or a low P_{O_2} but also can occur even in the absence of respiratory system or gas-exchange abnormalities. The sensation of increased effort or

---

Dyspnea is distinct from tachypnea, hyperventilation, and exertional fatigue.

Orthopnea, often associated with left ventricular failure, may accompany primary pulmonary disease.

The sensation of dyspnea probably has a number of underlying pathophysiologic mechanisms.

work of breathing is commonly experienced by patients who have increased resistance to airflow or abnormally stiff lungs. The sensation of chest tightness, frequently noted by patients with asthma, probably arises from intrathoracic receptors that are stimulated by bronchoconstriction. Because some disorders may produce breathlessness by more than one mechanism (e.g., asthma may have components of all three mechanisms), overlap or a mixture of these different sensations often occurs.

The differential diagnosis includes a broad range of disorders that result in dyspnea (Table 2-1). The disorders can be separated into the major categories of *respiratory disease* and *cardiovascular disease*. In addition, dyspnea may be present in conditions associated with *increased respiratory drive,* even in the absence of underlying respiratory or cardiovascular disease, or it may have an *anxiety-related* or *psychosomatic origin.*

The first major category consists of disorders at many levels of the respiratory system (airways, pulmonary parenchyma, pulmonary vasculature, pleura, and bellows) that can cause dyspnea. Airway diseases that cause dyspnea result primarily from obstruction to airflow, occurring anywhere from the upper airway to the large, medium, and small intrathoracic bronchi and bronchioles. *Upper airway obstruction,* which is defined here as obstruction above or including the vocal cords, is caused primarily by foreign bodies, tumors, edema (e.g., with anaphylaxis), and stenosis. A clue to upper airway obstruction is the presence of disproportionate difficulty during inspiration and an audible, prolonged gasping sound called *inspiratory stridor.* The pathophysiology of upper airway obstruction is discussed in Chapter 7.

Airways below the level of the vocal cords, from the trachea down to the small bronchioles, are more commonly involved with disorders that produce dyspnea. An isolated problem, such as an airway tumor, usually does not by itself cause dyspnea unless it occurs in the trachea or in a major bronchus. In contrast, diseases such as

Table 2-1

DIFFERENTIAL DIAGNOSIS OF DYSPNEA

RESPIRATORY DISEASE
Airway disease
  Asthma
  Chronic obstructive lung disease
  Upper airway obstruction
Parenchymal lung disease
  Acute respiratory distress syndrome
  Pneumonia
  Interstitial lung disease
Pulmonary vascular disease
  Pulmonary emboli
Pleural disease
  Pneumothorax
  Pleural effusion
"Bellows" disease
  Neuromuscular disease (e.g., polymyositis, myasthenia gravis, Guillain-Barré syndrome)
  Chest wall disease (e.g., kyphoscoliosis)
CARDIOVASCULAR DISEASE
Elevated pulmonary venous pressure
  Left ventricular failure
  Mitral stenosis
Decreased cardiac output
Severe anemia
INCREASED RESPIRATORY DRIVE
Hyperthyroidism
Pregnancy
ANXIETY/PSYCHOSOMATIC ORIGIN

asthma and chronic obstructive pulmonary disease have widespread effects throughout the tracheobronchial tree, with airway narrowing resulting from spasm, edema, secretions, or loss of radial support (see Chapter 4). With this type of obstruction, difficulty with expiration generally predominates over that with inspiration, and the physical findings associated with obstruction (wheezing, prolongation of airflow) are more prominent on expiration.

The category of pulmonary parenchymal disease includes disorders causing inflammation, infiltration, fluid accumulation, or scarring of the alveolar structures. Such disorders may be diffuse in nature, as with the many causes of interstitial lung disease, or they may be more localized, as occurs with a bacterial pneumonia.

Pulmonary vascular disease results in obstruction or loss of vessels in the lung. The most common acute type of pulmonary vascular disease is pulmonary embolism, in which one or many pulmonary vessels are occluded by thrombi originating in systemic veins. Chronically, vessels may be blocked by recurrent pulmonary emboli or by inflammatory or scarring processes that result in thickening of vessel walls or obliteration of the vascular lumen.

Two major disorders affecting the pleura may result in dyspnea: pneumothorax (air in the pleural space) and pleural effusion (liquid in the pleural space). With pleural effusions, a substantial amount of fluid must be present in the pleural space to result in dyspnea, unless the patient also has significant underlying cardiopulmonary disease or additional complicating features.

The term *bellows* is used here for the final category of respiratory-related disorders causing dyspnea. It refers to the pump system that works under the control of a central nervous system generator to expand the lungs and allow airflow. This pump system includes a variety of muscles (primarily but not exclusively diaphragm and intercostal) and the chest wall. Primary disease affecting the muscles, their nerve supply, or neuromuscular interaction, including polymyositis, myasthenia gravis, and Guillain-Barré syndrome, may result in dyspnea. Deformity of the chest wall, particularly kyphoscoliosis, produces dyspnea by several pathophysiologic mechanisms, not the least of which is the increased work of breathing. Disorders of the respiratory bellows are discussed in Chapter 19.

The second major category of disorders that produce dyspnea is cardiovascular disease. In the majority of cases, the feature that patients have in common is an elevated hydrostatic pressure in the pulmonary veins and capillaries that leads to a transudation or leakage of fluid into the pulmonary interstitium and alveoli. Left ventricular failure, from either ischemic or valvular heart disease, is the most common example. In addition, mitral stenosis, with increased left atrial pressure, produces elevated pulmonary venous and capillary pressures even though left ventricular function and pressure are normal. A frequent accompaniment of the dyspnea associated with these forms of cardiac disease is orthopnea, paroxysmal nocturnal dyspnea, or both. Although worsening of dyspnea in the supine position is not specific to pulmonary venous hypertension and can also be found in some patients with pulmonary disease, improvement of dyspnea in the supine position is a point against left ventricular failure as the causative factor.

The third category of conditions associated with dyspnea includes those characterized by increased respiratory drive but no underlying cardiopulmonary disease. Both thyroid hormone and progesterone augment respiratory drive, and patients with hyperthyroidism and pregnant women commonly complain of dyspnea. Dyspnea during pregnancy often starts before the abdomen is noticeably distended, indicating that diaphragmatic elevation from the enlarging uterus is not the primary explanation for the dyspnea.

Finally, dyspnea may be due to anxiety or other psychosomatic problems. Because the sensation of dyspnea is so subjective, any awareness of one's breathing may start a self-perpetuating problem. The patient breathes faster, becomes more aware of breathing, and finally has a sensation of frank dyspnea. At the extreme, a person can hyperventilate and lower arterial P_{CO_2} sufficiently to cause additional symptoms of lightheadedness and tingling, particularly of the fingers and around the mouth. Of course, patients who seem anxious or have a history of psychologic problems can also have lung disease. Similarly, patients with lung or heart disease can have dyspnea with a functional cause unrelated to their underlying disease process.

COUGH

Cough is a symptom that everyone has experienced at some point. It is a physiologic mechanism for clearing and protecting the airway and does not necessarily imply disease. Normally, cough is protective against food or other foreign material entering the airway. It also is responsible for aiding in the clearance of secretions produced within the tracheobronchial tree. Generally, mucociliary clearance is adequate to propel secretions upward through the trachea and into the larynx so that the secretions can be removed from the airway and swallowed. However, if the mucociliary clearance mechanism is temporarily damaged or not functioning well, or if the mechanism is overwhelmed by excessive production of secretions, then cough becomes an important additional mechanism for clearing the tracheobronchial tree.

Cough usually is initiated by stimulation of receptors (called *irritant receptors*) at a number of locations. Irritant receptor nerve endings are found primarily in the larynx, trachea, and major bronchi, particularly at points of bifurcation. However, sensory receptors are also located in other parts of the upper airway as well as on the pleura, the diaphragm, and even the pericardium. Irritation of these nerve endings initiates an impulse that travels via afferent nerves (primarily the vagus but also trigeminal, glossopharyngeal, and phrenic) to a poorly defined cough center in the medulla. The efferent signal is carried in the recurrent laryngeal nerve (a branch of the vagus), which controls closure of the glottis, and in phrenic and spinal nerves, which effect contraction of the diaphragm and the expiratory muscles of the chest and abdominal walls. The initial part of the cough sequence is a deep inspiration to a high lung volume, followed by closure of the glottis, contraction of the expiratory muscles, and opening of the glottis. When the glottis suddenly opens, contraction of the expiratory muscles and relaxation of the diaphragm produce an explosive rush of air at high velocity, which transports airway secretions or foreign material out of the tracheobronchial tree.

> Irritant receptors triggering cough are located primarily in larger airways.

The major causes of cough are listed in Table 2-2. Cough commonly results from an airway irritant, regardless of whether the person has respiratory system disease. The most common inhaled irritant is cigarette smoke. Noxious fumes, dusts, and chemicals also stimulate irritant receptors and result in cough. Secretions resulting from postnasal drip are a particularly common cause of cough, presumably triggering the symptom via stimulation of laryngeal cough receptors. Aspiration of gastric contents or upper airway secretions, which amounts to "inhalation" of liquid or solid material, can result in cough, the cause of which may be unrecognized if the aspiration has not been clinically apparent. In the case of gastroesophageal reflux, in which gastric acid flows retrograde into the esophagus, cough is due not only to aspiration of gastric contents from the esophagus or pharynx into the tracheobronchial tree but also to reflex mechanisms triggered by acid entry into the lower esophagus and mediated by the vagal nerve.

Cough caused by respiratory system disease derives mainly but not exclusively from disorders affecting the airway. Most commonly, viruses or other organisms (such as *Mycoplasma*, *Chlamydophila*, and *Bordetella pertussis*) producing upper respiratory

Table	2-2

DIFFERENTIAL DIAGNOSIS OF COUGH

AIRWAY IRRITANTS
Inhaled smoke, dusts, fumes
Aspiration
   Gastric contents
   Oral secretions
   Foreign bodies
Postnasal drip
AIRWAYS DISEASE
Upper respiratory tract infection
Postinfectious cough
Acute or chronic bronchitis
Eosinophilic bronchitis
Bronchiectasis
Neoplasm
External compression by node or mass lesion
Reactive airways disease (asthma)
PARENCHYMAL DISEASE
Pneumonia
Lung abscess
Interstitial lung disease
CONGESTIVE HEART FAILURE
MISCELLANEOUS
Drug-induced (angiotensin-converting enzyme inhibitors)

tract infections also affect parts of the tracheobronchial tree, and the airway inflammation results in a bothersome cough that lasts sometimes from weeks to months. Bacterial infections of the lung, either acute (pneumonia, acute bronchitis) or chronic (bronchiectasis, chronic bronchitis, lung abscess), generally have an airway component and an impressive amount of associated coughing. Space-occupying lesions in the tracheobronchial tree (tumors, foreign bodies, granulomas) and external lesions compressing the airway (mediastinal masses, lymph nodes, other tumors) commonly manifest as cough secondary to airway irritation. Hyperirritable airways with airway constriction, as in asthma, are frequently associated with cough, even when a specific inhaled irritant is not identified. The more readily recognized manifestations of asthma (wheezing and dyspnea) may not be apparent, and cough may be the sole presenting symptom. An entity of unknown etiology called *eosinophilic bronchitis,* characterized by eosinophilic inflammation of the airway in the absence of asthma, has also been identified as a cause of chronic cough.

Patients with pulmonary interstitial disease may have cough, probably owing more to secondary airway or pleural involvement, inasmuch as few irritant receptors are in the lung itself. In congestive heart failure, cough may be related to the same unclear mechanism operative in patients with interstitial lung disease, or it may be secondary to bronchial edema.

A variety of miscellaneous causes of cough, such as irritation of the tympanic membrane by wax or a hair or stimulation of one of the afferent nerves by osteophytes or neural tumors, have been identified but are not discussed in further detail here. With the widespread use of angiotensin-converting enzyme inhibitors (e.g., enalapril, lisinopril) for treatment of hypertension and congestive heart failure, cough has been recognized as a relatively common side effect of these agents. Because angiotensin-converting enzyme breaks down bradykinin and other inflammatory peptides, accumulation of bradykinin or other peptides in patients taking these inhibitors may be responsible by stimulating receptors capable of initiating cough. Of note, cough is a far less common side effect of angiotensin II receptor antagonists such as losartan. Finally, coughing may be a nervous habit that can be especially prominent when the patient is anxious, although the physician must not neglect the possibility of an organic cause.

The symptom of cough is generally characterized by whether it is productive or nonproductive of sputum. Virtually any cause of cough may be productive at times of small amounts of clear or mucoid sputum. However, thick yellow or green sputum indicates the presence of numerous leukocytes in the sputum, either neutrophils or eosinophils. Neutrophils may be present with just an inflammatory process of the airways or parenchyma, but they also frequently reflect the presence of a bacterial infection. Specific examples include bacterial bronchitis, bronchiectasis, lung abscess, and pneumonia. Eosinophils, which can be seen after special preparation of the sputum, often occur with bronchial asthma, whether or not an allergic component plays a role, and in the much less common entity of eosinophilic bronchitis.

> Yellow or green sputum reflects the presence of numerous leukocytes, either neutrophils or eosinophils.

In clinical practice, cough often is divided into three major temporal categories: acute, subacute, or chronic, depending on the duration of the symptom. *Acute cough,* defined by a duration of less than 3 weeks, is most commonly due to an acute viral infection of the respiratory tract, such as the common cold. *Subacute cough* is defined by a duration of 3 to 8 weeks, and *chronic cough* lasts 8 or more weeks. Whereas chronic bronchitis is a particularly frequent cause of cough in smokers, common causes of either subacute or chronic cough in nonsmokers are postnasal drip (also called *upper airway cough syndrome*), gastroesophageal reflux, and asthma. An important subacute cough is *postinfectious cough* that lasts for more than 3 weeks following an upper respiratory tract infection. It often is due to persistent airway inflammation, postnasal drip, or bronchial hyperresponsiveness (as seen with asthma). In all cases, however, the clinician must keep in mind the broader differential diagnosis of cough outlined in Table 2-2, recognizing that cough may be a marker and the initial presenting symptom of a more serious disease, such as carcinoma of the lung.

HEMOPTYSIS

Hemoptysis is coughing or spitting up blood derived from airways or the lung itself. When the patient complains of coughing or spitting up blood, whether the blood actually originated from the respiratory system is not always apparent. Other sources of blood include the nasopharynx (particularly in the common nosebleed), the mouth (even lip or tongue biting can be mistaken for hemoptysis), and the upper gastrointestinal tract (esophagus, stomach, and duodenum). The patient often can distinguish some of these causes of pseudohemoptysis, but the physician also should search by examination for a mouth or nasopharyngeal source.

The major causes of hemoptysis can be divided into three categories based on location: airways, pulmonary parenchyma, and vasculature (Table 2-3). Airway disease is the most common cause, with bronchitis, bronchiectasis, and bronchogenic carcinoma leading the list. Bronchial carcinoid tumor (formerly called *bronchial adenoma*), a less common neoplasm with variable malignant potential, also originates in the airway. In patients with acquired immunodeficiency syndrome, hemoptysis may be due to endobronchial (and/or pulmonary parenchymal) involvement with Kaposi's sarcoma.

> Diseases of the airways (e.g., bronchitis) are the most common causes of hemoptysis.

Parenchymal causes of hemoptysis frequently are infectious in nature: tuberculosis, lung abscess, pneumonia, and localized fungal infection (generally attributable to *Aspergillus* organisms) termed *mycetoma* ("fungus ball") or *aspergilloma*. Rarer causes of parenchymal hemorrhage are Goodpasture's syndrome, idiopathic pulmonary hemosiderosis, and Wegener's granulomatosis, some of which are discussed in Chapter 11.

Vascular lesions resulting in hemoptysis are generally related to problems with the pulmonary circulation. Pulmonary embolism, with either frank infarction or transient

Table 2-3
DIFFERENTIAL DIAGNOSIS OF HEMOPTYSIS

AIRWAYS DISEASE
Acute or chronic bronchitis
Bronchiectasis
Bronchogenic carcinoma
Bronchial carcinoid tumor (bronchial adenoma)
Other endobronchial tumors (Kaposi's sarcoma, metastatic carcinoma)
PARENCHYMAL DISEASE
Tuberculosis
Lung abscess
Pneumonia
Mycetoma ("fungus ball")
Miscellaneous
   Goodpasture's syndrome
   Idiopathic pulmonary hemosiderosis
   Wegener's granulomatosis
VASCULAR DISEASE
Pulmonary embolism
Elevated pulmonary venous pressure
   Left ventricular failure
   Mitral stenosis
Vascular malformation
MISCELLANEOUS/RARE CAUSES
Impaired coagulation
Pulmonary endometriosis

bleeding without infarction, often is a cause of hemoptysis. Elevated pressure in the pulmonary venous and capillary bed may also be associated with hemoptysis. Acutely elevated pressure, as in pulmonary edema, may have associated hemoptysis, commonly seen as pink- or red-tinged frothy sputum. Chronically elevated pulmonary venous pressure results from mitral stenosis, but this valvular lesion is a relatively infrequent cause of significant hemoptysis. Vascular malformations, such as arteriovenous malformations, may also be associated with coughing of blood.

Other miscellaneous etiologic factors in hemoptysis should be considered. Some of these belong in more than one of the aforementioned categories; others are included here because of their rarity. Cystic fibrosis affects both airways and pulmonary parenchyma. Although either component theoretically can cause hemoptysis, bronchiectasis (a common complication of cystic fibrosis) is most frequently responsible. Patients with impaired coagulation may rarely have pulmonary hemorrhage in the absence of other obvious causes of hemoptysis. An interesting but rare disorder is pulmonary endometriosis, in which implants of endometrial tissue in the lung can bleed coincident with the time of the menstrual cycle. Other causes are even more rare, and discussion of them is beyond the scope of this chapter.

CHEST PAIN

Chest pain as a reflection of respiratory system disease does not originate in the lung itself, which is free of sensory pain fibers. When chest pain does occur in this setting, its origin usually is the parietal pleura (lining the inside of the chest wall), the diaphragm, or the mediastinum, each of which has extensive innervation by nerve fibers capable of pain sensation.

Chest pain can be associated with pleural, diaphragmatic, or mediastinal disease.

For the parietal pleura or the diaphragm, an inflammatory or infiltrating malignant process generally produces the pain. When the diaphragm is involved, the pain commonly is referred to the shoulder. In contrast, pain from the parietal pleura usually is relatively well localized over the area of involvement. Pain involving the pleura or the diaphragm often is worsened on inspiration; in fact, chest pain that is particularly pronounced on inspiration is described as "pleuritic."

Inflammation of the parietal pleura producing pain often is secondary to pulmonary embolism or to pneumonia extending to the pleural surface. A pneumothorax may result in acute onset of pleuritic pain, although the mechanism is not clear inasmuch as an acute inflammatory process is unlikely to be involved. Some diseases, particularly connective tissue disorders such as lupus, may result in episodes of pleuritic chest pain from a primary inflammatory process involving the pleura. Inflammation of the parietal pleura as a result of a viral infection (e.g., viral pleurisy) is a common cause of pleuritic chest pain in otherwise healthy individuals.

Infiltrating tumor can produce chest pain by affecting the parietal pleura or adjacent soft tissue, bones, or nerves. In the case of malignant mesothelioma, the tumor arises from the pleura itself. In other circumstances, such as lung cancer, the tumor may extend directly to the pleural surface or involve the pleura after bloodborne (hematogenous) metastasis from a distant site.

A variety of disorders originating in the mediastinum may result in pain; they may or may not be associated with additional problems in the lung itself. These disorders of the mediastinum are discussed in Chapter 16.

REFERENCES

Dyspnea

American Thoracic Society: Dyspnea. Mechanisms, assessment, and management: a consensus statement, *Am J Respir Crit Care Med* 159:321–340, 1999.

Harver A, Mahler DA, Schwartzstein RM, Baird JC: Descriptors of breathlessness in healthy individuals: distinct and separable constructs, *Chest* 118:679–690, 2000.

Luce JM, Luce JA: Management of dyspnea in patients with far-advanced lung disease, *JAMA* 285:1331–1337, 2001.

Manning HL, Schwartzstein RM: Pathophysiology of dyspnea, *N Engl J Med* 333:1547–1553, 1995.

Scano G, Stendardi L, Grazzini M: Understanding dyspnea by its language, *Eur Respir J* 25:380–385, 2005.

Tobin MJ: Dyspnea: pathophysiologic basis, clinical presentation, and management, *Arch Intern Med* 150:1604–1613, 1990.

Cough

Gibson PG, Fujimara M, Niimi A: Eosinophilic bronchitis: clinical manifestations and implications for treatment, *Thorax* 57:178–182, 2002.

Irwin RS, Baumann MH, Bolser DC, et al: Diagnosis and management of cough: executive summary. ACCP evidence-based clinical practice guidelines, *Chest* 129:1S–23S, 2006.

Irwin RS, Madison JM: The diagnosis and treatment of cough, *N Engl J Med* 343:1715–1721, 2000.

Irwin RS, Madison JM: Symptom research on chronic cough: a historical perspective, *Ann Intern Med* 134:809–814, 2001.

Irwin RS, Madison JM: The persistently troublesome cough, *Am J Respir Crit Care Med* 165:1469–1474, 2002.

Israili ZH, Hall WD: Cough and angioneurotic edema associated with angiotensin-converting enzyme inhibitor therapy, *Ann Intern Med* 117:234–242, 1992.

Kwon NH, Oh MJ, Min TH, Lee BJ, Choi DC: Causes and clinical features of subacute cough, *Chest* 129:1142–1147, 2006.

Morice AH: The diagnosis and management of chronic cough, *Eur Respir J* 24:481–492, 2004.

Morice AH, McGarvey L, Pavord I, British Thoracic Society Cough Guideline Group: BTS guidelines: recommendations for the management of cough in adults, *Thorax* 61 (Suppl1): i1–i24, 2006.

Hemoptysis

Andersen PE: Imaging and interventional radiological treatment of hemoptysis, *Acta Radiol* 47:780–792, 2006.

Bidwell JL, Pachner RW: Hemoptysis: diagnosis and management, *Am Fam Physician* 72:1253–1260, 2005.

Cahill BC, Ingbar DH: Massive hemoptysis: assessment and management, *Clin Chest Med* 15:147–168, 1994.

Israel RH, Poe RH: Hemoptysis, *Clin Chest Med* 8:197–205, 1987.

Jean-Baptiste E: Clinical assessment and management of massive hemoptysis, *Crit Care Med* 28:1642–1647, 2000.

Santiago S, Tobias J, Williams AJ: A reappraisal of the causes of hemoptysis, *Arch Intern Med* 151:2449–2451, 1991.

Savale L, Parrot A, Khalil A, et al: Cryptogenic hemoptysis: from a benign to a life-threatening pathologic vascular condition, *Am J Respir Crit Care Med* 175:1181–1185, 2007.

Chest Pain

Branch WT Jr, McNeil BJ: Analysis of the differential diagnosis and assessment of pleuritic chest pain in young adults, *Am J Med* 75:671–679, 1983.

Cayley WE Jr: Diagnosing the cause of chest pain, *Am Fam Physician* 72:2012–2021, 2005.

Donat WE: Chest pain: cardiac and noncardiac causes, *Clin Chest Med* 8:241–252, 1987.

Lee TH, Goldman L: Evaluation of the patient with acute chest pain, *N Engl J Med* 342:1187–1195, 2000.

Winters ME, Katzen SM: Identifying chest pain emergencies in the primary care setting, *Prim Care* 33:625–642, 2006.

3

Evaluation of the Patient with Pulmonary Disease

EVALUATION ON A MACROSCOPIC LEVEL	Ultrasonography
	Bronchoscopy
Physical Examination	**EVALUATION ON A**
Chest Radiography	**MICROSCOPIC LEVEL**
Computed Tomography	Obtaining Specimens
Magnetic Resonance	Processing Specimens
Imaging	**ASSESSMENT ON A**
Lung Scanning	**FUNCTIONAL LEVEL**
Pulmonary Angiography and	Pulmonary Function Tests
Computed Tomographic	Arterial Blood Gases
Angiography	Exercise Testing

In evaluating the patient with pulmonary disease, the physician is concerned with three levels of evaluation: macroscopic, microscopic, and functional. The methods for assessing each of these levels range from simple and readily available studies to highly sophisticated and elaborate techniques requiring state-of-the-art technology.

Each level is considered here, with an emphasis on the basic principles and utility of the studies. Subsequent chapters repeatedly refer to these methods because they form the backbone of the physician's approach to the patient.

EVALUATION ON A MACROSCOPIC LEVEL

PHYSICAL EXAMINATION

The most accessible method for evaluating the patient with respiratory disease is the physical examination, which requires only a stethoscope; the eyes, ears, and hands of the examiner; and the examiner's skill in eliciting and recognizing abnormal findings. Because the purpose of this discussion is not to elaborate the details of a chest examination but to examine a few of the basic principles, the primary focus is on selected aspects of the examination and what is known about mechanisms that produce abnormalities.

Apart from general observation of the patient, precise measurement of the patient's respiratory rate, and interpretation of the patient's pattern of and difficulty with breathing, the examiner relies primarily on palpation and percussion of the chest and auscultation with a stethoscope. Palpation is useful for comparing the expansion of the two sides of the chest. The examiner can determine whether the two lungs are expanding symmetrically or if some process is affecting aeration much more on one side than on the other. Palpation of the chest wall also is useful for feeling the vibrations created by spoken sounds. When the examiner places a hand over an area of lung, vibration normally should be felt as the sound is transmitted to the chest wall. This vibration is called *vocal* or *tactile fremitus*. Some disease processes improve transmission of sound and augment the intensity of the vibration. Other conditions diminish transmission of sound and reduce the intensity of the vibration or eliminate it altogether. Elaboration of this concept of sound transmission and its relation to specific conditions is provided in the discussion of chest auscultation.

When percussing the chest, the examiner notes the quality of sound produced by tapping a finger of one hand against a finger of the opposite hand pressed closely to the patient's chest wall. The principle is similar to that of tapping a surface and judging whether what is underneath is solid or hollow. Normally, percussion of the chest wall overlying air-containing lung gives a resonant sound, whereas percussion over a solid organ such as the liver produces a dull sound. This contrast allows the examiner to detect areas with something other than air-containing lung beneath the chest wall, such as fluid in the pleural space (pleural effusion) or airless (consolidated) lung, each of which sounds dull to percussion. At the other extreme, air in the pleural space (pneumothorax) or a hyperinflated lung (as in emphysema) may produce a hyper-resonant or more "hollow" sound, approaching what the examiner hears when percussing over a hollow viscus, such as the stomach. Additionally, the examiner can locate the approximate position of the diaphragm by a change in the quality of the percussed note, from resonant to dull, toward the bottom of the lung. A convenient aspect of the whole-chest examination is the basically symmetric nature of the two sides of the chest; a difference in the findings between the two sides suggests a localized abnormality.

When auscultating the lungs with a stethoscope, the examiner listens for two major features: the quality of the breath sounds and the presence of any abnormal (commonly called *adventitious*) sounds. As the patient takes a deep breath, the sound of airflow can be heard through the stethoscope. When the stethoscope is placed over normal lung tissue, sound is heard primarily during inspiration, and the quality of the sound is relatively smooth and soft. These normal breath sounds heard over lung tissue are called *vesicular breath sounds*. There is no general agreement about where these sounds originate, but the source presumably is somewhere distal to the trachea and proximal to the alveoli.

When the examiner listens over consolidated lung—that is, lung that is airless and filled with liquid or inflammatory cells—the findings are different. The sound is louder and harsher, more hollow or tubular in quality, and expiration is at least as loud and as long as inspiration. Such breath sounds are called *bronchial breath sounds,* as opposed to the normal vesicular sounds. This difference in quality of the sound is due to the ability of consolidated lung to transmit sound better than normally aerated lung. As a result, sounds generated by turbulent airflow in the central airways (trachea and major bronchi) are transmitted to the periphery of the lung and can be heard through the stethoscope. Normally, these sounds are not heard in the lung periphery; they can be demonstrated only by listening near their site of origin—for example, over the upper part of the sternum or the suprasternal notch. When the stethoscope is placed over large airways that are not quite so central or over an area of partially consolidated lung, the breath sounds are intermediate in quality between bronchial and vesicular and therefore are termed *bronchovesicular.*

Better transmission of sound through consolidated rather than normal lung also can be demonstrated when the patient whispers or speaks. The enhanced transmission of whispered sound results in more distinctly heard syllables and is termed *whispered pectoriloquy.* Spoken words can be heard more distinctly through the stethoscope placed over the involved area, a phenomenon commonly called *bronchophony.* When

---

Goals of auscultation:
1. Assessment of breath sounds
2. Detection of adventitious sounds

Consolidated lung does not filter sound in the same way as does air-containing lung.

the patient says the vowel "E," the resulting sound through consolidated lung has a nasal "A" quality. This E-to-A change is termed *egophony.* All these findings are variations on the same theme—an altered transmission of sound through airless lung—and basically have the same significance.

Two qualifications are important in interpreting the quality of breath sounds. First, normal transmission of sound depends on patency of the airway. If a relatively large bronchus is occluded, such as by tumor, secretions, or a foreign body, airflow into that region of lung is diminished or absent, and the examiner hears decreased or absent breath sounds over the affected area. A blocked airway proximal to consolidated or airless lung also eliminates the increased transmission of sound described previously. Second, either air or fluid in the pleural space acts as a barrier to sound so that either a pneumothorax or a pleural effusion causes diminution of breath sounds.

The second major feature the examiner listens for is adventitious sounds. Unfortunately, the terminology for these adventitious sounds varies considerably among examiners; therefore, only the most commonly used terms are considered here: crackles, wheezes, and friction rubs. A fourth category, rhonchi, is used inconsistently by different examiners, thus decreasing its clinical usefulness for communicating abnormal findings.

Crackles, also called *rales,* are a series of individual clicking or popping noises heard with the stethoscope over an involved area of lung. Their quality can range from the sound produced by rubbing hairs together to that generated by opening a hook and loop (Velcro) fastener or crumpling a piece of cellophane. These sounds are "opening" sounds of small airways or alveoli that have been collapsed or decreased in volume during expiration because of fluid, inflammatory exudate, or poor aeration. On each subsequent inspiration, opening of these distal lung units creates the series of clicking or popping sounds heard either throughout or at the latter part of inspiration. The most common disorders producing rales are pulmonary edema, pneumonia, interstitial lung disease, and atelectasis. Although some clinicians believe the quality of the crackles helps to distinguish the different disorders, others think that such distinctions in quality are of little clinical value.

> Crackles, heard during inspiration, are "opening" sounds of small airways and alveoli.

Wheezes are high-pitched, continuous sounds that are generated by airflow through narrowed airways. Causes of such narrowing include airway smooth muscle constriction, edema, secretions, intraluminal obstruction, and collapse because of poorly supported walls. These individual pathophysiologic features are discussed in Chapters 4 through 7. For reasons that are also described later, the diameter of intrathoracic airways is less during expiration than inspiration, and wheezing generally is more pronounced or exclusively heard in expiration. However, because sufficient airflow is necessary to generate a wheeze, wheezing may no longer be heard if airway narrowing is severe. In conditions such as asthma and chronic obstructive pulmonary disease, wheezes are generally polyphonic, meaning that they are a combination of different musical pitches that start and stop at different times during the expiratory cycle. In contrast, wheezing sounds tend to be monophonic when they result from focal narrowing of the trachea or large bronchi. When the site of narrowing is the extrathoracic airway (e.g., in the larynx or the extrathoracic portion of the trachea), the term *stridor* is used to describe the inspiratory wheezinglike sound that results from such narrowing. The physiologic factors that relate the site of narrowing and the phase of the respiratory cycle that is most affected are described later in this chapter and shown in Figures 3-20 and 3-21.

> Wheezes reflect airflow through narrowed airways.

Although clinicians commonly use the term *rhonchi* when referring to sounds generated by secretions in airways, examiners use the term in somewhat different ways. The term is used to describe low-pitched continuous sounds that are somewhat coarser than high-pitched wheezing. It is also used to describe the very coarse crackles that often result from airway secretions. As a result, the term is frequently used to describe the variety of noises and musical sounds that cannot be readily classified within the more generally accepted categories of crackles and wheezes but that all appear to have airway secretions as a common underlying cause.

A *friction rub* is the term for the sounds generated by inflamed or roughened pleural surfaces rubbing against each other during respiration. A rub is a series of creaky or rasping sounds heard during both inspiration and expiration. The most common causes are primary inflammatory diseases of the pleura or parenchymal processes that extend out to the pleural surface, such as pneumonia and pulmonary infarction.

Table 3-1 summarizes some of the pulmonary findings commonly seen in selected disorders affecting the respiratory system. Many of these are mentioned again in subsequent chapters when the specific disorders are discussed in more detail.

Although the focus here is the chest examination itself as an indicator of pulmonary disease, other nonthoracic manifestations of primary pulmonary disease may be detected on physical examination. Briefly discussed here are clubbing (with or without hypertrophic osteoarthropathy) and cyanosis.

Clubbing is a change in the normal configuration of the nails and the distal phalanx of the fingers or toes (Fig. 3-1). Several features may be seen: (1) loss of the normal angle between the nail and the skin, (2) increased curvature of the nail, (3) increased sponginess of the tissue below the proximal part of the nail, and (4) flaring or widening of the terminal phalanx. Although several nonpulmonary disorders can result in clubbing (e.g., congenital heart disease with right-to-left shunting, endocarditis, chronic liver disease, inflammatory bowel disease), the most common causes clearly

Respiratory system diseases associated with clubbing:
1. Carcinoma of the lung (or mesothelioma of the pleura)
2. Chronic intrathoracic infection
3. Interstitial lung disease

are pulmonary. Occasionally, clubbing is familial and of no clinical significance. Carcinoma of the lung (or mesothelioma of the pleura) is the single leading etiologic factor. Other pulmonary causes include chronic intrathoracic infection with suppuration (e.g., bronchiectasis, lung abscess, empyema) and some types of interstitial lung disease. Uncomplicated chronic obstructive lung disease is not associated with clubbing, so the presence of clubbing in this setting should suggest coexisting malignancy or suppurative disease.

Clubbing may be accompanied by *hypertrophic osteoarthropathy*, characterized by periosteal new bone formation, particularly in the long bones, and arthralgias and arthritis of any of several joints. With coexistent hypertrophic osteoarthropathy, either pulmonary or pleural tumor is the likely cause of the clubbing because hypertrophic osteoarthropathy is relatively rare with the other causes of clubbing.

Table 3-1

TYPICAL CHEST EXAMINATION FINDINGS IN SELECTED CLINICAL CONDITIONS

Condition	Percussion	Fremitus	Breath Sounds	Voice Transmission	Crackles
Normal	Resonant	Normal	Vesicular (at lung bases)	Normal	Absent
Consolidation or atelectasis (with patent airway)	Dull	Increased	Bronchial	Bronchophony, whispered pectoriloquy, egophony	Present
Consolidation or atelectasis (with blocked airway)	Dull	Decreased	Decreased	Decreased	Absent
Emphysema	Hyperresonant	Decreased	Decreased	Decreased	Absent
Pneumothorax	Hyperresonant	Decreased	Decreased	Decreased	Absent
Pleural effusion	Dull	Decreased	Decreased*	Decreased*	Absent

*May be altered by collapse of underlying lung, which will increase transmission of sound.

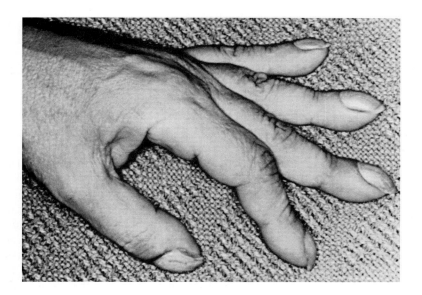

Figure 3-1. Clubbing in patient with carcinoma of lung. Curvature of nail and loss of angle between nail and adjacent skin can be seen.

The mechanism of clubbing and hypertrophic osteoarthropathy is not clear. It has been observed that clubbing is associated with an increase in digital blood flow, whereas the osteoarthropathy is characterized by an overgrowth of highly vascular connective tissue. Why these changes occur is a mystery. One interesting theory suggests an important role for stimuli coming through the vagus nerve, because vagotomy frequently ameliorates some of the bone and nail changes. Another theory proposes that megakaryocytes and platelet clumps, bypassing the pulmonary vascular bed and affecting the peripheral systemic circulation, release growth factors responsible for the soft-tissue changes of clubbing.

Cyanosis, the second extrapulmonary physical finding arising from lung disease, is a bluish discoloration of the skin (particularly under the nails) and mucous membranes. Whereas oxygenated hemoglobin gives lighter skin and all mucous membranes their usual pink color, a sufficient amount of deoxygenated hemoglobin produces cyanosis. Cyanosis may be either generalized, owing to a low Po_2 or low systemic blood flow resulting in increased extraction of oxygen from the blood, or localized, owing to low blood flow and increased O_2 extraction within the localized area. In lung disease the common factor causing cyanosis is a low Po_2, and several different types of lung disease may be responsible. The total amount of hemoglobin affects the likelihood of detecting cyanosis. In the anemic patient, if the total quantity of deoxygenated hemoglobin is less than the amount needed to produce the bluish discoloration, even a very low Po_2 may not be associated with cyanosis. In the patient with polycythemia, in contrast, much less depression of Po_2 is necessary before sufficient deoxygenated hemoglobin exists to produce cyanosis.

CHEST RADIOGRAPHY

The chest radiograph, which is largely taken for granted in the practice of medicine, is used not only in evaluating patients with suspected respiratory disease but also sometimes in the routine evaluation of asymptomatic patients. Of all the viscera, the lungs are the best suited for radiographic examination. The reason is straightforward: air in the lungs provides an excellent background against which abnormalities can stand out.

Additionally, the presence of two lungs allows each to serve as a control for the other so that unilateral abnormalities can be more easily recognized.

A detailed description of interpretation of the chest radiograph is beyond the scope of this text. However, a few principles can aid the reader in viewing films presented in this and subsequent chapters.

First, the appearance of any structure on a radiograph depends on the structure's density; the denser the structure, the whiter it appears on the film. At one extreme is air, which is radiolucent and appears black on the film. At the other extreme are metallic densities, which appear white. In between is a spectrum of increasing density from fat to water to bone. The viscera and muscles fall within the realm of water density tissues and cannot be distinguished in radiographic density from water or blood.

Second, in order for a line or an interface to appear between two adjacent structures on a radiograph, the two structures must differ in density. For example, within the cardiac shadow the heart muscle cannot be distinguished from the blood coursing within the chambers because both are of water density. In contrast, the borders of the heart are visible against the lungs, because the water density of the heart contrasts with the density of the lungs, which is closer to that of air. However, if the lung adjacent to a normally denser structure (e.g., heart or diaphragm) is airless, either because of collapse or consolidation, the neighboring structures are now both of the same density, and no visible interface or boundary separates them. This principle is the basis of the useful *silhouette sign*. If an expected border with an area of lung is not visualized or is not distinct, the adjacent lung is abnormal and lacks full aeration.

Chest radiographs usually are taken in two standard views—posteroanterior (PA) and lateral (Fig. 3-2). For a PA film, the x-ray beam goes from the back to the front of the patient, and the patient's anterior chest is adjacent to the film. The lateral view is taken with the patient's side against the film, and the beam is directed through the patient to the film. If a film cannot be taken with the patient standing and the chest adjacent to the film, as in the case of a bedridden patient, then an anteroposterior view is taken. For this view, which is generally obtained using a portable chest radiograph machine in the patient's hospital room, the film is placed behind the patient (generally between the patient's back and the bed), and the beam is directed through the patient from front to back. Lateral decubitus views, either right or left, are obtained with the patient in a side-lying position, with the beam directed horizontally. Decubitus views are particularly useful for detecting free-flowing fluid within the pleural space and therefore are often used when a pleural effusion is suspected.

Knowledge of radiographic anatomy is fundamental for interpretation of consolidation or collapse (atelectasis) and for localization of other abnormalities on the chest film. Lobar anatomy and the locations of fissures separating the lobes are shown in Figure 3-3. Localization of an abnormality often requires information from both the PA and lateral views, both of which should be taken and interpreted when an abnormality is being evaluated. As can be seen in Figure 3-3, the major fissure separating the upper (and middle) lobes from the lower lobe runs obliquely through the chest. Thus it is easy to be misled about location on the basis of the PA film alone; a lower lobe lesion may appear in the upper part of the chest, whereas an upper lobe lesion may appear much lower in position.

When a lobe becomes filled with fluid or inflammatory exudate, as in pneumonia, it contains water rather than air density and therefore is easily delineated on the chest radiograph. With pure consolidation the lobe does not lose volume, so it occupies its usual position and retains its usual size. An example of lobar consolidation on PA and lateral radiographs is shown in Figure 3-4.

In contrast, when a lobe has airless alveoli and collapses, it not only becomes more dense but also has features of volume loss characteristic for each individual lobe. Such

Both posteroanterior and lateral radiographs are often necessary for localization of an abnormality.

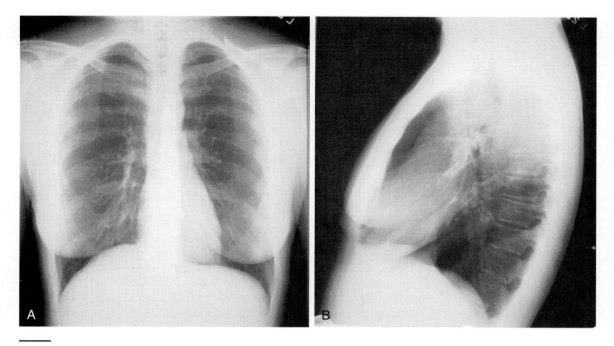

Figure 3-2. Normal chest radiograph. **A,** Posteroanterior view. **B,** Lateral view. Compare with Figure 3-3 for position of each lobe.

features of volume loss include change in position of a fissure or the indirect signs of displacement of the hilum, diaphragm, trachea, or mediastinum in the direction of the volume loss (Fig. 3-5). A common mechanism of atelectasis is occlusion of the airway leading to the collapsed region of lung, caused, for example, by a tumor, aspirated foreign body, or mucous plug. All the aforementioned examples reflect either pure consolidation or pure collapse. In practice, however, a combination of these processes often occurs, leading to consolidation accompanied by partial volume loss.

When the chest film shows a diffuse or widespread pattern of increased density within the lung parenchyma, it often is useful to characterize the process further, depending on the pattern of the radiographic findings. The two primary patterns are *interstitial* and *alveolar*. Although the naming of these patterns suggests a correlation with the type of pathologic involvement (i.e., interstitial, affecting the alveolar walls and the interstitial tissue; alveolar, involving filling of the alveolar spaces), such radiographic-pathologic correlations are often lacking. Nevertheless, many diffuse lung diseases are characterized by one of these radiographic patterns, and the particular pattern may provide clues about the underlying type or cause of disease.

An interstitial pattern generally is described as *reticular* or *reticulonodular*, consisting of an interlacing network of linear and small nodular densities. In contrast, an alveolar pattern appears more fluffy, and the outlines of air-filled bronchi coursing through the alveolar densities are often seen. This latter finding is called an *air bronchogram* and is due to air in the bronchi being surrounded and outlined by alveoli that are filled with fluid. This finding does not occur with a purely interstitial pattern. Examples of chest radiographs that show diffuse abnormality as a result of interstitial disease and alveolar filling are shown in Figures 3-6 and 3-7, respectively.

Diffuse increase in density on the radiograph often can be categorized as either alveolar or interstitial.

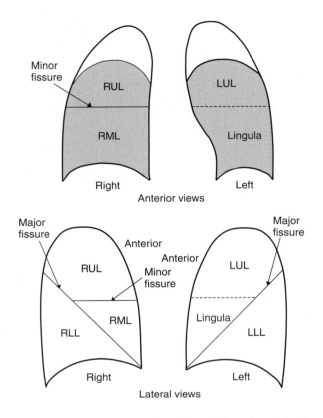

Figure 3-3. Lobar anatomy as seen from anterior and lateral views. In anterior views, *shaded regions* represent lower lobes and are behind upper and middle lobes. Lingula is part of the left upper lobe; *dashed line* between the two does not represent a fissure. LLL = Left lower lobe; LUL = left upper lobe; RLL = right lower lobe; RML = right middle lobe; RUL = right upper lobe.

Two additional terms used to describe patterns of increased density are worth mentioning. A *nodular* pattern refers to the presence of multiple discrete, typically spherical, nodules. A uniform pattern of relatively small nodules, several millimeters or less in diameter, is often called a *miliary* pattern, as can be seen with hematogenous (bloodborne) dissemination of tuberculosis throughout the lungs. Alternatively, the nodules can be larger (e.g., greater than 1 cm in diameter), as seen with hematogenous metastasis of carcinoma to the lungs. Another common term is *ground-glass,* which is used to describe a hazy, translucent appearance to the region of increased density. Although the term can be used to describe a region or a pattern of increased density on a plain chest radiograph, it is more commonly used when describing abnormalities seen on computed tomography (CT) of the chest.

Although the preceding focus on some typical abnormalities provides an introduction to pattern recognition on a chest radiograph, the careful examiner must also use a systematic approach in analyzing the film. A chest radiograph shows not only the lungs; radiographic examination also may reveal changes in bones, soft tissues, the heart, other mediastinal structures, and the pleural space.

COMPUTED TOMOGRAPHY

Within a relatively short time, computed tomography (CT) has revolutionized the field of diagnostic radiology. With this technique a narrow beam of x-rays is passed through the patient and sensed by a rotating detector on the other side of the patient.

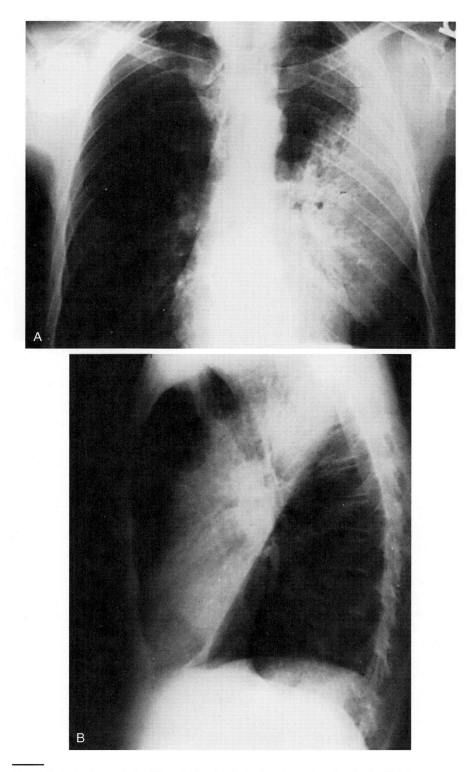

Figure 3-4. Posteroanterior **(A)** and lateral **(B)** chest radiographs of patient with left upper lobe consolidation attributable to pneumonia. The anatomic boundary is best appreciated on the lateral view, where it is easily seen that the normally positioned major fissure defines the lower border of consolidation (compare with Fig. 3-3). Part of the left upper lobe is spared. (Courtesy Dr. T. Scott Johnson.)

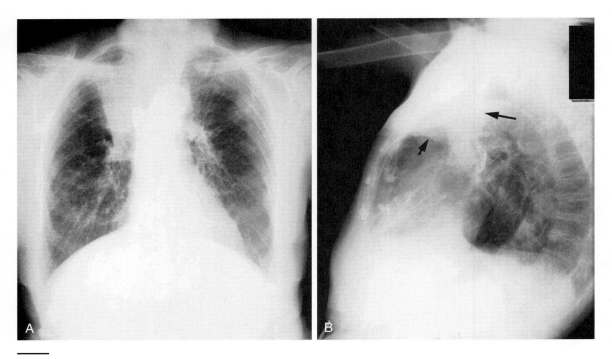

Figure 3-5. Posteroanterior **(A)** and lateral **(B)** chest radiographs demonstrating right upper lobe collapse. **A,** Displaced minor fissure outlines airless (dense) right upper lobe. **B,** Right upper lobe is outlined by elevated minor fissure *(short arrow)* and anteriorly displaced major fissure *(long arrow)*.

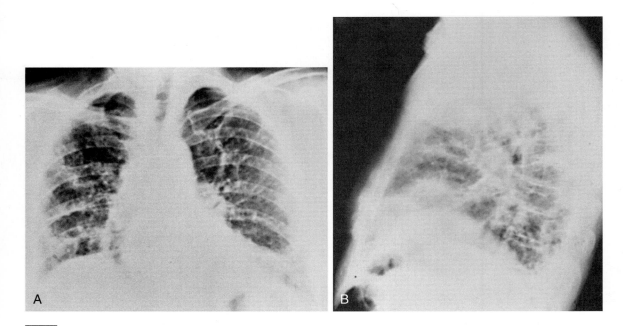

Figure 3-6. Posteroanterior **(A)** and lateral **(B)** chest radiographs of patient with interstitial lung disease. Reticulonodular pattern is present throughout but is most prominent in right lung and at base of left lung.

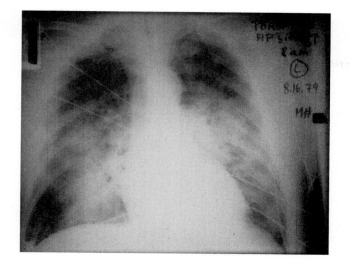

Figure 3-7. Chest radiograph showing a diffuse alveolar filling pattern, most prominent in the middle and lower lung fields.

The beam is partially absorbed within the patient, depending on the density of the intervening tissues. Computerized analysis of the information received by the detector allows a series of cross-sectional images to be constructed (Fig. 3-8). Use of different "windows" allows different displays of the collected data, depending on the densities of the structures of interest. With the technique of helical (spiral) CT scanning, the entire chest is scanned continuously (typically during a single breathhold and using multiple detectors) as the patient's body is moved through the CT apparatus (the gantry). If radiographic contrast is injected intravenously, images of the pulmonary arterial system obtained during helical scanning (CT angiography) can be used for detection of pulmonary emboli (see Chapter 13).

CT is particularly useful for detecting subtle differences in tissue density that cannot be distinguished by conventional radiography. In addition, the cross-sectional views obtained from the slices provide very different information from that provided by the vertical orientation of plain films.

> CT provides cross-sectional views of the chest and detects subtle differences in tissue density.

Chest CT has been used extensively in evaluating pulmonary nodules and the mediastinum. It also has been quite valuable in characterizing chest wall and pleural disease, and it now is frequently used for detecting pulmonary emboli through the technique of CT angiography. As the technology has advanced, CT has become progressively more useful in the diagnostic evaluation of various diseases affecting the pulmonary parenchyma and the airways. With high-resolution CT, the thickness of individual cross-sectional images is reduced to 1 to 2 mm instead of the traditional 5 to 10 mm. As a result, exceptionally fine detail can be seen, allowing earlier recognition of subtle disease and better characterization of specific disease patterns (Fig. 3-9).

Sophisticated software protocols now allow images obtained by CT scanning to be reconstructed and presented in any plane that best displays the abnormalities of interest. Additionally, it now is possible to produce three-dimensional images from the data acquired by CT scanning. For example, a three-dimensional view of the airways can be displayed in a manner resembling what is seen inside the airway lumen during bronchoscopy (described later in this chapter). This methodology creates an imaging tool that has been dubbed *virtual bronchoscopy.*

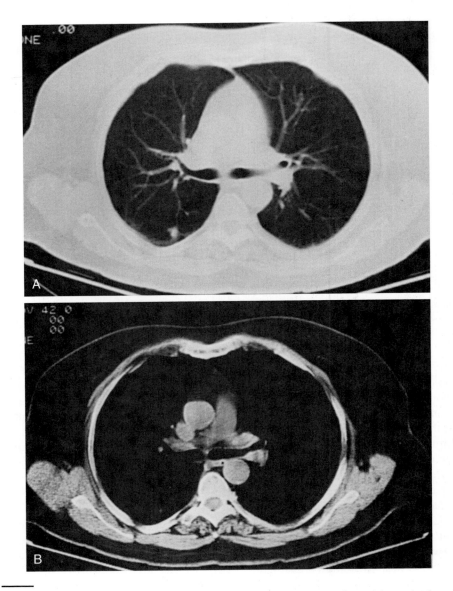

Figure 3-8. Cross-sectional slice from computed tomographic scan performed for evaluation of solitary peripheral pulmonary nodule. Nodule can be seen in posterior portion of right lung. The two images were taken using different "windows" at the same cross-sectional level. **A,** Settings were chosen to optimize visualization of the lung parenchyma. **B,** Settings were chosen to distinguish different densities of soft tissues, such as structures within the mediastinum.

MAGNETIC RESONANCE IMAGING

Another radiologic technique available for evaluation of intrathoracic disease is magnetic resonance imaging (MRI). The physical principles of MRI, which are complicated and beyond the training of most physicians and students, are discussed here briefly. The interested reader is referred to other sources for an in-depth discussion of the principles of MRI. In brief, the technique depends on the way that nuclei within a stationary magnetic field change their orientation and release energy delivered to them by a radiofrequency pulse. The time required to return to the baseline energy state can be analyzed by a complex computer algorithm and a visual image created.

In the evaluation of intrathoracic disease, MRI has several important features. First, flowing blood produces a "signal void" and appears black, so blood vessels can be readily

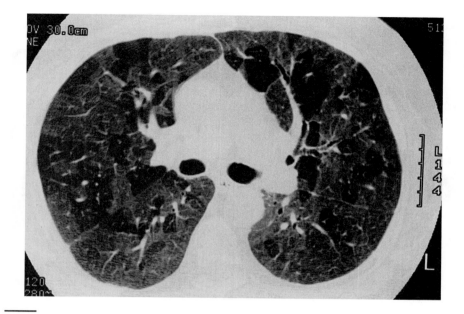

Figure 3-9. High-resolution computed tomographic scan of a patient with dyspnea and a normal chest radiograph. There are well-demarcated areas of lower density (normal lung) interspersed between hazy areas of increased ("ground-glass") density. Biopsy specimen showed findings of hypersensitivity pneumonitis.

distinguished from nonvascular structures without the need to use intravenous contrast agents. Second, images can be constructed in any plane so that the information obtained can be displayed as sagittal, coronal, or transverse (cross-sectional) views. Third, differences can be seen between normal and diseased tissues that are adjacent to each other, even when they are of the same density and therefore cannot be distinguished by routine radiography or CT. Some of these features are illustrated in Figure 3-10.

MRI scanning is expensive, so it generally is used when it can provide information not otherwise obtainable by less expensive, equally noninvasive means. Although MRI is newer than CT, it does not replace CT; rather, it often provides complementary diagnostic information. It can be a valuable tool in evaluating hilar and mediastinal disease as well as in defining intrathoracic disease that extends to the neck or the abdomen. On the other hand, it is less useful than CT in the evaluation of pulmonary parenchymal disease. However, knowledge about the power and the limitations of this technique continues to grow, and applications are likely to expand with further refinements in technology.

LUNG SCANNING

Injected or inhaled radioisotopes readily provide information about pulmonary blood flow and ventilation. Imaging of the γ radiation from these isotopes produces a picture showing the distribution of blood flow and ventilation throughout both lungs (Fig. 3-11). Other isotopes have been used for detecting and evaluating infectious, inflammatory, and neoplastic processes affecting the lungs.

Perfusion and Ventilation Scanning

For lung perfusion scanning, the most common technique involves injecting aggregates or microspheres of human albumin labeled with a radionuclide, usually technetium 99m, into a peripheral vein. These particles, which are approximately 10 to 60 μm in diameter, travel through the right side of the heart, enter the pulmonary vasculature, and become lodged in small pulmonary vessels. Only areas of the lung receiving perfusion

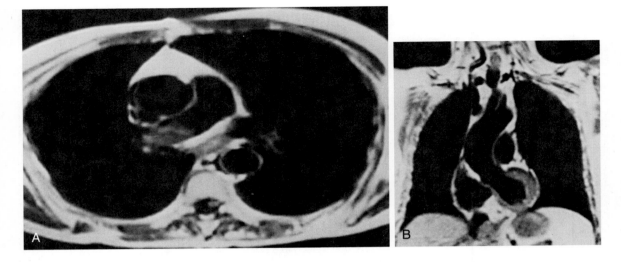

Figure 3-10. Magnetic resonance images of normal chest in cross-sectional **(A)** and coronal **(B)** views. Lumen of structures that contain blood appears black because flowing blood produces signal void.

from the pulmonary arterial system demonstrate uptake of the tracer, whereas nonperfused regions show no uptake of the labeled albumin.

For ventilation scanning, a gaseous radioisotope, usually xenon 133, is inhaled, and the sequential pictures obtained show how the gas distributes within the lung. Pictures obtained at different times after inhalation reveal information about gas distribution after the first breath (wash-in phase), after a longer time of breathing the gas (equilibrium phase), and after the patient again breathes air to eliminate the radioisotope (wash-out phase). Ventilation scanning shows which regions of the lungs are being ventilated and any significant localized problems with expiratory airflow and "gas trapping" of the radioisotope during the wash-out phase.

Perfusion and ventilation scans are performed chiefly for two reasons: detection of pulmonary emboli and assessment of regional lung function. When a pulmonary embolus occludes a pulmonary artery, blood flow ceases to the lung region normally supplied by that vessel, and a corresponding perfusion defect results. Generally, ventilation is preserved, and a ventilation scan does not show a corresponding ventilation defect. In practice, many pieces of information are considered in the interpretation of the scan, including the appearance of the chest radiograph and the size and distribution of the defects on the perfusion scan. These issues are discussed in greater detail in Chapter 13.

Scans to assess regional lung function are sometimes performed before surgery involving resection of a part of the lung, usually one or more lobes. By visualizing which areas of lung receive ventilation and perfusion, the physician can determine how much the area to be resected is contributing to overall lung function. When the scanning techniques are used in conjunction with pulmonary function testing, the physician can approximately predict postoperative pulmonary function, which is a guide to postoperative respiratory problems and impairment.

> Perfusion and ventilation lung scans are useful for detecting pulmonary emboli and evaluating regional lung function.

Gallium Scanning

A radioisotope occasionally used for detection and evaluation of infectious and inflammatory disorders affecting the lungs is gallium 67, in the form of gallium citrate. Gallium scanning has also been used for detection of *Pneumocystis jiroveci* (formerly called *Pneumocystis carinii*) in patients with acquired immunodeficiency syndrome (AIDS), although uptake of gallium can also be seen in a variety of other

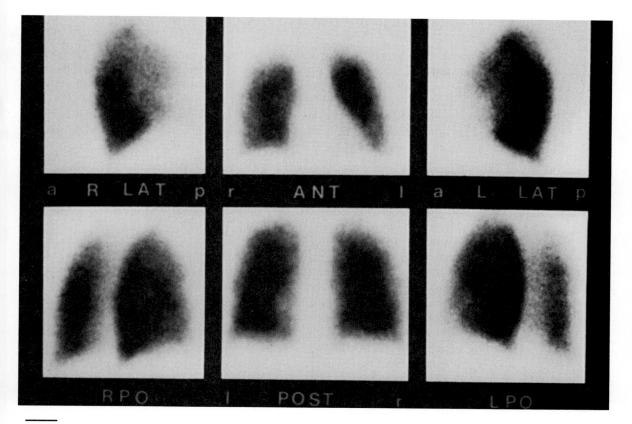

Figure 3-11. Normal perfusion lung scan shown in six views. a = Anterior; ANT = anterior view; l = left; LAT = lateral view; LPO = left posterior oblique view; p = posterior; POST = posterior view; r = right; RPO = right posterior oblique view. (Courtesy Dr. Henry Royal.)

opportunistic infections. Gallium scanning has also been used as a marker of inflammation and disease activity in patients with a variety of noninfectious inflammatory disorders affecting the lungs, but its use in this setting is controversial and now rare.

Fluorodeoxyglucose Scanning

On the basis of the principle that malignant tumors typically exhibit increased metabolic activity, scanning following injection of the radiolabeled glucose analogue 18-fluorodeoxyglucose (FDG) has been used as a way of identifying malignant lesions in the lungs and the mediastinum. Malignant cells, as a consequence of their increased uptake and use of glucose, take up the FDG but cannot metabolize it beyond the initial phosphorylation step, and the FDG is trapped within the cell. The radiolabeled FDG emits positrons, which are detected by positron emission tomography (PET) using a specialized imaging system, or by adapting a γ camera for imaging of positron-emitting radionuclides. PET imaging with FDG has been used primarily for evaluation of solitary pulmonary nodules and for staging of lung cancer, particularly for mediastinal lymph node involvement. However, the distinction between benign and malignant disease is not perfect, and false-negative and false-positive results can be seen with hypometabolic malignant lesions and highly active inflammatory lesions, respectively. PET scans can be performed in conjunction with CT scans, allowing coregistration and direct correlation of specific lesions visible on CT scan with their corresponding FDG uptake.

PULMONARY ANGIOGRAPHY AND COMPUTED TOMOGRAPHIC ANGIOGRAPHY

Although the perfusion lung scan provides useful information about pulmonary blood flow and traditionally was the first procedure performed to diagnose pulmonary embolism, it has limitations, particularly in patients with other forms of underlying lung disease. When the results of the perfusion scan were inconclusive, the physician often needed to investigate further with pulmonary angiography, a radiographic technique in which a catheter is guided from a peripheral vein, through the right atrium and ventricle, and into the main pulmonary artery or one of its branches. A radiopaque dye is injected, and the pulmonary arterial tree is visualized on a series of rapidly exposed chest films (Fig. 3-12). A clot in a pulmonary vessel appears either as an abrupt termination ("cutoff") of the vessel or as a filling defect within its lumen.

The pulmonary angiogram has other uses, including investigation of congenital vascular anomalies and invasion of a vessel by tumor. However, use of the angiogram in these situations is quite infrequent.

More recently, CT angiography, in which the pulmonary arterial system is visualized by helical CT scanning following injection of radiographic contrast into a peripheral vein, has been increasingly used in place of both perfusion lung scanning and traditional pulmonary angiography. Its use is attractive because it is more likely to be diagnostic than perfusion scanning, and it is less invasive than traditional pulmonary angiography. Although CT angiography is not as sensitive as traditional angiography for detecting emboli in relatively small pulmonary arteries, ongoing improvements in CT scanner technology have provided better identification of clots in progressively smaller pulmonary arteries.

ULTRASONOGRAPHY

The ability of different types of tissue to transmit sound and of tissue interfaces to reflect sound has made ultrasonography useful for evaluating a variety of body structures. A piezoelectric crystal generates sound waves, and the reflected echoes are detected and recorded by the same crystal. Images are displayed on a screen and can be captured for a permanent record.

The heart is the intrathoracic structure most frequently studied by ultrasonography, but the technique is also useful in evaluating pleural disease. In particular, ultrasonography is capable of detecting small amounts of pleural fluid and is often used to guide placement of a needle for sampling a small amount of this fluid. Additionally, it

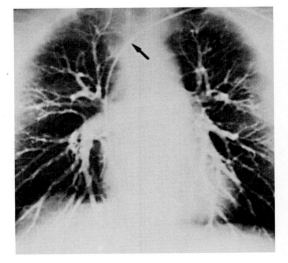

Figure 3-12. Normal pulmonary angiogram. Radiopaque dye was injected directly into pulmonary artery, and the pulmonary arterial tree is well visualized. Catheter used for injecting dye is indicated by *arrow*. (Courtesy Dr. Morris Simon.)

can detect walled-off compartments (loculations) within pleural effusions and distinguish fluid from pleural thickening.

Ultrasonography is capable of localizing the diaphragm and detecting disease immediately below the diaphragm, such as a subphrenic abscess. Ultrasonography is not useful for defining structures or lesions within the pulmonary parenchyma because the ultrasound beam penetrates air poorly.

BRONCHOSCOPY

Direct visualization of the airways is possible by bronchoscopy, originally performed with a hollow, rigid metal tube and now much more commonly with a thin flexible instrument (Fig. 3-13). The flexible instrument transmits images either via flexible fiberoptic bundles (traditional fiberoptic bronchoscope) or more recently, and now much more commonly, via a digital chip at the tip of the bronchoscope that displays the images on a monitor screen. Because the bronchoscope is flexible, the bronchoscopist can bend the tip with a control lever and maneuver into airways at least down to the subsegmental level.

The bronchoscopist can obtain an excellent view of the airways (Fig. 3-14) and collect a variety of samples for cytologic, pathologic, and microbiologic examination. Sterile saline can be injected through a small, hollow channel in the bronchoscope and suctioned back into a collection chamber. This technique, called *bronchial washing*, samples cells and, if present, microorganisms from the lower respiratory tract. When the bronchoscope is passed as far as possible and wedged into an airway before saline is injected, the washings are able to sample the contents of the alveolar spaces; this technique is called *bronchoalveolar lavage* (BAL).

With the flexible bronchoscope, airways are visualized and laboratory samples are obtained.

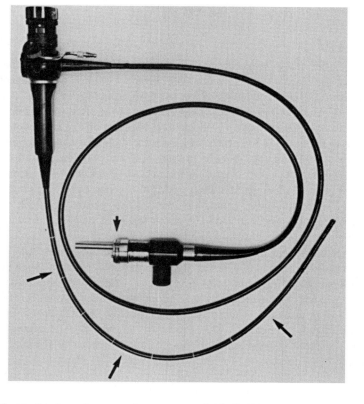

Figure 3-13. Flexible bronchoscope. *Long arrows* point to flexible part passed into patient's airways. *Short arrow* points to portion of bronchoscope connected to light source. Controls for clinician performing the procedure are shown at upper left.

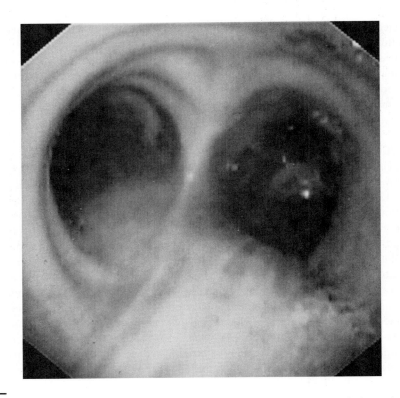

Figure 3-14. Airways as seen through a fiberoptic bronchoscope. At this level, the carina can be seen separating the right and left mainstem bronchi. A large endobronchial mass (squamous cell carcinoma of the lung) obstructs the right mainstem bronchus.

A long flexible wire instrument with a small brush at the tip can be passed through the hollow channel of the bronchoscope. The surface of a lesion within a bronchus can be brushed and the cells collected or smeared onto a slide for cytologic examination. Brushes are frequently passed into diseased areas of the lung parenchyma, and the material collected by the bristles is subjected to cytologic and microbiologic analysis.

A needle at the end of a long catheter passed through the bronchoscope can puncture an airway wall and sample cells from lymph nodes or lesions adjacent to the airway. This technique, called *transbronchial needle aspiration,* can be used to obtain malignant cells from mediastinal lymph nodes in the staging of known or suspected lung cancer. Using an ultrasound probe within the airway during bronchoscopy *(endobronchial ultrasound)* can help the bronchoscopist localize mediastinal lymph nodes that are external to the airway and therefore greatly assist with accurate placement of a needle into the node for transbronchial needle aspiration.

With a small biopsy forceps passed through the bronchoscope, the clinician can extract a biopsy specimen from a lesion visualized on the bronchial wall *(endobronchial biopsy).* When a fluoroscope is used to aid in passage of the forceps, the lung parenchyma is quite accessible after the forceps puncture a small bronchus and move out into the distal parenchyma. This procedure, known as a *transbronchial biopsy,* yields pieces of tissue that are small but have a sizable number of alveoli.

There are many indications for bronchoscopy, usually with a flexible instrument, although the rigid instrument is used under some circumstances. When appropriate, the flexible instrument is preferred because the procedure can be performed using only mild sedation and the patient need not be hospitalized. In contrast, rigid bronchoscopy is performed only under general anesthesia. Some indications for bronchoscopy include (1) evaluation of a suspected endobronchial malignancy; (2) sampling of an area of parenchymal disease by BAL, brushings, or biopsy; (3) evaluation of hemoptysis; and (4) removal of a foreign body (with special instruments that can be passed through the bronchoscope and are capable of retrieving objects). A variety of newer therapeutic modalities are being delivered to the airways via either flexible or rigid bronchoscopic techniques. These modalities include laser techniques for shrinking endobronchial tumors causing airway obstruction; placement of stents to maintain patency of airways having a compromised or obstructed lumen; procedures for dilation of strictures; placement of radioactive seeds directly into malignant airway lesions (brachytherapy); and delivery of electric current (electrocautery), low temperature (cryotherapy), or certain wavelengths of light (photodynamic therapy) to endobronchial masses. Deployment of these novel therapeutic opportunities has spawned a relatively new and rapidly evolving area of subspecialization within pulmonary medicine called *interventional pulmonology*.

During the past 40 years or so, bronchoscopy has become a common, useful technique in evaluating and managing pulmonary disease. Even though the physician who first suggested placing a tube into the larynx and bronchi was censured in 1847 for proposing a technique that is "an anatomical impossibility and an unwarrantable innovation in practical medicine," bronchoscopy generally is well tolerated and complications are infrequent.

EVALUATION ON A MICROSCOPIC LEVEL

Microscopy often provides the definitive diagnosis of pulmonary disease suggested by the history, physical examination, or chest radiograph. Several types of disorders are particularly amenable to diagnosis by microscopy: lung tumors (by either histology or cytology), pulmonary infection (by microscopic identification of a specific organism), and a variety of miscellaneous pulmonary diseases, particularly those affecting the interstitium of the lung (by histology). Frequently, when a diagnosis is uncertain, the same techniques are used to obtain samples that are processed both for histologic (or cytologic) examination and for identification of microorganisms. This section provides a discussion of how specimens are obtained and then considers how the specimens are processed.

OBTAINING SPECIMENS

The three main types of specimens the physician uses for microscopic analysis in diagnosing the patient with lung disease are (1) tracheobronchial secretions, (2) tissue from the lung parenchyma, and (3) fluid or tissue from the pleura. A number of methods are available for obtaining each of these types of specimens, and knowledge of the yield and the complications determines the most appropriate method.

The easiest way to obtain a specimen of tracheobronchial secretions is to collect sputum that is expectorated spontaneously by the patient. The sample can be used for identifying inflammatory or malignant cells and for staining (and culturing) microorganisms. Collecting sputum sounds simple, but it presents several potential problems. First, the patient may not have any spontaneous cough and sputum production. If this is the case, sputum frequently can be induced by having the patient inhale an irritating aerosol, such as hypertonic saline. Second, what is thought to be sputum originating from the tracheobronchial tree frequently is either nasal secretions or "spit" expectorated from the mouth or the back of the throat. Finally, as a result of passage through the mouth, even a good, deep sputum specimen is contaminated by the multiplicity of microorganisms that reside in the mouth. Because of this contamination, care is required in interpreting the results of sputum culture, particularly with regard to the normal flora of the upper respiratory tract. Despite these limitations, sputum remains a valuable resource when looking for malignancy and infectious processes such as bacterial pneumonia and tuberculosis.

Tracheobronchial secretions also can be obtained by two other routes: transtracheal aspiration and bronchoscopy. With transtracheal aspiration, a small plastic catheter is passed inside (or over) a needle inserted through the cricothyroid membrane and into the trachea. The catheter induces coughing, and secretions are collected either with or without the additional instillation of saline through the catheter. This technique avoids the problem of contamination by mouth and upper airway flora. It also allows collection of a sample even when the patient has no spontaneous sputum production. However, the technique is not without risk. Bleeding complications and, to a lesser extent, subcutaneous emphysema (air dissecting through tissues in the neck) are potentially serious sequelae. Because of these potential complications, the availability of alternative methods of sampling, and physicians' inexperience with the procedure, transtracheal aspiration is now rarely performed.

Bronchoscopy, generally with a flexible instrument, is a suitable way to obtain tracheobronchial secretions. It has the additional benefit of allowing visualization of the airways. Bronchoscopy has distinct advantages in collecting material for cytologic analysis because specimens can be collected from a localized area directly visualized with the bronchoscope. However, because the instrument passes through the upper respiratory tract, collection of specimens for culture is subject to contamination by upper airway flora. Specially designed systems with a protected brush can decrease contamination, and quantitating the bacteria recovered can be helpful in distinguishing upper airway contamination from true lower respiratory infection.

BAL has become an increasingly popular method for obtaining specimens from the lower respiratory tract. The fluid obtained by BAL has been used quite effectively for detecting *P. jiroveci*, particularly in patients with AIDS. In some interstitial lung diseases (see Chapters 9 and 11), analysis of the cellular and biochemical components of BAL may provide information that is useful diagnostically and for research about basic disease mechanisms.

As is true of tracheobronchial secretions, tissue specimens for microscopic examination can be collected in numerous ways. A brush or a biopsy forceps can be passed through a bronchoscope. The brush is often used to scrape cells from the surface of an airway lesion, but it also can be passed more distally into the lung parenchyma to obtain specimens directly from a diseased area. The biopsy forceps is used in a similar fashion to sample tissue either from a lesion in the airway (endobronchial biopsy) or from an area of disease in the parenchyma (transbronchial biopsy, so named because the forceps must puncture a small bronchus to sample the parenchyma). In the case of bronchial brushing, the specimen that adheres to the brush is smeared onto a slide for staining and microscopic examination. For both endobronchial and transbronchial biopsies, the tissue obtained can be fixed and sectioned, and slides can be made for subsequent microscopic examination.

A lesion or diseased area in the lung parenchyma can be reached with a needle through the chest wall. Depending on the type of needle used, a small sample may be aspirated or taken by biopsy. Bleeding and pneumothorax are potential complications, just as they are for a transbronchial biopsy with a bronchoscope.

Lung tissue is frequently obtained by a surgical procedure involving an approach through the chest wall. Traditionally, a surgeon made an incision in the chest wall, allowing direct visualization of the lung surface and removal of a small piece of lung tissue. This type of open lung biopsy has largely been supplanted by a less invasive procedure called *thoracoscopy* (or *video-assisted thoracic surgery*). Video-assisted thoracic surgery involves placement of a thoracoscope and biopsy instruments through small incisions in the chest wall; a high-quality image obtained through the

Tracheobronchial secretions are provided by
1. Expectorated sputum
2. Transtracheal aspiration
3. Flexible bronchoscopy

Lung biopsy specimens can be obtained by
1. Flexible bronchoscopy
2. Percutaneous needle aspiration or biopsy
3. Video-assisted thoracic surgery
4. Open surgical procedure

thoracoscope can be displayed on a monitor screen. The surgeon uses the video image as a guide for manipulating the instruments to obtain a biopsy sample of peripheral lung tissue or to remove a peripheral lung nodule.

Finally, fluid in the pleural space is frequently sampled in the evaluation of a patient with a pleural effusion. A small needle is inserted through the chest wall and into the pleural space, and fluid is withdrawn. The fluid can be examined for malignant cells and microorganisms. Chemical analysis of the fluid (see Chapter 15) often provides additional useful diagnostic information. A biopsy specimen of the parietal pleural surface (the tissue layer lining the pleural space) also may be obtained either blindly, with a special needle passed through the chest wall, or under direct visualization using a thoracoscope. The tissue can be used for microscopic examination and microbiologic studies.

PROCESSING SPECIMENS

Once the specimens are obtained, the techniques of processing and the types of examination performed are common to those used for many types of tissue and fluid specimens.

Diagnosis of pulmonary infections depends on smears and cultures of the material obtained, such as sputum, other samples of tracheobronchial secretions, or pleural fluid. The standard Gram stain technique often allows initial identification of organisms, and inspection may reveal inflammatory cells (particularly polymorphonuclear leukocytes) and upper airway (squamous epithelial) cells, the latter indicating contamination of sputum by upper airway secretions. Final culture results provide definitive identification of an organism, but the results must always be interpreted with the knowledge that the specimen may be contaminated and that what is grown is not necessarily causally related to the clinical problem.

Identification of mycobacteria, the causative agent for tuberculosis, requires special staining and culturing techniques. Mycobacteria are stained by agents such as carbolfuchsin or auramine-rhodamine, and the organisms are almost unique in their ability to retain the stain after acid is added. Hence, the expression *acid-fast bacilli* is used commonly when referring to mycobacteria. Frequently used staining methods are the Ziehl-Neelsen stain or a modification called the Kinyoun stain. A more sensitive and faster way to detect mycobacteria involves use of a fluorescent dye such as auraminerhodamine. Mycobacteria take up the dye and fluoresce and can be detected relatively easily even when present in small numbers. Because mycobacteria grow slowly, they may require 6 to 8 weeks for growth and identification on culture media.

Organisms other than the common bacterial pathogens and mycobacteria often require other specialized staining and culture techniques. Fungi may be diagnosed by special stains, such as methenamine silver or periodic acid–Schiff stains, applied to tissue specimens. Fungi also can be cultured on special media favorable to their growth. *Pneumocystis jiroveci*, a pathogen that is now classified as a unique category of fungi (see Chapter 25) and is most common in patients with impaired defense mechanisms, is stained in tissue and tracheobronchial secretions by methenamine silver, toluidine blue, or Giemsa stain. An immunofluorescent stain using monoclonal antibodies against *Pneumocystis* is particularly sensitive for detecting the organism in sputum and BAL fluid. The organism identified in 1976 as *Legionella pneumophila*, the causative agent of legionnaires' disease, can be diagnosed by silver impregnation or immunofluorescence staining. The organism also can be grown, with difficulty, on some special media.

Cytologic examination for malignant cells is available for expectorated sputum, specimens obtained by needle aspiration, bronchial washings or brushings obtained with a bronchoscope, and pleural fluid. A specimen can be smeared directly onto a

Specimens can be processed for staining and culture of microorganisms and for cytologic and histopathologic examination.

slide (as with a bronchial brushing), subjected to concentration (bronchial washings, pleural fluid), or digested (sputum) prior to being smeared on the slide. The slide then is stained by the Papanicolaou technique, and the cells are examined for findings suggestive or diagnostic of malignancy.

Pathologic examination of tissue sections obtained by biopsy is most useful for diagnosis of malignancy or infection as well as for a variety of other processes affecting the lungs and the pleura. In many circumstances, examination of tissue obtained by biopsy is the gold standard for diagnosis, although even biopsy results can show false-negative findings or yield misleading information.

Tissue obtained by biopsy is routinely stained with hematoxylin and eosin for histologic examination. A wide assortment of other stains is available that more or less specifically stain collagen, elastin, and a variety of microorganisms. Further discussion of the specific techniques and stains can be found in standard pathology textbooks.

There has been great interest in applying state-of-the-art molecular biologic techniques to respiratory specimens for diagnosis of certain types of respiratory tract infection. For example, the polymerase chain reaction uses specific synthetic oligonucleotide "primer" sequences and DNA polymerase to amplify DNA that is unique to a specific organism. If the particular target DNA sequence is present, even if only from a single organism, sequential amplification allows production of millions of copies, which can be detected by gel electrophoresis. This technique can be applied to samples such as sputum and BAL, providing an exquisitely sensitive test for identifying organisms such as mycobacteria, *P. jiroveci,* and cytomegalovirus. These newer molecular techniques are becoming more readily available and are likely to see increasing clinical use over time.

ASSESSMENT ON A FUNCTIONAL LEVEL

Pulmonary evaluation on a macroscopic or microscopic level aims at a diagnosis of lung disease, but neither can determine the extent to which normal functions of the lung are impaired. This final aspect of evaluation adds an important dimension to overall assessment of the patient because it reflects how much the disease may limit a patient's daily activities. The two most common methods for determining a patient's functional status are pulmonary function testing and evaluation of gas exchange (using either arterial blood gases or pulse oximetry). In addition, a variety of measurements taken during exercise can help to determine how much exercise a patient can perform and what factors contribute to any limitation of exercise. Many other types of functional studies are useful for clinical or research purposes, but they are not discussed in this chapter.

PULMONARY FUNCTION TESTS

Pulmonary function testing provides an objective method for assessing functional changes in a patient with known or suspected lung disease. With the results of tests that are widely available, the physician can answer several questions: (1) Does the patient have significant lung disease sufficient to cause respiratory impairment and to account for his or her symptoms? (2) What functional pattern of lung disease does the patient have—restrictive or obstructive disease?

In addition, serial evaluation of pulmonary function allows the physician to quantitate any improvement or deterioration in a patient's functional status. Information obtained from such objective evaluation may be essential in deciding when to treat a patient with lung disease and in assessing whether a patient has responded to therapy.

Preoperative evaluation of patients can be useful in predicting which patients are likely to have significant postoperative respiratory problems and which are likely to have adequate pulmonary function after lung resection.

Three main categories of information can be obtained with routine pulmonary function testing:

1. Lung volumes, which provide a measurement of the size of the various compartments within the lung
2. Flow rates, which measure maximal flow within the airways
3. Diffusing capacity, which indicates how readily gas transfer occurs from the alveolus to pulmonary capillary blood

Before examining how these tests indicate what type of functional lung disease a patient has, we briefly describe the tests themselves and how they are performed.

Lung Volumes. Although the lung can be subdivided into compartments in different ways, four volumes are particularly important (Fig. 3-15):

1. Total lung capacity (TLC): Total volume of gas within the lungs after a maximal inspiration
2. Residual volume (RV): Volume of gas remaining within the lungs after a maximal expiration
3. Vital capacity (VC): Volume of gas expired when going from TLC to RV
4. Functional residual capacity (FRC): Volume of gas within the lungs at the resting state, that is, at the end of expiration during the normal tidal breathing pattern

VC can be measured by having the patient exhale into a spirometer from TLC down to RV. By definition, the volume expired in this manner is the VC. However, because RV, FRC, and TLC all include the amount of gas left within the lungs even after a maximal expiration, these volumes cannot be determined simply by having the patient breathe into a spirometer. To quantitate these volumes, a variety of methods can measure one of these three volumes, and the other two volumes then can be calculated or derived from the spirometric tracing. Two methods are described here:

1. Dilution tests: A known volume of an inert gas (usually helium) at a known concentration is inhaled into the lungs. This gas is diluted by the volume of gas

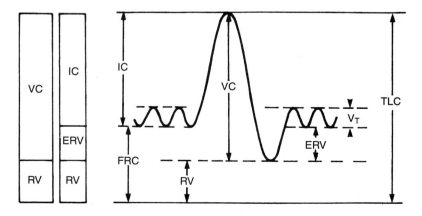

Figure 3-15. Subcompartments of lung (lung volumes). On the *right*, lung volumes are labeled on spirographic tracing. On the *left*, block diagrams show two ways that total lung capacity can be subdivided. ERV = Expiratory reserve volume; FRC = functional residual capacity; IC = inspiratory capacity; RV = residual volume; TLC = total lung capacity; VC = vital capacity; V_T = tidal volume.

Lung volumes are determined by spirometry and either gas dilution or body plethysmography.

already present within the lungs, and the concentration of expired gas (relative to inspired) therefore reflects the initial volume of gas in the lungs.

2. Body plethysmography: The patient, sitting inside an airtight box, performs a maneuver that causes expansion and compression of gas within the thorax. By quantitating volume and pressure changes and by applying Boyle's law, the volume of gas in the thorax can be calculated.

In many circumstances, dilution methods are adequate for determining lung volumes. However, for patients who have air spaces within the lung that do not communicate with the bronchial tree (e.g., bullae), the inhaled gas is not diluted in these noncommunicating areas, and the measured lung volumes determined by dilution methods are falsely low. In such situations, body plethysmography gives a more accurate reflection of intrathoracic gas volume inasmuch as it does not depend on ready communication of all peripheral air spaces with the bronchial tree.

Flow Rates. Measurement of flow rates on routine pulmonary function testing involves assessing airflow during maximal forced expiration, that is, with the patient blowing out as hard and as fast as possible from TLC down to RV. The volume expired during the first second of such a forced expiratory maneuver is called the *forced expiratory volume in 1 second* (FEV_1) (Fig. 3-16). When pulmonary function tests are interpreted, FEV_1 is routinely compared with VC, or with VC specifically measured during the forced expiratory maneuver called the *forced vital capacity* (FVC). In interpreting flow rates, the ratio between these two measurements (FEV_1/VC or FEV_1/FVC) is the most important number used to determine the presence of obstruction to airflow. Another parameter often calculated from the forced expiratory maneuver is the maximal midexpiratory flow rate (MMFR), which is the rate of airflow during the middle one-half of the expiration (between 25% and 75% of the volume expired during the FVC). MMFR is frequently called the forced expiratory flow (FEF) between 25% and 75% of

Maximal expiratory airflow is assessed by the FEV_1/FVC (or FEV_1/VC) ratio and MMFR ($FEF_{25\%-75\%}$).

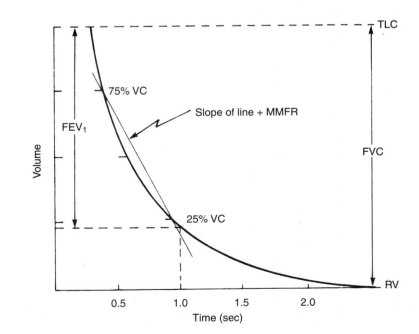

Figure 3-16. Forced expiratory spirogram. Volume is plotted against time while patient breathes out as hard and fast as possible from total lung capacity (TLC) to residual volume (RV). FEV_1 = Forced expiratory volume in 1 second; FVC = forced vital capacity; MMFR = maximal midexpiratory flow rate (also called forced expiratory flow from 25%-75% [$FEF_{25\%-75\%}$]); VC = vital capacity.

vital capacity ($FEF_{25\%-75\%}$). The MMFR or $FEF_{25\%-75\%}$ is a relatively sensitive index of airflow obstruction and may be abnormal when the FEV_1/FVC ratio is still preserved.

Diffusing Capacity. The diffusing capacity is a measurement of the rate of transfer of gas from the alveolus to hemoglobin within a capillary, measured in relation to the driving pressure of the gas across the alveolar-capillary membrane. Small concentrations of carbon monoxide are generally used for this purpose. Carbon monoxide combines readily with hemoglobin, and the rate of transfer of gas from the alveolus to the capillary depends on movement through the alveolar-capillary membrane and the amount of hemoglobin available for binding the carbon monoxide.

Although the diffusing capacity may be influenced to some extent by the thickness of the alveolar-capillary membrane, it is most dependent on the number of functioning alveolar-capillary units, that is, the surface area available for gas exchange, and the volume of blood (hemoglobin) in the pulmonary capillaries available to bind carbon monoxide. Because diffusing capacity may be depressed if a patient is anemic (owing to less available hemoglobin to bind carbon monoxide), the observed value is generally corrected for the patient's hemoglobin level. In practice, the diffusing capacity is commonly decreased in three categories of disease in which surface area for gas exchange is lost, pulmonary capillary blood volume is decreased, or both: (1) emphysema, (2) interstitial lung disease, and (3) pulmonary vascular disease. In disorders that affect only the airways and not pulmonary parenchymal tissue (e.g., asthma, chronic bronchitis), diffusing capacity is generally preserved. On the other hand, the diffusing capacity may be elevated in cases of recent intrapulmonary hemorrhage as a result of uptake of carbon monoxide by hemoglobin in the erythrocytes within the alveolar spaces.

> Diffusing capacity of carbon monoxide depends largely on the surface area for gas exchange and the pulmonary capillary blood volume.

Interpretation of Normality in Pulmonary Function Testing

Interpretation of pulmonary function tests necessarily involves a qualitative judgment about normality or abnormality on the basis of quantitative data obtained from these tests. To arrive at a relatively objective judgment, the patient's values are compared with normal standards established for each test based on measurements in large numbers of normal, nonsmoking control subjects. Separate regression equations for men and for women have been constructed to fit the data obtained from these normal control subjects. Separate race/ethnicity-specific equations are available because of slight differences in pulmonary function in normal individuals of different races and ethnicities. A "normal" or predicted value for a test in a given patient can be determined by inputting the patient's age and height into the appropriate regression equation.

The standards for determining what constitutes the "lower limits of normal" for a particular test vary among laboratories. Most laboratories now consider values below the bottom 5th percentile of a normal reference group (also called the "95% confidence interval") to be abnormal, whereas others consider an observed value to be abnormal if it is less than 80% of the predicted value. No matter which criteria are used, all the data must be considered to determine whether certain patterns are consistently present. Interpretation of any test in isolation, with the assumption that a patient with a value of 79% has lung disease but a patient with a value of 81% is disease free, is obviously dangerous.

The normal FEV_1/VC or FEV_1/FVC ratio is 0.70 or greater. An individual without lung disease should, during the first second of a maximal exhalation, be able to exhale at least 70% of the total volume exhaled. However, because the normal ratio can decrease with age, the actual value ideally should be considered abnormal if it is less than the 95% confidence interval for that patient's age.

Patterns of Pulmonary Function Impairment

In the analysis of pulmonary function tests, abnormalities usually are categorized as one of two patterns (or a combination of the two): (1) an *obstructive* pattern, characterized mainly by obstruction to airflow, and (2) a *restrictive* pattern, with evidence of decreased lung volumes but no airflow obstruction.

An obstructive pattern, as seen in patients with asthma, chronic bronchitis, and emphysema, consists of a decrease in rates of expiratory airflow and usually manifests as a decrease in MMFR and FEV_1/FVC ratio (Fig. 3-17). There is generally a high RV and an increased RV/TLC ratio, indicating air trapping owing to closure of airways during forced expiration (Fig. 3-18). Hyperinflation, reflected by an increased TLC, is often found, particularly in patients with either asthma or emphysema. Diffusing capacity tends to be decreased in patients who have loss of alveolar-capillary bed (as seen in emphysema) but not in those without loss of available surface area for gas exchange (as in chronic bronchitis and asthma).

The hallmark of restrictive disease is a reduction in lung volumes, whereas expiratory airflow is normal (see Fig. 3-18). Therefore, TLC, RV, VC, and FRC all tend to be reduced, whereas MMFR and FEV_1/FVC are preserved. In some patients with significant loss of volume resulting from restrictive disease, MMFR is decreased because less volume is available to generate a high flow rate. Interpreting a low MMFR in the face of significant restrictive disease is difficult unless MMFR is clearly decreased out of proportion to the decrease in lung volumes.

A wide variety of parenchymal, pleural, neuromuscular, and chest wall diseases can demonstrate a restrictive pattern. Certain clues are useful in distinguishing among these causes of restriction. For example, a decrease in the diffusing capacity for carbon monoxide suggests loss of alveolar-capillary units and points toward interstitial disease as the cause of the restrictive pattern. The finding of a relatively high RV can indicate either expiratory muscle weakness or a chest wall abnormality that makes the thoracic cage particularly stiff (noncompliant) at low volumes.

Although lung diseases often occur with one or the other of these patterns, a mixed picture of obstructive and restrictive disease can be present, making interpretation of

---

Patterns of impairment:
1. Obstructive: Diminished rates of expiratory airflow ($\downarrow FEV_1$/FVC, $\downarrow$MMFR)
2. Restrictive: Diminished lung volumes (especially $\downarrow$TLC) and preserved expiratory airflow

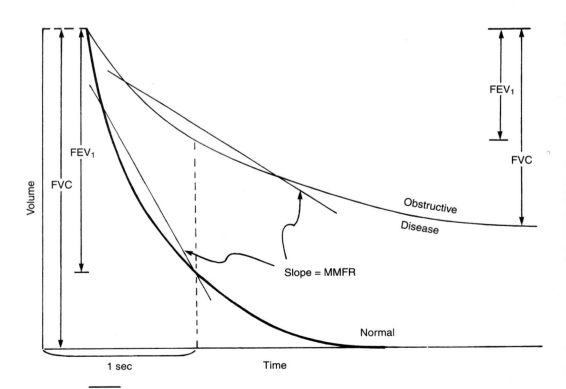

Figure 3-17. Forced expiratory spirograms in normal individual and patient with airflow obstruction. Note prolonged expiration and changes in forced vital capacity (FVC) and forced expiratory volume in 1 second (FEV_1) in patient with obstructive disease. MMFR = Maximal midexpiratory flow rate.

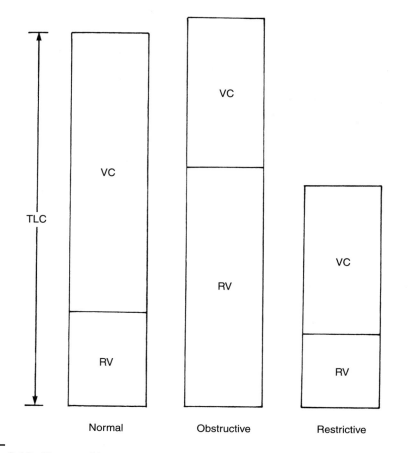

Figure 3-18. Diagram of lung volumes (total lung capacity [TLC] and subcompartments vital capacity [VC] and residual volume [RV]) in normal individual and patients with obstructive and restrictive disease.

the tests much more complex. These tests do not directly reflect a patient's overall capability for O_2 and CO_2 exchange, which is assessed by measurement of arterial blood gases.

A simplified guide to the interpretation of pulmonary function tests is presented along with several sample problems in Appendix B.

Other Tests

A significant amount of work was performed in the past to develop tests that detect early obstruction to airflow, particularly when it is due to small or peripheral airways obstruction. Such tests include maximal expiratory flow-volume loops, analysis of closing volume, and frequency-dependent dynamic compliance. Unfortunately, pathologic studies have shown that the correlation between tests of "small airways function" and the actual presence of disease in small airways (as demonstrated by histopathologic specimens) is inconsistent, making the value of these tests unclear. Despite this limitation, the maximal expiratory flow-volume loop is a test with sufficient routine clinical applicability to warrant a short discussion here.

The flow-volume loop is a graphic record of maximal inspiratory and maximal expiratory maneuvers. However, rather than the graph of volume versus time that is given with usual spirometric testing, the flow-volume loop has a plot of flow (on the Y-axis) versus volume (on the X-axis). Although the initial flows obtained during the early part of a forced expiratory maneuver are effort dependent, the flows during the latter part of the maneuver are effort independent and primarily reflect the mechanical properties of the lungs and the resistance to airflow.

In patients with evidence of airflow obstruction, flow rates at a given volume are decreased, often giving the curve a "scooped out" or coved appearance. The flow data obtained from maximal expiratory flow-volume loops can be interpreted quantitatively (comparing observed flow rates at specified volumes with predicted values) or qualitatively (visually analyzing the shape and concavity of the expiratory portion of the curve). When routine spirometric parameters reflecting airflow obstruction (MMFR, FEV_1/FVC) are abnormal, the flow-volume loop generally is abnormal. However, in patients with early airflow obstruction, perhaps localized to small airways, the contour of the terminal part of the expiratory curve may be abnormal even when the FEV_1/FVC ratio is normal. Examples of flow-volume loops in a normal patient and in a patient with obstructive lung disease are shown in Figure 3-19.

Another important application of flow-volume loops is for diagnosing and localizing upper airway obstruction. By analyzing the contour of the inspiratory and expiratory portions of the curve, the obstruction can be categorized as *fixed* or *variable*, as well as *intrathoracic* or *extrathoracic*. In a fixed lesion, changes in pleural pressure do not affect the degree of obstruction, and a limitation in peak airflow (a plateau) is seen on both the inspiratory and the expiratory portions of the curve. In a variable lesion the amount of obstruction is determined by the location of the lesion and by the effect of

> In obstructive lung disease, the expiratory portion of the flow-volume curve has a "scooped out" or coved appearance.

> Upper airway obstruction is characterized by maximal inspiratory and expiratory flow-volume curves.

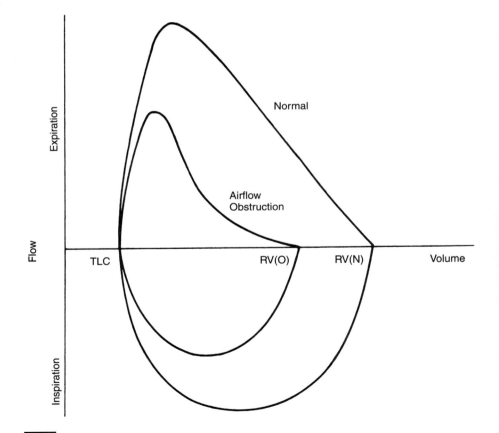

Figure 3-19. Flow-volume loops in normal individual and patient with airflow obstruction. Expiratory "coving" is apparent on tracing of patient with airflow obstruction. RV(N) = Residual volume in normal individual; RV(O) = residual volume in patient with obstructive disease; TLC = total lung capacity.

alterations in pleural and airway pressure with inspiration and expiration (Fig. 3-20). A variable intrathoracic lesion is characterized by expiratory limitation of airflow and a plateau on the expiratory portion of the flow-volume curve, whereas a variable extra-thoracic lesion demonstrates inspiratory limitation of airflow and a plateau on the inspiratory portion of the flow-volume curve (Fig. 3-21).

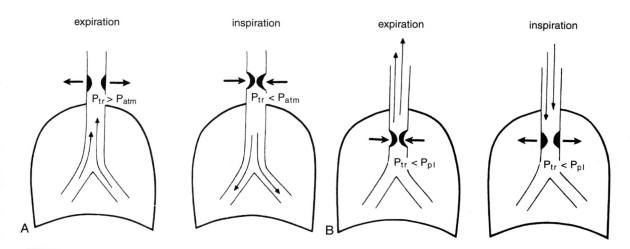

Figure 3-20. Effect of phase of respiration on upper airway obstruction. **A,** Variable extrathoracic obstruction. During forced inspiration, airway or tracheal pressure (P_{tr}) becomes more negative than surrounding atmospheric pressure (P_{atm}), and airway diameter decreases. During forced expiration, more positive intratracheal pressure distends airway and decreases magnitude of obstruction. **B,** Variable intrathoracic obstruction. Pleural pressure (Ppl) surrounds and acts on large intrathoracic airways, affecting airway diameter. During forced expiration, pleural pressure is markedly positive, and airway diameter is decreased. During forced inspiration, negative pleural pressure causes intrathoracic airways to be increased in size, and obstruction is decreased. (From Kryger M, Bode F, Antic R, Anthonisen N: Diagnosis of obstruction of the upper and lower airways. *Am J Med* 61:85–93, 1976, with permission from Excerpta Medica Inc.)

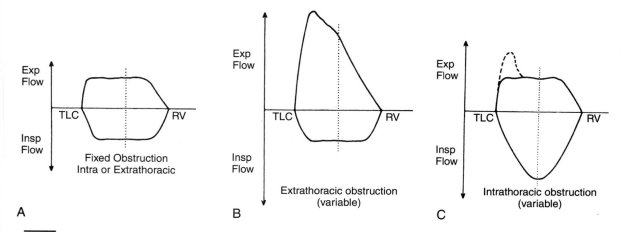

Figure 3-21. Maximal inspiratory and expiratory flow-volume curves in three types of upper airway obstruction. **A,** Fixed obstruction, either intrathoracic or extrathoracic. Obstruction is equivalent during inspiration and expiration so that maximal inspiratory and expiratory flows are limited to the same extent. **B,** Variable extrathoracic obstruction. Obstruction is more marked during inspiration, and only the inspiratory part of the curve demonstrates plateau. **C,** Variable intrathoracic obstruction. Obstruction is more marked during expiration, and only the expiratory part of the curve demonstrates a plateau. *Dashed line* represents a higher initial flow that is occasionally observed before plateau in intrathoracic obstruction. (From Kryger M, Bode F, Antic R, Anthonisen N: Diagnosis of obstruction of the upper and lower airways. *Am J Med* 61:85–93, 1976, with permission from Excerpta Medica Inc.)

A test of airflow that is commonly used in clinical practice, particularly in asthmatics as a method to follow severity of disease, is the *peak expiratory flow rate*. In performing this test, the patient blows out from TLC as hard as possible into a simple, readily available device that records the maximal (or peak) expiratory flow rate achieved. Patients with asthma frequently perform and record serial measurements of the test at home as a way of self-monitoring their disease. A significant drop in the peak flow rate from the usual baseline often indicates an exacerbation of the disease and the need for escalating or intensifying the therapeutic regimen.

ARTERIAL BLOOD GASES

Despite the extensive information provided by pulmonary function tests, they do not show the net effect of lung disease on gas exchange, which is easily assessed by studies performed on arterial blood. Arterial blood can be conveniently sampled by needle puncture of a radial artery or, less commonly and with more potential risk, of a brachial or femoral artery. The blood is collected into a heparinized syringe (to prevent clotting), and care is taken to expel air bubbles from the syringe and to analyze the sample quickly (or to keep it on ice until analyzed). Three measurements are routinely obtained: arterial Po_2, Pco_2, and pH.

Arterial Po_2 normally is between 80 and 100 mm Hg, but the expected value depends significantly on the patient's age and the simultaneous level of Pco_2 (reflecting alveolar ventilation, an important determinant of alveolar and, secondarily, arterial Po_2). From the arterial blood gases, the alveolar-arterial oxygen gradient ($AaDo_2$) can be calculated, as discussed in Chapter 1. Normally, the difference between alveolar and arterial Po_2 is less than 10 to 15 mm Hg, but again this value depends on the patient's age. The oxygen content of the blood does not begin to fall significantly until the arterial Po_2 drops below approximately 60 mm Hg (see Chapter 1). Therefore, an abnormally low Po_2 generally does not affect O_2 transport to the tissues until it drops below this level and the saturation falls.

The range of normal arterial Pco_2 is approximately 36 to 44 mm Hg, with a corresponding pH between 7.44 and 7.36. Respiratory and metabolic factors interact closely in determining these numbers and a patient's acid-base status. Pco_2 and pH should be interpreted simultaneously because both pieces of information are necessary to distinguish respiratory from metabolic abnormalities.

When Pco_2 rises acutely, carbonic acid is formed and the concentration of H^+ also rises; therefore pH falls. As a general rule, pH falls approximately 0.08 (or, rounded off, approximately 0.1) for each 10 mm Hg increase in Pco_2. Such a rise in Pco_2 with an appropriate decrease in pH indicates an *acute respiratory acidosis.* Conversely, a drop in Pco_2 resulting from hyperventilation, with the attendant increase in pH, indicates an *acute respiratory alkalosis.* With time (hours to days), the kidneys attempt to compensate for a prolonged respiratory acidosis by retaining bicarbonate (HCO_3^-) or by excreting bicarbonate in the case of a prolonged respiratory alkalosis. In either case the compensation returns the pH value toward but not entirely to normal, and the disturbance is termed a *chronic* (i.e., compensated) *respiratory acidosis* or *alkalosis.*

On the other hand, a patient who is producing too much (or excreting too little) acid has a *primary metabolic acidosis.* Conversely, an excess of HCO_3^- (equivalent to a decrease in H^+) defines a *primary metabolic alkalosis.* In the same way that the kidneys attempt to compensate for a primary respiratory acid-base disturbance, respiratory elimination of CO_2 is adjusted to compensate for metabolic acid-base disturbances. Hence, metabolic acidosis stimulates ventilation, CO_2 elimination, and a rise in the pH toward the normal level, whereas metabolic alkalosis suppresses ventilation and CO_2 elimination, and the pH falls toward the normal range.

In practice, the clinician considers three fundamental questions in defining all acid-base disturbances: (1) Is there an acidosis or alkalosis? (2) Is the primary disorder

Arterial Pco_2 and pH together determine the nature of an acid-base disorder and the presence or absence of compensation.

of respiratory or metabolic origin? (3) Is there evidence for respiratory or metabolic compensation? Table 3-2 summarizes the findings in the major types of acid-base disturbances. Unfortunately, matters are not always so simple in clinical practice, and it is quite common to see complex mixtures of acid-base disturbances in patients who have several diseases and are receiving a variety of medications.

A simplified guide to the interpretation of arterial blood gases is presented along with several sample problems in Appendix C.

Pulse Oximetry

Although direct measurement of arterial blood gases provides the best method for assessing gas exchange, it requires collection of blood by arterial puncture. Sampling of arterial blood is uncomfortable for patients, and a small but finite risk is associated with arterial puncture. As a result, pulse oximetry, a noninvasive method for assessing arterial oxygenation, has come into widespread use, particularly for hospitalized patients. The pulse oximeter is clipped onto a patient's finger, and specific wavelengths of light are passed through the finger. Oxygenated and deoxygenated hemoglobin have different patterns of light absorption, and measurement of the pulsatile absorption of light by arteriolar blood passing through the finger allows quantitation of the two forms of hemoglobin. However, certain limitations are inherent to pulse oximetry: (1) the oximeter measures O_2 saturation rather than Po_2, (2) no information is provided about CO_2 elimination and acid-base status, and (3) the results typically are inaccurate in the presence of an abnormal hemoglobin such as carboxyhemoglobin, as seen in carbon monoxide poisoning.

EXERCISE TESTING

Because limited exercise tolerance is frequently the most prominent symptom of patients with a variety of pulmonary problems, study of patients during exercise may provide valuable information about how much these patients are limited and why. Adding measurements of arterial blood gases during exercise provides an additional dimension and shows whether gas-exchange problems (either hypoxemia or hypercapnia) contribute to the impairment. Pulse oximetry is also commonly used during exercise, particularly because it is noninvasive; however, it provides less information than direct measurement of arterial blood gases.

Although any form of exercise is theoretically possible for the testing procedure, the patient usually is studied while exercising on a treadmill or a stationary bicycle. Measurements that can be made at various points during exercise include work output, heart rate, ventilation, O_2 consumption, CO_2 production, expired gas tensions, and

Table	3-2			

ACID-BASE DISTURBANCES

Condition	Pco_2	pH	HCO_3^-
Normal	36–44 torr	7.36–7.44	23–30 mEq/L
Respiratory acidosis			
No metabolic compensation	↑	↓	Normal (or ↑)
With metabolic compensation	↑	Lesser ↓	↑
Respiratory alkalosis			
No metabolic compensation	↓	↑	Normal (or ↓)
With metabolic compensation	↓	Lesser ↑	↓
Metabolic acidosis			
No respiratory compensation	Normal	↓	↓
With respiratory compensation	↓	Lesser ↓	↓
Metabolic alkalosis			
No respiratory compensation	Normal	↑	↑
With respiratory compensation	↑	Lesser ↑	↑

arterial blood gases. Analysis of these data often can distinguish whether ventilation, cardiac output, or problems with gas exchange (particularly hypoxemia) provide the major limitation to exercise tolerance. The results can guide the physician to specific therapy on the basis of the type of limitation found.

A simpler form of exercise that is often used to assess functional limitation is the 6-minute walk test. This test measures the distance that a patient is able to walk (not jog or run) in 6 minutes. However, the test does not provide any information about the mechanism of exercise limitation. Although this test does not distinguish limitation owing to lung disease from that attributable to other medical problems such as heart disease, peripheral vascular disease, or muscle weakness, it does provide an easily performed, objective measure of a patient's exercise tolerance and can be used to follow how a patient is doing over time, with or without treatment.

REFERENCES

PHYSICAL EXAMINATION

Dickinson CJ: The aetiology of clubbing and hypertrophic osteoarthropathy, *Eur J Clin Invest* 23:330–338, 1993.
Hansen-Flaschen J, Nordberg J: Clubbing and hypertrophic osteoarthropathy, *Clin Chest Med* 8:287–298, 1987.
Loudon R, Murphy RLH Jr: Lung sounds, *Am Rev Respir Dis* 130:663–673, 1984.
Loudon RG, Murphy RLH. Lung sounds. In Crystal RG, West JB, Barnes PJ, Weibel ER, editors: *The lung. Scientific foundations.* ed 2, Philadelphia, 1997, Lippincott-Raven, pp. 1383–1391.
Maitre B, Similowski T, Derenne J-P: Physical examination of the adult patient with respiratory diseases: inspection and palpation, *Eur Respir J* 8:1584–1593, 1995.
Marrie TJ, Brown N: Clubbing of the digits, *Am J Med* 120:940–941, 2007.
Martin L, Khalil H: How much reduced hemoglobin is necessary to generate central cyanosis? *Chest* 97:182–185, 1990.
Myers KA, Farquhar DRE: Does this patient have clubbing? *JAMA* 286:341–347, 2001.
Pasterkamp H, Kraman SS, Wodicka GR: Respiratory sounds. Advances beyond the stethoscope, *Am J Respir Crit Care Med* 156:974–987, 1997.

CHEST ROENTGENOGRAPHY

Chiles C: A radiographic approach to diffuse lung disease, *Radiol Clin North Am* 29:919–929, 1991.
Felson B: *Chest roentgenology,* Philadelphia, 1973, WB Saunders.
Fraser RS, Colman N, Müller NL, Paré PD editors: *Fraser and Paré's diagnosis of diseases of the chest,* vol I, ed 4, Philadelphia, 1999, WB Saunders.
Fraser R, Colman N, Müller N, Paré P: *Synopsis of diseases of the chest,* ed 3, Philadelphia, 2005, Elsevier.
Goodman LR: *Felson's principles of chest roentgenology: a programmed text,* ed 3, Philadelphia, 2007, WB Saunders.

COMPUTED TOMOGRAPHY

Ferretti GR, Bricault I, Coulomb M: Virtual tools for imaging of the thorax, *Eur Respir J* 18:381–392, 2001.
Müller NL: Advances in imaging, *Eur Respir J* 18:867–871, 2001.
Müller NL: Computed tomography and magnetic resonance imaging: past, present and future, *Eur Respir J* 19(suppl 35):3s–12s, 2002.
Naidich DP, Webb WR, Müller NL, Vlahos I, Krinsky GA, Kim EE: *Computed tomography and magnetic resonance of the thorax,* 4 ed. Philadelphia, 2007, Lippincott Williams & Wilkins.
Touliopoulos P, Costello P: Helical (spiral) CT of the thorax, *Radiol Clin North Am* 33:843–861, 1995.
Webb WR, Müller NL, Naidich DP: *High-resolution CT of the lung,* ed 3, Philadelphia, 2001, Lippincott Williams & Wilkins.

MAGNETIC RESONANCE IMAGING

Bittner RC, Felix R: Magnetic resonance (MR) imaging of the chest: state-of-the-art, *Eur Respir J* 11:1392–1404, 1998.
Hatabu H, Stock KW, Sher S, et al: Magnetic resonance imaging of the thorax. Past, present, and future, *Radiol Clin North Am* 38:593–620, 2000.

Müller NL: Computed tomography and magnetic resonance imaging: past, present and future, *Eur Respir J* 19(suppl 35):3s–12s, 2002.

Naidich DP, Webb WR, Müller NL, Vlahos I, Krinsky GA, Kim EE: *Computed tomography and magnetic resonance of the thorax*, Philadelphia, 2007, Lippincott Williams & Wilkins.

LUNG SCANNING

Gould MK, Maclean CC, Kuschner WG, Rydzak CE, Owens DK: Accuracy of positron emission tomography for diagnosis of pulmonary nodules and mass lesions. A meta-analysis, *JAMA* 285: 914–924, 2001.

Kramer EL, Divgi CR: Pulmonary applications of nuclear medicine, *Clin Chest Med* 12:55–75, 1991.

The PIOPED Investigators: Value of the ventilation/perfusion scan in acute pulmonary embolism, *JAMA* 263:2753–2759, 1990.

Vansteenkiste JF, Stroobants SG: The role of positron emission tomography with ^{18}F-fluoro-2-deoxy-D-glucose in respiratory oncology, *Eur Respir J* 17:802–820, 2001.

PULMONARY ANGIOGRAPHY AND COMPUTED TOMOGRAPHIC ANGIOGRAPHY

Greenspan RH: Pulmonary angiography and the diagnosis of pulmonary embolism, *Prog Cardiovasc Dis* 37:93–106, 1994.

Remy-Jardin M, Remy J: Spiral CT angiography of the pulmonary circulation, *Radiology* 212:615–636, 1999.

Ryu JH, Swensen SJ, Olson EJ, Pellikka PA: Diagnosis of pulmonary embolism with use of computed tomographic angiography, *Mayo Clin Proc* 76:59–65, 2001.

Stein PD, Fowler SE, Goodman LR, et al: Multidetector computed tomography for acute pulmonary embolism, *N Engl J Med* 354:2317–2327, 2006.

ULTRASONOGRAPHY

Beckh S, Bölcskei PL, Lessnau K-D: Real-time chest ultrasonography. A comprehensive review for the pulmonologist, *Chest* 122:1759–1773, 2002.

Rosenberg ER: Ultrasound in the assessment of pleural densities, *Chest* 84:283–285, 1983.

Yang PC, Luh KT, Chang DB, Wu HD, Yu CJ, Kuo SH: Value of sonography in determining the nature of pleural effusion: analysis of 320 cases, *AJR Am J Roentgenol* 159:29–33, 1992.

Yu C-J, Yang P-C, Chang D-B, Luh K-T: Diagnostic and therapeutic use of chest sonography: value in critically ill patients, *AJR Am J Roentgenol* 159:695–701, 1992.

BRONCHOSCOPY

Bolliger CT, Mathur PN: ERS/ATS statement on interventional pulmonology, *Eur Respir J* 19: 356–373, 2002.

Bolliger CT, Sutedja TG, Strausz J, Freitag L: Therapeutic bronchoscopy with immediate effect: laser, electrocautery, argon plasma coagulation and stents, *Eur Respir J* 27: 1258–1271, 2006.

Mehta AC, editor: Flexible bronchoscopy in the 21st century, *Clin Chest Med* 20:1–217, 1999.

Mehta AC, editor: Flexible bronchoscopy update, *Clin Chest Med* 22:225–379, 2001.

Seijo LM, Sterman DH: Interventional pulmonology, *N Engl J Med* 344:740–749, 2001.

Sheski FD, Mathur PN: Endobronchial ultrasound, *Chest* 133: 264–270, 2008.

Wahidi MM, Herth FJF, Ernst A: State of the art. Interventional pulmonology, *Chest* 131:261–274, 2007.

OBTAINING AND PROCESSING SPECIMENS

American Thoracic Society: Clinical role of bronchoalveolar lavage in adults with pulmonary disease, *Am Rev Respir Dis* 142:481–486, 1990.

American Thoracic Society Workshop: Rapid diagnostic tests for tuberculosis: what is the appropriate use? *Am J Respir Crit Care Med* 155:1804–1814, 1997.

Baughman RP, Conrado CE: Diagnosis of lower respiratory tract infections: what we have and what would be nice, *Chest* 113(suppl 3):219S–223S, 1998.

Epstein RL: Constituents of sputum: a simple method, *Ann Intern Med* 77:259–265, 1972.

Goldberg M, Unger M: Lung cancer. Diagnostic tools, *Chest Surg Clin North Am* 10: 763–779, 2000.

Health and Public Policy Committee, American College of Physicians: Diagnostic thoracentesis and pleural biopsy in pleural effusions, *Ann Intern Med* 103:799–802, 1985.

Kaiser LR, Shrager JB: Video-assisted thoracic surgery: the current state of the art, *AJR Am J Roentgenol* 165:1111–1117, 1995.

Larscheid RC, Thorpe PE, Scott WJ: Percutaneous transthoracic needle aspiration biopsy: a comprehensive review of its current role in the diagnosis and treatment of lung tumors, *Chest* 114: 704–709, 1998.

Leslie KO, Helmers RA, Lanza LA, Colby TV: Processing and evaluation of lung biopsy specimens, *Eur Respir Mon* 5(monograph 14):55–62, 2000.

Loddenkemper R: Thoracoscopy: state of the art, *Eur Respir J* 11:213–221, 1998.

Mayaud C, Cadranel J: A persistent challenge: the diagnosis of respiratory disease in the non-AIDS immunocompromised host, *Thorax* 55:511–517, 2000.

Murray PR, Washington JA II: Microscopic and bacteriologic analysis of expectorated sputum, *Mayo Clin Proc* 50:339–334, 1975.

Reynolds HY: Bronchoalveolar lavage, *Am Rev Respir Dis* 135:250–263, 1987.

Reynolds HY: Use of bronchoalveolar lavage in humans: past necessity and future imperative, *Lung* 178:271–293, 2000.

Salzman SH: Bronchoscopic techniques for the diagnosis of pulmonary complications of HIV infection, *Semin Respir Infect* 14:318–326, 1999.

Schluger NW, Rom WN: The polymerase chain reaction in the diagnosis and evaluation of pulmonary infections, *Am J Respir Crit Care Med* 152:11–16, 1995.

Soini H, Musser JM: Molecular diagnosis of mycobacteria, *Clin Chem* 47:809–814, 2001.

ASSESSMENT ON A FUNCTIONAL LEVEL

American Thoracic Society: Lung function testing: selection of reference values and interpretative strategies, *Am Rev Respir Dis* 144:1202–1218, 1991.

American Thoracic Society: Single-breath carbon monoxide diffusing capacity (transfer factor): recommendations for a standardized technique—1995 update, *Am J Respir Crit Care Med* 152:2185–2198, 1995.

American Thoracic Society: Standardization of spirometry—1994 update, *Am J Respir Crit Care Med* 152:1107–1136, 1995.

American Thoracic Society and American College of Chest Physicians: ATS/ACCP statement on cardiopulmonary exercise testing, *Am J Respir Crit Care Med* 167:211–277, 2003.

ATS statement: guidelines for the six-minute walk test, *Am J Respir Crit Care Med* 166:111, 2002.

Bates DV: *Respiratory function in disease*, ed 3, Philadelphia, 1989, WB Saunders.

Chupp GL, editor: Pulmonary function testing, *Clin Chest Med* 22:599–859, 2001.

Crapo RO: Pulmonary-function testing, *N Engl J Med* 331:25–30, 1994.

Evans SE, Scanlon PD: Current practice in pulmonary function testing, *Mayo Clin Proc* 78: 758-763, 2003.

Hughes JMB, Pride NB: In defence of the carbon monoxide transfer coefficient K_{CO} (T_L/V_A), *Eur Respir J* 17:168–174, 2001.

Hughes JMB, Pride NB, editors: *Lung function tests: physiological principles and clinical applications*, London, 2000, WB Saunders.

Jain P, Kavuru MS, Emerman CL, Ahmad M: Utility of peak expiratory flow monitoring, *Chest* 114: 861–876, 1998.

Jones NL: *Clinical exercise testing*, ed 4, Philadelphia, 1997, WB Saunders.

Miller MR, Crapo R, Hankinson J, et al: General considerations for lung function testing, *Eur Respir J* 26:153–161, 2005.

Narins RG, Emmett M: Simple and mixed acid-base disorders: a practical approach, *Medicine* 59: 161–187, 1980.

Palange P, Ward SA, Carlsen K-H, et al: Recommendations on the use of exercise testing in clinical practice, *Eur Respir J* 29: 185–209, 2007.

Pellegrino R, Viegi G, Brusasco V, et al: Interpretative strategies for lung function tests, *Eur Respir J* 26:948–968, 2005.

Quanjer PH, Lebowitz MD, Gregg I, Miller MR, Pedersen OF: Peak expiratory flow: conclusions and recommendations of a Working Party of the European Respiratory Society, *Eur Respir J Suppl* 24:2S–8S, 1997.

Raffin TA: Indications for arterial blood gas analysis, *Ann Intern Med* 105:390–398, 1986.

Shapiro BA, Peruzzi WT, Kozelowski-Templin R: *Clinical application of blood gases*, ed 5, St. Louis, 1994, Mosby.

Wasserman K: Diagnosing cardiovascular and lung pathophysiology from exercise gas-exchange, *Chest* 112:1091–1101, 1997.

Wasserman K, Hansen JE, Sue DY, Stringer WW, Shipp BJ: *Principles of exercise testing and interpretation: including pathophysiology and clinical applications*, ed 4, Philadelphia, 2004, Lippincott Williams & Wilkins.

Williams AJ: ABC of oxygen: assessing and interpreting arterial blood gases and acid-base balance, *BMJ* 317:1213–1216, 1998.

4

Anatomic and Physiologic Aspects of Airways

STRUCTURE	FUNCTION
Neural Control of Airways	Airway Resistance
	Maximal Expiratory Effort

In its transit from the nose or the mouth to the gas-exchanging region of the lung, air passes through the larynx and then along a series of progressively branching tubes, from the trachea down to the smallest bronchioles. In preparation for a discussion of diseases affecting the airways, this chapter describes the structure of these airways and then considers how they function.

STRUCTURE

The trachea, bronchi, and bronchioles down to the level of the terminal bronchioles constitute the *conducting airways*. Their functions are to transport gas and protect the distal lung from inhaled contaminants. Beyond the terminal bronchioles are the *respiratory bronchioles*. They mark the beginning of the *respiratory zone* of the lung, where gas exchange takes place. Respiratory bronchioles are considered part of the gas-exchanging region of lung because alveoli are present along their walls. With successive generations of respiratory bronchioles, more alveoli appear along the walls up to the site of the alveolar ducts, which are entirely "alveolarized" (Fig. 4-1). The discussion in this chapter is limited to the conducting airways and to those aspects of the more distal airways that affect air movement but not gas exchange. Alveolar structure is discussed further in Chapter 8.

The airways are composed of several layers of tissue (Fig. 4-2). Adjacent to the airway lumen is the mucosa, beneath which is a basement membrane separating the epithelial cells of the mucosa from the submucosa. Within the submucosa are mucous glands (the contents of which are extruded through the mucosa), smooth muscle, and loose connective tissue with some nerves and lymphatic vessels. Surrounding the submucosa is a fibrocartilaginous layer, which contains the cartilage rings that support several generations of airways. Finally, a layer of peribronchial tissue, with fat, lymphatics, vessels, and nerves, encircles the rest of the airway wall. Each of these layers is considered here, with a description of the component cells and the way the structure changes in the distal progression through the tracheobronchial tree.

The surface layer (mucosa) consists of pseudostratified, columnar epithelial cells, which appear to be several cells thick in the trachea and large bronchi (see Fig. 4-2, *A*). The ciliated cells, which are most superficial, are responsible for protecting the deeper airways by propelling tracheobronchial secretions (and inhaled particles) toward the

Conducting airways: Trachea, bronchi, bronchioles down to the level of terminal bronchioles. Respiratory zone: Respiratory bronchioles, alveolar ducts, and alveoli.

The mucosal layer of large airways consists of pseudostratified, ciliated columnar epithelial cells.

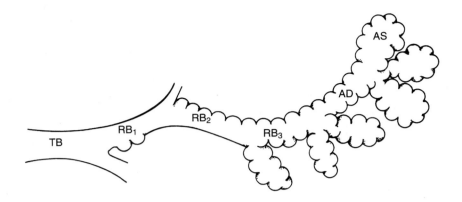

Figure 4-1. Schematic diagram of the most distal portion of the respiratory tree. Each terminal bronchiole (TB) supplies several generations of respiratory bronchioles (RB_1 through RB_3), which have progressively more respiratory (alveolar) epithelium lining their walls. Alveolar ducts (AD) are entirely lined by alveolar epithelium, as are alveolar sacs (AS). Region of lung distal to and supplied by terminal bronchiole is termed *acinus*. (From Thurlbeck WM: Chronic obstructive lung disease. In Sommers SC, editor: *Pathology annual*, vol 3, New York, 1968, Appleton-Century-Crofts.)

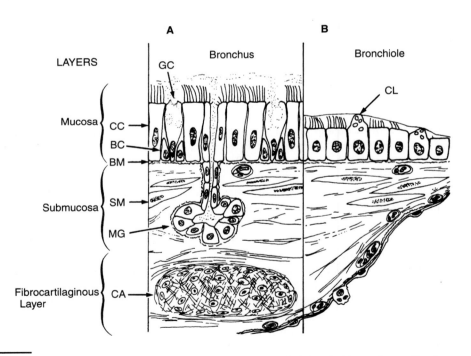

Figure 4-2. Schematic diagram of components of airway wall. **A,** Level of large airways (trachea and bronchi). **B,** Level of small airways (bronchioles). BC = Basal cell; BM = basement membrane; CA = cartilage; CC = ciliated columnar epithelial cell; CL = Clara cell; GC = goblet cell; MG = mucous gland; SM = smooth muscle. (Adapted from Weibel ER, Burri PH: Funktionelle aspekte der lungenmorphologie. In Fuchs WA, Voegeli E, editors: *Aktuelle probleme der roentgendiagnostik,* vol 2, Bern, 1973, Huber.)

pharynx. The cilia have the characteristic ultrastructure seen in other ciliated cells: a central pair of microtubules and an outer ring of nine double microtubules (see Fig. 22-1). Small side arms, called *dynein arms,* are found on the outer double microtubules. Their presence appears to be important for normal functioning of the cilia. Patients with cilia lacking the dynein side arms have impaired ciliary action and recurrent bronchopulmonary infections. Scattered between the ciliated epithelial cells are secretory cells called *goblet cells,* which produce and discharge mucus into the airway lumen. However, the goblet cells produce a relatively small proportion of total bronchial mucus, the largest portion of which is made by the bronchial mucous glands in the submucosa.

The surface epithelium appears to have other important functions that may be altered in certain clinical conditions. By virtue of tight junctions between epithelial cells at the luminal surface, the epithelium prevents access of inhaled foreign material to deeper levels of the airway wall. Whether a disturbance in this barrier function is important in asthma—perhaps by allowing inhaled foreign material to penetrate the epithelial surface—is not known with certainty. Another important function involves active transport of ions, particularly chloride, to maintain a favorable ionic environment in the mucous layer lining the airway wall. In cystic fibrosis, an abnormality in chloride transport by surface epithelial cells is believed to play a crucial role in the pathogenesis of the disease (see Chapter 7).

The deepest layer of epithelial cells, which abuts the basement membrane, includes cells called *basal cells.* The function of basal cells is to differentiate into and replenish the more superficial cells of the mucosa, either the ciliated cells or the secretory goblet cells. Another important cell type found in the basal layer of the surface epithelium is the *Kulchitsky* or *K cell,* which is believed to have a neuroendocrine function. These cells probably are part of the amine precursor uptake and decarboxylation system and therefore may be capable of producing amine products, polypeptide products, or both. In addition, K cells have cytoplasmic processes that extend to the luminal surface. As a result of these processes, K cells may be involved in sensing the composition of inspired gas and have been postulated to play a role in the regional control of ventilation and perfusion. These different cell types are important not only because of their normal physiologic roles but also because of the way they respond to airway irritation and their potential for becoming neoplastic.

The submucosal layer has two major components: *bronchial mucous glands* and *bronchial smooth muscle.* The mucous glands are the main source of bronchial secretions. A duct transports the secretions through the mucosa and discharges them into the airway lumen. As mentioned earlier, superficial goblet cells also produce mucus, which qualitatively appears to be identical to mucus formed by the bronchial mucous glands. However, why both sources of mucus exist and whether both, in fact, are necessary is unknown. Airway smooth muscle is present from the trachea down to the level of the bronchioles and even the alveolar ducts. Disturbances in the quantity and function of the smooth muscle are important in disease, particularly in the case of bronchial asthma.

Bronchial secretions are produced by submucosal glands and to a lesser extent by goblet cells in the mucosa.

The fibrocartilaginous layer is important because of the structural support that cartilage provides to the airways. The configuration of the cartilage varies significantly at different levels of the tracheobronchial tree, but the function at all levels probably is similar.

The preceding discussion describes the general structure of the airways. However, the structure varies considerably at different levels of the airway. Some of these differences are illustrated in Figure 4-2. In the progression distally through the tracheobronchial tree, the following changes are normally seen:

Airway structure changes considerably in the distal progression through the tracheobronchial tree.

1. The epithelial layer of cells becomes progressively thinner until there is a single layer of cuboidal cells at the level of the terminal bronchioles.
2. Goblet cells decrease in number until they disappear approximately at the level of the terminal bronchiole. In their place are dome-shaped cells, called *Clara cells,*

which project into the airway lumen. Although the function of the Clara cells is not known with certainty, they are believed to be involved in producing a liquid surface layer that coats the bronchiolar epithelium.

3. Mucous glands, which are present in the trachea and large bronchi, are most numerous in the medium-sized bronchi. They become progressively fewer in number more distally and are absent from the bronchioles.

4. Smooth muscle changes in configuration at different levels of the tracheobronchial tree. In the trachea and large bronchi, the muscle is found either as bands or as a spiral network, whereas in the smaller bronchi and bronchioles a continuous layer of smooth muscle encircles the airway. As airway size decreases distally in the tracheobronchial tree, smooth muscle generally occupies a larger portion of the total thickness of the airway wall. The proportion of smooth muscle to airway wall thickness becomes maximal at the level of the terminal bronchiole.

5. Cartilage also changes in configuration. In the trachea, the cartilaginous rings are horseshoe shaped, with the posterior aspect of the trachea being free of cartilage. In the bronchi, plates of cartilage become smaller and less numerous distally until cartilage is absent in the bronchioles.

The preceding discussion describes many of the structural features of normal airways. However, a variety of changes occur with chronic exposure to an irritant, such as cigarette smoke. Some of these changes, particularly in the epithelial cells, are important because of the potential for eventual malignancy (see Chapter 20). Other changes are apparent in the mucus-secreting structures (bronchial mucous glands and goblet cells) and are important features of chronic bronchitis. With chronic irritation the mucous glands hypertrophy; the goblet cells become more numerous and are found more distally than usual, even in the terminal bronchioles. The implications of these changes in disease states are discussed in Chapter 6.

NEURAL CONTROL OF AIRWAYS

The innervation (neural control) of airways is an important aspect of airway structure, with particular clinical relevance (see Chapter 5). Neural control of airways affects not only the contraction and relaxation of bronchial smooth muscle but also the activity of bronchial mucous glands. An understanding of the innervation, receptors, and mediators involved in neural control of airway function is important both because of the potential role of neural control in the pathogenesis of asthma and because of the well-established role of pharmacotherapy in stimulating or blocking airway receptors. The following discussion focuses on three components of the neural control of airways: the parasympathetic (cholinergic) system, the sympathetic (adrenergic) system, and the nonadrenergic inhibitory system (Fig. 4-3).

The parasympathetic nervous system provides the primary bronchoconstrictor tone to the airways. This innervation comes from branches of the vagus nerve; stimulation of these branches causes contraction of smooth muscle in the airway wall. In addition, vagal fibers innervate bronchial mucous glands and goblet cells, resulting in increased secretions from both components of the mucus-secreting apparatus. The receptors on smooth muscle and on the mucus-secreting apparatus are muscarinic cholinergic receptors; the neurotransmitter is acetylcholine. These cholinergic receptors are more dense in central than in peripheral airways. Identification of multiple muscarinic receptors, elucidation of a variety of effects on both airway smooth muscle and on nerves supplying smooth muscle, and evidence of "cross-talk" among muscarinic and adrenergic receptors have demonstrated that muscarinic receptor signaling actually is much more complicated, but the simplified schema just described provides a practical framework for later discussions about pathophysiology and treatment of airway diseases. The inhaled anticholinergic medications ipratropium and tiotropium

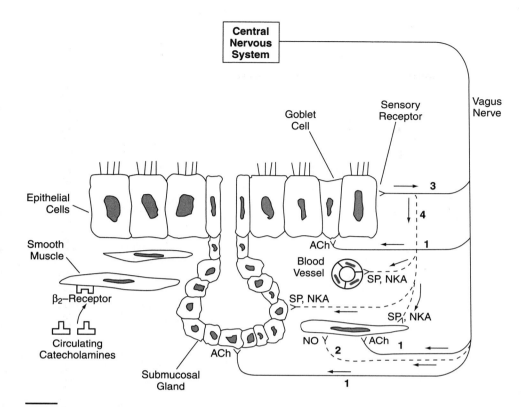

Figure 4-3. Schematic diagram of neural control of airways. Parasympathetic fibers innervating airway smooth muscle cells, submucosal glands, and goblet cells are labeled 1; nonadrenergic, noncholinergic innervation of airway smooth muscle cells is labeled 2; afferent innervation of airway epithelial cells is labeled 3; neural traffic along pathway labeled 4 goes to vagus nerve but also has effects on airway smooth muscle cells, submucosal glands, and blood vessels via local reflexes. ACh = Acetylcholine; NKA = neurokinin A; NO = nitric oxide; SP = substance P.

block the muscarinic cholinergic receptors, resulting in bronchodilation and decreased mucous production (see Chapter 6.)

A role for the sympathetic (adrenergic) nervous system in controlling airway tone is much less clear because there is sparse, if any, adrenergic innervation of human airways. Despite the paucity of innervation by sympathetic nerves, there are adrenergic, primarily β_2 receptors on bronchial smooth muscle. These receptors are stimulated by circulating catecholamines. When stimulated, β_2 receptors activate adenylate cyclase, increasing the intracellular concentration of cyclic adenosine monophosphate and causing relaxation of bronchial smooth muscle. In contrast, stimulation of the less important α-adrenergic receptors results in bronchoconstriction. Receptor density of β_2-adrenergic receptors is opposite that of cholinergic receptors; β_2-adrenergic receptors are more dense in peripheral than in central airways. Inhaled β-adrenergic agonists cause bronchodilation and are a critical part of asthma treatment (see Chapter 6).

A search for innervation of the airways with a smooth muscle relaxant (bronchodilating) effect has demonstrated a third component of neural control, often called the *nonadrenergic, noncholinergic inhibitory system*. These nerve fibers run in the vagal trunk, but when stimulated they cause bronchial smooth muscle to relax, not constrict. Evidence suggests that the bronchodilator transmitter for these nerves is nitric oxide.

Thus far only the neural output to (i.e., efferent control of) the airways has been discussed. In addition, there are airway receptors with sensory nerve innervation.

Parasympathetic innervation provides bronchoconstrictor tone to the airways; nonadrenergic inhibitory innervation provides bronchodilator tone. Adrenergic receptors are present on bronchial smooth muscle despite the absence of significant sympathetic innervation.

These receptors, which are located in the airway epithelial layer and are responsive to various chemical and mechanical stimuli, include myelinated cough ("irritant") receptors and unmyelinated C fibers. Neural traffic is carried from these sensory endings in afferent fibers of the vagus nerve. This sensory information not only is communicated to the central nervous system via the afferent vagal fibers but also is responsible for activation of local reflexes causing release of mediators called *tachykinins* from nerve endings in the airway wall. The tachykinins, which include substance P and neurokinin A, can cause bronchoconstriction, increased submucosal gland secretion, and increased vascular permeability (see Fig. 4-3). However, the magnitude of their importance in disease states (e.g., asthma) is not known with certainty.

FUNCTION

With each breath, air flows from the mouth, through the bronchial tree, to the regions of the lung responsible for gas exchange. In order to generate this flow of air during inspiration, the pressure must be lower in the alveoli than at the mouth because air flows from a region of higher pressure to one of lower pressure. The diaphragm and inspiratory muscles of the chest wall cause expansion of the chest and lungs, producing negative pressure in the pleural space and in the alveoli, thereby initiating airflow.

Flow in the airways can be considered analogous to the flow of current in an electrical system. However, rather than a voltage drop when electrons flow across a resistance, airways have a pressure difference between two points of airflow, and resistance to flow is provided primarily by the limited cross-sectional area of the airways themselves. The rate of airflow depends in part on the pressure difference between the two points and in part on the airway resistance. During inspiration, alveolar pressure is negative relative to mouth pressure (which is atmospheric), and air flows inward. In contrast, during expiration, alveolar pressure is positive relative to mouth pressure, and air flows outward from the alveoli toward the mouth.

AIRWAY RESISTANCE

The preceding description is comparatively simple; airflow is in fact a much more complex phenomenon. For instance, consider in more detail the problem of resistance. Normal airway resistance is approximately 0.5 to 2 cm $H_2O/L/s$, that is, a pressure difference of 0.5 to 2 cm H_2O between mouth and alveoli is required for air to flow at a rate of 1 L/s between these two points. Which airways provide most of the resistance? Although a single smaller airway provides more resistance to airflow than does a single larger airway, it does not follow that the aggregate of smaller airways provides the bulk of the resistance. In fact, the opposite is true. For example, even though the trachea is large, there is only one trachea, and the total cross-sectional area of the airways at this level is quite small. In contrast, at the level of small airways (e.g., less than 2 mm in diameter), the enormous number of these airways makes up for the small diameter of each one and results in a very large total cross-sectional area.

Table 4-1 lists the total cross-sectional area of the airways at different levels of the tracheobronchial tree. The major site of resistance (the smallest total cross-sectional area) is at the level of medium-sized bronchi. The small or peripheral airways, generally defined as airways less than 2 mm in diameter, contribute only approximately 10% to 20% of the total resistance. Hence, these airways frequently are called the "silent" zone, because disease in them can affect their size without significantly altering the total airway resistance. Unfortunately, despite a great deal of work by physiologists to develop methods capable of detecting increased resistance in small airways, the usefulness of such tests has not met original expectations. The correlation between these

Resistance to airflow in the tracheobronchial tree depends on the total cross-sectional area of the airways; therefore, large- and medium-sized airways provide greater resistance than do the more numerous small airways.

Table 4-1

AIRWAY NUMBERS AND DIMENSIONS

Name	Number	Diameter (mm)	Cross-sectional Area (cm^2)
Trachea	1	25	5
Main bronchi	2	11–19	3.2
Lobar bronchi	5	4.5–13.5	2.7
Segmental bronchi	19	4.5–6.5	3.2
Subsegmental bronchi	38	3–6	6.6
Terminal bronchi	1000	1	7.9
Terminal bronchioles	35,000	0.65	116
Terminal respiratory bronchioles	630,000	0.45	1000
Alveolar ducts and sacs	4×10^6	0.4	17,100
Alveoli	300×10^6	0.25–0.30	700,000 (surface area)

Adapted from Thurlbeck WM: Chronic obstructive lung disease. In Sommers SC, editor: *Pathology annual, vol. 3,* New York, 1968, Appleton-Century-Crofts.

functional studies and histopathologic confirmation of disease in small airways has been inconsistent; consequently, these tests are used infrequently.

MAXIMAL EXPIRATORY EFFORT

The next important aspect of the physiology of airflow is the distinction between normal breathing and forced or maximal respiratory efforts. A great deal of information can be obtained by looking at flow during a forced expiration, that is, breathing out from total lung capacity down to residual volume as hard and as fast as possible. In a discussion of this concept, it is useful to consider the flow-volume curve mentioned in Chapter 3 and shown again in Figure 4-4. In this figure, a series of expiratory curves shows the kind of flow rates generated by progressively greater expiratory efforts. Curve A shows expiratory flow with a relatively low effort, whereas curve D shows flow with a maximal expiratory effort.

During the first part of this curve, perhaps until approximately 30% of the vital capacity has been exhaled, the flow rate is quite dependent on the effort expended, that is, greater expiratory efforts cause a continuing increase of expiratory flow rates, which results from increased pleural pressure and thus an increased driving force for expiratory airflow. This region of the vital capacity during maximal expiratory flow is often termed the *effort-dependent portion.*

Below 70% of vital capacity comes a point at which we can no longer increase the flow rate with increasing effort. In other words, something other than our muscular strength (hence, other than the pleural pressure we can generate) limits flow. In fact, the limiting factor is a critical narrowing of the airways. When we try harder, all we do is compress the airway further, without any increase in the flow rate. This part of the flow-volume curve is frequently termed the *effort-independent portion* at which, beyond a certain level of effort, further effort does not result in an augmented flow rate.

During most of a forced expiration, flow is limited by critical narrowing of the airway; further effort does not result in augmented flow.

Two unanswered questions about maximal expiratory flow remain. First, why does critical narrowing of the airways occur so that increasing effort proves fruitless in augmenting flow? Second, at what level in the airways does this critical narrowing occur? Answers to these questions, which have been of great interest to pulmonary physiologists, must be distilled from a large amount of theory and research.*

---

*This discussion uses a model based on the *equal pressure point* concept. A different model, based on *wave speed theory,* probably provides a more accurate conceptual framework for expiratory flow limitation, but it is far more complicated and beyond the scope of this discussion.

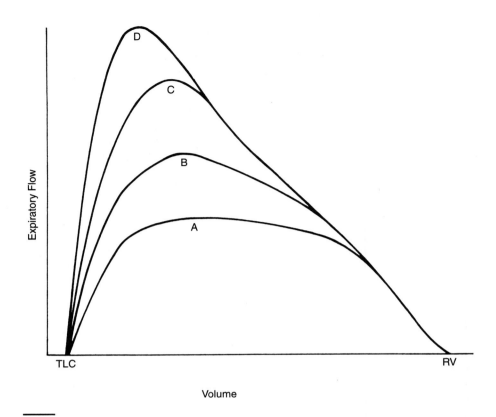

Figure 4-4. Expiratory flow-volume curves with progressively greater effort. Curve A represents the least effort; curve D represents maximal expiratory effort. On the downsloping part of the curve, beyond the point at which approximately 30% of the vital capacity has been exhaled, flow is limited by the mechanical properties of the airways and lungs, not by muscular effort. RV = Residual volume; TLC = total lung capacity.

Airway diameter depends on the level of the airway in the tracheobronchial tree, airway smooth muscle tone, traction on the airway from surrounding lung tissue, and internal and external pressures on the airway.

During a forced expiration, there are several determinants of airway diameter. First and most obvious is the inherent size of the airway, which depends on its level in the tracheobronchial tree and the tone of the airway smooth muscle. In disease, smooth muscle tone may be increased (as in asthma), or secretions in the airway may narrow the lumen (as in asthma or chronic bronchitis). Second is the amount of radial traction exerted by surrounding lung tissue on the airway walls. Airways are not isolated structures but are surrounded by a supporting framework of alveolar walls that are constantly "pulling" or "tethering" the airways open. When lung parenchyma is destroyed, as in emphysema, the airways lose some of their normal support and are more likely to collapse (see Chapter 6). Third, and perhaps most difficult to understand, is the combination of pressures acting on the airway from without and from within. This balance of pressures is crucial in determining whether a particular airway remains open or closed during a forced expiration.

The external pressure acting on an airway is determined to a large extent by pleural pressure (Fig. 4-5). When pleural pressure is strongly positive, as with a forced expiration, the airway becomes compressed. It is only because of a counteracting pressure within the airways that they are able to remain open in the face of a strongly positive external pressure. Two factors contribute to this counteracting internal airway pressure: (1) the elastic recoil of the lungs and (2) pleural pressure transmitted to the alveoli and airways. Figure 4-5 shows that the alveolar wall is like a stretched balloon trying to expel its air. In the same way that a balloon, in trying to collapse, exerts pressure on the air inside, the alveolar wall has its elastic recoil that exerts pressure on the gas within. This

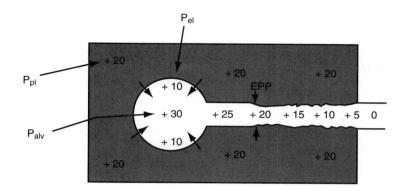

Figure 4-5. Schematic diagram of the equal pressure point concept during a forced (maximal) expiration. Alveolus and its airway are shown inside the box, which represents pleural space. Alveolar pressure (P_{alv}) has two contributing components: pleural pressure (P_{pl}) and elastic recoil pressure of lung (P_{el}). In this diagram, P_{pl} = 20 cm H_2O, and P_{el} = 10 cm H_2O. Therefore, P_{alv}, which is the sum of P_{pl} and P_{el}, is 30 cm H_2O.

pressure results in flow through the airways; however, as mentioned earlier, flow through an airway must result in a pressure drop along the airway. At a certain point along the airway, the pressure falls enough so that pressure within the airway becomes equal to the pressure outside the airway (i.e., pleural pressure). This point is called the *equal pressure point.* If the amount of effort, that is, the amount of pleural pressure, is increased, the pressure is exerted both on the alveolus and externally on the airway wall. The driving pressure (i.e., the difference between alveolar pressure and the pressure at the equal pressure point) remains the elastic recoil pressure of the lung. With additional effort the increased alveolar driving pressure is exactly balanced by the increased external pressure on the airway (see Fig. 4-5). This increased external pressure promotes airway collapse. As a net result, the elastic recoil pressure, not the pleural pressure produced by a maximal expiratory effort, is the important determinant of maximal expiratory flow, at least in the effort-independent or latter part of a forced expiration. Subsequent chapters show that in diseases with altered elastic recoil, maximal expiratory flow rates are affected by this change in the effective driving pressure for airflow.

The final question to be addressed here is the level at which this critical narrowing (i.e., the equal pressure point) occurs. The answer depends on the lung volume. The equal pressure point does not remain at a constant position all along the flow-volume curve going toward residual volume. At higher lung volumes, the elastic recoil pressure is greater (the alveoli are stretched more), and a longer distance separates the alveoli from the equal pressure point. At lung volumes above functional residual capacity, this critical point of narrowing is within relatively large airways, segmental bronchi or larger. At lower lung volumes, the elastic recoil pressure is lower, the distance from alveoli to the equal pressure point is smaller, and critical narrowing occurs more peripherally. Because maximal airflow depends on elastic recoil and the resistance of the airways peripheral ("upstream") to the equal pressure point, the resistance of the small airways is a larger component of the upstream resistance at small lung volumes and therefore is a greater determinant of maximal expiratory flow at lower volumes along the flow-volume curve.

In summary, flow through the tracheobronchial tree reflects a combination of factors: airway size, support or radial traction exerted by the surrounding lung parenchyma, and driving pressure provided by the elastic recoil of the lung. Although pleural pressure contributes to the driving pressure for airflow, it also exerts a counterbalancing external pressure on the airway, promoting airway collapse. Later discussion of specific disorders will show how these different factors are interrelated as determinants of maximal expiratory airflow and how they can be altered in disease states.

At the equal pressure point, internal and external pressures on the airway are equal. The net driving pressure from the alveolus to the equal pressure point is the elastic recoil pressure of the lung.

The equal pressure point moves peripherally (toward smaller airways) as lung volume decreases during a forced expiration; hence the resistance of small airways limits maximal expiratory flow more at low than at high lung volumes.

REFERENCES

Barnes PJ: Airway pharmacology. In Mason RJ, Broaddus VC, Murray JF, Nadel JA, editors: *Textbook of respiratory medicine,* ed 4, Philadelphia, 2005, WB Saunders, pp. 235–279.

Barnes PJ: Neural control of airway smooth muscle. In Crystal RG, West JB, Weibel ER, Barnes PJ, editors: *The lung: scientific foundations,* ed 2, Philadelphia, 1997, Lippincott-Raven, pp. 1269–1285

Barnes PJ: Neurogenic inflammation in the airways, *Respir Physiol* 125:145–154, 2001.

Canning BJ, Fischer A: Neural regulation of airway smooth muscle tone, *Respir Physiol* 125:113–127, 2001.

Drazen JM, Gaston B, Shore SA: Chemical regulation of pulmonary airway tone, *Annu Rev Physiol* 57: 151–170, 1995.

Finkbeiner WE: Physiology and pathology of tracheobronchial glands, *Respir Physiol* 118:77–83, 1999.

Gail DB, Lenfant CJM: Cells of the lung: biology and clinical implications, *Am Rev Respir Dis* 127:366–387, 1983.

Hall IP: Second messengers, ion channels and pharmacology of airway smooth muscle, *Eur Respir J* 15: 1120–1127, 2000.

Leslie KO, Wick MR: Lung anatomy. In Leslie KO, Wick MR, editors: *Practical pulmonary pathology. A diagnostic approach,* Philadelphia, 2005, Churchill Livingstone, pp. 1–17.

Proskocil BJ, Fryer AD: β_2-agonist and anticholinergic drugs in the treatment of lung disease, *Proc Am Thorac Soc* 2:305–310, 2005.

Schwartzstein RM, Parker MJ: *Respiratory physiology: a clinical approach,* Philadelphia, 2006, Lippincott Williams & Wilkins.

Wanner A, Matthias S, O'Riordan TG: Mucociliary clearance in the airways, *Am J Respir Crit Care Med* 154:1868–1902, 1996.

Weibel ER: *The pathway for oxygen,* Cambridge, MA, 1984, Harvard University Press, pp. 272–382.

West JB: *Respiratory physiology—the essentials,* ed 7, Philadelphia, 2005, Lippincott Williams & Wilkins.

Asthma

Chapter 4 discussed the normal structure of airways and considered several aspects of airway function. The most common disorders disrupting the normal structure and function of the airways—asthma and chronic obstructive pulmonary disease—are discussed here and in Chapter 6, respectively. Several other miscellaneous diseases affecting airways are covered in Chapter 7.

Asthma is a condition characterized by episodes of reversible airway narrowing, associated with contraction of smooth muscle within the airway wall. It is a common disorder that affects approximately 3% to 5% of the population. Although asthma can occur in any age group, it is particularly common in children and young adults and probably is the most common chronic disease in these age groups.

The primary feature that patients with asthma appear to have in common is *hyperresponsiveness* of the airways, that is, an exaggerated response of airway smooth muscle to a wide variety of stimuli. The hyperresponsiveness likely is due to underlying airway inflammation with a variety of types of inflammatory cells, especially eosinophils. The particular constellation of stimuli triggering the attacks often varies among patients, but the net effect (bronchoconstriction) is qualitatively similar. Because asthma is, by definition, a disease with at least some reversibility, the patient experiences exacerbations (attacks) interspersed between intervals of diminished symptoms or symptom-free periods. During an attack, the diagnosis usually is straightforward. During a symptom-free period, the diagnosis may be more difficult to make and may require provocation or challenge tests to induce airway constriction.

> Asthma is characterized by hyperreactivity of the airways and reversible episodes of bronchoconstriction.

ETIOLOGY AND PATHOGENESIS

Despite the high prevalence of asthma in the general population and the many advances that have been made in treating the manifestations of the disease, a great deal about its etiology and pathogenesis remains speculative. This section focuses on two major questions: (1) What causes certain people to have airways that hyperreact to various stimuli? (2) What is the sequence of events from the time of exposure to the stimulus until the time of clinical response?

PREDISPOSITION TO ASTHMA

Potential factors that may predispose an individual to developing asthma are either inherited or acquired. There has been significant interest in and investigation of genetic and environmental factors that may contribute to the development of asthma, but the roles of these factors and their possible interactions have not been fully elucidated.

Genetics

A substantial proportion of patients with asthma have an underlying history of allergies (allergic rhinitis and eczema) along with accompanying markers for allergic disease, such as positive skin tests and elevated immunoglobulin E (IgE) levels. In these patients, the asthma frequently is exacerbated by exposure to various allergens to which the patients have been previously sensitized. Patients with an allergic component to their asthma often have a strong family history of asthma or other allergies, suggesting that genetic factors may play a role in the development of asthma as well as the underlying allergic diathesis (often called *atopy*). However, no simple pattern of mendelian inheritance suggesting a single gene as responsible for either atopy or asthma has been identified.

Epidemiologic studies have confirmed an increased frequency of asthma and atopy in first-degree relatives of asthmatic subjects compared with control subjects, and studies in twins indicate a much higher concordance for asthma in monozygotic than in dizygotic twins. Attempts to identify chromosomal regions carrying genes associated with asthma have found a number of such regions, particularly on the long arm of chromosomes 5, 11, and 12 (5q, 11q, and 12q, respectively) and on the short arm of chromosome 6 (6p). Examples of candidate genes proposed to be involved in the predisposition to asthma include the β-subunit gene of the high-affinity receptor for IgE (on chromosome 11q), a gene cluster for production of various cytokines (on chromosome 5q) and the gene encoding the β_2-adrenergic receptor (on chromosome 5q). More recently, a disintegrin and matrix metalloproteinase gene called ADAM33 on the short arm of chromosome 20 (20p) has attracted interest as a major candidate gene for asthma and bronchial hyperresponsiveness. Despite these intriguing associations, there is general agreement that the genetic influences in asthma are complex and that multiple genes, gene products, and environmental exposures likely interact in the pathogenesis of the disease.

Acquired (Environmental) Factors

A variety of environmental factors that might predispose an individual to develop asthma, most likely interacting with one or more genetic factors, have been proposed. Exposure to allergens, possibly at a critical time during childhood, may be an important environmental factor. Some of these allergens are common environmental allergens, such as those derived from house dust mites, domestic animals, and cockroaches. These allergens are found indoors, often concentrated in bedding and carpets, and are present throughout the year.

Another potential environmental factor is maternal cigarette smoking. An increased risk for early-onset asthma is found in children whose mothers smoke, possibly related to increasing the immune responsiveness of the child. Finally, viral respiratory tract infections precipitate airway inflammation and trigger acute exacerbations of asthma, but their potential role as an inducer or cause of asthma in the absence of other factors is controversial. One theory suggests that early childhood viral infections are causally associated with later development of asthma. A contrary view (the so-called "hygiene hypothesis") suggests that respiratory infections during childhood protect against development of asthma by shifting the immunologic profile of helper T (T_H) cells toward a T_H1 response (responsible for cellular defense) and away from a T_H2 response (which mediates allergic inflammation).

AIRWAY INFLAMMATION AND BRONCHIAL HYPERRESPONSIVENESS

The association between asthma and allergies is significant but not universal. Many individuals with asthma have no other evidence of atopy and do not experience exacerbations as a result of antigen exposure. In this group, asthma attacks often are precipitated by other stimuli, as will be described later. However, the feature that both groups of patients—those with and those without an allergic background, sometimes referred to as "extrinsic" and "intrinsic" asthmatic patients, respectively—have in common is hyperresponsiveness of their airways to a variety of stimuli. When exposed to such stimuli, the airways often demonstrate bronchoconstriction, which can be measured as an increase in airway resistance or a decrease in forced expiratory flow rates.

The histologic feature that accompanies this hyperresponsiveness and is thought to be a critical component of its pathogenesis is *airway inflammation*. Airway inflammation, especially with eosinophils and lymphocytes, has been found on postmortem examination in persons with asthma who died of their disease as well as on bronchial biopsy specimens obtained from patients with mild asthma. Another typical finding is evidence of what has been called "airway remodeling," which likely results from chronic airway inflammation and the associated production and release of a multitude of mediators, including growth factors. Such remodeling changes include epithelial damage, airway fibrosis, and smooth muscle hyperplasia. These histologic findings, particularly the increase in airway smooth muscle, may be partly responsible for the hyperresponsiveness that can be documented in such persons with asthma, even when they are free of obvious bronchospasm.

No single factor or cell appears to be responsible for asthma; rather, a complex and interrelated series of events, including cellular infiltration, cytokine release, and airway remodeling, likely culminates in airway hyperresponsiveness and episodes of airflow obstruction (Fig. 5-1). A variety of mediators released from inflammatory cells can

> Although many asthmatic patients have allergies, some do not, and the overall relationship between allergies and asthma is not clear.

> Airway inflammation and epithelial injury may contribute to nonspecific bronchial hyperresponsiveness.

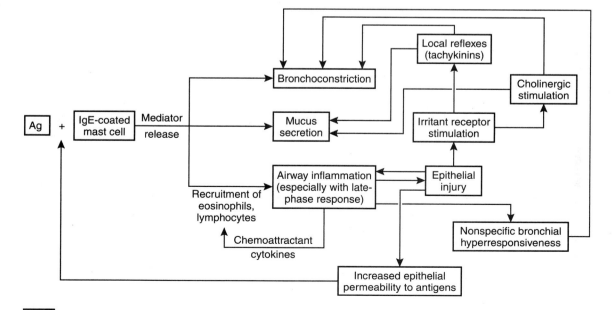

Figure 5-1. Schematic diagram of events in pathogenesis of antigen-induced asthma. Hypothetical series of complex interactions is shown, focusing on bronchoconstriction, mucus secretion, and airway inflammation. Ag = Antigen; IgE = immunoglobulin E.

alter the extracellular milieu of bronchial smooth muscle, increasing its responsiveness to bronchoconstrictive stimuli. Mediators that have been proposed to play such a role include prostaglandin and leukotriene products of arachidonic acid metabolism. Some cytokine mediators released from inflammatory cells have various effects on other inflammatory cells, thus perpetuating the inflammatory response. For example, lymphocytes of the T_H2 phenotype, which are thought to be a prominent component of the inflammatory response in asthma, release interleukin (IL)-5, which has a chemoattractant effect for eosinophils. IL-5 also stimulates the growth, activation, and degranulation of eosinophils. IL-4, another cytokine released from T_H2 lymphocytes, exerts a different type of proinflammatory effect by activating B lymphocytes, enhancing synthesis of IgE and promoting differentiation of T_H2 cells.

> Mediators from inflammatory cells may recruit and activate other inflammatory cells and may promote epithelial injury.

Mediators released from inflammatory cells may produce tissue damage that contributes to the pathogenesis of asthma. For example, when eosinophils degranulate, they release several toxic proteins from their granules, such as major basic protein and eosinophil cationic protein. These and other eosinophil products may contribute to the epithelial damage found in the asthmatic airway. Once the epithelium is injured or denuded, its barrier function is disrupted, allowing access of inhaled material to deeper layers of the mucosa. Additionally, the epithelial cells themselves may become actively involved in amplifying the inflammatory process (through production of cytokine and chemokine mediators) and in perpetuating airway edema (through vasodilation mediated by release of nitric oxide, leukotrienes, and prostaglandins). Finally, sensory nerve endings in the airway epithelial layer may become exposed, triggering a reflex arc and release of tachykinin mediators, such as substance P and neurokinin A, as shown in pathway 4 of Fig. 4-3. These peptide mediators, released at bronchial smooth muscle, submucosal glands, and blood vessels, are capable of causing bronchoconstriction and airway edema.

COMMON PROVOCATIVE STIMULI

A substantial amount is known about the sequence of events from the time of exposure to a stimulus until the clinical response of bronchoconstriction in asthmatic persons. Four stimuli that can result in bronchoconstriction are considered here: (1) allergen (antigen) exposure, (2) inhaled irritants, (3) respiratory tract infection, and (4) exercise.

> Common stimuli that precipitate bronchoconstriction in the asthmatic patient are the following:
> 1. Exposure to an allergen
> 2. Inhaled irritants
> 3. Respiratory tract infection
> 4. Exercise

Allergen Exposure

The pathogenetic mechanisms leading to bronchoconstriction are best defined for allergen-induced asthma. Allergens to which an asthmatic person may be sensitized are widespread throughout nature. Although patients and clinicians often first consider seasonal outdoor allergens, such as pollen, many indoor allergens may play a more critical role. These allergens include antigens from house dust mites (*Dermatophagoides* and others), domestic animals, and cockroaches. When an asthmatic person has IgE antibody against a particular antigen, the antibody binds to high-affinity IgE receptors on the surface of tissue mast cells and circulating basophils (see Fig. 5-1). If that particular antigen is inhaled, it binds to and cross-links IgE antibody (against the antigen) bound to the surface of mast cells in the bronchial lumen. The mast cell then is activated, leading to release of preformed as well as newly synthesized mediators. The mediators released from the mast cell induce bronchoconstriction and increase the permeability of the airway epithelium, allowing the antigen access to the much larger population of specific IgE-containing mast cells that are deeper within the epithelium. Binding of antigen to antibody on this larger population of mast cells again initiates a sequence of events leading to release of chemical mediators capable of inducing bronchoconstriction and inflammation. Several mediators have been recognized (Table 5-1), but the discussion here is limited to the few that have been primarily implicated in the pathogenesis of allergic asthma. The major mediators include histamine and leukotrienes.

Table 5-1
POTENTIAL CHEMICAL MEDIATORS IN ASTHMA

Histamine
Leukotrienes (LTC$_4$, LTD$_4$, LTE$_4$)
Platelet-activating factor
Prostaglandins (PGD$_2$)
Eosinophil chemotactic factor of anaphylaxis
Neutrophil chemotactic factor of anaphylaxis
Bradykinin
Serotonin
Kallikrein

Histamine

This relatively small (molecular weight 111) compound is found preformed within the mast cell and is released on exposure to the appropriate antigen. Histamine has several effects that may be important in asthma, including contraction of bronchial smooth muscle, augmentation of vascular permeability with formation of airway edema, and stimulation of irritant receptors (which can trigger a reflex neurogenic pathway via the vagus nerve, causing secondary bronchoconstriction). Despite these varied effects, the fact that the clinical manifestations of asthma do not respond to antihistamines suggests that histamine is not the most important chemical mediator involved.

Leukotrienes

The leukotrienes include a series of compounds (LTC$_4$, LTD$_4$, and LTE$_4$) that formerly were called slow-reacting substance of anaphylaxis (SRS-A). Unlike histamine, the leukotrienes are not preformed in the mast cell but are synthesized after antigen exposure and then released. To some extent, their actions are similar to those of histamine; they also have a direct bronchoconstrictor action on smooth muscle and can increase vascular permeability. The leukotrienes are synthesized from arachidonic acid (also the precursor for prostaglandins) but along a different pathway involving a lipoxygenase enzyme as opposed to the cyclooxygenase enzyme used for prostaglandin synthesis (Fig. 5-2). LTC$_4$ and LTD$_4$, in particular, are extraordinarily potent bronchoconstrictors, and they may have an important role in the pathogenesis of bronchial asthma. An interesting sidelight is provided by knowledge that some persons with asthma experience exacerbations of their disease after taking aspirin or other nonsteroidal antiinflammatory drugs. These drugs are known inhibitors of the cyclooxygenase enzyme and may result in preferential shifting of the pathway shown in Figure 5-2 toward production of the bronchoconstrictor leukotrienes.

The role of the other mediators listed in Table 5-1 in the pathogenesis of asthma is less clear. Platelet-activating factor has been proposed to play a role in the recruitment of eosinophils to the lung. In addition, platelet-activating factor activates eosinophils, stimulating them to release proteins toxic to airway epithelial cells.

Late-Phase Asthmatic Response

The airway response to antigen challenge, as measured by changes in forced expiratory volume in 1 second (FEV$_1$), appears to be more complicated and involves more than just the rapid, mediator-induced bronchoconstriction seen within the first half hour following exposure. In many patients, the return of FEV$_1$ to normal is followed by a secondary, delayed fall in FEV$_1$ occurring hours after antigen exposure and lasting up to days (Fig. 5-3). The delayed fall in FEV$_1$ is accompanied histologically by inflammatory changes in the airway wall. At the same time, bronchial hyperresponsiveness to nonspecific stimuli, such as histamine or methacholine, can be demonstrated.

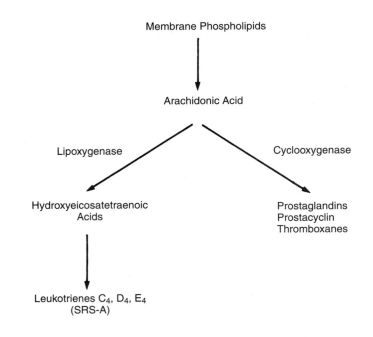

Figure 5-2. Outline of pathway for formation of leukotrienes (slow-reacting substance of anaphylaxis [SRS-A]) and prostaglandins. Aspirin and other nonsteroidal antiinflammatory drugs are inhibitors of the enzyme cyclooxygenase.

It now appears that this "late-phase response," as it has been called, depends on the presence of antigen-specific IgE. Presumably, release of mediators after allergen binding to IgE-coated mast cells results in the influx of inflammatory cells, especially eosinophils, into the airway wall. Experimental data suggest that this airway inflammation is responsible for the nonspecific bronchial hyperresponsiveness seen at the time of the late-phase response.

Inhaled Irritants

Inhaled irritants, such as cigarette smoke, inorganic dusts, and environmental pollutants, are common precipitants of bronchoconstriction in asthmatic persons. These airborne irritants appear to stimulate *irritant receptors* located primarily in the walls of the larynx, trachea, and large bronchi. Stimulation of the receptors initiates a reflex arc that travels to the central nervous system and back to the bronchi via the vagus nerve. This efferent vagal stimulation of the bronchi completes the reflex arc and induces bronchoconstriction. As mentioned in the discussion about chemical mediators, histamine is capable of stimulating irritant receptors, and at least part of its bronchoconstrictive effect may be mediated indirectly via stimulation of the irritant receptors.

Respiratory Tract Infection

Respiratory tract infection is a factor for patients with nonallergic as well as allergic asthma. Viral infections are the most common causes in this category, but bacterial infections of the tracheobronchial tree also can be implicated. The mechanism by which respiratory infections precipitate bronchoconstriction in asthmatic persons is not entirely clear but likely is related to epithelial damage and airway inflammation. Potential consequences of epithelial injury include release of mediators from inflammatory cells, stimulation of irritant receptors, and nonspecific bronchial hyperresponsiveness.

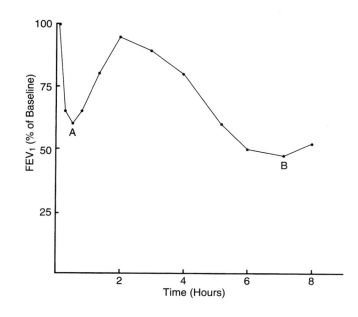

Figure 5-3. Response of forced expiratory volume in 1 second (FEV$_1$) after antigen challenge in patient who demonstrates a biphasic response. Early bronchoconstrictive response is at point A. Slower onset, late-phase asthmatic response is at point B.

Exercise

Exercise can frequently provoke bronchoconstriction in patients with hyperreactive airways. The crucial factor in the pathogenesis appears to be heat movement from the airway wall, resulting in cooling of the airway. During exercise, individuals have a high minute ventilation, and the large amounts of relatively cool and dry inspired air must be warmed and humidified by the tracheobronchial mucosa. When the air is warmed and humidified, water evaporates from the epithelial surface, resulting in cooling of the airway epithelium. The phenomenon of exercise-induced bronchoconstriction can be reproduced by having an asthmatic person voluntarily breathe cold, dry air at a high minute ventilation. Inhalation of warm, saturated air at the same minute ventilation does not produce a similar effect. The mechanism that links airway cooling and drying with bronchoconstriction is less clear. Alteration of the ionic environment after drying of the mucosa, mediator release, hyperemia of the mucosa following airway rewarming, and stimulation of irritant receptors all have been proposed as mechanisms, but none is universally accepted.

Airway cooling is important in exercise-induced bronchoconstriction.

As might be expected from the description of exercise-induced bronchoconstriction, inhalation of cold air during the winter months can be responsible for asthma exacerbations or worsening of symptoms in selected patients. The mechanism of airway narrowing in these patients following inhalation of cold air is also believed to be due to airway cooling and drying and therefore is analogous to the mechanism of exercise-induced bronchoconstriction.

PATHOLOGY

Information about pathologic findings in asthma often has been obtained at autopsy studies and thus represents the consequences of particularly severe disease. In these cases, marked overdistention of the lungs is seen, and the airways are occluded by thick, tenacious mucous plugs. Information regarding the histologic appearance of the airways in patients with stable, mild disease has also become available. Examination of the airways by microscopy demonstrates the following findings of variable severity that are apparent in both mild and more severe disease:

1. Edema and cellular infiltrates within the bronchial wall, especially with eosinophils and lymphocytes
2. Epithelial damage, with a "fragile" appearance of the epithelium and with detachment of the surface epithelial cells from the basal cells
3. Hypertrophy and hyperplasia of the smooth muscle layer
4. Thickening of the epithelial basement membrane
5. Enlargement of the mucus-secreting apparatus, with hypertrophy of mucous glands and an increased number of goblet cells

As described earlier in this chapter, the presence of histologic abnormalities presumably contributes to the nonspecific bronchial hyperresponsiveness in patients, even when they are free of an acute attack. In addition to the bronchial hyperresponsiveness that results from airway inflammation and remodeling, the more long-standing structural changes that characterize airway remodeling contribute to the component of persisting airflow obstruction that can be seen in some asthmatics.

PATHOPHYSIOLOGY

The pathophysiologic features of asthma largely follow from the pathologic abnormalities. Contraction of smooth muscle in the bronchial walls, mucosal edema, and secretions within the airway lumen all contribute to a decreased airway diameter, which increases airway resistance. The pathologic changes are present at many levels of the tracheobronchial tree, from large airways down to the peripheral airways less than 2 mm in diameter.

As a result of narrowed airways with increased resistance, patients have difficulty with airflow during both inspiration and expiration. However, because intrathoracic airways are subjected to relatively negative external pressure (transmitted from negative pleural pressure) during inspiration, lumen size is larger during the inspiratory phase of the respiratory cycle. During expiration, relatively positive pleural pressure is transmitted to intrathoracic airways, thus decreasing their diameter. Therefore, greater difficulty with airflow on expiration than on inspiration is characteristic of asthma, as it is of any of the diseases that cause obstruction or narrowing of airways within the thorax. The greatest difficulty with expiration occurs when the patient is asked to perform a forced expiration, that is, to breathe out as hard and as fast as possible. With a forced expiration, pleural pressure becomes much more positive, thereby promoting airway closure and air trapping.

> In asthma and other diseases associated with obstruction of intrathoracic airways, airflow is most compromised during expiration.

The effects of increased airway resistance are readily seen by measuring pulmonary function in asthmatic persons. Pulmonary function studies performed during an attack show decreases in forced expiratory flow rates as well as evidence of air trapping. On the forced expiratory spirogram, patients generally exhibit a decrease in both forced vital capacity (FVC) and FEV_1, with the decrease in FEV_1 usually more pronounced than the decrease in FVC. Hence, the ratio FEV_1/FVC, which reflects the proportion of FVC that can be exhaled during the first second, is decreased. In addition, the maximal midexpiratory flow rate is diminished.

> Pulmonary function tests in patients with asthma generally demonstrate decreased FEV_1, FVC, and FEV_1/FVC ratio. Air trapping and hyperinflation are demonstrated by increases in RV, FRC, and sometimes TLC.

Measurement of lung volumes shows evidence of air trapping, with increases in functional residual capacity (FRC), residual volume (RV), and sometimes total lung capacity (TLC). Of all these lung volumes, the most impressive increase is seen in RV. RV, which is the volume left in the lungs at the end of a maximal exhalation, may be greater than 200% of the predicted value. The increase in RV is believed to be at least partly due to premature airway closure as a result of smooth muscle constriction, mucous plugs, and inflammatory changes of the mucosa.

Whether TLC truly increases and how the increase occurs are not entirely clear. Two main factors determine TLC: (1) inspiratory muscles act to expand the chest and (2) elastic recoil of the lung acts to decrease lung volume. Some evidence suggests that elastic recoil is decreased during acute asthma attacks; alternatively, it has been suggested that inspiratory muscle strength (or the efficiency of contraction) is increased.

FRC, the resting point of the lungs after a normal expiration, may be increased for at least two reasons. First, because more time is required for expiration when airways are obstructed, patients may not have sufficient time before the next breath to fully exhale the volume from the previous breath. This phenomenon, sometimes called *dynamic hyperinflation,* is a problem particularly when the asthmatic person is breathing at a rapid respiratory rate. Another reason for the increase in FRC is related to persistent activity of the inspiratory muscles during expiration, maintaining lung volume at a higher than expected level throughout expiration.

The focus so far has been on pulmonary function and physiologic abnormalities seen with a typical asthmatic attack. Between attacks, pulmonary function, as measured by FEV_1 and FVC, often returns to normal. However, even when a person is not having an acute attack, subtle abnormalities in pulmonary function may be present, such as a decrease in maximal midexpiratory flow rate and mild increase in RV. These abnormalities may reflect some residual disease in the small airways of the lung, frequently the last region to become normal after an attack.

A subgroup of asthmatic persons, generally those with long-standing disease, have pulmonary function that does not return to normal. Instead, they have easily demonstrable physiologic abnormalities (e.g., abnormal FEV_1 and FVC) that persist between attacks. Even though asthma is generally characterized by reversible episodes of airflow obstruction, these persons appear also to have a component of irreversible disease. Nevertheless, they still generally experience episodes of reversible airflow obstruction and worsening of expiratory flow rates superimposed upon whatever irreversible disease is present.

The increased resistance to airflow in asthma exerts a toll on gas exchange, which is generally disturbed during acute attacks. The most common pattern of arterial blood gases consists of a low Po_2 accompanied by a low Pco_2 (respiratory alkalosis). The mechanism for the hypoxemia is ventilation-perfusion mismatch. The increased airway resistance in asthma is not evenly distributed, such that some airways are affected more than others. Therefore, inspired air is not distributed evenly but tends to go to less diseased areas. However, blood flow remains relatively preserved in the regions that are ventilating poorly. The regions of low ventilation-perfusion ($\dot{V}/\dot{Q}$) ratio contribute blood with a low Po_2 that cannot be compensated for by increases in the $\dot{V}/\dot{Q}$ ratio from other regions of the lung (see Chapter 1).

Despite the abnormal Po_2, persons are able to hyperventilate, and Pco_2 usually is low. The stimulus or mechanism for the hyperventilation is not clear. During an acute asthma attack, activation of irritant receptors may stimulate ventilation, or other reflexes originating in the airways, lung, or chest wall may stimulate ventilation. Pco_2 that increases to either a normal or a frankly elevated level often means worsening airflow obstruction or a tiring individual who is no longer able to maintain normal or high minute ventilation in the face of significant airflow obstruction. Thus, the clinician should view a normal or high Pco_2 as a serious warning sign.

The most common pattern of arterial blood gases in asthma is low Po_2 (attributable primarily to $\dot{V}/\dot{Q}$ mismatch) and low Pco_2.

CLINICAL FEATURES

Onset of asthma occurs most frequently during childhood and young adulthood, although asthma can develop for the first time in older patients. In many patients, particularly those in whom asthma started before age 16 years, the disease eventually regresses, and patients are no longer subject to repeated episodes of reversible airway obstruction.

The symptoms most commonly noted by patients during an exacerbation of asthma are cough, dyspnea, wheezing, and chest tightness. Patients do not necessarily have a classic presentation with several or all of these complaints but may merely have an unexplained cough or breathlessness on exertion. In some cases, patients can clearly identify a precipitating factor for an attack, such as exposure to an allergen, respiratory tract infection, exercise, exposure to cold air, emotional stress, or exposure to irritating dusts, fumes, or odors. In other cases, no precipitant can be identified. Exposures in the workplace, related to proteins or other chemicals to which the patient may be sensitized, are important precipitants in a subgroup of patients who are said to have *occupational asthma*. Some asthmatic persons are particularly sensitive to ingestion of aspirin, which is believed to favor production of leukotrienes from arachidonic acid. Some patients with aspirin sensitivity also have nasal polyps, leading to a well-recognized triad of asthma, aspirin sensitivity, and nasal polyposis (sometimes referred to as *triad asthma* or *Samter's syndrome*). Other nonsteroidal antiinflammatory drugs (which also inhibit the cyclooxygenase enzyme) also can produce bronchoconstriction in patients who are aspirin sensitive.

On examination, patients experiencing an asthma attack usually have tachypnea and, on auscultation of the chest, prolonged expiration and evidence of wheezing. The wheezing is generally more prominent during expiration than inspiration and may be triggered by having the patient exhale forcefully. Although the tendency is to equate wheezing and asthma, the presence of wheezing does not necessarily indicate a diagnosis of asthma. Wheezing reflects only airflow through narrowed airways; it also can be seen in such diverse disorders as congestive heart failure and chronic obstructive pulmonary disease or in the case of a foreign body in the airway. On the other hand, not all asthmatic persons wheeze. It is a common observation that severe asthma may be associated with no wheeze at all if airflow is too impaired to generate an audible wheeze.

During a particularly severe attack that is refractory to treatment with bronchodilators, persons with asthma are said to be in *status asthmaticus*. These patients present difficult therapeutic challenges, may require assisted ventilation, and may even die as a result of the acute attack.

The overall severity of an individual's asthma can be characterized on the basis of the frequency of exacerbations, nocturnal symptoms, and magnitude of abnormality and variability in pulmonary function. The features used to define four categories of severity (mild intermittent asthma, mild persistent asthma, moderate persistent asthma, and severe persistent asthma) are listed in Table 5-2.

DIAGNOSTIC APPROACH

A clinical history of reversible episodes of bronchoconstriction often is crucial to the diagnosis of asthma. Other helpful features in the history include other evidence for atopy (e.g., hay fever or eczema) or a family history of allergies or asthma. Physical examination demonstrating wheezes during an attack often provides confirmatory evidence for airway obstruction.

The chest radiograph, although sometimes useful for ruling out other causes of wheezing or complications of asthma, is generally not particularly helpful in the diagnosis. It usually shows normal findings but may demonstrate hyperinflation with relatively large lung volumes.

If the patient is producing sputum, microscopic examination of the sputum frequently shows many eosinophils on the smear. An increased percentage of eosinophils

---

Major symptoms during an acute asthma attack are the following:
1. Cough
2. Dyspnea
3. Wheezing
4. Chest tightness

Despite its prominence, the presence of wheezing is not synonymous with asthma and merely reflects airflow through narrowed airways.

Table 5-2

CLASSIFICATION OF ASTHMA BY SEVERITY: CLINICAL ASPECTS AND TREATMENT

Asthma Severity	Clinical Features Before Treatment	Nighttime Symptoms	Lung Function	Treatment
Mild intermittent	• Symptoms no more than twice per week • No interference with normal activity • Exacerbations brief	• No more than twice per month	• FEV$_1$ >80% predicted • FEV$_1$/FVC normal	• Inhaled short-acting β$_2$ agonist as needed
Mild persistent	• Symptoms more than twice per week but less than once per day • Minor limitation with normal activity	• Three or four times per month	• FEV$_1$ or PEFR >80% predicted • FEV$_1$/FVC normal	• Antiinflammatory therapy (inhaled corticosteroid) • Alternative: sustained-release theophylline, leukotriene modifier, or cromoglycate • Inhaled short-acting β$_2$ agonist as needed
Moderate persistent	• Daily symptoms • Daily use of inhaled short-acting β$_2$ agonist • Some limitation with normal activity • Exacerbations at least twice per week; may last days	• More than once per week but not nightly	• FEV$_1$ >60% but <80% predicted • FEV$_1$/FVC reduced 5%	• Low-dose inhaled corticosteroid plus long-acting β$_2$ agonist OR • Medium-dose inhaled corticosteroid
Severe persistent	• Continual symptoms • Extremely limited with normal activity • Frequent exacerbations	• Often nightly	• FEV$_1$ <60% predicted • FEV$_1$/FVC reduced >5%	• Medium- or high-dose inhaled corticosteroid plus long-acting β$_2$ agonist • Consider short course of oral corticosteroid

Adapted from National Asthma Education and Prevention Program: *Guidelines for the diagnosis and management of asthma: Expert panel report 3*, Bethesda, MD, 2007, National Institutes of Health, NIH publication 08-4051.

FEV$_1$ = Forced expiratory volume in 1 second; PEFR = peak expiratory flow rate.

in peripheral blood also is common, even when the asthma has no clear relationship to allergies.

The clinical usefulness of skin testing and inhalation testing with allergens in an attempt to identify antigens to which the patient is sensitized is controversial. Unfortunately, these tests do not necessarily correlate with each other and do not establish that antigens causing positive test results are responsible for exacerbations of asthma.

Although the diagnosis of asthma usually is made on the basis of clinical features, spirometry, and response to therapy, other types of provocation tests are sometimes used to make or confirm the diagnosis of asthma. These tests rely on the principle that asthmatic persons have hyperreactive airways. Therefore, when tested with inhalation of methacholine (a cholinergic agent) or histamine, persons with asthma respond with bronchoconstriction to comparatively small doses of either agent. Inhalation of cold air at high minute ventilations with P_{CO_2} kept constant (termed *isocapnic hyperpnea*) also can be used as a challenge test to induce transient bronchoconstriction in patients in whom the diagnosis of asthma is uncertain.

Measurement of pulmonary function, especially FEV_1 and FVC, is particularly useful in the patient with suspected or known asthma. Documentation of reversible airflow obstruction, either during attacks or with a challenge test, frequently is sufficient to make the diagnosis. In practice, the diagnosis of asthma is most commonly made by the history of episodic dyspnea, wheezing, or cough, with documentation of reversible airflow obstruction by pulmonary function testing.

Patients can conveniently test their own pulmonary function through measurement of the peak expiratory flow rate. Such testing is particularly useful for monitoring the course of the disease and alerting the patient to adjust the medication regimen, seek attention from a physician, or both. In addition, the efficacy of treatment or changes in the therapeutic regimen can readily be assessed by serial measurement of the peak expiratory flow rate.

> A diagnosis of asthma includes a history of episodic dyspnea, wheezing, or cough, along with reversible airflow obstruction documented by pulmonary function testing.

TREATMENT

The major categories of drugs used to treat asthma are those that dilate smooth muscle of the bronchial wall and those that have an antiinflammatory action. Agents targeted at blocking production or activity of specific mediators also are used, and a monoclonal antibody against IgE has become available. The main categories of drugs used to treat asthma are listed in Table 5-3. Several of the drugs are also used for treatment of other types of pulmonary disease, particularly chronic obstructive pulmonary disease, and are mentioned in other chapters.

BRONCHODILATORS

The most common bronchodilator agents used for treatment of asthma are the sympathomimetic agents, which act on β_2 receptors from activate adenylate cyclase and increase intracellular cyclic adenosine monophosphate (cAMP). Increased levels of cAMP in bronchial smooth muscle, resulting specifically from stimulation of β_2 receptors, activate protein kinase A, which phosphorylates several regulatory proteins that mediate bronchodilation. β stimulation also increases intracellular cAMP in mast cells, inhibiting release of chemical mediators that, secondarily, cause bronchoconstriction. Specific examples of available sympathomimetic drugs are listed in Table 5-3. The preferred agents have action that is limited primarily to stimulation of β_2 receptors, in order to avoid some of the adverse cardiac effects induced by stimulation of β_1 receptors. Currently, the β_2-specific agents most commonly used are albuterol (short-acting β_2 agonist) and salmeterol (long-acting β_2 agonist), and the typical route

> Sympathomimetic agents increase intracellular cAMP by activating adenylate cyclase. Preferred agents preferentially stimulate β_2 receptors and decrease potential adverse cardiac effects caused by stimulation of β_1 receptors.

Table 5-3

DRUG THERAPY IN ASTHMA

	Examples	Possible Routes of Administration	Mechanism of Action
BRONCHODILATORS			
Sympathomimetics	Epinephrine Metaproterenol Terbutaline Albuterol Salmeterol Formoterol Arformoterol	Inhaled, oral, parenteral (depending on particular drug)	↑cAMP via stimulation of adenylate cyclase
Xanthines	Theophylline Aminophylline	Oral Oral, parenteral	?↑cAMP via inhibition of phosphodiesterase; ? antiinflammatory
Anticholinergics	Ipratropium Tiotropium	Inhaled	Blockade of cholinergic (bronchoconstrictor) effect on airways
ANTIINFLAMMATORY DRUGS			
Corticosteroids	Prednisone Methylprednisolone	Systemic (oral or parenteral, depending on particular drug)	Decreased inflammatory response in airways; ? additional mechanisms
	Beclomethasone Triamcinolone Flunisolide Fluticasone Budesonide	Inhaled	
Cromolyn		Inhaled	Inhibition of mediator release from mast cells; ? additional mechanisms
Nedocromil		Inhaled	? Similar to cromolyn
DRUGS DIRECTED AT SPECIFIC TARGETS			
5-Lipoxygenase inhibitors	Zileuton	Oral	Decreased production of leukotrienes
Leukotriene antagonists	Zafirlukast Montelukast	Oral	Leukotriene D_4 receptor antagonism
Anti-IgE antibody	Omalizumab	Parenteral	Binds circulating IgE antibody

cAMP = Cyclic adenosine monophosphate; IgE = immunoglobulin E.

of administration is inhalation. Although some sympathomimetic agents can be given orally or parenterally, the inhaled route is preferred because it has fewer systemic side effects and provides direct delivery to the site of action in the airways.

Short-acting inhaled β_2 agonists, such as albuterol, usually are used on an as-needed basis to reverse an acute episode of bronchoconstriction. They may be the only agents needed to control the patient's asthma when episodes are infrequent. The newest β_2 agonists salmeterol, formoterol, and arformoterol are long acting (approximately 12 hours) and are not appropriate for as-needed use to treat acute symptoms. Short-acting β_2-agonist drugs can used prophylactically before activities or exposure to stimuli that are known to precipitate bronchoconstriction. As the severity of asthma increases so that more frequent or regular use of an inhaled β_2 agonist is required, addition of an antiinflammatory agent (see the following section) is important.

The second class of bronchodilator agents, the methylxanthines, is used much less frequently than β_2 agonists. The methylxanthines, of which theophylline is the prototype, are generally believed to act by inhibiting the enzyme phosphodiesterase (PDE), which normally is responsible for metabolic degradation of cAMP. When degradation

Methylxanthines (aminophylline, theophylline) increase cAMP by inhibiting the enzyme PDE, which degrades cAMP. This mechanism is arguably responsible for bronchodilation.

is inhibited, the levels of cAMP in smooth muscle and mast cells increase, resulting again in bronchodilation and decreased mediator release from mast cells. However, the serum levels of methylxanthines needed to inhibit PDE are higher than those actually achieved in patients, so whether PDE inhibition is the major or exclusive mechanism of the action of theophylline as a bronchodilator is uncertain. In addition, theophylline may have a component of antiinflammatory activity, mediated by inhibition of the PDE IV isozyme in inflammatory cells. Theophylline is available only for oral administration, whereas aminophylline (a water-soluble salt of theophylline) can be given either orally or intravenously. Because methylxanthines can be administered only systemically (as opposed to locally in the airway), systemic side effects (gastrointestinal, cardiac, neurologic) are more problematic than with the inhaled sympathomimetic agents. This is an important reason why methylxanthines now are used relatively infrequently compared with inhaled β_2 agonists.

The third class of bronchodilator agents, also used less frequently than β_2 agonists in patients with asthma, consists of drugs that have an anticholinergic action. The anticholinergic agents dilate bronchial smooth muscle by decreasing bronchoconstrictor cholinergic tone to airways. Ipratropium, available as an aerosol for inhalation, is the primary short-acting example of this class of agents. It is formally approved in the United States only for use in chronic obstructive lung disease (see Chapter 6), not in asthma. The major use of ipratropium for asthma has been as adjunctive therapy to inhaled β_2 agonists in patients during an acute asthma attack. Tiotropium, a long-acting anticholinergic agent, is approved for and frequently used in patients with chronic obstructive lung disease, but it is neither approved for nor commonly used in patients with asthma.

ANTIINFLAMMATORY DRUGS

The second major category of drugs used to treat asthma includes the antiinflammatory agents: corticosteroids, disodium cromoglycate (cromolyn), and nedocromil. Corticosteroids have been used for years for treatment of asthma. They suppress the inflammatory response by decreasing the number of eosinophils and lymphocytes infiltrating the airway and decrease the production of a number of inflammatory mediators. However, despite the general rationale for use of corticosteroids, many aspects of their antiinflammatory action are unknown. The glucocorticoids are thought to bind to a cytoplasmic receptor that is present in nearly all cell types. After the receptor binds to its glucocorticoid ligand, it moves to the cell nucleus, where it interacts with transcription factors, such as activator protein-1 and nuclear factor-κB, which regulate the transcription of other target genes. Important target genes whose transcription is suppressed by the action of glucocorticoids include a variety of inflammatory cytokines (e.g., IL-1, IL-3, IL-4, IL-5, IL-6, and tumor necrosis factor-α), the inducible form of nitric oxide synthase, and an inducible form of cyclooxygenase.

Because airway inflammation is believed to play an important role in the pathogenesis of asthma, particularly in the patient with more frequent attacks or more persistent airflow obstruction, corticosteroids have assumed a central role in the management of many cases of asthma. By decreasing airway inflammation, steroids are thought to ameliorate the underlying disease process in asthma, not just the bronchoconstriction resulting from airway inflammation.

Steroids have an important place in both management of acute asthma attacks and maintenance therapy for disease requiring more than just infrequent use of a β_2-agonist bronchodilator. Frequently, steroids such as prednisone or methylprednisolone are started at high doses during an acute attack and then are tapered relatively rapidly. Because of the potential for significant adverse effects with long-term use of systemic (oral) steroids, chronic administration of oral steroids is avoided if the asthma can be

---

Systemic and inhaled corticosteroids have an important role in acute therapy and preventive management, respectively.

managed with other modes of therapy. Foremost among these alternative forms of therapy are inhaled forms of corticosteroids, which deliver the drug locally to the airway and have minimal systemic absorption and limited side effects. Inhaled steroids are now the preferred form of "controller" or preventive therapy for patients with asthma not adequately managed with infrequent use of a β-agonist inhaler.

Other antiinflammatory drugs used for treatment of asthma are disodium cromoglycate (cromolyn) and nedocromil. Their mode of action traditionally has been thought to be inhibition of mediator release from mast cells. However, this mechanism has been disputed, and alternative mechanisms have been proposed, including inhibitory effects on other types of inflammatory cells or on the action of tachykinins. Both cromolyn and nedocromil are given in inhaled form. Neither drug is a bronchodilator, so neither is useful for treatment of acute attacks. Rather, they are generally given as ongoing medication, with the goal of preventing future exacerbations.

> Antiinflammatory therapy is important when treatment of asthma requires more than infrequent use of an inhaled β_2 agonist.

AGENTS WITH SPECIFIC TARGETED ACTION

Agents are available that block the synthesis or action of a single type of mediator, specifically the leukotrienes. Interestingly, these agents appear to be effective for only some patients with asthma. It is believed that underlying patient-related genetic factors affect the likelihood of a positive response. Specific agents that modify leukotrienes or leukotriene pathways include zafirlukast and montelukast, which antagonize the action of LTD_4 at its receptor, and zileuton, which inhibits the enzyme 5-lipoxygenase and thus limits leukotriene production. On the basis of their mode of action, drugs that either block the synthesis of leukotrienes or antagonize their action have a particularly important role in patients who are sensitive to aspirin or other nonsteroidal antiinflammatory drugs.

The newest agent for treatment of asthma is omalizumab, a monoclonal antibody to IgE. On the basis of the principle that IgE is an important component of the pathobiology of allergic asthma, the drug was developed to block the binding of IgE to receptors on mast cells. However, omalizumab is administered every 2 to 4 weeks by subcutaneous injection in a health care setting (e.g., outpatient medical office) and is extremely expensive. Its use has been limited to selected patients with particularly severe asthma who have elevated levels of IgE and require chronic therapy with systemic corticosteroids.

BRONCHIAL THERMOPLASTY

Bronchial thermoplasty is a new procedure performed via a flexible bronchoscope in which thermal energy is delivered to the airways in an effort to reduce airway smooth muscle mass. Some preliminary studies have suggested that the procedure can produce sustained benefit in patients with moderate asthma, but experience is limited. Further trials are underway and should better define the optimal role of this procedure in the management of asthma.

MANAGEMENT STRATEGY

At present, the overall strategy for management of asthma commonly proceeds in the following manner. A patient with relatively infrequent attacks, with symptom-free periods, and with normal pulmonary function between attacks is managed with inhaled short-acting sympathomimetics (β_2 agonists). These drugs are used on an as-needed basis, that is, both for management of bronchospasm once it occurs and before exposure to stimuli often known to precipitate attacks (e.g., exercise and allergen exposure). These general guidelines are summarized in Table 5-2 according to the categories of clinical severity of disease.

When a patient's asthma cannot be managed successfully with infrequent use of a β_2-agonist inhaler, then an antiinflammatory agent is generally added as maintenance (ongoing) therapy to suppress the underlying airway inflammation. Inhaled corticosteroids are used most frequently and appear to be the most effective agents in this class, although cromolyn and nedocromil are alternatives, especially when allergens appear to have a prominent role in triggering exacerbations. Agents affecting leukotriene synthesis or action are increasingly being used, but their effectiveness in a given patient is unpredictable.

If therapy must be escalated beyond the above measures because of inadequate control, then addition of a regularly used, long-acting inhaled β_2 agonist (e.g., salmeterol) is the preferred option, although addition of an antileukotriene agent, escalation of the dose of inhaled corticosteroids, or addition of the methylxanthine theophylline are other options. When patients have a significant acute attack or an attack that occurs despite adequate therapy as described, intensive bronchodilator therapy plus a short course of systemic steroids are generally effective. Particularly severe asthma exacerbations (i.e., *status asthmaticus*) often require high doses of intravenous corticosteroids along with aggressive bronchodilator therapy. Patients with respiratory failure may require intubation and mechanical ventilation.

For patients in whom allergen exposure is an exacerbating factor for their asthma, allergen avoidance is a fundamental component of the management regimen. Environmental control measures to minimize allergen exposure include removing carpets, encasing mattresses and pillows in allergen-impermeable covers (to minimize dust mite exposure), and removing pets from the home (to minimize exposure to animal antigens). Immunotherapy with repeated injections of antigen extract is sometimes used to desensitize the patient to the offending allergen, but its efficacy in patients with asthma is controversial and not generally accepted.

Because of the availability of effective forms of therapy, patients with asthma are generally capable of leading normal lives with relatively little or no alteration in their daily activities. However, not all patients with asthma are so fortunate. Refractory disease, persistent airflow obstruction, and rapid development of life-threatening attacks are some extreme examples of asthma that pose a continuing challenge to physicians caring for these patients.

REFERENCES

REVIEWS

Holgate ST, Polosa R: The mechanisms, diagnosis, and management of severe asthma in adults, *Lancet* 368:780–793, 2006.

Kraft M, editor: Asthma, *Clin Chest Med* 27:1–147, 2006.

Moore WC, Peters SP: Update in asthma 2006, *Am J Respir Crit Care Med* 175:649–654, 2007.

National Asthma Education and Prevention Program: *Guidelines for the diagnosis and management of asthma. Expert Panel Report 3*, Bethesda, MD, 2007, National Institutes of Health, NIH publication 08-4051.

Pinnock H, Shah R: Asthma, *BMJ* 334: 847–850, 2007.

ETIOLOGY AND PATHOGENESIS

Barnes PJ: Neurogenic inflammation in the airways, *Respir Physiol* 125:145–154, 2001.

Bousquet J, Jeffery PK, Busse WW, Johnson M, Vignola AM: Asthma. From bronchoconstriction to airways inflammation and remodeling, *Am J Respir Crit Care Med* 161:1720–1745, 2000.

Busse WW, Lemanske RF Jr: Asthma, *N Engl J Med* 344:350–362, 2001.

Cookson WOC: Asthma genetics, *Chest* 121:7S–13S, 2002.

Fixman ED, Stewart A, Martin JG: Basic mechanisms of development of airway structural changes in asthma, *Eur Respir J* 29:379–389, 2007.

Gern JE, Busse WW: The role of viral infections in the natural history of asthma, *J Allergy Clin Immunol* 106:201–212, 2000.

Holgate ST, Yang Y, Haitchi HM, et al: The genetics of asthma. ADAM33 as an example of a susceptibility gene, *Proc Am Thorac Soc* 3:440–443, 2006.

Holgate ST, Davies DE, Powell RM, Howarth PH, Haitchi HM, Holloway JW: Local genetic and environmental factors in asthma disease pathogenesis: chronicity and persistence mechanisms, *Eur Respir J* 29:793–803, 2007.

Jacoby DB: Virus-induced asthma attacks, *JAMA* 287:755–761, 2002.

Martinez FD: Genes, environments, development and asthma: a reappraisal, *Eur Respir J* 29:179–184, 2007.

Platts-Mills TA, Rakes G, Heymann PW: The relevance of allergen exposure to the development of asthma in childhood, *J Allergy Clin Immunol* 105:S503–S508, 2000.

Thomson NC, Chaudhuri R, Livingston E: Asthma and cigarette smoking, *Eur Respir J* 24:822,–833 2004.

CLINICAL FEATURES AND DIAGNOSTIC APPROACH

Beach J, Russell K, Blitz S, et al: A systematic review of the diagnosis of occupational asthma, *Chest* 131:569–578, 2007.

Cherniack RM: Physiologic diagnosis and function in asthma, *Clin Chest Med* 16:567–581, 1995.

Corrao WM, Braman SS, Irwin RS: Chronic cough as the sole presenting manifestation of bronchial asthma, *N Engl J Med* 300:633–637, 1979.

Johnston NW, Sears MR: Asthma exacerbations. 1: Epidemiology, *Thorax* 61:722–728, 2006.

Martin RJ: Nocturnal asthma: circadian rhythms and therapeutic interventions, *Am Rev Respir Dis* 147: S25–S28, 1993.

McFadden ER Jr, Gilbert IA: Exercise-induced asthma, *N Engl J Med* 330:1362–1367, 1994.

McFadden ER Jr, Kiser R, DeGroot WJ: Acute bronchial asthma: relations between clinical and physiologic manifestations, *N Engl J Med* 288:221–225, 1973.

Naureckas ET, Solway J: Mild asthma, *N Engl J Med* 345:1257–1262, 2001.

Pratter MR, Irwin RS: The clinical value of pharmacologic bronchoprovocation challenge, *Chest* 85:260–265, 1984.

Scanlon PD, Beck KC: Methacholine inhalation challenge, *Mayo Clin Proc* 69:1118–1119, 1994.

Singh AM, Busse WW: Asthma exacerbations. 2: Etiology, *Thorax* 61:809–816, 2006.

TREATMENT

Aldington S, Beasley R: Asthma exacerbations. 5: Assessment and management of severe asthma in adults in hospital, *Thorax* 62:447–458, 2007.

Barnes PJ: Airway pharmacology. In Mason RJ, Murray JF, Broaddus VC, Nadel JA, editors: *Textbook of respiratory medicine*, ed 4, Philadelphia, 2005, WB Saunders, pp. 235–279.

Barnes PJ: Inhaled glucocorticoids for asthma, *N Engl J Med* 332:868–875, 1995.

Busse WW: Long- and short-acting β_2-adrenergic agonists, *Arch Intern Med* 156:1514–1520, 1996.

Corbridge TC, Hall JB: The assessment and management of adults with *status asthmaticus*, *Am J Respir Crit Care Med* 151:1296–1316, 1995.

Glassroth J: The role of long-acting β-agonists in the management of asthma: analysis, meta-analysis, and more analysis, *Ann Intern Med* 144:936–937, 2006.

Horiuchi T, Castro M: The pathobiologic implications for treatment. Old and new strategies in the treatment of chronic asthma, *Clin Chest Med* 21:381–395, 2000.

Kamada AK, Szefler SJ, Martin RJ, et al: Issues in the use of inhaled glucocorticoids, *Am J Respir Crit Care Med* 153:1739–1748, 1996.

Leff AR: Regulation of leukotrienes in the management of asthma: biology and clinical therapy, *Annu Rev Med* 52:1–14, 2001.

O' Byrne PM, Parameswaran K: Pharmacological management of mild or moderate asthma, *Lancet* 368: 794–803, 2006.

Peters-Golden M, Henderson WR: Leukotrienes, *N Engl J Med* 357: 1841–1854, 2007.

Prussin C, Metcalfe DD: Update on the management of asthma, *Adv Intern Med* 46:31–50, 2001.

Salvi SS, Krishna MT, Sampson AP, Holgate ST: The anti-inflammatory effects of leukotriene-modifying drugs and their use in asthma, *Chest* 119:1533–1546, 2001.

Strunk RC, Bloomberg GR: Omalizumab for asthma, *N Engl J Med* 354:2689–2695, 2006.

6

Chronic Obstructive Pulmonary Disease

ETIOLOGY AND PATHOGENESIS
  Smoking
  Environmental Pollution
  Infection
  Genetic Factors
PATHOLOGY
PATHOPHYSIOLOGY
  Functional Abnormalities in
    Airways Disease
	Functional Abnormalities in
	    Emphysema
	  Mechanisms of Abnormal
	    Gas Exchange
	  Pulmonary Hypertension
	  Two Types of Presentation
	CLINICAL FEATURES
	DIAGNOSTIC APPROACH
	TREATMENT

The term *chronic obstructive pulmonary disease* (COPD) refers to chronic disorders that disturb airflow, whether the most prominent process is within the airways or within the lung parenchyma. The two disorders generally included in this category are chronic bronchitis and emphysema. Although the pathophysiology of airflow obstruction is different in the two disorders, patients frequently have features of both; thus, it is appropriate to discuss them together. Although asthma could logically also be in this category, it is discussed in Chapter 5 because the term COPD, as commonly used, does not usually include bronchial asthma.

Other terms synonymous with COPD are chronic airflow limitation, chronic airflow obstruction, chronic obstructive airways disease, and chronic obstructive lung disease. Because COPD is the term in most common use, it is used here as well. Emphysema is discussed in this section of the textbook dealing with airway disease, even though the most obvious and visible pathologic manifestations of emphysema affect the lung parenchyma.

Chronic bronchitis is a clinical diagnosis used for patients with chronic cough and sputum production. The condition has certain pathologic features, but the diagnosis refers to the specific clinical presentation. For epidemiologic purposes, a more formal definition has been used, one requiring the presence of a chronic productive cough on most days during at least 3 months per year for 2 or more consecutive years. However, for clinical purposes, the physician does not necessarily adhere to this formal time requirement. Patients with chronic bronchitis frequently have periods of worsening or exacerbation, often precipitated by respiratory tract infection. Unlike patients with asthma, however, patients with pure chronic bronchitis usually have residual clinical disease even between exacerbations, and their disease is not primarily one of airway hyperreactivity. The diagnosis of *asthmatic bronchitis* is often given to patients with chronic bronchitis and a prominent component of airway hyperreactivity because features of both chronic bronchitis and asthma are present.

> Chronic bronchitis is a diagnosis made on the basis of chronic cough and sputum production.

In contrast to the clinical diagnosis of chronic bronchitis, emphysema is formally a pathologic diagnosis, although certain clinical and laboratory features are also highly suggestive of the disease. Pathologically, emphysema is characterized by destruction of lung parenchyma and enlargement of air spaces distal to the terminal bronchiole. The region of the lung from the respiratory bronchioles down to the alveoli is involved, and determination of the particular type of emphysema depends on the pattern of destruction within the acinus. Antemortem diagnosis of emphysema obviously does not have the kind of confirmation offered by postmortem examination of the lung, but indirect support for the diagnosis is still useful and reasonably reliable.

Because chronic bronchitis and emphysema coexist to a variable extent in different patients, the broader term COPD is frequently more accurate. That these two disorders are tied so closely together is not surprising. A single etiologic factor—cigarette smoking—is primarily responsible for both processes. Inflammation induced by cigarette smoke, from the large airways down to the alveolar walls of the pulmonary parenchyma, is believed to be the common thread that ties together many of the varied manifestations of COPD. Throughout this chapter, specific reference is made to chronic bronchitis or to emphysema because some of the clinical and pathophysiologic features are distinct enough to warrant separate consideration. However, patients frequently do not fit neatly into these separate diagnostic categories.

The public health problems posed by COPD are enormous. It has been estimated that 16 million Americans have COPD. The condition is the fourth most common cause of death and is responsible for approximately 110,000 deaths per year in the United States. Morbidity in terms of chronic symptoms, days lost from work, and permanent disability is even more staggering. Unlike many diseases encountered by the physician, COPD is preventable in the majority of cases because the main etiologic factor is well established and is totally avoidable. Fortunately, since 1964, when the first Surgeon General's report on smoking and health was published, the prevalence of smoking in the United States has decreased from 40% to approximately 22%. Nevertheless, there are still more than 45 million current smokers and a large reservoir of former smokers who have placed themselves at high risk for COPD and other smoking-related diseases. It is important to note that the vast majority of smokers start smoking in their teens and early twenties; thus, smoking avoidance programs are most effective when aimed at this age group. Worldwide, an increasing prevalence of smoking in developing countries is contributing to the World Health Organization's prediction that COPD will be the third most common cause of death in the year 2020.

> Emphysema is a diagnosis made on the basis of destruction of lung parenchyma and enlargement of air spaces distal to the terminal bronchiole.

ETIOLOGY AND PATHOGENESIS

Several factors have been implicated in the cause of COPD, including smoking, environmental pollution, infection, and genetics. Of these four factors, smoking is clearly the most important and the one that will receive most attention here. Yet the fact that symptomatic COPD develops in only approximately 20% of smokers suggests that other factors modify the risk. One other well-defined risk factor is discussed in detail in this section: the inherited deficiency of the protein α_1-antitrypsin. Other potential risk factors are discussed only briefly.

> Smoking is the key etiologic factor for chronic bronchitis. Environmental pollutants and respiratory tract infection cause exacerbations but generally have an insignificant etiologic role.

SMOKING

Smoking affects the lung at multiple levels: the bronchi, the bronchioles, and the pulmonary parenchyma. In the larger airways—the bronchi—smoking has a prominent effect on the structure and function of the mucus-secreting apparatus, the bronchial mucous glands. An increase in the number and size of the glands is responsible for excessive mucus within the airway lumen. The airway wall becomes thickened because of the hypertrophied and hyperplastic mucous glands as well as an influx of inflammatory cells (especially macrophages, neutrophils, and cytotoxic [CD8$^+$] T lymphocytes) into the airway wall. Thickening of the wall diminishes the size of the airway lumen, and mucus within the lumen further compromises its patency. Release of a variety of mediators from the inflammatory cells, including leukotriene B$_4$, interleukin-8, and tumor necrosis factor-α, contributes to tissue damage and amplifies the inflammatory process in both the airways and the lung parenchyma. Similarly, oxidative stress, occurring as a result of reactive oxygen species present in cigarette smoke or released from inflammatory cells, contributes to the overall pathologic process.

At the same time that more mucus is produced in the larger airways, clearance of the mucus is altered by effects of cigarette smoke on the cilia lining the bronchial lumen. Structural changes in cilia after long-term exposure to cigarette smoke have been well documented, and functional studies have demonstrated impaired mucociliary clearance as a consequence of cigarette smoking.

The combined effects of smoking on mucus production, mucociliary clearance, and airway inflammation easily explain the epidemiologic data demonstrating a significant correlation between cigarette smoking and the symptoms of chronic bronchitis: cough and sputum production. Pipe and cigar smoking are also predisposing factors in the development of chronic bronchitis, but the risk is significantly less than that from cigarette smoking, probably because pipe and cigar smoke is generally not inhaled as extensively.

Small airways (bronchioles less than approximately 2 mm in diameter) are prominently affected by smoking. Smoking induces bronchiolar narrowing, inflammation, and fibrosis, with resulting airflow obstruction. These changes in the small airways or bronchioles are believed to be responsible for much of the airflow obstruction demonstrable in patients with mild COPD (discussed later under Pathophysiology).

> Cigarette smoking is responsible for most cases of emphysema. Deficiency of serum α_1-antitrypsin is a predisposing factor for emphysema in a small proportion of cases.

In the pulmonary parenchyma, smoking results in the eventual development of emphysema. An understanding of the concepts about how smoking leads to the destruction of alveolar walls, which is characteristic of emphysema, requires familiarity with the *protease-antiprotease hypothesis*. According to this theory, emphysema results from destruction of the connective tissue matrix of alveolar walls by proteolytic enzymes (proteases) released by inflammatory cells in the alveoli. Studies in animals have demonstrated that injection of several proteolytic (i.e., capable of breaking down protein) enzymes into the airways of animals results in pathologic and physiologic changes similar to those of clinical emphysema.

The particular proteolytic enzymes thought to contribute to emphysema are those capable of breaking down elastin, a complex structural protein found in the walls of alveoli. Elastase, one of several enzymes within the category of serine proteases, appears to be the most important of the proteolytic enzymes. Neutrophils are the major source of elastase within the lungs; therefore the enzyme is commonly called *neutrophil elastase*. If elastase were allowed to exert its proteolytic effect on elastin whenever it was released from a neutrophil, destruction of this important structural protein of the alveolar wall would ensue. Fortunately, an inhibitor of neutrophil elastase, usually called α_1-antitrypsin but also sometimes called α_1-antiprotease or α_1-protease inhibitor, normally is present in the lung. It is believed that a balance between neutrophil elastase and its inhibitor prevents diffuse destruction of the alveolar walls. When this balance is disturbed, either by an increase in neutrophil elastase activity or by a decrease in antielastase activity, damage to elastin and to the alveolar wall can result, with eventual production of emphysema.

> Theories claim that proteolytic enzymes (especially elastase) are balanced by α_1-antitrypsin. Disturbance of this balance in favor of proteolytic enzymes, attributable to smoking or a deficiency of α_1-antitrypsin, may result in emphysema.

In smokers, the balance between elastase and antielastase is thought to be disturbed in more than one way by cigarette smoke. First, an increased number of neutrophils can be found in the lungs of smokers, thus providing a source for increased amounts of neutrophil elastase. Second, evidence indicates that oxidants derived from cigarette smoke and from inflammatory cells can oxidize a critical amino acid residue of α_1-antitrypsin at or near the site where the protease inhibitor binds to elastase. Oxidation of this amino acid interferes with the inhibitory activity of α_1-antitrypsin, again tipping the balance in favor of increased elastase activity. Hence, cigarette smoking may be a compound insult, increasing the amount of neutrophil elastase in the lung and decreasing the normal inhibitory mechanism that serves to limit uncontrolled elastin breakdown by the enzyme. This pathogenetic sequence hypothesized for the development of emphysema is summarized in Figure 6-1.

In addition to degrading elastin in the alveolar wall, neutrophil elastase, when released in the airways, stimulates secretion of mucus. The primary defense against the action of neutrophil elastase in the airway is provided by secretory leukoprotease inhibitor, an antiprotease produced by airway epithelial and mucus-secreting cells.

Elastase is not the only proteolytic enzyme that has been implicated in the development of smoking-related damage and emphysema. Recent interest has focused on an additional group of enzymes called the *matrix metalloproteinases,* which are produced by macrophages and neutrophils and are capable of breaking down a variety of structural components of the alveolar wall. Like the relationship between elastase and its inhibitor α_1-antitrypsin, the matrix metalloproteinases have a number of natural inhibitors, appropriately called *tissue inhibitors of matrix metalloproteinases.* Because of the influx of neutrophils and macrophages induced by cigarette smoke, it is believed that an increased burden of matrix metalloproteinases may result from smoking, potentially overwhelming the capability of the metalloproteinase inhibitors and contributing to the breakdown of alveolar walls.

ENVIRONMENTAL POLLUTION

Other factors implicated in the pathogenesis of COPD (environmental pollution, infection, and genetics) are quantitatively much less important than smoking. Air pollution is important primarily because of its potential for causing exacerbations of preexisting disease, not for initiating COPD. However, occupational exposure to pollutants or organic antigens (e.g., in miners or agricultural workers, respectively) does appear to be an important factor contributing to COPD, particularly chronic bronchitis. Additionally, in developing countries, environmental exposure to pollutants, as occurs with cooking in confined spaces, may play a role in the development of COPD.

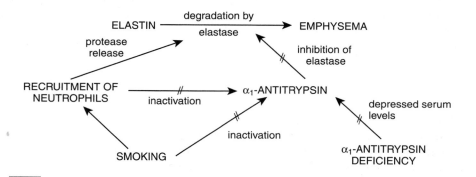

Figure 6-1. Schematic diagram of hypothesized relationship between elastase and α_1-antitrypsin (also called α_1-protease inhibitor), indicating how smoking and α_1-antitrypsin deficiency alter the balance, leading to degradation of elastin.

INFECTION

Similarly, infections do not initiate the disease, but they do cause transient worsening of symptoms and pulmonary function in patients with preexisting COPD. Of the different types of respiratory tract infection, viral infection appears to be responsible for a large number of clinical exacerbations of symptoms. Bacterial infections probably play a less important role but can cause superinfection of patients already harboring an acute viral infection.

An interesting additional role for infection is suggested by data indicating that childhood respiratory tract infections may increase the risk for subsequent development of COPD. This may be one of the factors helping to explain why the development of COPD is not uniform in all smokers. Childhood respiratory infection might contribute to the later risk for development of COPD by affecting lung growth and function during childhood. The smoker who starts with a lower level of function because of childhood respiratory infections may be more likely to suffer functionally important consequences from heavy smoking in later life.

GENETIC FACTORS

Genetic factors presumably contribute to the risk for development of COPD, but the nature of the predisposition is poorly defined. The one hereditary factor that has been best established as predisposing to emphysema is deficiency of the serum protein α_1-antitrypsin. α_1-Antitrypsin is a glycoprotein of the serine protease inhibitor (serpin) family that is produced by the liver and normally circulates in blood. Minor changes in the *SERPINA1* gene, which codes for α_1-antitrypsin, produce alterations in the structure of the protein that can be detected by biochemical methods. More than 100 different alleles of α_1-antitrypsin have been identified. Each person has two genes coding for α_1-antitrypsin, one of maternal origin and one of paternal origin. The normal (and most common) allele is the *M* allele, and the normal complement of two *M* genes is called *MM*. A person with the *MM* genotype has approximately 200 mg/dL of the *M* type of protease inhibitor circulating in the blood. With one of the variant alleles, termed *Z*, the amino acid sequence of the protein is slightly altered, impairing secretion of the protein from its site of production in the liver. Hence, the abnormal protein remains in globules in the liver, where it may result in liver disease, and only small amounts enter the blood. Individuals who are homozygous for the *Z* gene (i.e., with the *ZZ* genotype) have circulating levels of α_1-antitrypsin that are approximately 15% of normal, or 30 mg/dL. Heterozygotes, with one *M* and one *Z* gene (the *MZ* genotype), have intermediate levels of circulating α_1-antitrypsin, in the range from 50% to 60% of normal levels.

> The most important form of α_1-antitrypsin deficiency is associated with the *ZZ* genotype.

The *ZZ* genotype is a strong risk factor for premature development of emphysema, particularly if the individual is a smoker. Emphysema frequently develops as early as the third or fourth decade of life in persons with the *ZZ* genotype (who are commonly said to have α_1-antitrypsin deficiency because of low serum levels). As mentioned earlier, the structural integrity of alveolar walls appears to depend on the balance between elastin degradation by elastase and protection from this destruction afforded by α_1-antitrypsin. In patients with α_1-antitrypsin deficiency, lack of the elastase inhibitor is believed to permit elastase action to proceed in an unchecked fashion, and early development of emphysema is the consequence.

Another factor of interest, one that presumably is at least partially genetically determined, is the degree of the patient's preexisting bronchial hyperresponsiveness. Data support the hypothesis that accelerated decline in lung function occurs in patients who have greater levels of bronchial responsiveness. However, this is an area of controversy, in part because the potential for smoking to induce changes in bronchial responsiveness makes it difficult to determine cause-and-effect relationships.

PATHOLOGY

Much of the pathology in chronic bronchitis relates to mucus and the mucus-secreting apparatus in the airways. Mucus-secreting glands and goblet cells are responsible for the production of bronchial secretions, but the mucous glands are the more important source (see Chapter 4). In chronic bronchitis, enlargement (hypertrophy and hyperplasia) of the mucus-secreting glands has been objectively assessed by comparing the relative thickness of the mucous glands with the total thickness of the airway wall. This ratio, known as the *Reid index,* is increased in patients with chronic bronchitis. In general, the number of goblet cells in the airways is increased as well, and these particular cells are abundant in airways more peripheral than usual. As a result of these alterations in the mucus-secreting apparatus, the quantity of airway mucus is increased, and the composition likely is altered as well. In practice, the secretions found in patients often are thick and more viscous than usual. The bronchial walls demonstrate evidence of an inflammatory process, with cellular infiltration and variable degrees of fibrosis.

Chronic bronchitis is characterized by enlargement of the mucus-secreting glands and an increased number of goblet cells.

In the smaller airways (e.g., bronchioles), inflammation, fibrosis, intraluminal mucus, and an increase in goblet cells all contribute to a decrease in luminal diameter. Because the resistance of airways varies inversely with the fourth power of the radius, even small changes in bronchiolar size may result in major impairment to airflow at the level of the small airways. These pathologic changes in the small airways are thought to be the primary cause of airflow obstruction in patients with mild COPD.

In patients with severe chronic airflow obstruction, the most important process responsible for airflow obstruction is emphysema. As mentioned earlier, the pathology of emphysema is characterized by destruction of alveolar walls and enlargement of terminal air spaces (Fig. 6-2). Several types of emphysema have distinct pathologic

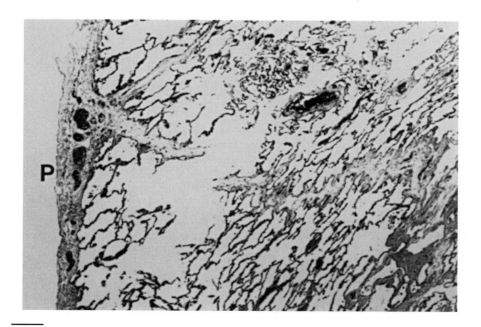

Figure 6-2. Low-power photomicrograph shows localized region of emphysema in left half of figure, adjacent to pleural surface (P). Because emphysema here is localized, destruction of alveolar walls and enlargement of terminal air spaces can be contrasted with appearance of normal lung in right half of figure. (Courtesy Dr. Earl Kasdon.)

features, primarily dependent on the distribution of the lesions. The most important types are panacinar (panlobular) emphysema and centriacinar (centrilobular) emphysema (Fig. 6-3). Panacinar emphysema is characterized by a relatively uniform involvement of the acinus, the region beyond the terminal bronchiole, including respiratory bronchioles, alveolar ducts, and alveolar sacs. Examination of a section of lung with panacinar emphysema shows that the damage in an involved area is relatively diffuse (Fig. 6-4). Typically, the lower zones of the lung are more involved than the upper zones. Panacinar emphysema is the usual type of emphysema described in patients who have α_1-antitrypsin deficiency, although the condition is not limited to this clinical setting.

> Pathologic changes from smoking often start in small airways, predating the advanced findings associated with chronic bronchitis and emphysema.

In centrilobular emphysema, the predominant involvement and dilation are found in the proximal part of the acinus, namely, the respiratory bronchiole. The appearance of a lung section with centrilobular emphysema is different from that with panacinar emphysema. In centrilobular emphysema, the involvement in an affected area seems to be more irregular, with apparently spared alveolar tissue between the dilated respiratory bronchioles at the center of the acinus (Fig. 6-5). This type of emphysema is the typical form seen in smokers. It is reasonable to speculate that the prominent involvement focused around the respiratory bronchiole is a consequence of an extension of the bronchiolar inflammation in mild COPD.

PATHOPHYSIOLOGY

Underlying a discussion of the pathophysiology of COPD is the fact that cigarette smoking affects the large airways, the small airways, and the pulmonary parenchyma. The pathophysiologic consequences resulting from disease at each of these levels contribute to the overall clinical picture of COPD. In addition, the degree of airway reactivity, which probably is affected by genetic and environmental factors, appears to modify the clinical expression of disease in a given patient. This section simplifies, summarizes, and places into a conceptual framework some of the information regarding structure-function correlations for each of these aspects of COPD.

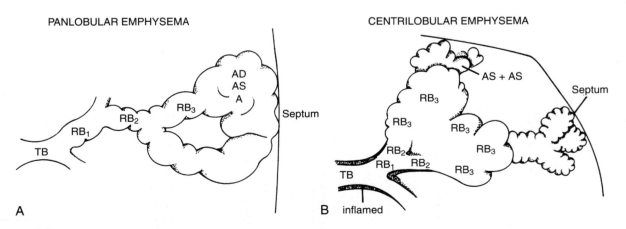

Figure 6-3. Diagram of panlobular **(A)** and centrilobular **(B)** emphysema. In panlobular (panacinar) emphysema, enlargement of air spaces is relatively uniform throughout acinus. In centrilobular (centriacinar) emphysema, enlargement of air spaces is primarily at the level of respiratory bronchioles. A = Alveolus; AD = alveolar duct; AS = alveolar sac; RB$_1$, RB$_2$, RB$_3$ = three generations of respiratory bronchioles; TB = terminal bronchiole. (From Thurlbeck WM: Chronic obstructive lung disease. In Sommers SC, editor: *Pathology annual,* vol 3, New York, 1968, Appleton-Century-Crofts.)

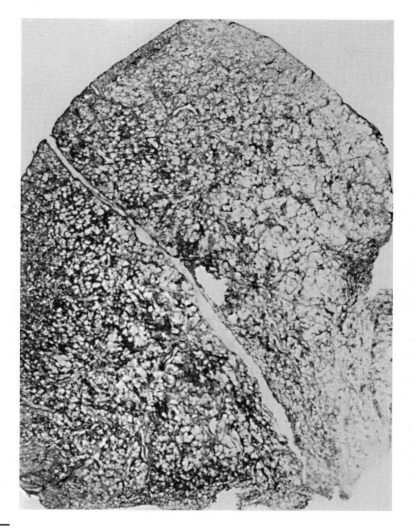

Figure 6-4. Mounted section of whole lung shows diffuse involvement seen with panacinar emphysema. (From Thurlbeck WM: *Chronic airflow obstruction in lung disease,* Philadelphia, 1976, WB Saunders.)

FUNCTIONAL ABNORMALITIES IN AIRWAY DISEASE

In the larger airways (the bronchi), an increase in the mucus-secreting apparatus and the amount of mucus produced results in the symptoms of excessive cough and sputum production characteristic of chronic bronchitis. A decrease in the size of the large airways as a result of secretions, an increase in the mucus-secreting apparatus, and inflammation might be expected to correlate well with the degree of airflow obstruction, but this does not necessarily appear to be the case. Some patients with typical symptoms of chronic bronchitis do not exhibit abnormally high resistance or changes in other measurements of airflow. When airflow obstruction exists, in general additional pathologic factors, either in the small airways (inflammation and fibrosis) or the pulmonary parenchyma (emphysema), are critical for the presence of obstruction. In relatively mild airflow obstruction associated with chronic bronchitis, disease in the small airways often makes an important contribution to airflow obstruction. When airflow obstruction is more marked, coexisting emphysema is often the primary reason for the obstruction.

Coexistent small airways disease, emphysema, or both contribute significantly to decreased expiratory flow rates in chronic bronchitis.

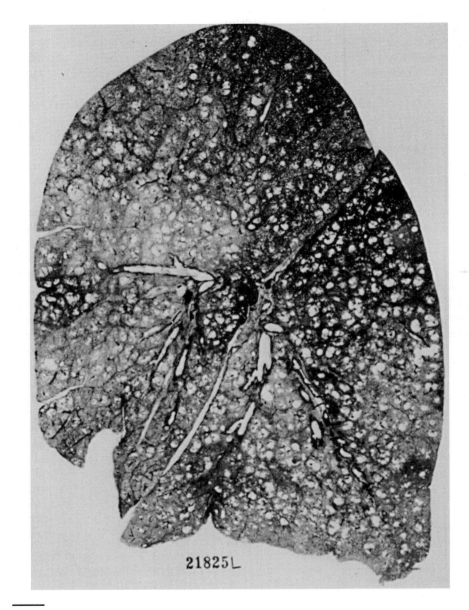

Figure 6-5. Mounted section of whole lung shows centrilobular emphysema. Adjacent to emphysematous spaces (which represent dilated respiratory bronchioles) are spared areas of lung parenchyma (representing alveolar ducts and alveolar spaces). (From Thurlbeck WM: Internal surface area and other measurements in emphysema, *Thorax* 22:483–496, 1967. BMJ Publishing Group.)

In patients who have a component of airway hyperreactivity contributing to their disease, the clinical expression often is more like asthmatic bronchitis. Airway smooth muscle constriction adds more reversible airflow obstruction than is typically seen in the patient without airway hyperreactivity.

The common problem produced by the processes affecting airways is a decrease in the overall cross-sectional area of the airways. Airways resistance (Raw) is potentially increased by anything that compromises the lumen of the airways, such as intraluminal secretions; bronchospasm; or thickening of the airway wall caused by edema, inflammatory cells, fibrosis, or enlargement of the mucus-secreting apparatus. When disease is located primarily in the peripheral airways and is mild, the functional consequences may be relatively subtle. Because the peripheral airways contribute only approximately 10% to 20% of overall airways resistance, total resistance is preserved unless the small airways disease is considerable or additional disease affects the larger airways.

As another consequence of airways disease, expiratory flow rates, including forced expiratory volume in 1 second (FEV_1), FEV_1/forced vital capacity (FVC) ratio, and maximal midexpiratory flow rate (MMFR), are generally decreased. Use of inhaled bronchodilators may or may not result in significantly improved flow rates. Patients with asthmatic bronchitis and greater airways reactivity generally have the most striking improvement in flow rates after receiving an inhaled bronchodilator.

Before a discussion of how lung volumes change in patients having the airway disease associated with COPD, it is useful to review the factors that determine the major lung volumes, namely, total lung capacity (TLC), functional residual capacity (FRC), and residual volume (RV). TLC is the point at which the force of the inspiratory muscles acting to expand the lungs is equaled by the elastic recoil of the respiratory system (primarily lung recoil) resisting expansion (see Chapter 1). At FRC, the resting point of the respiratory system, there is a balance between the elastic recoil of the lungs and the elastic recoil of the chest wall, which are acting in opposite directions—the lungs inward and the chest wall outward. The determinants of RV depend to some extent on age. In a normal young person, RV is the point at which the relatively stiff chest wall can be compressed no further by the expiratory muscles. With increasing age, a sufficient number of airways close at low lung volumes to limit further expiration, and airway closure is an important determinant of RV. In disease states in which airways are likely to close at low lung volumes, airway closure is associated with an elevated RV, even in young patients.

In patients with pure airway disease, TLC theoretically remains relatively close to normal because neither the elastic recoil of the lung nor inspiratory muscle strength is altered. Similarly, FRC should remain normal because the recoil of the lung and the recoil of the chest wall are unchanged. However, if expiration is prolonged and the respiratory rate is high, then the patient may not have sufficient time during expiration to reach the normal resting end-expiratory point. In this case, FRC is increased. RV is generally also increased with these processes that involve airways because the narrowing and occlusion of small airways by secretions and inflammation result in air trapping during expiration.

FUNCTIONAL ABNORMALITIES IN EMPHYSEMA

Although emphysema (i.e., destruction of alveolar walls) leads to decreased expiratory flow rates, the pathophysiology is different from the situation in pure airway disease. The primary problem in emphysema is loss of elastic recoil (i.e., loss of the lung's natural tendency to resist expansion). One consequence of decreased elastic recoil is a decreased driving pressure that expels air from the alveoli during expiration. A simple analogy is a balloon filled with air, in which the elastic recoil is the "stiffness" of the balloon. With a given volume of air inside an unsealed balloon, a stiffer balloon will expel air more rapidly than will a less stiff balloon. An emphysematous lung is like a less stiff balloon: a smaller than normal force drives air out of the lungs during expiration.

Loss of driving pressure is not the only consequence of emphysema. There is also an indirect effect on the collapsibility of airways. Normally, outward traction is exerted on the walls of airways by a supporting structure of tissue from the lung parenchyma. When the alveolar tissue is disrupted, as in emphysema, the supporting structure for the airways is diminished, and less radial traction is exerted to prevent airway collapse (Fig. 6-6). During a forced expiration, the strongly positive pleural pressure promotes

In emphysema, decreased expiratory flow rates are largely due to loss of elastic recoil of the lung, resulting in the following:
1. Lower driving pressure for expiratory airflow
2. Loss of radial traction on the airways provided by supporting alveolar walls, thus promoting airway collapse during expiration

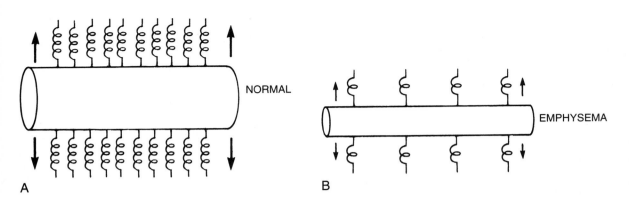

Figure 6-6. Schematic diagram of radial traction exerted by alveolar walls (represented as springs), acting to keep airways open. The normal situation is shown in **A**, and loss of radial traction, as seen in emphysema, is shown in **B**.

collapse. Airways lacking an adequate supporting structure are more likely to collapse (and have diminished flow rates and air trapping) than are normally supported airways.

The decrease in elastic recoil in emphysema also alters the compliance curve of the lung and the measured lung volumes. The compliance curve relates transpulmonary pressure and the associated volume of gas within the lung (see Chapter 1). Because an emphysematous lung has less elastic recoil (i.e., is less stiff), it resists expansion less than does its normal counterpart. Therefore, the compliance curve is shifted upward and to the left, and the lung has more volume at any particular transpulmonary pressure (Fig. 6-7). TLC is increased because loss of elastic recoil results in a smaller force opposing the action of the inspiratory musculature. FRC also is increased because the balance between the outward recoil of the chest wall and the inward recoil of the lung is shifted in favor of the chest wall. As in bronchitis, RV is substantially increased in emphysema because poorly supported airways are more susceptible to closure during a maximal expiration.

MECHANISMS OF ABNORMAL GAS-EXCHANGE

In obstructive lung disease, many of the observed pathologic changes affecting airflow are not uniformly distributed. For example, in chronic bronchitis some airways are extensively affected by secretions and plugging, whereas others remain relatively uninvolved. Therefore, ventilation is not uniformly distributed throughout the lung. Regions of the lung supplied by more diseased airways receive diminished ventilation in comparison with regions supplied by less diseased airways. Although there may be a compensatory decrease in blood flow to underventilated alveoli, the compensation is not totally effective, and inequalities and mismatching of ventilation and perfusion result. This type of ventilation-perfusion disturbance, with some areas of lung having low ventilation-perfusion ratios and contributing desaturated blood, leads to arterial hypoxemia.

Carbon dioxide elimination is impaired in some patients with obstructive lung disease. The mechanism of alveolar hypoventilation and CO_2 retention is less clear than the mechanism of hypoxemia. Several factors probably contribute, including increased work of breathing (resulting from impaired airflow), abnormalities of central ventilatory drive, and ventilation-perfusion mismatch creating some areas with high ventilation-perfusion ratios that effectively act as dead space.

An additional problem, fatigue of inspiratory muscles, has received attention as a factor contributing to acute CO_2 retention when affected patients are in respiratory

In obstructive lung disease, nonuniformity of the disease process results in $\dot{V}/\dot{Q}$ mismatch and hypoxemia.

Mechanisms that contribute to alveolar hypoventilation and CO_2 retention in obstructive lung disease are the following:
1. Increased work of breathing
2. Abnormalities of ventilatory drive
3. $\dot{V}/\dot{Q}$ mismatch
4. Decreased effectiveness of the diaphragm

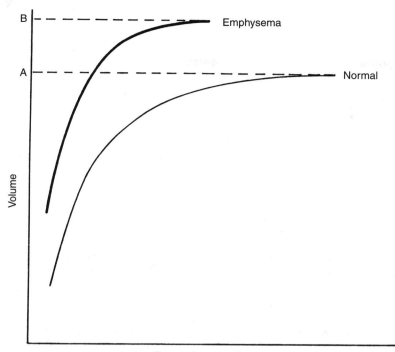

Figure 6-7. Compliance curve of lung in emphysema compared with that of normal lung. In addition to shift of curve upward and to left, total lung capacity in emphysema (point B on volume axis) is greater than normal total lung capacity (point A). In pure chronic bronchitis without emphysema, the compliance curve is normal.

failure (see Chapter 19). The importance of diaphragmatic fatigue in the stable patient with chronic hypercapnia is less certain. However, it is clear that contraction of the diaphragm, the major muscle of inspiration, is less efficient and less effective in patients with obstructive lung disease. When FRC is increased, the diaphragm is lower and flatter, and its fibers are shortened even before the initiation of inspiration. A shortened, flattened diaphragm is at a mechanical disadvantage compared with a longer, curved diaphragm, and it is less effective as an inspiratory muscle.

PULMONARY HYPERTENSION

A potential complication of COPD is the development of pulmonary hypertension (i.e., high pressures within the pulmonary arterial system). Long-standing pulmonary hypertension places an added workload onto the right ventricle, which hypertrophies and eventually may fail. The term *cor pulmonale* is used to describe disease of the right ventricle secondary to lung disease (either COPD or other forms of lung disease); this topic is discussed in Chapter 14. The primary feature of COPD that leads to pulmonary hypertension and eventually to cor pulmonale is hypoxia. A decrease in Po_2 is a strong stimulus to constriction of pulmonary arterioles (see Chapter 12). If the hypoxia is corrected, the element of pulmonary vasoconstriction may be reversible, although vascular remodeling from chronic hypoxia may not fully reverse.

Several other but less important factors that may contribute to elevated pulmonary artery pressure are hypercapnia, polycythemia, and reduction in area of the pulmonary

The major cause of pulmonary hypertension in COPD is hypoxia. Additional factors include hypercapnia, polycythemia, and destruction of the pulmonary vascular bed.

vascular bed. Hypercapnia, like hypoxia, is capable of causing pulmonary vasoconstriction. To a large extent, this effect may be mediated by the change in pH resulting from an increase in Pco_2. An elevation in hematocrit (i.e., polycythemia) is often found in the chronically hypoxemic patient, producing increased blood viscosity and contributing to elevated pulmonary artery pressure. Finally, in emphysema, the destruction of alveoli is accompanied by a loss of pulmonary capillaries. Therefore, in extensive disease, the limited pulmonary vascular bed may result in a high resistance to blood flow and consequently an increase in pulmonary artery pressure.

TWO TYPES OF PRESENTATION

Two presentations of obstructive lung disease are *pink puffer* (type A) and *blue bloater* (type B), but a clear distinction between their underlying processes is an oversimplification.

In practice, clinicians have often distinguished two pathophysiologic types of COPD, termed *type A* and *type B*, or, more colloquially, *pink puffer* and *blue bloater,* respectively. Originally, type A (pink puffer) physiology was associated with underlying emphysema, and type B (blue bloater) physiology was equated with chronic bronchitis. Although the association with a particular pathologic process appears to be an oversimplification, the pathophysiologic types of presentation can provide a helpful conceptual framework and are sometimes useful clinically. In most cases, a patient does not fall clearly into one or the other category but has some features suggestive of both.

The patient with type A disease is referred to as a pink puffer because (1) arterial Po_2 tends to be reasonably well preserved so that the patient is "pink," that is, the patient is not cyanotic, and (2) dyspnea and high minute ventilation are prominent features, with the patient appearing to be working hard to get air, that is, the patient is "puffing." Not only is Po_2 not markedly decreased, but Pco_2 is not abnormally high. On the basis of the general (although oversimplified) concept that emphysema is the primary process in these patients, relative preservation of Po_2 may be related to a simultaneous and matched loss of ventilation and perfusion when alveolar walls are destroyed. Because gas-exchange abnormalities are not a striking feature of patients with type A disease, significant hypoxia is absent and therefore does not provide a prominent stimulus for significant pulmonary hypertension. In addition, an elevated hematocrit value, often a result of hypoxemia, is not seen.

The patient with type B disease, on the other hand, is characterized by major problems with gas exchange, namely, hypoxemia and hypercapnia. This patient is termed a *blue bloater* because (1) cyanosis can result from significant hypoxemia and (2) the patient frequently is obese and can have peripheral edema resulting from right ventricular failure. Again, on the basis of the oversimplified concept that patients with type B disease have primarily chronic bronchitis, it is reasonable to attribute hypoxemia to ventilation-perfusion mismatch. Presumably, regions of lung supplied by diseased airways are underventilated, while perfusion is relatively preserved. Ventilation-perfusion mismatch results in arterial hypoxemia because of desaturated blood coming from areas with a low ventilation-perfusion ratio. As discussed earlier, several mechanisms may contribute to the development of CO_2 retention, although the primary differences explaining why type A patients do not retain CO_2 and type B patients often do are not entirely clear. As a consequence of the gas-exchange abnormalities (particularly a decrease in Po_2) in type B patients, pulmonary hypertension, cor pulmonale, and elevated hematocrit values (secondary polycythemia) commonly accompany the clinical picture.

Despite the common association of type B pathophysiology with the symptoms of chronic bronchitis, patients frequently also have pathologic evidence of emphysema, particularly of the centrilobular variety. How much of the clinical picture is secondary to bronchitis and how much is secondary to coexisting centrilobular emphysema are difficult to determine.

CLINICAL FEATURES

Symptoms most commonly experienced by patients with COPD include dyspnea and cough, frequently with sputum production. Dyspnea is the most prominent symptom in patients with type A pathophysiology; type B patients generally complain of chronic cough and sputum production. Most patients have features of both types; however, some patients with COPD are symptom free, and the diagnosis is determined on the basis of pulmonary function tests.

Frequently, patients have a certain level of chronic symptoms but their disease course is punctuated by periods of exacerbation. The precipitating factor producing an exacerbation is often a respiratory tract infection, particularly of viral origin. In addition, bacteria may be chronically present in the tracheobronchial tree, which normally should be sterile, and an acute bacterial infection, often attributable to acquisition of a new strain of the colonizing bacteria, can sometimes be implicated in acute exacerbations. Other factors that cause acute deterioration in patients include exposure to air pollutants, bronchospasm (particularly if patients have a superimposed asthmatic component to their disease), and congestive heart failure. When exacerbations are severe, patients may go into frank respiratory failure, a complication that is discussed in Chapter 27.

> The precipitating factor for an exacerbation of COPD is often a viral infection.

In addition to chronic symptoms of dyspnea, cough, or both, which may worsen during periods of acute exacerbation, patients may experience secondary cardiovascular complications of their lung disease (i.e., cor pulmonale). As mentioned, the patient with type B physiology is more susceptible to this complication than is the type A patient.

On physical examination, patients with type A physiology often appear thin (if not cachectic), and they frequently lean forward and rest on extended arms. This position allows fixation of one end of the shoulder and neck muscles, allowing them to function more effectively as accessory muscles of respiration. These patients are not cyanotic and do not demonstrate peripheral edema characteristic of right ventricular failure. In contrast, patients with type B disease often are obese and sometimes cyanotic but generally appear to be in less respiratory distress than their type A counterparts.

Examination of the chest often discloses an increased anteroposterior diameter, indicating hyperinflation of the lungs. Patients may be using accessory muscles of respiration, such as the sternocleidomastoid and trapezius muscles, and the intercostal muscles may retract with each inspiration. When diaphragmatic excursion is assessed by percussion of the lung bases during inspiration and expiration, diminished movement is noted. Breath sounds are generally decreased in intensity, and expiration is prolonged. Wheezing may be heard but unfortunately does not necessarily reflect reversible bronchospasm. Although some patients do not wheeze on their normal tidal breathing, they do so when asked to give a forced exhalation. In patients with chronic bronchitis and profuse airway secretions, coarse gurgling sounds labeled as rhonchi are frequently appreciated. When cor pulmonale is present, with or without frank right ventricular failure, patients have the cardiac findings described in Chapter 14.

Smoking not only is the primary factor that initiates COPD; it is a major risk factor that determines the prognosis of a patient's illness. Patients who continue to smoke appear to have the greatest further deterioration of pulmonary function over time. Respiratory tract infections may cause acute deterioration but do not appear to affect the rate at which pulmonary function is lost. Nonetheless, infections are the most important cause of acute mortality in patients with COPD, pointing to the need for influenza and pneumococcal vaccination as well as rapid, appropriate treatment of bacterial respiratory infections.

> Continuation of smoking is a major risk factor affecting the prognosis of COPD.

A wide spectrum of severity is characteristic of COPD; therefore the morbidity from the disease varies tremendously among patients. Patients with mild disease are able to continue their usual work and lifestyle with minimal, if any, changes. Patients with severe disease are quite limited in their capacity for any exertion, are subject to frequent hospitalizations, and may have a life expectancy of less than 5 years.

DIAGNOSTIC APPROACH

In most cases, the diagnosis of COPD is made with a combination of history and physical examination. Chronic bronchitis is actually a clinical diagnosis, and the history is particularly crucial. Although emphysema is formally a pathologic diagnosis, a lung biopsy is not performed to make the diagnosis. Pathologic confirmation is generally obtained only at postmortem examination, if one is performed.

A valuable study on a macroscopic level for assessing the lungs of patients with COPD is the chest radiograph. Patients with chronic bronchitis alone frequently have a normal chest radiograph. Minor changes of increased markings through the lungs may be present, but determining whether they can be attributed to coexisting emphysema is difficult. When cor pulmonale develops in these patients, secondary cardiac changes may also be seen, indicative of right ventricular hypertrophy or dilation.

> Characteristic radiographic findings in the more frequently recognized arterial deficiency pattern of COPD are the following:
> 1. Large lung volumes
> 2. Flat diaphragms
> 3. Increased anteroposterior diameter
> 4. Loss of vascular markings

In patients with emphysema, two radiographic patterns are well described. In the first pattern, which is the most frequently recognized, patients have hyperinflation, with large lung volumes, flat diaphragms, an increased retrosternal air space, and an increased anteroposterior diameter (seen on the lateral view). In addition, a paucity of vascular markings in the lung results from destruction of alveolar septa and enlargement of alveolar spaces. This pattern is known as the *arterial deficiency* pattern of emphysema because of the changes in vascular markings; it often is associated with underlying panacinar emphysema (Fig. 6-8). In patients with α_1-antitrypsin deficiency and early onset of emphysema, the arterial deficiency pattern is quite striking in the lower lobes, where there may be almost a complete loss of vascular markings.

The second radiographic pattern seen in patients with emphysema is termed the *increased markings* pattern. In this pattern, the radiograph shows prominent lung markings and may give evidence of pulmonary hypertension and cor pulmonale. Patients with this type of presentation often have clinical chronic bronchitis and type B physiology, and their radiographic findings probably are related to coexistent centrilobular emphysema.

High-resolution computed tomography is recognized as a more sensitive imaging method than chest radiograph for detecting emphysema. However, because it is expensive and rarely changes the management plan in this setting, it should not be considered part of the usual diagnostic evaluation for these patients.

> Pulmonary function tests in COPD show the following:
> 1. Airflow obstruction (decreased FVC, FEV$_1$, FEV$_1$/FVC, MMFR)
> 2. Air trapping (increased RV, FRC, and often TLC)
> 3. Diffusing capacity generally decreased in emphysema, normal in chronic bronchitis

The most useful physiologic adjuncts in evaluating patients with COPD are pulmonary function tests and arterial blood gas analysis. Pulmonary function tests demonstrate airflow obstruction, with decreases in FVC, FEV$_1$, FEV$_1$/FVC ratio, and MMFR. Measurements of lung volume generally give evidence of air trapping, with an elevation in RV. In patients whose lung compliance is increased (i.e., in patients with emphysema), TLC is generally elevated. FRC is elevated as a result of either increased compliance (decreased elastic recoil) in emphysema or insufficient expiratory time in the face of significant airflow obstruction. Whether emphysema is present can be indirectly assessed by measuring the diffusing capacity for carbon monoxide. In patients with emphysema, in whom the surface area for gas exchange is lost, the diffusing capacity typically is decreased. In pure airway disease (e.g., chronic bronchitis without emphysema), the diffusing capacity is generally normal.

The results of arterial blood gas analysis depend to a large extent on the pathophysiologic type of disease. In fact, blood gas determination is an important criterion

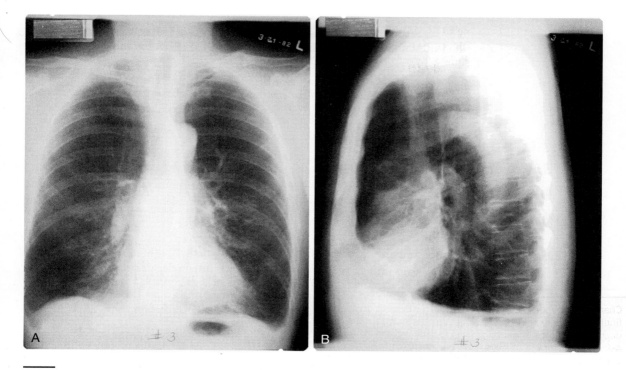

Figure 6-8. Chest radiographs of patient with severe chronic obstructive pulmonary disease showing arterial deficiency pattern of emphysema. Lungs are hyperinflated, diaphragms are low and flat (in this case they are actually inverted on lateral film), and there is paucity of vascular markings. **A,** Posteroanterior view. **B,** Lateral view.

for classifying the patient into one of the two pathophysiologic categories. Patients with type A pathophysiology have a normal or mildly decreased arterial Po_2 and a normal or slightly decreased arterial Pco_2. Patients with type B physiology have more strikingly abnormal blood gas values, often with marked hypoxemia as well as CO_2 retention. With chronic elevation in Pco_2, the kidneys retain bicarbonate in an attempt to compensate and return the pH toward normal. With acute exacerbations of COPD, hypoxemia frequently worsens and CO_2 retention becomes more pronounced so that the pH may drop from the stable compensated value.

Many of the clinical features characterizing patients with type A and those with type B pathophysiology are summarized in Table 6-1.

> Type B patients are more hypoxemic than are type A patients and often have hypercapnia.

TREATMENT

Several modalities of treatment, used either individually or in combination, are available for patients with COPD. Although bronchoconstriction in patients with COPD is considerably less than that in patients with bronchial asthma, bronchodilators remain an important part of the treatment of many patients with COPD. The agents used are identical to those discussed in Chapter 5, including sympathomimetic agents (β_2 agonists), anticholinergic drugs, and methylxanthines. Short-acting inhaled β_2 agonists (e.g., albuterol), short-acting anticholinergic agents (e.g., ipratropium), or both are most commonly used as needed for patients with mild disease who require only infrequent therapy. For patients with more severe disease who require regular therapy, either a long-acting β_2 agonist (e.g., salmeterol, formoterol, arformoterol), a long-acting anticholinergic agent (e.g., tiotropium), or both are commonly used, although regular

Table 6-1

CLINICAL DISTINCTIONS BETWEEN TYPE A AND TYPE B PATHOPHYSIOLOGY

FEATURE	TYPE A	TYPE B
Commonly used name	Pink puffer	Blue bloater
Disease association	Predominantly emphysema	Predominantly bronchitis
Major symptom	Dyspnea	Cough and sputum
Appearance	Thin, wasted, not cyanotic	Obese, cyanotic
Po_2	↓	↓↓
Pco_2	Normal or ↓	Normal or ↑
Elastic recoil of lung	↓	Normal
Diffusing capacity	↓	Normal
Hematocrit	Normal	Often ↑
Cor pulmonale	Infrequent	Common

use of short-acting agents is an alternative. The methylxanthine theophylline is another option, but concern for systemic side effects often relegates it to a secondary role in comparison with the inhaled bronchodilators.

Use of corticosteroids in patients with COPD is evolving and dependent on the clinical setting. A 10- to 14-day course of systemic corticosteroids is frequently administered at the time of an acute exacerbation, and most studies suggest a benefit of improved pulmonary function and reduced treatment failure in this setting. On the other hand, only a minority of patients with chronic, stable, but severe disease shows improved pulmonary function after a regimen of oral corticosteroids. Inhaled corticosteroids have little use in the setting of acute exacerbations of COPD. However, they are increasingly being used in patients with moderate to severe COPD who have frequent exacerbations because some evidence indicates that inhaled corticosteroids may reduce the frequency or severity of exacerbations.

Patients with COPD who develop an acute respiratory tract infection or patients with an exacerbation of their disease without a clear precipitant often are treated with antibiotics. The primary usefulness of antibiotics is treatment of bacterial infections; however, a bacterial cause is difficult to document with certainty, and many exacerbations are thought to be either noninfectious or triggered by viral respiratory infections. In practice, patients frequently are treated with antibiotics when a change in the quantity, color, and/or thickness of sputum in comparison with the usual pattern of sputum production is noted, regardless of whether a bacterial infection is present. Of the potential bacterial pathogens, those most frequently implicated are *Streptococcus pneumoniae, Haemophilus influenzae,* and *Moraxella catarrhalis.* As a result, the choice of antibiotic should provide coverage for these organisms.

An important adjunct to therapy is administration of supplemental O_2 to patients with significant hypoxemia (i.e., arterial Po_2 55 mm Hg or less). Fortunately, the Po_2 of hypoxemic patients with COPD usually responds quite well to even relatively small amounts of supplemental O_2 (range 24%–28% O_2). A low flow rate of O_2 (1–2 L/min), given by nasal prongs, is an effective, well-tolerated method for achieving these concentrations of inspired O_2. Oxygen is particularly important in patients with pulmonary hypertension and in those with secondary polycythemia because each of these complications is largely caused by hypoxemia and responsive to treatment for it. Evidence suggests that long-term survival of hypoxemic patients with COPD can be improved by chronic administration of supplemental O_2. Administration of supplemental O_2 is the only form of current therapy capable of altering the natural history and improving the long-term survival of these patients.

The goal of O_2 therapy is to shift Po_2 into the range in which hemoglobin is almost fully saturated (i.e., Po_2 greater than 60–65 mm Hg). Ideally, O_2 saturation should be

Modalities available for treatment of COPD are the following:
1. Bronchodilators
2. Antibiotics
3. Corticosteroids
4. Supplemental oxygen
5. Exercise rehabilitation
6. Chest physiotherapy
7. Surgery (selected cases)

well maintained on a continuous basis, throughout the day and night. In some patients with COPD who are not significantly hypoxemic during the day, a substantial drop in Po_2 and O_2 saturation can occur at night. In these patients, nocturnal O_2 theoretically may be of benefit, although this has not been proven.

For patients in whom airway secretions cause significant symptoms, chest physiotherapy and postural drainage are sometimes used to help mobilize and clear the secretions. These techniques use percussion of the chest wall to loosen secretions and induce cough, followed by positional changes to allow gravity to aid in drainage of secretions. However, the usefulness of chest physiotherapy and postural drainage is not generally accepted because outcome studies have not clearly supported their benefit.

In the small subgroup of patients with COPD who have α_1-antitrypsin deficiency, therapy is available in the form of intravenous α_1-antitrypsin concentrate prepared from pooled human plasma. The rationale for this therapy is to replace the deficient protease inhibitor and attempt to inhibit or prevent unchecked proteolytic destruction of alveolar tissue. Although intravenous infusions of α_1-antitrypsin have been shown to increase concentrations of this antiprotease in alveolar epithelial lining fluid, whether such replacement therapy alters the accelerated decline in pulmonary function is not definitively known.

In patients with impaired exercise tolerance secondary to COPD, a rehabilitation program focusing on education and a regimen of exercise training often is quite beneficial. Most patients participating in such a program report an improved sense of well-being at the same time they experience an improvement in exercise tolerance. Educating the patient about and assisting the patient with smoking cessation are absolutely critical parts of any comprehensive therapeutic program. Pharmacologic assistance to ameliorate the effects of nicotine withdrawal, using nicotine replacement therapy, bupropion, or varenicline, often is a valuable component of smoking cessation efforts. Vaccination against influenza and pneumococcus is indicated for all patients as a preventive strategy and as a component of the overall therapeutic regimen.

Two surgical approaches have been used for patients with severe COPD who remain markedly symptomatic despite optimal therapy. One approach, *lung volume reduction surgery,* initially sounds counterintuitive because it involves removing portions of both lungs from patients whose pulmonary reserve is marginal at best. However, two interesting pathophysiologic rationales underlie this approach. First, removal of some lung tissue diminishes overall intrathoracic volume, allowing the flattened and foreshortened diaphragm to return toward its normal position and resume its usual curved configuration. A flattened, foreshortened diaphragm is an inefficient respiratory muscle, and the changes in its position and shape following surgery facilitate its effectiveness during inspiration. Second, when the most diseased regions of lung are selectively removed (i.e., the regions with the least elastic recoil), the overall elastic recoil of the lung improves. Lung elastic recoil is an important determinant of expiratory flow and airway collapse, and improving the elastic recoil has secondary benefits on airway patency and expiratory flow. Although lung volume reduction surgery is a novel and potentially attractive approach, it appears to be beneficial only in well-selected patients. Critical aspects of patient selection include the severity of disease and the anatomic distribution of emphysematous changes.

The other surgical approach to treatment of end-stage COPD is *lung transplantation.* However, this is not a practical approach for large numbers of individuals because of the resources needed, the shortage of donor organs, and the age of most patients with COPD. Patients whose emphysema is due to α_1-antitrypsin deficiency, in whom the disease occurs at an early age, may be a particularly appropriate subgroup to consider for lung transplantation.

When acute respiratory failure supervenes as a part of COPD, mechanical ventilation may be necessary to support gas exchange and maintain acceptable arterial blood gas values. Such ventilatory assistance with intermittent positive pressure may be delivered via either a mask (noninvasive positive-pressure ventilation) or an endotracheal tube. More detailed information about the treatment of acute respiratory failure superimposed on chronic disease of the obstructive variety is covered in Chapter 27. Mechanical ventilation is discussed in Chapter 29.

REFERENCES

REVIEWS

Barnes PJ: Chronic obstructive pulmonary disease, *N Engl J Med* 343:269–280, 2000.

Celli BR, MacNee W; ATS/ERS Task Force: Standards for the diagnosis and treatment of patients with COPD: a summary of the ATS/ERS position paper, *Eur Respir J* 23:932–946, 2004.

Rabe KF, Beghé B, Luppi F, Fabbri LM: Update in chronic obstructive lung disease 2006, *Am J Respir Crit Care Med* 175:1222–1232, 2007.

Rabe KF, Hurd S, Anzueto A, et al: Global strategy for the diagnosis, management, and prevention of chronic obstructive pulmonary disease. GOLD executive summary, *Am J Respir Crit Care Med* 176: 532–555, 2007.

Siafakas NM, editor: Management of chronic obstructive pulmonary disease, *Eur Respir Mon* 11 (monograph 38):1–475, 2006.

Thurlbeck WM: *Chronic airflow obstruction in lung disease,* Philadelphia, 1976, WB Saunders.

ETIOLOGY AND PATHOGENESIS

Antó JM, Vermeire P, Vestbo J, Sunyer J: Epidemiology of chronic obstructive pulmonary disease, *Eur Respir J* 17:982–994, 2001.

Barnes PJ, Shapiro SD, Pauwels RA: Chronic obstructive pulmonary disease: molecular and cellular mechanisms, *Eur Respir J* 22:672–688, 2003.

Carrell RW, Lomas DA: Alpha$_1$-antitrypsin deficiency—a model for conformational diseases, *N Engl J Med* 346:45–53, 2002.

Hogg JC, Senior RM: Pathology and biochemistry of emphysema, *Thorax* 57:830–834, 2002.

Köhnlein T, Welte T: Alpha-1 antitrypsin deficiency: pathogenesis, clinical presentation, diagnosis, and treatment. *Am J Med* 121:3–9, 2008.

O'Donnell R, Breen D, Wilson S, Djukanovic R: Inflammatory cells in the airways in COPD, *Thorax* 61:448–454, 2006.

Saetta M, Turato G, Maestrelli P, Mapp CE, Fabbri LM: Cellular and structural bases of chronic obstructive pulmonary disease, *Am J Respir Crit Care Med* 163:1304–1309, 2001.

Stoller JK, Aboussouan LS: Alpha-1-antitrypsin deficiency, *Lancet* 365:2225–2236, 2005.

CLINICAL FEATURES

Celli BR, Barnes PJ: Exacerbations of chronic obstructive pulmonary disease, *Eur Respir J* 29:1224–1238, 2007.

Cleverley JR, Müller NL: Advances in radiologic assessment of chronic obstructive pulmonary disease, *Clin Chest Med* 21:653–663, 2000.

Currie GP, Legge JS: ABC of chronic obstructive pulmonary disease. Diagnosis, *BMJ* 332:1261–1263, 2006.

Mannino DM, Watt G, Hole D, et al: The natural history of chronic obstructive pulmonary disease, *Eur Respir J* 27:627–643, 2006.

Müller NL, Coxson H: Imaging the lungs in patients with chronic obstructive pulmonary disease, *Thorax* 57:982–985, 2002.

Sapey E, Stockley RA: COPD exacerbations. 2: Aetiology, *Thorax* 61:250–258, 2006.

White AJ, Gompertz S, Stockley RA: The aetiology of exacerbations of chronic obstructive pulmonary disease, *Thorax* 58:73–80, 2003.

TREATMENT

Alsaeedi A, Sin DD, McAlister FA: The effects of inhaled corticosteroids in chronic obstructive pulmonary disease: a systematic review of randomized placebo-controlled trials, *Am J Med* 113:59–65, 2002.

Barr RG, Bourbeau J, Camargo CA, Ram FSF: Tiotropium for stable chronic obstructive pulmonary disease: a meta-analysis, *Thorax* 61:854–862, 2006.

Ferguson GT: Update on pharmacologic therapy for chronic obstructive pulmonary disease, *Clin Chest Med* 21:723–738, 2000.

Fishman A, Martinez F, Naunheim K, et al: National Emphysema Treatment Trial Research Group: A randomized trial comparing lung-volume-reduction surgery with medical therapy for severe emphysema, *N Engl J Med* 348:2059–2073, 2003.

Flaherty KR, Martinez FJ: Lung volume reduction surgery for emphysema, *Clin Chest Med* 21:819–849, 2000.

McCrory DC, Brown C, Gelfand SE, Bach PB: Management of acute exacerbations of COPD. A summary and appraisal of published evidence, *Chest* 119:1190–1209, 2001.

McEvoy CE, Niewoehner DE: Corticosteroids in chronic obstructive pulmonary disease. Clinical benefits and risks, *Clin Chest Med* 21:739–752, 2000.

Qaseem A, Snow V, Shekelle P, et al: Diagnosis and management of stable chronic obstructive pulmonary disease: a clinical practice guideline from the American College of Physicians, *Am Intern Med* 147: 633–638, 2007.

Ranney L, Melvin C, Lux L, McClain E, Lohr KN: Systematic review: smoking cessation intervention strategies for adults and adults in special populations, *Ann Intern Med* 145:845–856, 2006.

Ries AL, Bauldoff GS, Carlin BW, et al: Pulmonary rehabilitation: joint ACCP/AACVPR evidence-based clinical practice guidelines, Chest 131(suppl):4S–42S, 2007.

· Rodríguez-Roisin R: COPD exacerbations. 5: Management, *Thorax* 61:535–544, 2006.

Singh JM, Palda VA, Stanbrook MB, Chapman KR: Corticosteroid therapy for patients with acute exacerbations of chronic obstructive pulmonary disease, *Arch Intern Med* 162:2527–2536, 2002.

Stoller JK: Acute exacerbations of chronic obstructive pulmonary disease, *N Engl J Med* 346:988–994, 2002.

Tonnesen P, Carrozzi L, Fagerström KO, et al: Smoking cessation in patients with respiratory diseases: a high priority, integral component of therapy, *Eur Respir J* 29:390–417, 2007.

Wilson R: Bacteria, antibiotics and COPD, *Eur Respir J* 17:995–1007, 2001.

7

Miscellaneous Airway Diseases

BRONCHIECTASIS
    Etiology and Pathogenesis
    Pathology
    Pathophysiology
    Clinical Features
    Diagnostic Approach
    Treatment
CYSTIC FIBROSIS
    Etiology and Pathogenesis
    Pathology

    Pathophysiology
    Clinical Features
    Diagnostic Approach
    Treatment
UPPER AIRWAY DISEASE
    Etiology
    Pathophysiology
    Clinical Features
    Diagnostic Approach
    Treatment

This chapter considers several disorders that affect airways, chosen because of their clinical or physiologic importance. The first of these disorders, bronchiectasis, is a disease that was much more common in the past. The availability of effective antibiotics for control of respiratory tract infections has made this problem less prevalent and has diminished its clinical consequences. The second disorder, cystic fibrosis, is a genetic disease that generally manifests in childhood and is notable for the often devastating clinical consequences that ensue. Abnormalities of the upper airway (which for our purposes here includes the airway at or above the level of the trachea) are discussed briefly to acquaint the reader with the physiologic principles that allow detection of these disorders.

BRONCHIECTASIS

Bronchiectasis is an irreversible dilation of airways caused by inflammatory destruction of airway walls. Because the most common etiologic factor is infection, which triggers the destructive inflammatory process, the extent of the bronchiectasis in a patient depends on the location and extent of the underlying infection. In some cases, bronchiectasis is localized to a specific region of the lung. In other cases, the process involves more than one area or even is diffuse, involving a large portion of both lungs.

ETIOLOGY AND PATHOGENESIS

> Prior infection, obstruction, or both are the most common problems leading to bronchiectasis.

Infection and impairment of drainage (frequently attributable to obstruction) are the two underlying problems that contribute to the development of dilated or bronchiectatic airways. The responsible infection(s) may be viral or bacterial. Years ago, measles and pertussis (whooping cough) pneumonia were common problems resulting in bronchiectasis. Currently, a variety of other viral and bacterial infections often are responsible; important examples are tuberculosis and *Mycobacterium avium* complex. At times, inflammation resulting from hypersensitivity to fungal organisms is the underlying cause, as with *allergic bronchopulmonary aspergillosis.* This condition, found almost exclusively in patients with clinically apparent asthma or cystic fibrosis, is characterized by colonization of airways with *Aspergillus* organisms and by thick mucous plugs and bronchiectasis in relatively proximal airways.

When an airway is obstructed, a superimposed infection may develop behind the obstruction, causing destruction of the airway wall and leading to bronchiectasis. Tumors, thick mucus, or foreign bodies commonly cause bronchial obstruction, resulting in bronchiectasis.

Another factor that plays a role in some patients is a defect in the ability of the airway to clear itself of, or protect itself against, bacterial pathogens (see Chapter 22). Such a defect predisposes a person to recurrent infections and eventually to airway dilation and bronchiectasis. The abnormality may involve inadequate humoral immunity and insufficient antibody production (hypogammaglobulinemia) or defective leukocyte function. Another problem that has received significant attention is dyskinetic cilia syndrome, in which ciliary dysfunction affects the ability of the ciliary blanket that lines the airway to clear bacteria and protect the airway against infection. The ciliary dysfunction is not limited to the lower airways; it also affects the nasal mucosa and, in males, may affect sperm motility and hence fertility. Pathologically, the dynein arms that are a characteristic feature of the ultrastructure of cilia are frequently absent in this disorder. One specific syndrome associated with bronchiectasis and ciliary dysfunction is *Kartagener's syndrome,* which includes a triad of sinusitis, bronchiectasis, and situs inversus (usually discovered because of the presence of dextrocardia).

> Abnormalities of ciliary structure and function can result in recurrent infections and bronchiectasis.

PATHOLOGY

The primary pathologic feature of bronchiectasis is evident on gross inspection of the airways, which are markedly dilated in the involved region (Fig. 7-1). Three specific patterns of dilation have been described: cylindrical (appearing as uniform widening of the involved airways), varicose (having irregularly widened airways resembling varicose veins), and saccular bronchiectasis (characterized by widening of peripheral airways in a balloonlike fashion). These terms are still used when describing radiographic patterns but are much less relevant clinically. The dilated airways are generally filled with a considerable amount of secretions, which may be grossly purulent. Microscopic changes of the bronchial wall epithelium, consisting of ulceration and squamous metaplasia, are seen.

As a result of the exuberant inflammatory changes in the bronchial wall, the blood supply, provided by the bronchial arteries, is increased. The arteries enlarge and increase in number, and new anastomoses may form between the bronchial and pulmonary artery circulations. Inflammatory erosion or mechanical trauma at the site of these vascular changes often is responsible for the hemoptysis seen frequently in patients with bronchiectasis.

> Vessels from the bronchial arterial circulation supplying a bronchiectatic region are often a source of bleeding and hemoptysis.

Coexisting disease in the remainder of the tracheobronchial tree is common. Other areas of bronchiectasis may be present, or generalized changes of chronic bronchitis may be seen (see Chapter 6).

PATHOPHYSIOLOGY

Once the airways have become irreversibly dilated, their defense mechanisms against infection are disturbed. The normal propulsive action of cilia in the involved area is lost, even if it was intact before development of bronchiectasis. Bacteria colonize the

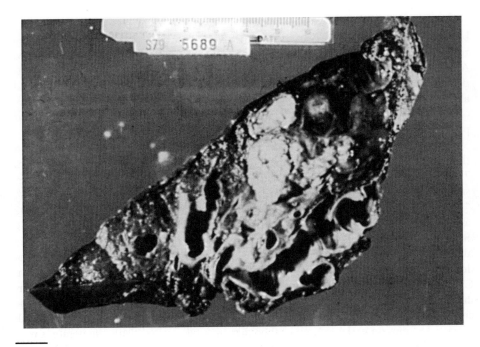

Figure 7-1. Surgically removed specimen of lung shows extensive bronchiectasis. Some of the grossly dilated airways are filled with large amounts of mucoid and purulent material.

enlarged airways, and secretions pool in the dilated sacs of patients with saccular bronchiectasis. Cough becomes much less effective at clearing secretions because of the abnormally collapsible airways. In many cases the relationship established between the colonizing bacteria and the host is relatively stable over time, but the course may be punctuated by acute exacerbations of airway infection.

Functionally, patients with a localized area of bronchiectasis are not impaired to the same extent as patients with generalized obstructive lung disease. Measurement of pulmonary function may reveal surprisingly few, if any, abnormalities. When seen, functional abnormalities are the result of either extensive bronchiectasis involving a large area of one or both lungs or coexistent generalized airway disease, primarily chronic bronchitis.

CLINICAL FEATURES

Common clinical features of bronchiectasis are the following:
1. Cough
2. Copious and purulent sputum
3. Hemoptysis
4. Localized rales or rhonchi
5. Clubbing

The most prominent symptoms in patients with bronchiectasis generally are cough and copious sputum production. The sputum may be frankly purulent and tenacious, and often the profuse amount of yellow or green sputum production raises the physician's suspicion of bronchiectasis. However, not all patients with bronchiectasis have significant sputum production. It has been estimated that approximately 10% to 20% of patients are free of copious sputum production; these patients are said to have "dry" bronchiectasis.

The other frequent symptom in patients with bronchiectasis is hemoptysis, which may be massive and life threatening. Hypertrophied bronchial artery circulation to the involved area is responsible for this symptom in the majority of cases.

Physical examination of the patient with bronchiectasis may reveal few abnormalities, even over the area of involvement. On the other hand, the examiner may hear strikingly abnormal findings, such as wheezes, rales, or rhonchi, in a localized area. Clubbing is frequently present. Although the mechanism is not clear, clubbing is thought to be associated with the chronic suppurative process.

Whether arterial blood gas values are abnormal in these patients often depends on the extent of involvement and the presence or absence of underlying chronic bronchitis. With well-localized disease, both Po_2 and Pco_2 may be normal. At the other extreme, patients may exhibit the blood gas changes seen in patients with the type B pattern of chronic obstructive lung disease, namely, hypoxemia and hypercapnia. Cor pulmonale may subsequently develop.

DIAGNOSTIC APPROACH

The diagnosis of bronchiectasis usually is suggested by a history of copious sputum production, hemoptysis, or both. Evaluation on a macroscopic level generally includes a chest radiograph, which often reveals nonspecific abnormalities in the involved area. The radiograph may show an area of increased markings, crowded vessels, or "ring" shadows corresponding to dilated or saccular airways. However, none of the findings on the routine radiograph is considered diagnostic of bronchiectasis.

Currently, computed tomography (CT) is the initial procedure generally used to define the presence, location, and extent of bronchiectasis (Fig. 7-2). High-resolution CT (with sections 1–2 mm thick) provides excellent detail and is particularly useful for detecting subtle bronchiectasis. In the past, the definitive diagnosis depended on bronchography, a radiographic procedure in which an inhaled opaque contrast material was used to outline part of the tracheobronchial tree (Fig. 7-3). This procedure is uncomfortable, can induce bronchospasm, and is rarely performed today.

Evaluation on a microscopic level is not particularly helpful for patients with presumed bronchiectasis, except for examination of the sputum for microorganisms, particularly during an acute exacerbation of the disease. Patients with bronchiectasis frequently become colonized and infected with *Pseudomonas aeruginosa,* and the finding of this otherwise relatively unusual pathogen may be a clue to the presence of

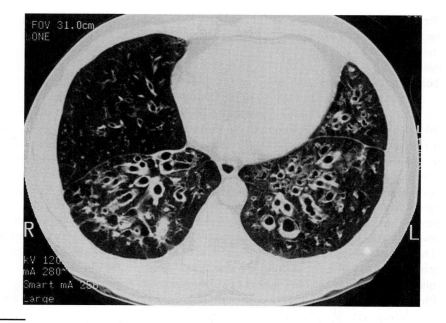

Figure 7-2. High-resolution computed tomographic scan of bronchiectasis shows dilated airways in both lower lobes and in the lingula. When seen in cross section, the dilated airways have a ringlike appearance.

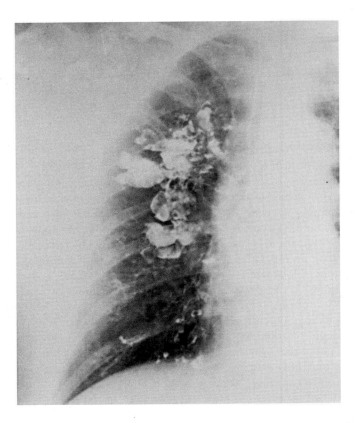

Figure 7-3. Bronchogram of patient with extensive saccular bronchiectasis, primarily in the right upper lobe.

underlying bronchiectasis. The findings on functional evaluation were discussed in the sections on pathophysiology and clinical features.

TREATMENT

Treatment of bronchiectasis includes bronchopulmonary drainage, antibiotics, and bronchodilators. Surgical therapy with resection of the diseased area is infrequent.

The three major aspects of treatment of bronchiectasis are antibiotics, bronchopulmonary drainage (clearance of airway secretions), and bronchodilators. Antibiotics are used in various ways. Some patients are treated only when the quantity or appearance of the sputum clearly changes. Other patients, especially those who have severe disease and frequent exacerbations, are given a regimen of intermittent or even continuous antibiotics in an attempt to control chronic infection. Oral agents such as amoxicillin and trimethoprim-sulfamethoxazole, which are effective against many strains of *Streptococcus pneumoniae* and *Haemophilus influenzae,* are often used in patients with bronchiectasis. Inhaled tobramycin is sometimes used prophylactically to diminish the growth of gram-negative organisms. When these patients are infected with *Pseudomonas* organisms, treatment is generally more difficult. Oral fluoroquinolones such as ciprofloxacin have become useful therapy for *Pseudomonas* infection as an alternative to parenteral antibiotics, but secondary development of resistance to this class of antibiotics is common. Infection with *Mycobacterium avium* complex requires prolonged therapy with multiple drugs (see Chapter 24). Chest physical therapy and positioning to allow better drainage of secretions (postural drainage) are frequently used for patients with copious sputum. Alternatively, inflatable vests or mechanical vibrators on the chest are increasingly being used to facilitate clearance of secretions.

Bronchodilators may be useful in patients with coexisting airway obstruction that is at least partially reversible. Inhaled DNAse has been used to decrease the viscosity of pulmonary secretions in patients with cystic fibrosis (see section on cystic fibrosis) but has not proven effective in bronchiectasis resulting from other causes.

In the past, surgery was used for many patients with localized bronchiectasis. Because medical therapy frequently is effective in limiting symptoms and impairment, resection of the diseased area now is performed much less frequently. In general, surgery is reserved for selected patients who have significant, poorly controlled symptoms attributable to a single localized area and who do not have other areas of bronchiectasis or significant evidence of generalized chronic obstructive pulmonary disease.

CYSTIC FIBROSIS

Cystic fibrosis is the most common lethal genetic disease affecting the white population. It is inherited as an autosomal recessive trait and is present in approximately 1 in 2500 live births. Manifestations of the disease usually are seen in childhood, although increasingly more cases are being recognized in adults, and children with the disease are living longer into adulthood. The clinical presentation is dominated by severe lung disease and pancreatic insufficiency resulting from thick and tenacious secretions produced by exocrine glands.

ETIOLOGY AND PATHOGENESIS

Two major abnormalities are recognized as responsible for the clinical expression of cystic fibrosis. The first abnormality relates to the quality of secretions produced by various exocrine glands. The secretions are thick and tenacious and block the tubes into which the secretions are normally deposited (especially airways and pancreatic ducts). Second, the sweat produced by affected patients has an abnormal electrolyte composition (specifically, elevated concentrations of sodium, chloride, and potassium). These abnormalities in the composition of sweat have proved to be crucial in diagnosing the disorder.

The techniques of molecular biology have identified the basic genetic defect in the majority of patients with cystic fibrosis. On the long arm of chromosome 7 resides the gene coding for a 1480-amino-acid protein called the *cystic fibrosis transmembrane conductance regulator* (CFTR). This protein appears to play a critical role in normal chloride transport across the apical surface of epithelial cells. Because of a three-nucleotide deletion in most patients with cystic fibrosis, a single phenylalanine residue is missing at position 508 (called the ΔF508 deletion), resulting in abnormal chloride transport across cell membranes. Working by mechanisms that are not fully elucidated, the impermeability of epithelial cells to chloride transport is thought to be responsible for both the high electrolyte concentrations in sweat and the abnormally thick secretions produced by exocrine glands. Although the ΔF508 mutation is responsible for approximately 70% of cases of cystic fibrosis, more than 1250 different cystic fibrosis mutations have been identified.

Major defects in cystic fibrosis are the following:
1. Production of thick, tenacious secretions from exocrine glands
2. Elevated concentrations of sodium, chloride, and potassium in sweat

PATHOLOGY

The pathologic findings in cystic fibrosis appear to result from obstruction of ducts or tubes by tenacious secretions. In the pancreas, obstruction of the ducts eventually produces fibrosis, atrophy of the acini, and cystic changes. In the airways, thick mucous plugs appear in the bronchi, obstructing both airflow and normal drainage of the tracheobronchial tree. Early in the course of the disease, airway changes are found predominantly in the bronchioles, which are plugged and obliterated by the secretions. Later, the findings are more extensive. Superimposed areas of pneumonitis appear, and frank bronchiectasis and areas of abscess formation may be found. Cardiac complications of cor pulmonale frequently occur, and pathologic examination of the heart shows evidence of right ventricular hypertrophy.

PATHOPHYSIOLOGY

In the pancreas, the pathologic process leads to exocrine pancreatic insufficiency, with maldigestion and malabsorption of foodstuffs, particularly fat and the fat-soluble vitamins A, D, E, and K. Diabetes mellitus may develop in later stages. In the lung, the major problem is recurrent episodes of tracheobronchial infection and bronchiectasis resulting from bronchial obstruction and defective mucociliary transport. In addition, evidence suggests that the CFTR mutation contributes to airway infection by altering the binding and clearance of microorganisms by airway epithelial cells, and the altered chloride concentration of airway fluid appears to impair the activity of antimicrobial peptides (especially human β-defensin-1). The major organisms that eventually colonize the airways are *Staphylococcus aureus* and *P. aeruginosa*. Difficulty with these organisms seems to be entirely the result of local (airway) host defense mechanisms; the humoral immune system (i.e., the ability to form antibodies) appears to be intact.

As a result of airway obstruction, functional changes characteristic of obstructive airways disease and air trapping develop. Patients also exhibit the pathophysiologic changes seen in type B patients with chronic obstructive pulmonary disease, that is, ventilation-perfusion mismatch, hypoxemia (sometimes with CO_2 retention), pulmonary hypertension, and cor pulmonale.

> Major clinical problems from cystic fibrosis are the following:
> 1. Pancreatic insufficiency
> 2. Recurrent episodes of tracheobronchial infection
> 3. Bronchiectasis
> 4. Intestinal obstruction
> 5. Sterility in males

CLINICAL FEATURES

Approximately 10% to 20% of patients with cystic fibrosis develop their first clinical problem in the neonatal period, manifested as intestinal obstruction with thick meconium (the newborn's intestinal contents composed of ingested amniotic fluid). This obstruction is called *meconium ileus*. The remainder of patients usually have a childhood presentation, manifested as pancreatic insufficiency, recurrent bronchial infections, or both. Occasionally, patients are first diagnosed when they are adults. Almost all males with the disease are sterile because of congenital absence of the vas deferens. Females are capable of having children, but their fertility rate is decreased.

Physical examination of patients with cystic fibrosis reveals the findings expected with severe airflow obstruction and plugging of airways by secretions. Wheezing and coarse rales or rhonchi occur frequently, and clubbing is common.

Several complications may develop as a result of the disease. Pneumothorax and hemoptysis, which may be massive, can be major problems in management. Eventually, frank respiratory insufficiency and cor pulmonale develop. Although most patients live into adult life when good care has been provided, their life span is significantly reduced.

> Serious complications of cystic fibrosis are the following:
> 1. Pneumothorax
> 2. Massive hemoptysis
> 3. Respiratory insufficiency
> 4. Cor pulmonale

DIAGNOSTIC APPROACH

Definitive diagnosis of cystic fibrosis is made by the combination of compatible clinical features and one of the following: (1) identification of mutations known to cause cystic fibrosis in both CFTR genes, (2) characteristic abnormalities in measurements of nasal mucosal electrical potential difference, or (3) abnormal sweat electrolytes. The concentrations of sodium, chloride, and potassium are elevated in sweat from these patients, and a sweat chloride concentration greater than 60 mEq/L is generally considered diagnostic. Only individuals homozygous for the cystic fibrosis gene demonstrate this abnormality; heterozygous carriers have normal sweat electrolytes. Identification of heterozygotes (i.e., carriers of the cystic fibrosis gene) and in utero detection of homozygotes are possible with current DNA probe techniques.

The chest radiograph often shows an increase in markings and the findings of bronchiectasis described in the previous section (Fig. 7-4). Evidence of focal pneumonitis may be seen during the course of the disease.

Functional assessment of these patients early in the disease shows evidence of obstruction of small airways. As the disease progresses, evidence of more generalized airway obstruction (decreased forced expiratory volume in 1 second [FEV_1], forced vital capacity [FVC], and FEV_1/FVC ratio) and air trapping (increased residual volume [RV]/total lung capacity [TLC] ratio) is seen. The elastic recoil of the lung is generally preserved, and TLC most commonly is within the normal range. Because emphysematous changes generally are not seen in patients with cystic fibrosis and the alveolar–capillary interface remains relatively preserved, most frequently the diffusing capacity is relatively normal. Arterial blood gas values often indicate hypoxemia, and hypercapnia may be seen as the disease progresses.

> Diagnosis of cystic fibrosis is made by demonstration of an elevated concentration of sweat chloride, a culprit mutation in the CFTR gene, or an abnormal electrical potential difference in the nasal mucosa.

TREATMENT

Therapy for cystic fibrosis is based on an attempt to diminish the clinical consequences and to manage complications when they occur. Other than a sustained focus on adequate nutrition, the principles of therapy are similar to those used for

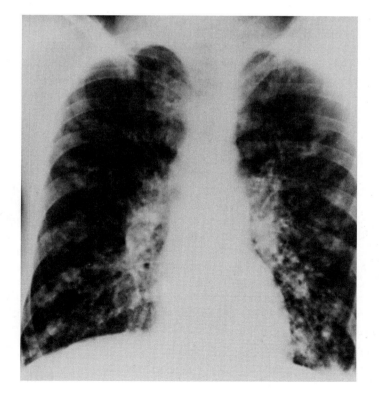

Figure 7-4. Posteroanterior chest radiograph of a patient with cystic fibrosis shows diffuse increase in markings throughout both lungs. These findings represent extensive fibrotic changes and bronchiectasis. (Courtesy Dr. Mary Ellen Wohl.)

bronchiectasis: bronchopulmonary drainage (using chest physical therapy and postural drainage, a flutter valve, or a vibrating vest), antibiotics, and bronchodilators. Agents used to decrease the viscosity of the sputum appear to offer benefit in some patients. In particular, because DNA released from inflammatory cells contributes significantly to the viscosity of mucus, inhalation of recombinant deoxyribonuclease (DNase) has been used to degrade DNA, decrease mucus viscosity, and improve clearance of secretions. Inhaled hypertonic saline also may be useful as a mucolytic agent. Oral macrolide antibiotics such as azithromycin may offer some benefit that is believed related to their antiinflammatory effects rather than their antimicrobial properties.

Although current forms of therapy have significantly improved prognosis in cystic fibrosis, the natural history still is one of progressive pulmonary dysfunction and eventual death as a result of the disease or its complications. Despite initial concern about lung transplantation in these patients because of their chronic pulmonary infection, experience with bilateral lung transplantation suggests posttransplantation survival is similar to that of other patients undergoing this procedure.

With identification of the genetic basis for the disease in the majority of patients had come hope that gene therapy would provide a means for reversing the primary defect as well as the characteristic abnormality in airway secretion. Unfortunately, initial enthusiasm for gene therapy as a "cure" for cystic fibrosis has been tempered by difficulty finding an effective and nontoxic method (vector) for delivering the gene to the airway and achieving sufficient and durable expression of the normal gene.

UPPER AIRWAY DISEASE

The obstructive diseases considered so far affect primarily the airways below the level of the main carina, that is, the bronchi and the bronchioles. In contrast to disease of these lower airways, a variety of other disorders affect the pharynx, larynx, and trachea and produce what is termed *upper airway obstruction*. The discussion of these disorders includes a brief consideration of representative etiologic factors and some of the tests used to make the diagnosis. In particular, use of the flow-volume loop to define the location of upper airway obstruction is considered.

ETIOLOGY

The upper airway can be affected by either acute problems or those following a more subacute or chronic course. On an acute basis, the larynx probably is the major area subject to obstruction. Potential causes include infection (epiglottitis, which often is due to *Haemophilus influenzae*), thermal injury and the resulting laryngeal edema from smoke inhalation, aspiration of a foreign body, laryngeal edema from an allergic (anaphylactic) reaction, or physical trauma associated with endotracheal intubation.

On a chronic basis, the upper airway may be partially obstructed by hypertrophy of the tonsils, by tumors (particularly of the trachea), by strictures of the trachea (often resulting from prior instrumentation of the trachea), or by vocal cord paralysis. Some patients are subject to recurrent episodes of upper airway obstruction during sleep; this entity is one variety of what is termed *sleep apnea syndrome*, which is considered further in Chapter 18.

PATHOPHYSIOLOGY

The resistance of a tube to airflow varies inversely to the fourth power of the radius; hence, even small changes in airway size may produce dramatic changes in resistance and in the work of breathing. If the airways under consideration were always stiff or if a disorder did not allow any flexibility in the size of the airway, then inspiration and expiration would be impaired by the same amount, and the flow rate generated during inspiration would be essentially identical to the flow rate during expiration. This type of obstruction is termed a *fixed* obstruction.

On the other hand, if airway diameter changes during the respiratory cycle, then the greatest impairment to airflow occurs when the airway diameter is smallest. This type of obstruction is termed a *variable* obstruction. If the obstruction is located within the thorax, then changes in pleural pressure during the respiratory cycle affect the size of the airway and therefore the magnitude of the obstruction. During a forced expiration, the positive pleural pressure causes airway narrowing, making the obstructing lesion more critical. In contrast, during inspiration, the airways increase their diameter, and the effects of a partial obstruction are less pronounced (see Fig. 3-20).

If the obstruction is located above the level of the thorax (i.e., outside the thorax), then changes in pleural pressure are not directly transmitted to the airway in question. Rather, the negative airway pressure during inspiration tends to create a vacuumlike effect on extrathoracic upper airways, narrowing them and augmenting the effect of any partial obstruction. During expiration the pressure generated by the flow of air from the intrathoracic airways tends to widen the extrathoracic airways and to decrease the net effect of a partially obstructing lesion (see Fig. 3-20).

> The location and respiratory variability of an upper airway obstruction affect the appearance of the flow-volume curve and the findings on physical examination.

CLINICAL FEATURES

Patients with upper airway obstruction may have dyspnea or cough. On physical examination they may have evidence of flow through narrowed airways. If the lesion is variable and intrathoracic, the primary difficulty with airflow occurs during expiration, and patients demonstrate expiratory wheezing. If the lesion is variable and extrathoracic, obstruction is more marked during inspiration, and patients frequently manifest inspiratory stridor, a high-pitched, monophonic, continuous inspiratory sound often best heard over the trachea. With acute upper airway obstruction, such as that seen with inhalation of a foreign body, anxiety and respiratory distress often are apparent, signaling a medical emergency. In patients with epiglottitis, respiratory distress often is accompanied by sore throat, change in voice, dysphagia, and drooling.

DIAGNOSTIC APPROACH

In the evaluation of suspected disorders of the upper airway, radiography and direct visualization provide the most useful information about the macroscopic appearance of the airway. Lateral neck radiographs or CT scans of the upper airway may reveal the localization, extent, and character of a partially obstructing lesion. A CT scan may offer particularly useful information by providing a cross-sectional view of the airways from the larynx down to the carina. Direct visualization of the upper airway may be obtained by laryngoscopy or bronchoscopy, which may reveal the presence of edema, vocal cord paralysis, or an obstructing lesion such as a tumor. However, direct visualization of the airways by these techniques is not without risk. The instrument used occupies part of the already compromised airway and may induce airway spasm or swelling that further obstructs the airway. This is especially true in cases of suspected epiglottitis, in which direct visualization should not be attempted unless the examiner is prepared to perform an emergency tracheostomy.

Functional assessment of the patient with presumed upper airway obstruction can be useful in quantifying and localizing the obstruction because the functional consequences of a fixed versus a variable obstruction and an extrathoracic versus an intrathoracic obstruction are quite different. To understand these differences, the flow-volume loop and the principles discussed in the pathophysiology section must be understood. This type of physiologic evaluation is appropriate for chronic upper airway obstruction, not for acute, life-threatening obstruction.

When a fixed lesion is causing a relatively critical obstruction, maximal flow rates generated during inspiration and expiration are approximately equal, and a "plateau" marks both the inspiratory and expiratory parts of the flow-volume curve. When the lesion is variable, the effect of the obstruction depends on whether the lesion is intrathoracic or extrathoracic. With an intrathoracic obstruction, critical narrowing occurs during expiration, and the expiratory part of the flow-volume curve displays a plateau. With an extrathoracic obstruction, the expiratory part of the loop is preserved, and the inspiratory portion displays the plateau. A schematic diagram of the flow-volume loops observed in these types of upper airway obstruction is shown in Figure 3-21.

TREATMENT

Because many different types of disorders result in upper airway obstruction, treatment varies greatly depending on the underlying problem, particularly its acuteness and severity. In acute, severe upper airway obstruction, an emergency procedure such as endotracheal intubation or tracheostomy may be necessary to maintain a patent airway. A procedure such as bronchoscopic laser therapy or airway stenting also may be used. Discussion of each disorder and further consideration of management can be found in other textbooks and in some articles listed in the references.

REFERENCES

BRONCHIECTASIS

Barker AF: Bronchiectasis, *N Engl J Med* 346:1383–1393, 2002.
Cartier Y, Kavanagh PV, Johkoh T, Mason AC, Müller NL: Bronchiectasis: accuracy of high-resolution CT in the differentiation of specific diseases, *AJR Am J Roentgenol* 173:47–52, 1999.
Cohen M, Sahn SA: Bronchiectasis in systemic disease, *Chest* 116:1063–1074, 1999.
Fujimoto T, Hillejan L, Stamatis G: Current strategy for surgical management of bronchiectasis, *Ann Thorac Surg* 72:1711–1715, 2001.
Keistinen T, Saynajakangas O, Tuuponen T, Kivela SL: Bronchiectasis: an orphan disease with a poorly-understood prognosis, *Eur Respir J* 10:2784–2787, 1997.
Kumar NA, Nguyen B, Maki D: Bronchiectasis: current clinical and imaging concepts, *Semin Roentgenol* 36:41–50, 2001.
Lillington GA: Dyskinetic cilia and Kartagener's syndrome. Bronchiectasis with a twist, *Clin Rev Allergy Immunol* 21:65–69, 2001.
Pasteur MC, Helliwell SM, Houghton SJ, et al: An investigation into causative factors in patients with bronchiectasis, *Am J Respir Crit Care Med* 162:1277–1284, 2000.
Rosen MJ: Chronic cough due to bronchiectasis: ACCP evidence-based clinical practice guidelines, *Chest* 129(1 suppl):122s–131s, 2006.

CYSTIC FIBROSIS

Boyle MP: Adult cystic fibrosis, *JAMA* 298: 1787–1793, 2007.
Fiel SB, editor: Cystic fibrosis, *Clin Chest Med* 19:423–567, 1998.
Liou TG, Adler FR, Cahill BC, et al: Survival effect of lung transplantation among patients with cystic fibrosis, *JAMA* 286:2683–2689, 2001.
Mehta A: CFTR: more than just a chloride channel, *Pediatr Pulmonol* 39:292–298, 2005.
Pier GB, Grout M, Zaidi TS, et al: Role of mutant CFTR in hypersusceptibility of cystic fibrosis patients to lung infections, *Science* 271:64–67, 1996.
Pitt BR: CFTR trafficking and signaling in respiratory epithelium, *Am J Physiol Lung Cell Mol Physiol* 281: L13–L15, 2001.
Ratjen F, Doring G: Cystic fibrosis, *Lancet* 361:681–689, 2003.
Rowe SM, Miller S, Sorscher EJ: Mechanisms of disease: cystic fibrosis, *N Engl J Med* 352:1992–2001, 2005.
Rubin BK: Emerging therapies for cystic fibrosis lung disease, *Chest* 115:1120–1126, 1999.

Stern RC: The diagnosis of cystic fibrosis, *N Engl J Med* 336:487–491, 1997.

Wine JJ: The genesis of cystic fibrosis lung disease, *J Clin Invest* 103:309–312, 1999.

UPPER AIRWAY DISEASE

Ernst A, Feller-Kopman D, Becker HD, Mehta AC: Central airway obstruction, *Am J Respir Crit Care Med* 169:1278–1297, 2004.

Limper AH, Prakash UBS: Tracheobronchial foreign bodies in adults, *Ann Intern Med* 112:604–609, 1990.

Mayo-Smith MF, Spinale JW, Donskey CJ, et al: Acute epiglottis. An 18-year experience in Rhode Island, *Chest* 108: 1640–1647, 1995.

Miller WT: Obstructive diseases of the trachea, *Semin Roentgenol* 36:21–40, 2001.

Proctor DF: The upper airways—II: the larynx and trachea, *Am Rev Respir Dis* 115:315–342, 1977.

Rafanan AL, Mehta AC: Stenting of the tracheobronchial tree, *Radiol Clin North Am* 38:395–408, 2000.

Seijo LM, Sterman DH: Interventional pulmonology, *N Engl J Med* 344:740–749, 2001.

8

Anatomic and Physiologic Aspects of the Pulmonary Parenchyma

ANATOMY	PHYSIOLOGY

Chapters 8 through 11 focus on the region of the lung directly involved in gas exchange, often called the *pulmonary parenchyma*. This region includes the alveolar walls and spaces (with the alveolar–capillary interface) at the level of the alveolar sacs, ducts, and respiratory bronchioles. Although the broad group of disorders involving these structures traditionally has been described under the rubric of *interstitial lung disease*, the term *diffuse parenchymal lung disease* is increasingly used and more accurately reflects the breadth of the pathologic involvement.

This chapter provides a description of the normal anatomy of the gas-exchanging region of the lung and some aspects of its normal physiology. Chapters 9 through 11 focus on specific disorders, generally subacute or chronic, the main pathologic features of which appear to reside within the alveolar wall. Pneumonia, acute lung injury (acute respiratory distress syndrome), and diseases of the pulmonary vasculature are deliberately excluded because of their different pathologic appearance and are considered separately in other parts of this text.

Chapter 9 provides an overview of the diffuse parenchymal lung diseases, emphasizing how disturbances in alveolar structure are closely linked with aberrations in function. Although a wide variety of disorders affect the alveolar wall, many of the pathophysiologic features are common to a large number of individual diseases. Knowledge of these general pathophysiologic features and their effects on the normal function of the lung is useful for understanding the consequences of individual disease entities. For specific diseases with special characteristics, a consideration of these individual features is included.

ANATOMY

For the lung to function efficiently as a gas-exchanging organ, a large surface area should be available where O_2 can be taken up and CO_2 released. At the alveolar wall, where gas exchange occurs, an extensive network of capillaries coursing through and coming into close contact with alveolar gas facilitates the exchange. In the normal lung the capillaries are closely apposed to the alveolar lumen, and there is little tissue extraneous to the gas-exchanging process (Fig. 8-1).

The surface of the alveolar walls (the region bordering the alveolar lumen) is lined by a continuous layer of epithelial cells. Two different types of these lining epithelial

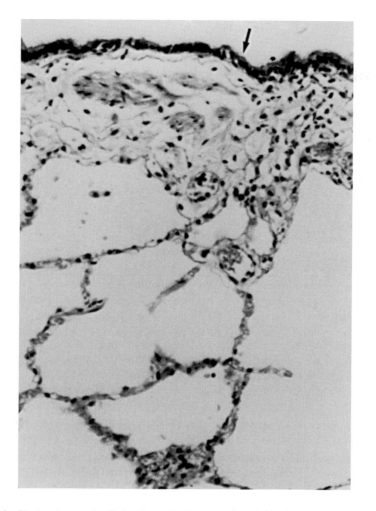

Figure 8-1. Photomicrograph of alveolar walls shows a normal thin, lacy appearance. At top of photo is bronchial lumen, lined by bronchial epithelial cells *(arrow)*. Peribronchial tissue lies between bronchial epithelium and alveolar walls. (Courtesy Dr. Earl Kasdon.)

cells, called *type I* and *type II cells,* can be identified. Type I cells are less numerous than type II cells. They have impressively long cytoplasmic extensions that line more than 95% of the alveolar surface (Fig. 8-2). Type I cells function as a barrier preventing free movement of material, such as fluid, from the alveolar wall into the alveolar lumen. Although they have few cytoplasmic organelles, increasing evidence indicates that type I cells play an important role in the regulation of ion and fluid balance in the lung, in part because they cover such a large part of the alveolar surface area.

Type I alveolar epithelial cells have long cytoplasmic processes that line almost the entire alveolar surface.

The second lining epithelial cell is the type II cell. Type II cells have three well-defined functions: synthesis of surfactant, alveolar epithelial repair, and ion and fluid transport. In contrast to type I cells, type II epithelial cells have a cuboidal shape and often bulge into the alveolar lumen. Because they do not have long cytoplasmic extensions, type II cells cover less than 5% of the alveolar surface. The more numerous type II cells have many cytoplasmic organelles (mitochondria, rough endoplasmic reticulum, Golgi apparatus), which relate to their important synthetic role.

Type II cells produce surfactant, are important in the reparative process for type I cells, and are active in ion and fluid transport.

The primary product of the type II cells is *surfactant.* Specific inclusion bodies within the type II cells, termed *lamellar inclusions,* appear to be the packaged form of

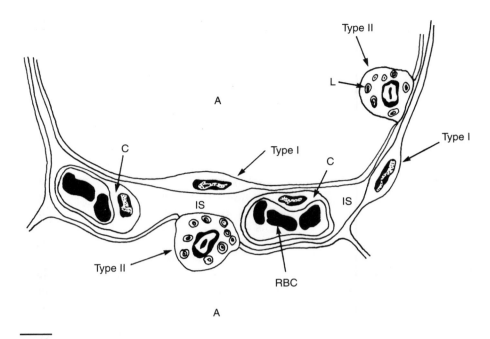

Figure 8-2. Schematic diagram of normal alveolar structure. Type I and type II epithelial cells line the alveolar wall. Type I cells are relatively flat and are characterized by long cytoplasmic processes. Type II cells are cuboidal. Two capillaries are shown. A = Alveolar space; C = capillary endothelial cells; IS = interstitial space (relatively acellular region of the alveolar wall); L = type II cell cytoplasmic lamellar bodies, the source of surfactant; RBC = erythrocytes in the capillary lumen.

surfactant that eventually is released into the alveolar lumen. Surfactant is composed of a high proportion of lipids as well as associated proteins and carbohydrates that are necessary for effective function. Surfactant acts like a detergent, reducing the surface tension of the alveoli. It stabilizes the alveolus in the same way that a bubble is prevented from collapsing by a detergent material, thereby preventing microatelectasis (alveolar collapse on a microscopic level). Four types of protein are associated with surfactant: surfactant protein A, B, C, and D (SP-A, SP-B, SP-C, and SP-D, respectively). The function of surfactant in maintaining a low surface tension is critically dependent on the hydrophobic proteins SP-B and SP-C. Although SP-A and SP-D also affect surface tension, they additionally have an important role in the innate immunity of the lung.

Type II cells have a significant role in maintenance and repair of the injured alveolar epithelium. Type I epithelial cells are quite susceptible to a variety of injurious agents, whether the agents reach the alveolar wall via the airways or the bloodstream. When type I cells are damaged, the reparative process involves hyperplasia of the type II cells and eventual differentiation into cells with the characteristics of type I cells. Normally, this orderly process results in some hyperplastic type II cells undergoing apoptosis, while the remainder transdifferentiate into thin, delicate, type I cells. As discussed in Chapter 11, defects in this process have been identified in idiopathic pulmonary fibrosis, a devastating disease of progressive parenchymal scarring.

The third function of type II cells is regulation of alveolar fluid via transepithelial sodium and chloride transport. Proper regulation of ion and fluid balance requires an intact epithelium. Inhibition of this function occurs during inflammation and probably contributes to the edema formation seen in acute lung injury.

Type II cells are involved in the synthesis of a number of other proteins. They have been reported to elaborate several growth factors and cytokines, cytokine receptors, and proteins involved in innate immunity, such as β defensins. These additional activities of type II cells are areas of active research.

Pulmonary capillaries course through the alveolar walls as part of an extensive network of intercommunicating vessels. Unlike the alveolar epithelial cells, which are quite impermeable under normal circumstances, junctions between capillary endothelial cells permit passage of small-molecular–weight proteins. The importance of the permeability features of the alveolar epithelial and capillary endothelial cells will become apparent in the discussion of acute respiratory distress syndrome in Chapter 28 because this disorder is characterized by increased permeability and leakage of fluid and protein into alveolar spaces.

The alveolar epithelial and capillary endothelial cells rest on a basement membrane. At some regions of the alveolar wall, nothing stands between the epithelial and endothelial cells other than the basement membranes, which are fused to form a single structure. At other regions, the *interstitial space,* which consists of relatively acellular material (see Fig. 8-2), intervenes. The major components of the interstitial space are collagen, elastin, proteoglycans, a variety of macromolecules involved with cell–cell and cell–matrix interactions, some nerve endings, and some fibroblastlike cells. There are also small numbers of lymphocytes as well as cells that appear to be in a transition state between blood monocytes and alveolar macrophages (which are derived from circulating monocytes).

Within the alveolar lumen a thin layer of liquid covers the alveolar epithelial cells. This extracellular alveolar lining layer is composed of an aqueous phase immediately adjacent to the epithelial cells, covered by a surface layer of lipid-rich surfactant produced by the type II epithelial cells. The alveolar lining layer also contains alveolar macrophages, a type of phagocytic cell important in protecting the distal lung against bacteria and in clearing inhaled particulate matter. Alveolar macrophages and the innate immunity of the lung are discussed further in Chapter 22.

PHYSIOLOGY

Some of the physiologic principles relating to the pulmonary parenchyma were covered briefly in Chapter 1. This chapter further discusses two topics that are important in the pathophysiologic abnormalities resulting from diffuse parenchymal lung disease. This section reviews gas exchange at the alveolar-capillary level, followed by a discussion of how disturbances within the pulmonary parenchyma affect the mechanical properties of the lung.

Gas exchange between the alveolus and the capillary depends on passive diffusion of gas from a region of higher partial pressure to one of lower partial pressure. As discussed in Chapter 1, the Po_2 in the alveolus normally is approximately 100 mm Hg, and in the blood entering the pulmonary capillary is approximately 40 mm Hg. This difference results in a driving pressure for O_2 to diffuse from the alveolus to the pulmonary capillary, where it binds with hemoglobin within the erythrocyte. The barrier to diffusion—which includes the thin cytoplasmic extension of the type I cell, the basement membrane of type I and capillary endothelial cells, and the capillary endothelial cell itself—is extremely thin, measuring approximately 0.5 μm. Some areas of the alveolar wall also contain a thin layer of interstitium, but presumably diffusion and gas exchange occur preferentially at the thinnest region, where the interstitium is sparse or absent.

Although the rate of gas transfer across the alveolar-capillary interface depends on the thickness of the barrier, O_2 uptake by the blood is usually complete early during the transit through the capillaries. The total time spent by a red blood cell traveling through the pulmonary capillaries is approximately 0.75 second, and equilibration

Oxygen uptake and CO_2 elimination at the alveolar-capillary interface are completed early during transit of an erythrocyte through the pulmonary vascular bed.

with O_2 occurs within the first third of this time. Therefore, extra time is available for diffusion should disease affect the alveolar-capillary interface and impair the normal process of diffusion. Carbon dioxide diffuses much more readily than does O_2; therefore, even more ample reserve time is available for its diffusion.

Consequently, although diffuse parenchymal lung diseases do affect gas exchange, impaired diffusion across an abnormal alveolar-capillary interface is not a primary contributor to the disturbance in gas exchange when the patient is at rest. However, when a patient exercises and increases cardiac output, blood flows more rapidly through the pulmonary capillaries, and the combination of a diffusion impairment and less time for diffusion of oxygen may lead to hypoxemia. This issue is considered further in Chapter 9 as part of the discussion of abnormalities in gas exchange in patients with diseases affecting the alveolar wall.

Another important aspect of physiology relating to the lung parenchyma is compliance or, more simply, the stiffness of the lung. As stated in Chapter 1, the lung is elastic and behaves like a balloon or a rubber band in terms of resisting expansion. Pressure must be exerted through the airway to inflate the lung; conversely, negative pressure can be applied around the lung to cause it to expand. For any given volume of air in the lungs, a certain pressure is required to achieve this degree of inflation, and a curve can be drawn relating volume on the Y-axis to pressure on the X-axis (see Fig. 1-3, *A*). Because the net pressure producing expansion is the difference between the pressure exerted on the alveoli (via the airway) and the absolute pressure outside the lung, the term *transpulmonary pressure* is used to describe this distending pressure. In vivo, when the lung is sitting within the chest, the pressure outside the

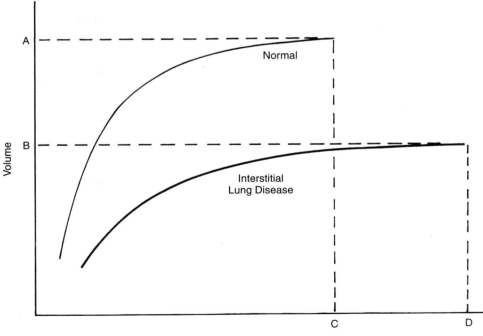

Figure 8-3. Compliance curve of lung in interstitial lung disease compared with that of normal lung. In addition to shift of the curve downward and to right, total lung capacity (TLC) in interstitial lung disease *(point B on volume axis)* is characteristically less than normal TLC *(point A)*. Maximal pressure at TLC is called *maximal static recoil pressure* (Pst_{max}), represented for normal lung and lung with interstitial disease by points C and D, respectively. (Compare with Fig. 6-7.)

lung is pleural pressure. If a lung is removed and studied in isolation, the pressure outside the lung is atmospheric pressure.

The normal compliance relationship between volume and pressure in the lung is a curve that flattens out at high distending pressures when the lung reaches its upper limit of expansion. At this point the elastic tissues of the lung can be stretched no further, and additional pressure does not add volume to the lung.

Diseases affecting the alveolar walls commonly disturb this pressure–volume relationship, making the lung either more stiff (more resistant to expansion) or less stiff (easier to expand). For the stiffer, less compliant lung, the compliance curve is shifted to the right, that is, a lower volume is achieved for any given transpulmonary pressure. Most of the diseases discussed in this section, which are included in the category of diffuse parenchymal lung disease, affect the compliance of the lung in this way (Fig. 8-3). In contrast, as discussed in Chapter 6 and illustrated in Figure 6-7, patients with emphysema, whose lungs are less resistant to expansion (i.e., are more compliant), have compliance curves that are shifted to the left. This principle of compliance is important in pulmonary physiology. Chapters 1 and 6 alluded to the role of compliance in determining lung volumes measured by pulmonary function testing, particularly total lung capacity and functional residual capacity. This principle is cited again Chapter 9, which discusses the pathophysiology of diseases that affect the alveolar walls.

> The compliance curve of the lung in interstitial lung disease is shifted downward and to the right.

REFERENCES

ANATOMY

Mason RJ: Biology of alveolar type II cells, *Respirology* 11:S12–S15, 2006.

Rooney SA: The surfactant system and lung phospholipid biochemistry, *Am Rev Respir Dis* 131:439–460, 1985.

Schneeberger EE: Alveolar type I cells. In Crystal RG, West JB, Weibel ER, Barnes PJ, editors: *The lung: scientific foundations,* ed 2, Philadelphia, 1997, Lippincott-Raven, pp. 535–542.

Weibel ER: *The pathway for oxygen,* Cambridge, MA, 1984, Harvard University Press.

Weibel ER, Crystal RG: Structural organization of the pulmonary interstitium. In Crystal RG, West JB, Weibel ER, Barnes PJ, editors: *The lung: scientific foundations,* ed 2, Philadelphia, 1997, Lippincott-Raven, pp. 685–695.

Whitsett JA, Weaver TE: Hydrophobic surfactant proteins in lung function and disease, *N Engl J Med* 347:2141–2148, 2002.

Whitsett JA: Surfactant proteins in innate host defense of the lung, *Biol Neonate* 88:175–180, 2005.

PHYSIOLOGY

Schwartzstein RM, Parker MJ: *Respiratory physiology: a clinical approach,* Philadelphia, 2006, Lippincott Williams & Wilkins.

West JB: *Respiratory physiology—the essentials,* ed 7, Baltimore, 2005, Lippincott Williams & Wilkins.

9

Overview of Diffuse Parenchymal Lung Diseases

PATHOLOGY
    Pathology of Idiopathic Interstitial
      Pneumonias
    End-Stage Diffuse Parenchymal
      Lung Disease
PATHOGENESIS
PATHOPHYSIOLOGY
    Decreased Compliance
    Decrease in Lung Volumes

Impairment of Diffusion
Abnormalities in Small Airways
    Function
Disturbances in Gas Exchange
Pulmonary Hypertension
CLINICAL FEATURES
DIAGNOSTIC APPROACH
TREATMENT

A large group of disorders affects the alveolar wall in a fashion that ultimately may lead to diffuse scarring or fibrosis. These disorders traditionally have been referred to as *interstitial lung diseases,* although the term is somewhat of a misnomer (see Chapter 8). The interstitium formally refers only to the region of the alveolar wall exclusive of and separating the alveolar epithelial and the capillary endothelial cells. However, interstitial lung diseases affect all components of the alveolar wall: epithelial cells, endothelial cells, and cellular and noncellular components of the interstitium. In addition, the disease process often extends into the alveolar spaces and therefore is not limited to the alveolar wall. Many authors now prefer the expression *diffuse parenchymal lung disease,* which is the term generally used in this book. For practical purposes, however, the reader should recognize that the expressions *diffuse parenchymal lung disease* and *interstitial lung disease* typically refer to the same group of disorders causing inflammation and fibrosis of alveolar structures.

There are more than 150 diffuse parenchymal lung diseases. Table 9-1 lists the most common of these disorders, grouped by broad categories according to whether the underlying etiology of the disease is currently known or unknown. A third category of "mimicking disorders" is included, in recognition of the fact that a number of additional well-defined clinical problems can produce diffuse parenchymal abnormalities on chest radiograph. Even though these mimicking disorders often are not included in traditional lists of diffuse parenchymal lung diseases, the clinician must remember to consider these mimicking disorders in the appropriate clinical settings.

Knowing about all these diseases is difficult even for the pulmonary specialist, so the novice in pulmonary medicine cannot be expected to amass knowledge regarding each individual entity. Rather, the reader is urged first to develop an understanding of

Table 9-1		
CLASSIFICATION OF SELECTED DIFFUSE PARENCHYMAL LUNG DISEASES		

Known Etiology
Resulting from inhaled inorganic dusts (pneumoconiosis, e.g., asbestosis, silicosis)
Caused by organic antigens (hypersensitivity pneumonitis)
Iatrogenic (drugs, radiation pneumonitis)
Unknown Etiology
Idiopathic interstitial pneumonias
Associated with connective tissue (systemic rheumatic) disease
Sarcoidosis
Less common
    Pulmonary Langerhans cell histiocytosis
    Lymphangioleiomyomatosis
    Goodpasture's syndrome
    Wegener's granulomatosis*
    Chronic eosinophilic pneumonia
    Pulmonary alveolar proteinosis
Mimicking Disorders
Congestive heart failure
Disseminated carcinoma (lymphangitic carcinomatosis)
Pulmonary infection (e.g., *Pneumocystis,* viral pneumonia)

*Typically associated with focal or multifocal disease rather than diffuse disease.

the pathologic, pathogenetic, pathophysiologic, and clinical features that are common to these disorders. This chapter, which covers these areas, refers to individual diseases only when necessary. Chapters 10 and 11 focus on the major types of diffuse parenchymal lung disease. Chapter 10 discusses disorders associated with an identifiable etiologic agent. Approximately 35% of patients with diffuse parenchymal lung disease are in this category. Chapter 11 discusses diseases for which a specific etiologic agent has not been identified. The majority of patients with diffuse parenchymal lung disease belong in this second category. These chapters cover only a small number of the described types of diffuse parenchymal disease; the goal throughout is to consider those disorders that the reader most likely will encounter. Included in the discussion of diseases of unknown etiology in Chapter 11 are several disorders that affect the lung parenchyma but do not characteristically have diffuse findings on chest radiograph. Examples of diseases in which the findings are more typically focal (or multifocal, with more than one area of involvement) include Wegener's granulomatosis and cryptogenic organizing pneumonia.

The diseases covered in these three chapters are primarily *chronic* (or sometimes *subacute*) diseases affecting the alveolar structures. Another group of diseases is associated with acute injury to various components of the alveolus. These latter disorders, which are of clinical importance as causes of acute respiratory failure, are discussed in Chapter 28.

PATHOLOGY

Typically, the diffuse parenchymal lung diseases, regardless of cause, have two major pathologic components: an inflammatory process in the alveolar wall and alveolar spaces (sometimes called an *alveolitis*) and a scarring or fibrotic process (Fig. 9-1). Both features frequently occur simultaneously, although the relative proportions of inflammation and fibrosis vary with the particular cause and duration of disease. The general presumption has been that active inflammation is the primary process and

Diffuse parenchymal (interstitial) lung diseases are characterized pathologically by alveolitis and fibrosis.

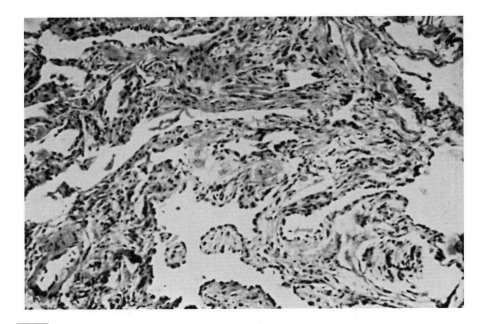

Figure 9-1. Photomicrograph of interstitial lung disease shows markedly thickened alveolar walls. Cellular inflammatory process and fibrosis are present. Compare with appearance of normal alveolar walls in Figure 8-1.

that fibrosis follows as a secondary feature. Idiopathic pulmonary fibrosis is a major exception to this generalization. As discussed in Chapter 11, the primary process in this disorder appears to be epithelial cell injury and fibrosis (representing an abnormal repair of injury) rather than alveolar inflammation (see section on pathogenesis).

When an active alveolitis is present, a variety of inflammatory cells (e.g., macrophages, lymphocytes, neutrophils, eosinophils, and plasma cells) infiltrate the alveolar wall. Individual types of diffuse parenchymal lung disease may be associated with a prominence of a particular one of these cell types, such as eosinophils in chronic eosinophilic pneumonia. In addition to the presence of inflammatory cells, other characteristic pathologic features that help define a specific disorder may be associated with the alveolitis. These individual patterns are useful in, and in many cases critical to, the diagnosis of a specific pathologic entity.

One of the most important pathologic features associated with several of the diffuse parenchymal lung diseases is the *granuloma*. A granuloma is a localized collection of cells called *epithelioid histiocytes*, which are essentially tissue cells of the phagocytic or macrophage series (Fig. 9-2). These cells are generally accompanied by T lymphocytes within the granuloma and often forming a rim around it. When cellular necrosis is present in the center of a granuloma, the entity is termed a "caseating" granuloma. However, diffuse parenchymal lung diseases are associated almost exclusively with "noncaseating" granulomas, that is, granulomas in which the central area is not necrotic. In contrast, caseating granulomas are characteristically seen in infectious diseases, especially tuberculosis (see Chapter 24, section on pathology). The granuloma typically also has multinucleated giant cells, which result from fusion of several phagocytic cells into a single large cell with abundant cytoplasm and many nuclei (see Fig. 9-2). Examples of diffuse parenchymal lung disease in which granulomas are part of the pathologic process include sarcoidosis and hypersensitivity pneumonitis. Granulomas are often considered to reflect some underlying immune process, specifically an immune reaction to an exogenous agent. In the case of hypersensitivity

Interstitial diseases with granulomas include sarcoidosis and hypersensitivity pneumonitis.

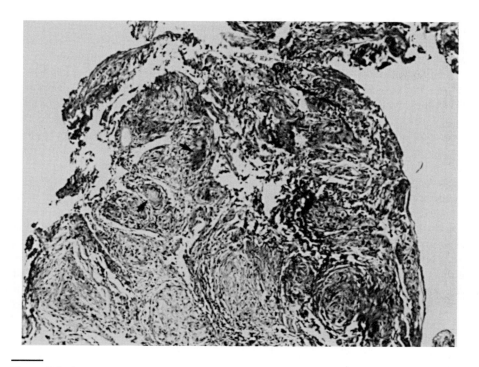

Figure 9-2. Low-power photomicrograph of transbronchial lung biopsy sample from patient with sarcoidosis. Numerous confluent granulomas throughout the entire specimen obliterate normal pulmonary architecture. Two multinucleated giant cells are marked by arrows. (Courtesy Dr. Earl Kasdon.)

pneumonitis, many agents have been identified. However, in the case of sarcoidosis, no specific exogenous agent has been identified. Granulomas in the lung have many other causes (e.g., tuberculosis, certain fungal infections, and foreign bodies), but they are not covered here because the granulomas are generally not associated with diffuse parenchymal lung disease.

PATHOLOGY OF IDIOPATHIC INTERSTITIAL PNEUMONIAS

The *idiopathic interstitial pneumonias* represent a subgroup of diffuse parenchymal lung disease. Pathologists and clinicians have spent considerable time and effort trying to refine the description and categorization of this subgroup. These disorders display variable amounts of nonspecific inflammation and fibrosis, and they lack granulomas or other specific pathologic features characteristic of other, previously well-defined diseases. Classification of the idiopathic interstitial pneumonias and determination of whether the various pathologic appearances represent different diseases or different stages or parts of the spectrum of a single disease have been subject to uncertainty and confusion. Although the field is still evolving, this chapter attempts to present a simplified framework based on current pathologic and clinical concepts about these disorders.

This chapter discusses seven pathologic entities subsumed under the broad term *idiopathic interstitial pneumonias:* (1) usual interstitial pneumonia, (2) desquamative interstitial pneumonia, (3) respiratory bronchiolitis interstitial lung disease, (4) nonspecific interstitial pneumonia, (5) acute interstitial pneumonia, (6) cryptogenic organizing pneumonia, and (7) lymphocytic interstitial pneumonia. This section briefly describes the pathologic characteristics defining these seven entities. Chapter 11 focuses on a

Some pathologic categories subsumed under the idiopathic interstitial pneumonias include the following:
1. Usual interstitial pneumonia (UIP)
2. Desquamative interstitial pneumonia (DIP)
3. Respiratory bronchiolitis interstitial lung disease (RBILD)
4. Nonspecific interstitial pneumonia (NSIP)
5. Acute interstitial pneumonia (AIP)
6. Cryptogenic organizing pneumonia (COP)
7. Lymphocytic interstitial pneumonia (LIP)

broader consideration of the more important clinical counterparts of some of these pathologic entities. An important clinical branch point is distinguishing between UIP and the other conditions because UIP typically carries a much worse prognosis.

Usual interstitial pneumonia (UIP) is characterized by patchy areas of parenchymal fibrosis and interstitial inflammation interspersed between areas of relatively preserved lung tissue (Fig. 9-3). Fibrosis is the most prominent component of the pathology, with focal collections of proliferating fibroblasts called *fibroblastic foci.* The fibrosis often is associated with *honeycombing,* which represents cystic air spaces that result from retraction of the surrounding fibrotic lung tissue. The inflammatory process in the alveolar walls is nonspecific and typically composed of a variety of cell types, including lymphocytes, macrophages, and plasma cells. Hyperplasia of type II pneumocytes (alveolar epithelial cells) presumably reflects an attempt to replenish damaged type I cells. By far the most important of the clinical disorders associated with the histopathologic pattern of UIP is *idiopathic pulmonary fibrosis (IPF),* and the terms are often used synonymously. However, the pathologic appearance of UIP also can result from exposure to certain inhaled dusts (especially asbestos), from a number of drug-induced lung diseases, and as a form of parenchymal lung disease associated with some systemic rheumatic (connective tissue) diseases. Remember that the term UIP refers to the histologic pattern seen under the microscope, whereas IPF refers to the clinical disease associated with idiopathic UIP.

Desquamative interstitial pneumonia (DIP) is a more homogeneous-appearing process than UIP and is characterized by large numbers of intraalveolar mononuclear cells. Although originally thought to represent desquamated alveolar epithelial cells (hence the name desquamative interstitial pneumonia), these cells now are known to be intraalveolar macrophages. A less prominent component of the histology is inflammation within alveolar walls, and associated fibrosis is minimal. In contrast to UIP, the process is temporally uniform, and architectural distortion is minimal. Based on a

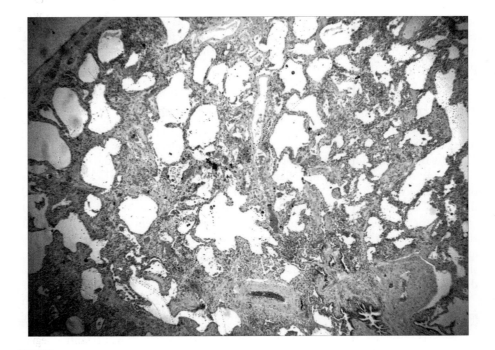

Figure 9-3. Low-power photomicrograph of usual interstitial pneumonia shows the heterogeneity of the fibrotic and inflammatory process. (Courtesy Dr. Olivier Kocher.)

strong association of this histologic pattern with a history of smoking as well as an apparent overlap with smoking-induced inflammation of respiratory bronchioles with pigmented macrophages, smoking is believed to be an important underlying etiology for this pathologic pattern.

Respiratory bronchiolitis interstitial lung disease (RBILD) and DIP are related. In general, RBILD is also associated with pigmented macrophages, which are present within the lumen of respiratory bronchioles. However, in contrast to DIP, interstitial inflammation is not present. RBILD nearly always is associated with smoking. The most important clinical intervention is assisting patients to successfully quit smoking. At times, the distinction between RBILD and DIP is difficult and somewhat arbitrary.

The most prominent histopathologic component of *nonspecific interstitial pneumonia* (NSIP) is a mononuclear cell infiltrate within the alveolar walls. In contrast to UIP, the process appears relatively uniform, and fibrosis is variable but generally less apparent. In the past, this pattern was often not separated from UIP, and its inclusion in many clinical studies of idiopathic pulmonary fibrosis (IPF) served to confound our understanding of the natural history and treatment of IPF. The histologic pattern of NSIP can be idiopathic, but it also can occur in association with a number of the connective tissue diseases.

Acute interstitial pneumonia (AIP) is believed to represent the organizing or fibrotic stage of diffuse alveolar damage, which is the histologic pattern seen in the acute respiratory distress syndrome (ARDS) (see Chapter 28). In most cases of ARDS, an inciting cause is apparent, whereas in AIP, no initiating trigger for ARDS can be identified. The histology shows fibroblast proliferation and type II pneumocyte hyperplasia in the setting of what appears to be organizing diffuse alveolar damage.

Cryptogenic organizing pneumonia (COP) is characterized by organizing fibrosis (also referred to as "granulation tissue") in small airways associated with a mild degree of chronic interstitial inflammation. Intraluminal airway involvement is a key feature and distinguishes COP from the other idiopathic interstitial pneumonias. The histologic picture is termed *bronchiolitis obliterans with organizing pneumonia (BOOP)*. Although the terms *cryptogenic organizing pneumonia* and *bronchiolitis obliterans with organizing pneumonia* are sometimes used interchangeably, the former term is applied to the clinical disease associated with the idiopathic form of the latter. The histologic pattern of BOOP may also be associated with specific known causes, such as infections, toxic inhalants, and connective tissue diseases.

Lymphocytic interstitial pneumonia (LIP) is characterized by infiltration in the alveolar walls and interstitium by lymphocytes and plasma cells. LIP is part of a spectrum of pulmonary lymphoproliferative disorders that range from benign scattered areas of lymphocyte infiltration to malignant lymphomas. This histologic pattern is most commonly associated with Sjögren's syndrome or with human immunodeficiency virus infection (especially in children). Some cases are idiopathic, which explains why LIP is included in the classification of idiopathic interstitial pneumonias.

The most recent international consensus conferences have classified COP and LIP as idiopathic interstitial pneumonias. In older literature and depending on the authority, the classification of these two conditions is variable.

END-STAGE DIFFUSE PARENCHYMAL LUNG DISEASE

When diffuse parenchymal lung disease has been present for a fairly long time and is associated with significant fibrosis, any distinctive features of a prior alveolitis often are lost. For example, any of the granulomatous lung diseases may no longer demonstrate the characteristic granulomas after sufficient time has elapsed and a substantial degree of fibrosis has developed. Therefore, at a certain point all the diffuse parenchymal lung diseases, if sufficiently severe and chronic, follow a final common pathway toward *end-stage* diffuse parenchymal lung disease. Along with severe fibrosis, the lung at end stage exhibits a great deal of distortion that can be seen both grossly and microscopically, with areas of contraction and other areas showing formation of cystic spaces. In many cases, the result is "honeycomb lung," in which the dense scarring and intervening cystic regions make areas of the lung resemble a honeycomb (Fig. 9-4).

PATHOGENESIS

A great deal of research during the last two decades attempted to clarify the pathogenetic sequence of events in various types of diffuse parenchymal lung disease. However, in most cases what initiates these diseases remains unknown, and our understanding of the cellular and biochemical events producing inflammation and fibrosis remains mostly at the descriptive level. This section outlines the general scheme of events thought to be operative in the production of parenchymal inflammation and fibrosis. Chapters 10 and 11 discuss specific diseases and provide additional information believed to be relevant to the pathogenesis of each disease. The general scheme outlined here has features similar to that of other forms of lung injury described elsewhere in this book (e.g., emphysema in Chapter 6 and acute respiratory distress syndrome in Chapter 28). A fundamental but unanswered question is what determines whether an injurious agent eventually leads to emphysema, acute lung injury (with acute respiratory distress syndrome), or chronic parenchymal inflammation and fibrosis.

Figure 9-5 summarizes the general sequence of events presumed to be common to many of the diffuse parenchymal lung diseases. The events can be divided into three stages: initiation, propagation, and final pathologic consequences. Each of these stages is considered in turn.

Pathogenetic features of interstitial lung disease are the following:
1. Initiation—by antigens, toxins
2. Propagation—with inflammatory cells, proteases, cytokines
3. Final pathologic consequence—fibrosis

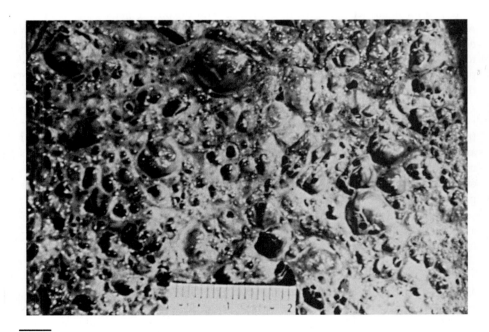

Figure 9-4. Appearance of honeycomb lung from patient with severe interstitial lung disease. Many cystic areas are seen between bands of extensively scarred and retracted pulmonary parenchyma.

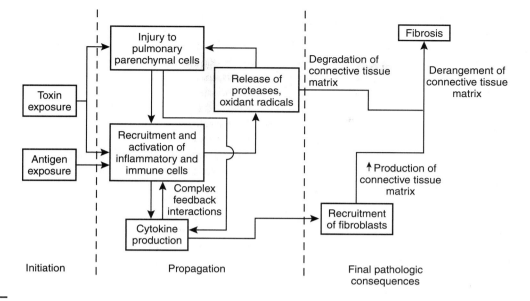

Figure 9-5. Schematic diagram illustrates general aspects of pathogenesis of the diffuse parenchymal lung diseases.

The initiating stimulus for the diffuse parenchymal lung diseases is generally believed to be either a toxin or an antigen. The most obvious presumed toxins include some of the inhaled inorganic dusts (e.g., asbestos) responsible for producing the pneumoconioses. Inhaled antigens have been best identified as the cause of chronic hypersensitivity pneumonitis. In sarcoidosis and perhaps in idiopathic pulmonary fibrosis, exposure to one or more antigens may initiate the disease, but no specific antigens have been identified.

After exposure to an initiating stimulus occurs, a complex series of interrelated events is responsible for propagation of the disease. At the microscopic level the consequence of these propagating events is inflammation, a hallmark of many of the diffuse parenchymal lung diseases. Toxins may be directly injurious to pulmonary parenchymal (alveolar epithelial) cells, whereas either toxins or antigens may result in activation and recruitment of inflammatory and immune cells. Inflammatory cells can release a variety of mediators, such as proteolytic enzymes or toxic oxygen radicals, which can secondarily further injure pulmonary parenchymal cells. In addition, a wide variety of cytokine mediators, produced by epithelial, inflammatory, and immune cells, have been identified. These cytokines have complex secondary effects on other inflammatory and immune cells, often acting either to amplify or diminish the inflammatory response.

Some of the cytokines (e.g., transforming growth factor-β and platelet-derived growth factor) are capable of recruiting and stimulating the replication of fibroblasts, which are critical for the eventual production of new connective tissue. Action of proteases from inflammatory cells may also be responsible for degradation of connective tissue components. The combination of new synthesis and degradation of connective tissue defines the derangement of the connective tissue matrix that is seen histologically as fibrosis, the final pathologic consequence of interstitial lung disease. In idiopathic pulmonary fibrosis, the most recent (and now prevailing) concept is that alveolar epithelial injury results in epithelial cell expression of cytokine mediators that promote fibrogenesis, and that inflammation, although present in variable degrees, is not the critical trigger for the development of fibrosis.

PATHOPHYSIOLOGY

With minor exceptions and variations, the pathophysiologic features of the chronic diffuse parenchymal lung diseases are similar and therefore are discussed here as a single group. As a result of the inflammation and fibrosis affecting the alveolar walls, the following abnormalities are generally seen (Fig. 9-6): (1) decreased compliance (increased stiffness) of the lung, (2) generalized decrease in lung volumes, (3) impairment of diffusion, (4) abnormalities in small airway function without generalized airflow obstruction, (5) disturbances in gas exchange, usually consisting of hypoxemia without CO_2 retention, and (6) in some cases pulmonary hypertension. Each of these features is briefly considered in turn.

DECREASED COMPLIANCE

The distensibility of the lungs is altered significantly by processes involving inflammation and fibrosis of the alveolar walls. The lungs become much stiffer, have a greatly increased elastic recoil, and therefore require greater distending (transpulmonary) pressures to achieve any given lung volume. The pressure-volume or compliance curve is shifted to the right (see Fig. 8-3), and at total lung capacity (TLC) a much higher elastic recoil pressure is found than in normal lungs. This maximal pressure at TLC is termed the *maximal static recoil pressure of the lung* (Pst_{max}). Because wider swings in transpulmonary pressure are required to achieve a normal tidal volume during inspiration, the patient's work of breathing is increased. As a result, patients with diffuse parenchymal lung disease tend to breathe with smaller tidal volumes but with increased respiratory frequency. This method allows the patient to expend less energy per breath but maintain adequate alveolar ventilation.

> Compliance curves in diffuse parenchymal lung disease are shifted downward and to the right, reflecting increased stiffness of the lung.

DECREASE IN LUNG VOLUMES

Early in the course of diffuse parenchymal lung disease, the lung volumes may be normal. However, in most cases some reduction in lung volumes is seen shortly thereafter, including a reduction in TLC, vital capacity (VC), functional residual capacity (FRC), and, to a lesser extent, residual volume (RV). The decreases in TLC, FRC, and RV are direct consequences of the change in lung compliance. At TLC, the force generated by the inspiratory muscles is balanced by the inward elastic recoil of the lung.

> Lung volumes are characteristically decreased in interstitial lung disease.

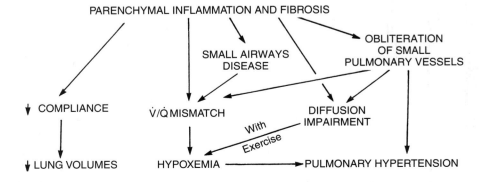

Figure 9-6. Schematic diagram illustrates interrelationships between various pathologic and physiologic features of interstitial lung disease.

Because the recoil pressure is increased, this balance is achieved at a lower lung volume or lower TLC. At FRC, the outward recoil of the chest wall is balanced by the inward elastic recoil of the lung. The balance is achieved at a lower lung volume or lower FRC because of the greater elastic recoil of the lung. As discussed in Chapter 1, RV is primarily determined by the strength of the expiratory muscles; however, a small component is determined by the inward elastic recoil of the lungs. Because the elastic recoil is greater in diffuse parenchymal lung disease, the RV is slightly smaller. Generally, TLC is reduced more than RV; therefore, it follows that VC (representing the difference between TLC and RV) also is decreased.

IMPAIRMENT OF DIFFUSION

Measurement of diffusion by the usual techniques involving carbon monoxide typically shows a decrease in the diffusing capacity. Although thickening of the alveolar-capillary interface (because of interstitial inflammation and fibrosis) might be expected to be responsible for this decrease, it is not the major factor. Rather, the processes of inflammation and fibrosis destroy a portion of the alveolar-capillary interface and reduce the surface area available for gas exchange. This decrease in surface area appears to be mainly responsible for the observed diffusion abnormality.

Diffusing capacity is reduced, with destruction of a portion of the alveolar-capillary interface and reduced surface area for gas exchange.

ABNORMALITIES IN SMALL AIRWAYS FUNCTION

Large airways generally function normally in these patients, and the forced expiratory volume in 1 second to forced vital capacity ratio usually is normal or even increased. However, frequently the pathologic process occurring in the alveolar walls also affects small airways within the lung. Light microscopy commonly demonstrates inflammation and fibrosis in the peribronchiolar regions, with narrowing of the lumen of the small airways or bronchioles. Tests of small airways function often show the physiologic effects of this narrowing. The clinical importance of small airways dysfunction in the absence of larger airways abnormalities is uncertain, but it is likely that ventilation-perfusion ($\dot{V}/\dot{Q}$) mismatching and hypoxemia are consequences. Evidence of more significant airflow obstruction may be seen in a few of the disorders causing diffuse parenchymal lung disease. This relatively infrequent problem sometimes results from severe fibrosis and airway distortion.

Small airways function often is disturbed in interstitial lung disease. Large airways function generally is preserved.

DISTURBANCES IN GAS EXCHANGE

The gas-exchange consequences of diffuse parenchymal lung disease most frequently consist of hypoxemia without CO_2 retention or, in fact, with hypocapnia. Although a diffusion block once was proposed as the cause of the hypoxemia, most evidence supports $\dot{V}/\dot{Q}$ mismatch as the major contributor to hypoxemia. The pathologic process in the alveolar walls is uneven, and normal matching of ventilation and perfusion is disrupted. In patients with small airways disease, dysfunction at this level probably also contributes to $\dot{V}/\dot{Q}$ mismatch and hypoxemia. Characteristically, patients with interstitial lung disease become even more hypoxemic with exercise. Although the entire mechanism of the fall in Po_2 with exercise is complex, diffusion limitation appears to be a contributing factor. The combination of impaired diffusion and decreased transit time of the red blood cell during exercise may prevent complete equilibration of Po_2 in pulmonary capillary blood with alveolar Po_2. Despite the often profound hypoxemia in patients with severe pulmonary fibrosis, Pco_2 is generally normal or low because patients are able to increase minute ventilation sufficiently to compensate for a decrease in tidal volume and for any additional dead space. Elevation of Pco_2 does not generally occur until the very late stages of the disease.

Arterial blood gases in interstitial lung disease generally show hypoxemia (resulting from $\dot{V}/\dot{Q}$ mismatch) and normal or decreased Pco_2. Po_2 falls even further with exercise.

PULMONARY HYPERTENSION

Eventually, pulmonary hypertension and cor pulmonale often develop in patients with severe interstitial lung disease. Rarely, the cause of pulmonary hypertension is a primary process affecting pulmonary vessels in addition to the alveolar walls. More frequently, the process in the alveolar walls is the cause of pulmonary hypertension. The two main contributing factors are (1) hypoxemia and (2) obliteration of small pulmonary vessels by the fibrotic process within the alveolar walls. During exercise, pulmonary hypertension becomes even more marked; this is due partly to worsening hypoxemia and partly to limited ability of the pulmonary capillary bed to distend and recruit new vessels to handle the exercise-induced increase in cardiac output.

Pulmonary hypertension is common in severe interstitial lung disease, resulting from hypoxemia and obliteration of small pulmonary vessels.

CLINICAL FEATURES

Patients with diffuse parenchymal lung disease most commonly have dyspnea as the presenting symptom. The dyspnea is noticed initially on exertion but with severe disease may be experienced even at rest. Cough, usually nonproductive, may be present. On physical examination, auscultation of the chest characteristically reveals dry crackles or rales, which often are most prominent at the bases of the lungs. Clubbing may be present, particularly with certain types of interstitial lung disease. If cor pulmonale develops, cardiac physical findings may be associated with pulmonary hypertension and right ventricular hypertrophy.

Chest examination often is notable for crackles, particularly at the lung bases.

DIAGNOSTIC APPROACH

The chest radiograph is the most important means for making the initial macroscopic assessment of diffuse parenchymal lung disease. The characteristic radiographic picture is an interstitial pattern, described as either *reticular* (increased linear markings) or *reticulonodular* (increased linear and small nodular markings; see Fig. 3-6). The interstitial pattern is believed to reflect a process involving the alveolar walls, although histopathology often indicates that the process extends into alveolar spaces as well. Absence of radiographic abnormalities does not exclude the presence of interstitial disease. Entirely normal chest radiographic findings have been reported in up to 10% of patients. The pattern on chest radiograph is not particularly useful for gauging the relative amounts of inflammation versus fibrosis, each of which may result in a similar pattern. The reticular or reticulonodular changes are frequently diffuse throughout both lung fields, although individual causes of interstitial lung disease may be more likely to result in either an upper or a lower lung field predominance of the abnormal markings. In addition to the interstitial pattern, certain diseases may reveal other associated findings on chest radiograph, such as hilar adenopathy or pleural disease. These additional features noted with some diseases are discussed in Chapters 10 and 11.

A reticular or reticulonodular pattern on chest radiograph is characteristic of interstitial lung disease; however, up to 10% of patients have normal radiographic findings.

With long-standing and severe disease, the lungs may become grossly distorted. In addition, regions of cyst formation between scarred and retracted areas of lung may occur (see Fig. 9-4). A corresponding pattern of honeycombing on chest radiograph may be apparent. Cor pulmonale may be suspected on chest radiograph by the presence of right ventricular enlargement, best seen on the lateral view.

High-resolution computed tomography of the chest has assumed an increasing role in the evaluation of diffuse parenchymal lung disease (see Fig. 3-9). Because of the quality of images of the pulmonary parenchyma, early changes of interstitial lung disease that are not evident on routine chest radiography can often be seen by high-resolution computed tomography. In addition, the specific pattern of abnormality on a high-resolution computed tomographic scan may be suggestive of a particular underlying diagnosis such as IPF and may help to distinguish inflammation from fibrosis.

Despite the importance of the macroscopic evaluation, making a diagnostic distinction between the different types of diffuse parenchymal lung disease usually requires investigation at the microscopic or histologic level. A variety of biopsy procedures have been used to obtain tissue specimens from the lung, which are subjected to several routine staining techniques. The most frequently used biopsy procedures for this purpose are thoracoscopic lung biopsy and transbronchial biopsy (via flexible bronchoscopy). Thoracoscopic biopsy often is the more appropriate of the two procedures for obtaining a sufficiently large specimen of tissue for examination. However, when sarcoidosis (or certain other forms of interstitial disease) is suspected, transbronchial biopsy is a particularly suitable initial procedure.

Another procedure for sampling the cell population of the alveolitis is *bronchoalveolar lavage*. A flexible bronchoscope is placed as distally as possible into an airway, and an irrigation or lavage of fluid through the bronchoscope allows collection of cells from the alveolar spaces. These cells are thought to be representative of the cell populations that are responsible for the alveolitis. Although this technique has been useful as a relatively noninvasive means of obtaining cells for research studies on interstitial lung disease, its clinical usefulness for making a diagnosis or for sequential evaluation of disease activity is limited.

Findings on functional assessment of the patient with interstitial lung disease were reviewed in the section on pathophysiology. Briefly, patients have a restrictive pattern on pulmonary function testing, with decreased lung volumes and preserved airflow. Diffusing capacity usually is reduced, which is indicative of loss of surface area for gas exchange. Hypoxemia is usually (although not necessarily) present, and Po_2 falls even further with exercise. Hypercapnia is rarely a feature of the disease. When it occurs, hypercapnia usually reflects preterminal disease or an additional unrelated process.

TREATMENT

Treatment considerations vary among the diseases. In general, patients with interstitial disease either do not respond well to any form of treatment or respond to immunosuppressive agents (e.g., corticosteroids, cyclophosphamide) to a variable extent. The rationale for immunosuppressive therapy is to reduce the alveolitis component of the disease; the fibrosis is generally considered irreversible. Other interesting therapeutic approaches involve targeting specific growth factors, cytokines, or oxidants that are involved in the inflammatory and fibrotic process within the lungs. However, these approaches are investigational at present. Specific aspects of treatment are covered in the discussion of individual diseases in Chapters 10 and 11.

Corticosteroids and other immunosuppressive agents are used for decreasing the inflammatory component of a number of the diffuse parenchymal lung diseases.

REFERENCES

American Thoracic Society and European Respiratory Society: Idiopathic pulmonary fibrosis: diagnosis and treatment, *Am J Respir Crit Care Med* 161:646–664, 2000.

American Thoracic Society and European Respiratory Society: American Thoracic Society/European Respiratory Society international multidisciplinary consensus classification of the idiopathic interstitial pneumonias, *Am J Respir Crit Care Med* 165:277–304, 2002.

British Thoracic Society: The diagnosis, assessment and treatment of diffuse parenchymal lung disease in adults, *Thorax* 54(suppl 1):S1–S30, 1999.

Demedts M, du Bois RM, Nemery B, Verleden GM, editors: Interstitial lung diseases: a clinical update, *Eur Respir J* 18(suppl 32):1s–133s, 2001.

Gibson GJ: Interstitial lung diseases: pathophysiology and respiratory function, *Eur Respir Mon* 5(monograph 14):15–28, 2000.

Glaspole I, Conron M, du Bois RM: Clinical features of diffuse parenchymal lung disease, *Eur Respir Mon* 5(monograph 14):1–14, 2000.

Lama VN, Martinez FJ: Resting and exercise physiology in interstitial lung diseases, *Clin Chest Med* 25:435–453, 2004.

Leslie KO: Pathology of interstitial lung disease, *Clin Chest Med* 25:657–703, 2004.

Pipavath S, Godwin JD: Imaging of interstitial lung disease, *Clin Chest Med* 25:455–465, 2004.

Ryu JH, Olson EJ, Midthun DE, Swensen SJ: Diagnostic approach to the patient with diffuse lung disease, *Mayo Clin Proc* 77:1221–1227, 2002.

Schwarz MI, King TE Jr, editors: *Interstitial lung disease,* ed 4, Hamilton, Ontario, 2003, BC Decker.

Selman M, King TE Jr, Pardo A: Idiopathic pulmonary fibrosis: prevailing and evolving hypotheses about its pathogenesis and implications for therapy, *Ann Intern Med* 134:136–151, 2001.

Visscher DW, Myers, JL: Histologic spectrum of idiopathic interstitial pneumonias, *Proc Am Thorac Soc* 3:322–329, 2006.

Wells AU, Hogaboam CM: Update in diffuse parenchymal lung disease 2006, *Am J Respir Crit Care Med* 175:655–660, 2007.

Wittram C: The idiopathic interstitial pneumonias, *Curr Probl Diagn Radiol* 33:189–199, 2004.

Wolff G, Crystal RG: Biology of pulmonary fibrosis. In Crystal RG, West JB, Weibel ER, Barnes PJ, editors: *The lung: scientific foundations,* ed 2, Philadelphia, 1997, Lippincott-Raven, pp. 2509–2524.

10

Diffuse Parenchymal Lung Diseases Associated with Known Etiologic Agents

DISEASES CAUSED BY INHALED INORGANIC DUSTS Silicosis Coal Worker's Pneumoconiosis Asbestosis Berylliosis	**HYPERSENSITIVITY PNEUMONITIS** **DRUG-INDUCED PARENCHYMAL LUNG DISEASE** **RADIATION-INDUCED LUNG DISEASE**

This chapter focuses on several of the major categories of diffuse parenchymal (interstitial) lung disease for which an etiologic agent has been identified. The general principles discussed in Chapter 9 apply to most of these conditions, and the features emphasized here are those peculiar to or characteristic of each cause. Considering the vast number of diffuse parenchymal lung diseases, this chapter only scratches the surface of information available. When a physician is confronted with a patient having a particular type of interstitial lung disease, it is best to relearn the details of the disease at that time.

DISEASES CAUSED BY INHALED INORGANIC DUSTS

Many types of interstitial lung disease caused by inhalation of inorganic dusts have been identified; the term *pneumoconiosis* is used for these conditions. Examples of the many responsible agents include silica, asbestos, coal, talc, mica, aluminum, and beryllium. In most cases, contact has occurred for a prolonged time as a result of occupational exposure. In some of these diseases, the parenchymal process progresses even in the absence of continued exposure.

For an inhaled inorganic dust to initiate an alveolitis, it must be deposited at an appropriate area of the lower respiratory tract. If particle size is too large or too small, deposition tends to be in the upper airway or in the larger airways of the tracheobronchial tree. Particles with a diameter of approximately 0.5 to 5 μm are most likely to deposit in the respiratory bronchioles or the alveoli.

No effective treatment is available for interstitial lung disease caused by most inhaled inorganic dusts. Therefore, the important issues facing physicians are recognition and prevention of these disorders. Total avoidance of exposure is the optimal form of prevention, but when exposure is necessary, appropriate precautions with effective masks or respirators are essential.

Particles with a diameter of 0.5 to 5 μm are most likely to be deposited in respiratory bronchioles or alveoli.

Four types of pneumoconiosis are briefly considered here: silicosis, coal worker's pneumoconiosis, asbestosis, and berylliosis. For information about the numerous other agents, consult the more detailed references at the end of this chapter.

SILICOSIS

Silicosis is the interstitial lung disease resulting from exposure to silica (silicon dioxide). Of several crystalline forms of silica, quartz is the one most frequently encountered, usually as a component of rock or sand. Persons at risk include sandblasters, rock miners, quarry workers, and stonecutters. In most cases, development of disease requires at least 20 years of exposure. However, with particularly heavy doses of inhaled silica, as are found in sandblasters, much shorter periods are sufficient.

> The pulmonary effects of silica may be related to a toxic effect on alveolar macrophages.

Although the pathogenesis of silicosis is not known with certainty, theories have centered around the potential toxicity of silica for macrophages. Silica particles in the lower respiratory tract are engulfed and ingested by alveolar macrophages. Freshly cut silica particles are more pathogenic than are older particles. This property is thought to be due to the increased redox potential of the fresh surface, which is highly reactive. After engulfing the silica particle, the macrophage is activated and releases inflammatory mediators, including tumor necrosis factor-α (TNF-α), interleukin-1, and arachidonic acid metabolites. The macrophages eventually are destroyed, and toxic silica particles are released that are capable of repeating the process after they are reingested by other macrophages. With their activation and destruction, the macrophages release chemical mediators that initiate or perpetuate an alveolitis, eventually leading to development of fibrosis. Pathologically, the inflammatory process initially is localized around the respiratory bronchioles but eventually becomes more diffuse throughout the parenchyma. Generally, characteristic acellular nodules, called *silicotic nodules,* which are composed of connective tissue, are seen (Fig. 10-1). At first the nodules are small and discrete. With disease progression they become larger and may coalesce.

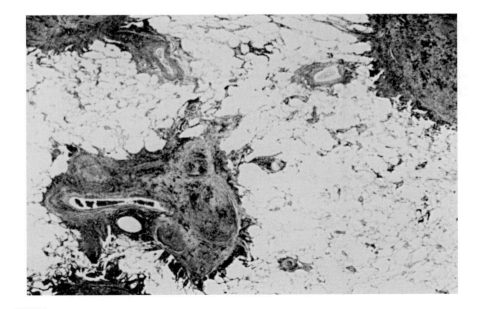

Figure 10-1. Low-power micrograph of silicotic lung shows characteristic appearance of silicotic nodules. (From Morgan WKC, Seaton A: *Occupational lung diseases,* Philadelphia, 1975, WB Saunders.)

Silicotic nodules are believed to be areas in which the cycle of macrophage ingestion, activation, destruction, and release of the toxic silica particles occurs.

Initially, the radiographic appearance of silicosis is notable for small, rounded opacities or nodules. At this point the patient is said to have *simple pneumoconiosis*. When the nodules become larger and coalescent, the pneumoconiosis is called *complicated,* for which the term *progressive massive fibrosis* has also been used (Fig. 10-2). As a general rule, in patients with silicosis the upper lung zones are affected more heavily than are the lower zones. Enlargement of the hilar lymph nodes, which frequently calcify, may be seen.

In addition to the potential problem of progressive pulmonary involvement and eventual respiratory failure, patients with silicosis are particularly susceptible to infections with mycobacteria, perhaps because of impaired macrophage function. The specific organisms may be either *Mycobacterium tuberculosis,* the etiologic agent for tuberculosis, or other species of mycobacteria, often called *atypical* or *nontuberculous mycobacteria* (see Chapter 24).

> Silicosis is a predisposing factor for secondary infections by mycobacteria.

COAL WORKER'S PNEUMOCONIOSIS

Individuals who have worked as part of the coal mining process and have been exposed to large amounts of coal dust are at risk for development of *coal worker's pneumoconiosis* (CWP). In comparison with silica, coal dust is a less fibrogenic material, and the tissue reaction is much less marked for equivalent amounts of dust deposited in the lungs.

> Tissue reaction to inhaled coal dust is much less than that to silica.

The pathologic hallmark of CWP is the coal macule, which is a focal collection of coal dust surrounded by relatively little tissue reaction in terms of either cellular infiltration or fibrosis (Fig. 10-3). The initial lesions tend to be distributed primarily around respiratory bronchioles. Small associated regions of emphysema, termed *focal emphysema,* may be seen.

As with silicosis, the disease often is separated into *simple* and *complicated* forms. In simple CWP the chest radiograph consists of relatively small and discrete densities that

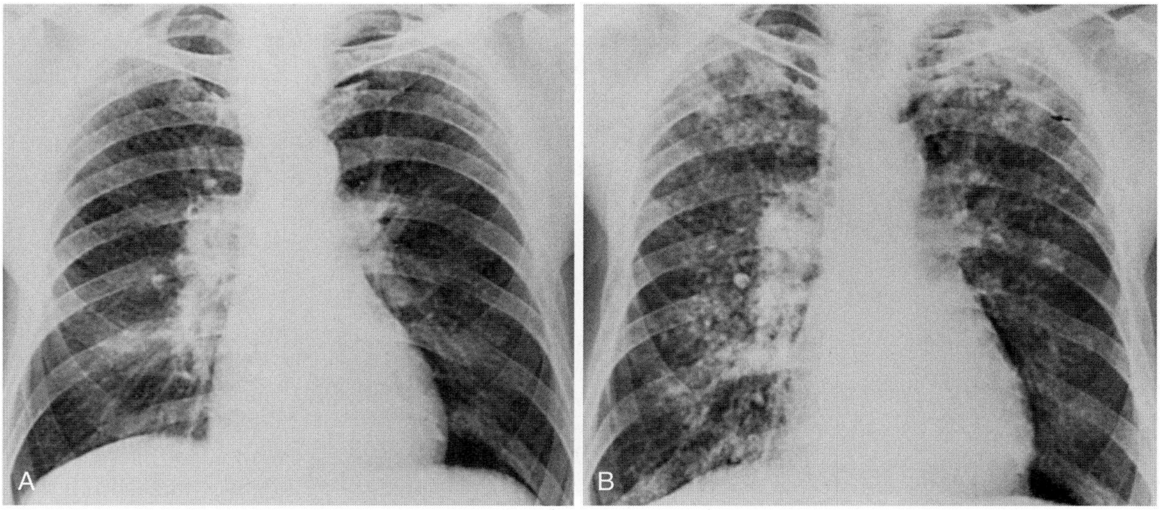

Figure 10-2. Radiographic appearance of **(A)** simple and **(B)** complicated silicosis in the same patient. **A,** Small nodules are present throughout both lungs, particularly in the upper zones. A reticular component is seen as well. **B,** Nodules have become larger and are coalescent in upper zones. One of the confluent shadows on the left shows cavitation *(arrow).* Interval between radiographs shown in A and B is 11 years. (From Fraser RG, Müller NL, Colman N, Paré PD: *Diagnosis of diseases of the chest,* vol 4, 4th ed, Philadelphia, 1999, WB Saunders.)

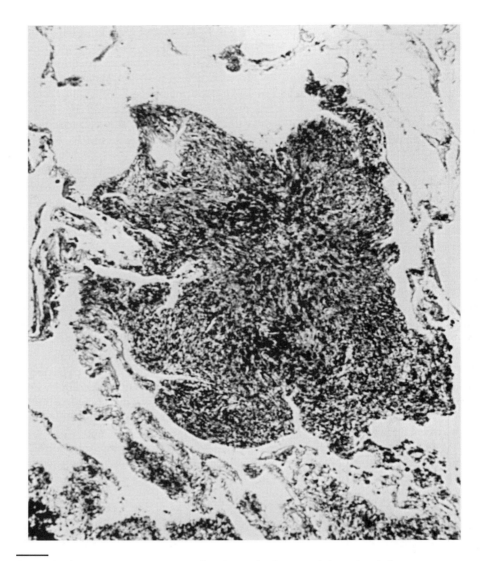

Figure 10-3. Histologic appearance of coal macule shows coal dust, dust-laden macrophages, and relatively small amounts of fibrous reaction. (From Morgan WKC, Seaton A: *Occupational lung diseases*, Philadelphia, 1975, WB Saunders.)

Symptoms and pulmonary function changes in coal worker's pneumoconiosis (CWP) occur primarily in patients with progressive massive fibrosis.

usually are more nodular than linear. In this phase of the disease, patients have few symptoms, and pulmonary function usually is relatively preserved. In later stages of the disease, to which only a small minority of individuals progress, chest radiographic findings and clinical symptoms are more pronounced. With extensive disease and coalescent opacities on chest radiograph, patients are said to have complicated disease, also called *progressive massive fibrosis*.

Why complicated disease develops in some patients with CWP is not entirely clear. At one time, it was speculated that patients with progressive massive fibrosis had also been exposed to toxic amounts of silica and that the simultaneous silica exposure was responsible for most of the fibrotic process. However, although some patients do have a mixed form of pneumoconiosis from both coal dust and silica exposure, progressive massive fibrosis can result from coal dust in the absence of concomitant exposure to silica. More recently, genetic polymorphisms have been identified that may help to explain the different clinical responses to inhalational exposures.

ASBESTOSIS

Asbestos has been widely used because of its thermal and fire resistance. It is a fibrous derivative of silica, termed a *fibrous silicate*. It is a naturally occurring mineral that, because of its long narrow shape, can be woven into cloth. Among the health hazards it presents are the development of diffuse interstitial fibrosis and the potential for inducing several types of neoplasm, particularly bronchogenic carcinoma and mesothelioma. These latter problems are discussed in Chapters 20 and 21, respectively. The term *asbestosis* should be reserved for the interstitial lung disease that occurs as a result of asbestos exposure.

Individuals at risk for development of asbestosis include insulation, shipyard, and construction workers as well as persons who have been exposed by working with brake linings. Even though the health hazards of asbestos are well recognized and the use of asbestos has been curtailed in industrialized countries, workers still may be exposed in the course of remodeling or reinsulating pipes or buildings in which asbestos had been used. In addition, asbestos still presents a major health issue in many developing countries. The duration of exposure necessary for development of asbestosis usually is more than 10 to 20 years but can vary depending on the intensity of the exposure.

One theory for the pathogenesis of asbestosis suggests that asbestos fibers activate macrophages and induce the release of mediators that attract other inflammatory cells, including neutrophils, lymphocytes, and more alveolar macrophages. Unlike silica, asbestos probably is not cytotoxic to macrophages. That is, it does not seem to destroy or "kill" macrophages in the way that silica does. The mechanism of the often significant fibrotic reaction that occurs with asbestos may be related to the release of mediators from macrophages (e.g., fibronectin, insulin-like growth factor-I, and platelet-derived growth factor) that can promote fibroblast recruitment and replication. An area of active research involves studying the effects of asbestos fibers on initiating abnormalities in alveolar epithelial cell apoptosis and proliferation.

The earliest microscopic lesions appear around respiratory bronchioles, with an alveolitis that progresses to peribronchiolar fibrosis. The fibrosis subsequently becomes more generalized throughout the alveolar walls and can become quite marked. Areas of the lung that are heavily involved by the fibrotic process include the lung bases and the subpleural regions.

A characteristic finding of asbestos exposure is the *ferruginous body,* which is a rod-shaped body with clubbed ends (Fig. 10-4) that appears yellow-brown in stained tissue. Ferruginous bodies represent asbestos fibers that have been coated by macrophages with an iron–protein complex. Although large numbers of these structures are commonly seen by light microscopy in patients with asbestosis, not all such coated fibers are asbestos, and ferruginous bodies may be seen even in the absence of parenchymal lung disease. Uncoated asbestos fibers, which are long and narrow, cannot be seen by light microscopy and require electron microscopy for detection.

The chest radiograph in patients with asbestosis shows a pattern of linear streaking that is generally most prominent at the lung bases (Fig. 10-5). In advanced cases the findings may be quite extensive and associated with cyst formation and honeycombing. Commonly, there is evidence of associated pleural disease, either in the form of diffuse pleural thickening or localized plaques (which may be calcified) or, much less frequently, in the form of pleural effusions. Because asbestos is a predisposing factor in the development of malignancies of the lung and pleura, either of these complications may be seen on the chest radiograph.

In asbestosis, microscopic examination of lung tissue often shows large numbers of ferruginous bodies.

Pulmonary complications of asbestos exposure are the following:
1. Interstitial lung disease (asbestosis)
2. Diffuse pleural thickening
3. Localized pleural plaques
4. Pleural effusions
5. Lung cancer
6. Pleural malignancy (mesothelioma)

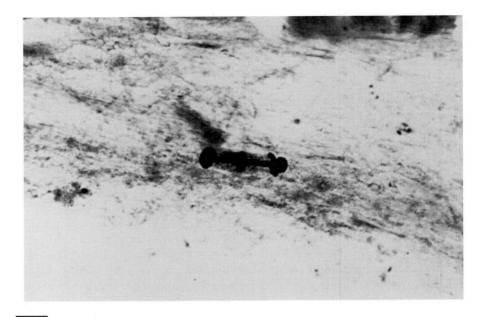

Figure 10-4. High-power photomicrograph of ferruginous body. Rod-shaped body with clubbed ends represents "coated" asbestos fiber. (Courtesy Dr. Earl Kasdon.)

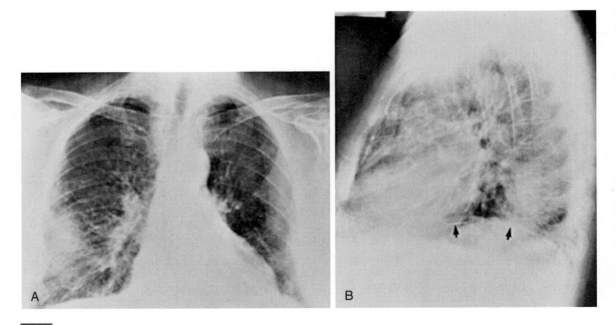

Figure 10-5. Chest radiograph of patient with parenchymal and pleural disease secondary to asbestos exposure. Interstitial markings are increased at lung bases, and extensive pleural thickening is present. Diaphragmatic calcification, which strongly suggests prior asbestos exposure, is highlighted by arrows. **A,** Posteroanterior view. **B,** Lateral view.

The clinical, pathophysiologic, and diagnostic features of asbestosis usually follow the general description of interstitial lung disease discussed in Chapter 9. However, of the pneumoconioses already discussed, asbestosis is much more likely on physical examination to be associated with clubbing than is either silicosis or CWP.

BERYLLIOSIS

Berylliosis is a pneumoconiosis that results from inhalation of the metal dust beryllium. The disease initially was described in individuals who make fluorescent light bulbs, but more recent cases involve workers in the aerospace, nuclear weapons, and electronics industries and in other industries in which beryllium is used. The histologic appearance of disease caused by beryllium is quite different from that seen with the other pneumoconioses described earlier. Instead, the pathologic reaction is found in the lungs as well as hilar and mediastinal lymph nodes, and it involves formation of granulomas resembling those seen in sarcoidosis.

A great deal of research has been performed to elucidate the pathogenesis of berylliosis, which is known to represent a cellular immune (delayed hypersensitivity) response to beryllium. Lymphocytes harvested from blood or from bronchoalveolar lavage fluid of patients with berylliosis demonstrate transformation (i.e., proliferation) when exposed to beryllium salts in vitro. Not only does this "beryllium lymphocyte transformation test" confirm the pathogenesis of the disease, but it also serves as a useful diagnostic test in individuals with a clinical picture consistent with berylliosis. In addition, sensitization to beryllium can be demonstrated in some workers before the onset of clinical disease, a finding that may be important for prevention or early intervention to arrest progression from subclinical to clinical disease.

Whether beryllium interacts directly with T lymphocytes or whether the metal first must bind to antigenic peptides is not known. Whatever the mechanism, the particular pattern of cytokine release by lymphocytes following exposure to beryllium suggests a response by the T_H1 helper T cell class of $CD4^+$ lymphocytes. Studies also suggest a genetic susceptibility to development of the disease in response to exposure to beryllium. One form of this susceptibility is identified by the presence of glutamate in position 69 of the human leukocyte antigen DPB1 molecule.

Clinically and radiographically, the disease closely mimics sarcoidosis (see Chapter 11). Specifically, patients with berylliosis demonstrate granulomatous inflammation in multiple organ systems, especially the pulmonary parenchyma and intrathoracic lymph nodes.

> Berylliosis, which resembles sarcoidosis in many respects, represents a cellular immune response to beryllium.

HYPERSENSITIVITY PNEUMONITIS

In *hypersensitivity pneumonitis*, immunologic phenomena directed against an antigen are responsible for the production of interstitial lung disease. This disorder is sometimes referred to as *extrinsic allergic alveolitis*.

The antigens that induce the series of immunologic events are inhaled particulates and aerosol antigens from a variety of sources. Almost all the antigens are derived from microorganisms, plant proteins, and animal proteins. Exposure often is related either to the patient's occupation or to some avocation. The first of the hypersensitivity pneumonitides described was *farmer's lung*, which is due to antigens from microorganisms (thermophilic actinomycetes) that may be present on moldy hay. The list of antigens and types of exposure is quite extensive and includes entities such as air conditioner or humidifier lung (caused by antigens from microorganisms contaminating a forced air system) and bird breeder's or bird fancier's lung (attributable to avian proteins).

> Hypersensitivity pneumonitis represents an immunologic response to an inhaled organic antigen.

Interestingly, even when a large number of individuals are exposed to a given antigen by virtue of their occupation or avocation, disease develops in only a small percentage. Studies indicate that polymorphisms in TNF-α are important in determining the development of bird breeder's lung. Clearly, additional factors, perhaps genetic, determine who will contract the disease, but these factors are not yet identified.

Despite much research, we do not yet have a complete understanding of the pathogenesis of hypersensitivity pneumonitis. However, a type IV immune reaction (cell-mediated or delayed hypersensitivity, mediated by T lymphocytes) causing a lymphocytic alveolitis is known to be of prime importance in producing the disease. A type III (immune complex disease) mechanism plays a contributory role, especially early in the disease process. Evidence suggests that T lymphocytes in the lower respiratory tract become sensitized to the particular organic antigen. They then may release soluble cytokines that attract macrophages and possibly induce them to form granulomas in the lung. Antigen–antibody immune complexes also may be involved, with binding of complement and the resulting production of chemotactic factors and activation of macrophages.

Pathologic examination of the lung in patients with hypersensitivity pneumonitis reveals an alveolitis composed primarily of lymphocytes (especially cytotoxic/suppressor CD8+ cells) and macrophages, as well as the presence of granulomas. The granulomas often are poorly formed, unlike the well-defined granulomas characteristic of sarcoidosis (see Chapter 11). Often the pathologic changes have a peribronchiolar prominence, thus accounting for the frequent physiologic evidence for obstruction of small airways.

Clinically, hypersensitivity pneumonitis manifests in different ways, ranging from acute episodes of dyspnea, cough, fever, and infiltrates on chest radiograph, occurring approximately 4 to 6 hours after exposure to the offending antigen, to a chronic form of diffuse parenchymal lung disease. The latter presentation is more insidious. The patient often reports gradual onset of shortness of breath and cough, along with systemic symptoms of fatigue, loss of appetite, and weight loss. Long-term antigen exposure has been occurring in these circumstances, and because acute episodes are not necessarily an important feature, the patient does not associate the symptoms with any particular exposure.

Unlike the acute form, the chronic form of hypersensitivity pneumonitis behaves like other forms of interstitial lung disease. Unless the physician is attuned to the possibility that hypersensitivity to an antigen in the environment might be responsible for the patient's lung disease, the entity may easily be missed, and exposure to the antigen may continue.

With an acute episode of hypersensitivity pneumonitis, the chest radiograph shows patchy or diffuse infiltrates. As the disease becomes chronic, the abnormality may take on a more nodular quality, eventually appearing as the reticulonodular pattern characteristic of the other chronic interstitial lung diseases. In the chronic form of disease, an upper lobe predominance to the radiographic changes is often seen. High-resolution chest CT scanning may be particularly helpful in suggesting the diagnosis, often demonstrating a mosaic ground-glass pattern (see Fig. 3-9).

The diagnosis is more likely to be considered if the patient gives a history of acute episodes, which either occur by themselves or punctuate a more chronic illness. Historic features concerning the patient's occupation, hobbies, and other environmental exposures may provide valuable clues for detecting the responsible factor. One standard diagnostic test is a search for precipitating antibodies to the common organic antigens known to cause hypersensitivity pneumonitis. Unfortunately, false-positive and false-negative results for precipitins may cause diagnostic confusion. For example, the finding of precipitins to thermophilic actinomycetes, the agent responsible for

Hypersensitivity pneumonitis occurs either with acute episodes 4 to 6 hours after exposure to the offending antigen or with the more insidious course of chronic interstitial lung disease.

farmer's lung, is relatively common in healthy farmers without any evidence of the disease. In addition, making a diagnosis of hypersensitivity pneumonitis by the finding of precipitins requires that the responsible antigen be included in the panel of antigens tested. If a lung biopsy is performed for diagnosis of interstitial lung disease, findings on microscopic examination may suggest this entity.

The best treatment is avoidance of exposure. Unfortunately, the chronic form of the disease often leads to irreversible changes in the lung that persist even after exposure is terminated. Corticosteroids are sometimes administered to patients with persistent disease, but the results are variable.

DRUG-INDUCED PARENCHYMAL LUNG DISEASE

As the list of available pharmacologic agents expands every year, so does the list of potential complications. The lung is certainly one of the target organs for these adverse effects, and diffuse parenchymal lung disease is a particularly important (although not the only) manifestation of drug toxicity. Each drug cannot be considered in detail here, nor can a complete list of the growing number of drugs that have been implicated be provided. However, this chapter briefly discusses the general principles of drug-induced parenchymal lung disease and the major agents responsible.

The largest single category of drugs associated with disease of the alveolar wall includes the chemotherapeutic or cytotoxic agents, that is, those drugs designed primarily as antitumor agents. Individual drugs that have been commonly implicated in the development of lung disease are bleomycin, mitomycin, busulfan, cyclophosphamide, methotrexate, and the nitrosoureas, although several others have been described in smaller numbers of cases. In general, the risk of developing interstitial lung disease increases with higher cumulative doses of a particular agent. However, occasional cases with even relatively low cumulative doses are described. In most cases, interstitial lung disease develops in a period ranging from 1 month to several years after use of the agent. Busulfan is particularly notable for late development of complications, often several years after onset of therapy.

> Chemotherapeutic and cytotoxic agents are the largest category of drugs associated with interstitial lung disease.

The pathogenesis of chemotherapy-induced diffuse parenchymal lung disease often appears to involve either direct toxicity to normal lung parenchymal cells, especially epithelial cells, or oxidant injury induced by generation of toxic oxygen radicals. One exception is methotrexate, for which hypersensitivity mechanisms may also play a role. When oxidant damage is involved, as with bleomycin, other agents that promote formation of oxygen free radicals, such as radiation therapy or high concentrations of inhaled oxygen, can augment the injury caused by the chemotherapeutic agent.

The pathologic appearance of interstitial lung disease caused by cytotoxic agents frequently is notable for the presence of atypical, bizarre-appearing type II alveolar epithelial cells with large hyperchromatic nuclei. When this feature is associated with the other usual findings of interstitial lung disease, the pathologist should suspect that a chemotherapeutic agent may be responsible. In conjunction with its presumed difference in pathogenesis, methotrexate does not produce the same degree of epithelial cell atypia as do the other cytotoxic agents. In contrast, granulomas, consistent with a hypersensitivity mechanism, are frequently seen.

> Cytotoxic drug-induced interstitial lung disease shows atypical, bizarre-appearing alveolar type II epithelial cells.

Clinically, fever is a common accompaniment to the respiratory symptoms associated with drug-induced interstitial lung disease. An increase in eosinophils in peripheral blood is often noted in patients with methotrexate-induced lung disease.

For those patients receiving these drugs in whom pulmonary infiltrates develop, often associated with fever, several diagnostic considerations routinely arise. In addition to the possibility of drug toxicity is concern about infection (because host defenses are generally impaired by the drug or by the underlying malignancy), dissemination of the malignancy through the lung, bleeding into the lung, and, in patients who have received radiation therapy, toxic effects from the irradiation. When the diagnosis is not clear, a lung biopsy often is performed, primarily to rule out an infectious process. If atypical epithelial cells but no infectious agents are found, a drug-induced process is suspected.

For patients who are believed to have a cytotoxic drug-related interstitial lung disease, the particular chemotherapeutic agent generally is discontinued. Steroids may be administered, but, as with their use in other diffuse parenchymal diseases, the results are variable.

Several drugs that are not chemotherapeutic agents have been implicated in the development of parenchymal lung disease. Nitrofurantoin, an antibiotic, has been associated with both acute and chronic reactions. The acute problem, which presumably is a hypersensitivity phenomenon, often is characterized by pulmonary infiltrates, pleural effusions, fever, and eosinophilia in peripheral blood. The chronic problem, which does not appear to be related to prior acute episodes, is characterized by a nonspecific interstitial pneumonitis and fibrosis akin to that of the other interstitial pneumonitides.

Therapy with injections of gold, which is used in rheumatoid arthritis, has been associated with development of interstitial lung disease. The diagnosis here may be confusing because the underlying disease (rheumatoid arthritis) also can be associated with alveolitis and pulmonary fibrosis.

Amiodarone-induced lung disease is an important cause of either focal or diffuse pulmonary infiltrates.

The commonly used antiarrhythmic agent amiodarone has been associated with clinically significant parenchymal lung disease in approximately 5% to 10% of treated patients. Amiodarone pulmonary toxicity is dose related and may be fatal. In addition to nonspecific inflammation and fibrosis, the pathologic appearance of amiodarone-induced interstitial lung disease is notable for macrophages that appear foamy because of cytoplasmic phospholipid inclusions. However, similar foamy macrophages with cytoplasmic inclusions have been found in autopsy specimens of lung tissue from amiodarone-treated patients without interstitial inflammation and fibrosis. This finding suggests that the phospholipid inclusions may only be a marker of amiodarone use and may not necessarily be directly responsible for the other pathologic and clinically important pulmonary consequences of amiodarone. Radiographically, patients with amiodarone-induced lung disease can develop either focal or diffuse infiltrates. CT scanning commonly shows a relatively high density of the infiltrates, resulting from a high iodine content within the amiodarone molecule.

A large number of drugs have been linked with the development of an illness that resembles systemic lupus erythematosus, and patients with this "drug-induced lupus" may have parenchymal lung disease as one manifestation. In addition, a variety of drugs have been associated with pulmonary infiltrates and peripheral blood eosinophilia. This constellation of pulmonary infiltrates with eosinophilia, of which drugs are just one of several possible causes, is often abbreviated as the *PIE* syndrome.

RADIATION-INDUCED LUNG DISEASE

Interstitial lung disease is a potential complication of radiation therapy for tumors within the thorax or in close proximity to it, particularly lymphoma (Hodgkin's disease) and carcinoma of the breast or lung. It is estimated that signs and symptoms of clinically apparent injury will develop in 5% to 15% of patients whose radiation therapy includes exposure of portions of normal lung. However, radiographic changes in the absence of symptoms are seen even more frequently, in 20% to 70% of exposed patients.

Radiation-induced pulmonary disease generally is divided into two phases: early pneumonitis and late fibrosis. The acute phase of radiation pneumonitis develops approximately 1 to 3 months after completion of a course of therapy, depending to a large extent on the total dose and the volume of lung irradiated. The later stage of radiation fibrosis may directly follow earlier radiation-induced pneumonitis, may occur after a symptom-free latent interval, or occasionally may develop without any prior clinical evidence of acute pneumonitis. Fibrosis, when it occurs, does so generally 6 to 12 months after radiation therapy has been completed.

> Radiation-induced lung disease includes an early period of radiation pneumonitis and a later period of radiation fibrosis.

Although the pathogenesis of radiation-induced lung disease is not entirely known, toxicity to capillary endothelial cells and, to a lesser extent, to type I alveolar epithelial cells is believed to be the primary mode of injury, perhaps mediated by oxygen-derived free radicals. In the period preceding chronic fibrosis, an alveolitis probably contributes directly to the development of fibrotic changes. The possibility of hypersensitivity playing a role in the pathogenesis of the alveolitis has been suggested by the finding of increased lymphocytes in the bronchoalveolar fluid of the nonirradiated lung in patients with radiation-induced pneumonitis.

Early pathologic changes include swelling of endothelial cells, interstitial edema, mononuclear cell infiltrates, and atypical hyperplastic epithelial cells. Subsequent changes during the fibrotic stage consist of progressive fibrosis (indistinguishable from pulmonary fibrosis of other causes) and sclerosis of small vessels, with obliteration of a major portion of the capillary bed in the involved area.

Clinically, patients may have fever with the acute pneumonitis in conjunction with respiratory symptoms, and distinguishing radiation pneumonitis from an atypical pneumonia is often difficult. On chest radiograph, the acute pneumonitis is usually characterized by an infiltrate that conforms in shape and location to the region of lung irradiated. Chest CT scanning may be particularly useful, both because it may detect subtle abnormalities earlier than can be seen on chest radiograph and because the cross-sectional views readily show the correspondence of the radiographic abnormalities to the radiation ports. However, for reasons that are unclear, additional changes outside the field of radiation may develop in some patients. The pattern of chronic radiation fibrosis is an increase in interstitial markings, again generally corresponding in location to the irradiated region of lung, often with associated volume loss. The acute changes of the pneumonitis are potentially reversible, whereas the chronic fibrotic changes generally are permanent.

> The interstitial pattern in radiation-induced lung disease generally conforms in distribution to the region of lung irradiated.

Diagnostic considerations usually are similar to those for drug-induced parenchymal lung disease. A history of recent irradiation occurring at the appropriate time is crucial to the diagnosis. In addition, the finding of radiographic changes that conform to the radiation port, often with a relatively sharp cutoff, is strongly suggestive of the diagnosis.

Corticosteroids are frequently used to treat radiation-induced pneumonitis, often with reasonably good results. When the chronic changes of fibrosis have supervened, corticosteroids are much less effective.

REFERENCES

DISEASES CAUSED BY INHALED INORGANIC DUSTS

American Thoracic Society: Adverse effects of crystalline silica exposure, *Am J Respir Crit Care Med* 155:761–765, 1997.

American Thoracic Society: Diagnosis and initial management of nonmalignant diseases related to asbestos, *Am J Respir Crit Care Med* 170:691–715, 2004.

Amicosante M, Fontenot AP: T cell recognition in chronic beryllium disease, *Clin Immunol* 121:134–143, 2006.

Beckett WS: Occupational respiratory diseases, *N Engl J Med* 342:406–413, 2000.

Castranova V, Vallyathan V: Silicosis and coal workers' pneumoconiosis, *Environ Health Perspect* 108(suppl):675–684, 2000.

Chong S, Lee KS, Chung MJ, Han J, Kwon OJ, Kim TS: Pneumoconiosis: comparison of imaging and pathologic findings, *Radiographics* 26:59–77, 2006.

Cohen R, Velho V: Update on respiratory disease from coal mine and silica dust, *Clin Chest Med* 23: 811–826, 2002.

Glazer CS, Newman LS: Occupational interstitial lung disease, *Clin Chest Med* 25:467–478, 2004.

Hessel PA, Gamble JF, McDonald JC: Asbestos, asbestosis, and lung cancer: a critical assessment of the epidemiological evidence, *Thorax* 60:433–436, 2005.

Kamp DW, Weitzman SA: The molecular basis of asbestos-induced lung injury, *Thorax* 54:638–652, 1999.

Mapp CE, editor: Occupational lung disorders, *Eur Respir Mon* 4(monograph 11):1–355, 1999.

Mossman BT, Churg A: Mechanisms in the pathogenesis of asbestosis and silicosis, *Am J Respir Crit Care Med* 157:1666–1680, 1998.

Mossman BT, Gee JBL: Asbestos-related diseases, *N Engl J Med* 320:1721–1730, 1989.

Newman LS: Immunology, genetics, and epidemiology of beryllium disease, *Chest* 109:40S–43S, 1996.

Rom WN, Travis WD, Brody AR: Cellular and molecular basis of the asbestos-related diseases, *Am Rev Respir Dis* 143:408–422, 1991.

Ross MH, Murray J: Occupational respiratory disease in mining, *Occup Med (Lond)* 54:304–310, 2004.

Saltini C, Amicosante M: Beryllium disease, *Am J Med Sci* 321:89–98, 2001.

Yucesoy B, Luster MI: Genetic susceptibility in pneumoconiosis, *Toxicol Lett* 168:249–254, 2007.

HYPERSENSITIVITY PNEUMONITIS

Bertorelli G, Bocchino V, Olivieri D: Hypersensitivity pneumonitis, *Eur Respir Mon* 5(monograph 14): 120–136, 2000.

Fink JN: Clinical features of hypersensitivity pneumonitis, *Chest* 89:193S–195S, 1986.

Fink JN, Ortega HG, Reynolds HY, et al: Needs and opportunities for research in hypersensitivity pneumonitis, *Am J Respir Crit Care Med* 171:792–798, 2005.

Rose C, King TE Jr: Controversies in hypersensitivity pneumonitis, *Am Rev Respir Dis* 145:1–2, 1992.

Salvaggio JE, deShazo RD: Pathogenesis of hypersensitivity pneumonitis, *Chest* 190S–193S, 1986.

Selman M: Hypersensitivity pneumonitis: a multifaceted deceiving disorder, *Clin Chest Med* 25:531–547, 2004.

Silva CI, Churg A, Müller NL: Hypersensitivity pneumonitis: spectrum of high-resolution CT and pathologic findings, *AJR Am J Roentgenol* 188:334–344, 2007.

Trentin L, Facco M, Semenzato G: Hypersensitivity pneumonitis, *Eur Respir Mon* 4(monograph 11): 301–319, 1999.

DRUG-INDUCED PARENCHYMAL LUNG DISEASE

Camus P, Bonniaud P, Fanton A, Camus C, Baudaun N, Foucher P: Drug-induced and iatrogenic infiltrative lung disease, *Clin Chest Med* 25:479–519, 2004.

Camus P, Martin WJ, Rosenow EC: Amiodarone pulmonary toxicity, *Clin Chest Med* 25:65–75, 2004.

Cooper JAD Jr, White DA, Matthay RA: Drug-induced pulmonary disease, *Am Rev Respir Dis* 133:321–340, 488–505, 1986.

Dunn M, Glassroth J: Pulmonary complications of amiodarone toxicity, *Prog Cardiovasc Dis* 31:447–453, 1989.

Flieder DB, Travis WD: Pathologic characteristics of drug-induced lung disease, *Clin Chest Med* 25:37–45, 2004.

Foucher P, Biour M, Blayac JP, et al: Drugs that may injure the respiratory system, *Eur Respir J* 10:265–279, 1997.

Imokawa S, Colby TV, Leslie KO, Helmers RA: Methotrexate pneumonitis: review of the literature and histopathological findings in nine patients, *Eur Respir J* 15:373–381, 2000.

Limper AH: Chemotherapy-induced lung disease, *Clin Chest Med* 25:53–64, 2004.

Lock BJ, Eggert M, Cooper JA: Infiltrative lung disease due to noncytotoxic agents, *Clin Chest Med* 25:47–52, 2004.

Silva CI and Müller N: Drug-induced lung diseases: most common reaction patterns and corresponding high-resolution CT manifestations, *Semin Ultrasound CT MR* 27:111–116, 2006.

Sleijfer S: Bleomycin-induced pneumonitis, *Chest* 120:617–624, 2001.

RADIATION-INDUCED LUNG DISEASE

Abratt RP, Morgan GW, Silvestri G, Willcox P: Pulmonary complications of radiation therapy, *Clin Chest Med* 25:167–177, 2004.

Cameron EH, Crystal RG: Radiation-induced lung injury. In Crystal RG, West JB, Weibel ER, Barnes PJ, editors: *The lung: scientific foundations,* ed 2, Philadelphia, 1997, Lippincott-Raven, pp. 2647–2651.

Gibson PG, Bryant DH, Morgan GW, et al: Radiation-induced lung injury: a hypersensitivity pneumonitis? *Ann Intern Med* 109:288–291, 1988.

Gross NJ: Pulmonary effects of radiation therapy, *Ann Intern Med* 86:81–92, 1977.

Movsas B, Raffin TA, Epstein AH, Link CJ Jr: Pulmonary radiation injury, *Chest* 111:1061–1076, 1997.

Tsoutsou PG, Koukourakis ML: Radiation pneumonitis and fibrosis: mechanisms underlying its pathogenesis and implications for future research, *Int J Radiat Oncol Biol Phys* 66:1281–1293, 2006.

Diffuse Parenchymal Lung Diseases of Unknown Etiology

IDIOPATHIC PULMONARY FIBROSIS	**MISCELLANEOUS DISORDERS INVOLVING THE PULMONARY PARENCHYMA**
OTHER IDIOPATHIC INTERSTITIAL PNEUMONIAS	Pulmonary Langerhans Cell Histiocytosis
PULMONARY PARENCHYMAL INVOLVEMENT COMPLICATING CONNECTIVE TISSUE DISEASE	Lymphangioleiomyomatosis
	Goodpasture's Syndrome
	Wegener's Granulomatosis
SARCOIDOSIS	Chronic Eosinophilic Pneumonia
	Pulmonary Alveolar Proteinosis

Approximately 65% of patients with diffuse parenchymal lung disease are victims of a process for which no etiologic agent has been identified, even though a specific name may be attached to the disease entity. Included in this category of disease are idiopathic pulmonary fibrosis, pulmonary fibrosis associated with connective tissue disease, sarcoidosis, pulmonary Langerhans cell histiocytosis, and a variety of other disorders. Many general aspects of these problems were discussed in Chapter 9. This chapter focuses on the specific diseases and their particular characteristics.

IDIOPATHIC PULMONARY FIBROSIS

Although the name *idiopathic pulmonary fibrosis* (IPF) has often been used nonspecifically to describe fibrotic interstitial lung disease without an identifiable diagnosis, most clinicians and investigators believe that IPF represents a specific disease entity. This chapter adopts that assumption and considers pulmonary fibrosis associated with an underlying connective tissue disease as a separate entity. Other names that have been used interchangeably with IPF are cryptogenic fibrosing alveolitis and usual interstitial pneumonia. The latter term now is generally used as a description of the pathologic pattern associated with IPF, a pattern that occasionally is seen in clinical settings other than IPF.

As implied by the name, IPF does not yet have a recognizable inciting agent. Whether the primary agent, if one exists, reaches the lung via the airways or the bloodstream has not been determined. The theory behind the pathogenesis of IPF has changed considerably over the past several years. For many years the prevailing thought was that exposure to an unknown agent (perhaps an antigen leading to formation of antigen–antibody complexes) led to alveolar inflammation, which was perpetuated by release of chemotactic factors from inflammatory cells. The ongoing inflammation was believed to be responsible for subsequent development of fibrosis.

Over the past several years, a newer conceptual framework has emerged. According to the newer theory, alveolar inflammation does not play a critical role in the eventual development of fibrosis. Rather, fibrosis is believed to result directly from alveolar epithelial injury and is thought to be a manifestation of abnormal wound healing within the lung parenchyma. According to the newer paradigm, injury to alveolar epithelial cells (still from an unidentified source or agent) is the primary initiating event. Whereas injury to type I alveolar epithelial cells normally would be followed by a repair process that includes proliferation of type II cells and differentiation into type I cells, this repair process is impaired, at least in part because of disruption of the basement membrane, which normally is important for the reepithelialization process. At the same time, alveolar epithelial cells express a variety of profibrotic cytokines and growth factors, including platelet-derived growth factor (PDGF) and transforming growth factor-β1 (TGF–β1), which enhance fibroblast migration and proliferation. Fibroblastic foci develop at sites of alveolar injury and appear to be responsible for increased extracellular matrix deposition. This process is summarized in Figure 11-1.

Clinically, the most common age at presentation of patients with IPF is between 50 and 70 years. The onset of the disease is generally insidious. The symptoms are similar to those of other interstitial lung diseases; dyspnea is the most prominent complaint. In addition to the classic finding of dry crackles or rales on physical examination, patients frequently have evidence of clubbing of the digits.

The chest radiograph shows an interstitial (reticular or reticulonodular) pattern that is generally bilateral and relatively diffuse but typically is more prominent at the bases of the lungs (see Fig. 3-6). Neither pleural effusions nor hilar enlargement is found on the radiograph. High-resolution computed tomographic (HRCT) scanning often has a

> Idiopathic pulmonary fibrosis is thought to represent a dysregulated pattern of fibrosis in response to alveolar epithelial injury.

> The chest radiograph in IPF demonstrates a diffuse interstitial pattern without pleural disease or hilar enlargement.

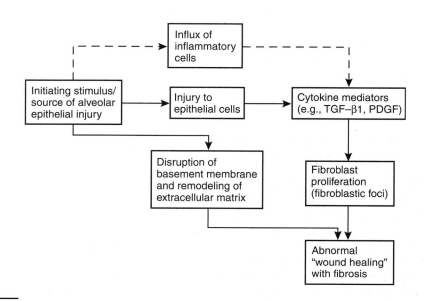

Figure 11-1. Proposed pathogenetic sequence in idiopathic pulmonary fibrosis. Dotted lines indicate that, although there is an influx of inflammatory cells, this is not thought to be a primary component of the pathogenesis. PDGF = Platelet-derived growth factor; TGF-β1 = transforming growth factor-β1.

characteristic appearance, showing interstitial densities that are patchy, peripheral, subpleural, and associated with small cystic spaces (Fig. 11-2). The pattern of small cystic peripheral abnormalities on HRCT is termed *honeycombing* and indicates irreversible fibrosis. Many patients have serologic abnormalities, such as a positive test result for antinuclear antibodies, which are generally found in patients with autoimmune or connective tissue disease. However, in the absence of other suggestive clinical features, these abnormalities are thought to be nonspecific and not indicative of an underlying rheumatologic disease.

The diagnosis is definitively made by surgical lung biopsy, but only in the appropriate clinical setting when other etiologic factors for interstitial lung disease cannot be identified. Some patients are too frail for lung biopsy, and if HRCT scan shows the classic pattern of honeycombing, the diagnosis can be made with relative certainty without a lung biopsy. The histologic expression of IPF is in the form of usual interstitial pneumonia (UIP) (see Fig. 9-3), and patients who have a pathologic pattern more compatible with desquamative interstitial pneumonia or nonspecific interstitial pneumonia (see Chapter 9 and the section on other idiopathic interstitial pneumonias) should not be considered to have IPF. Granulomas should not be seen on an IPF biopsy specimen. If they are found, granulomas indicate the presence of another disorder.

From the time of clinical presentation, patients have a relatively poor prognosis; mean survival ranges from 2 to 5 years. Corticosteroids frequently are used to treat patients with IPF. Cytotoxic and other immunosuppressive agents, especially azathioprine or cyclophosphamide, have been used in conjunction with steroids in many cases. Unfortunately, the response of IPF to both steroids and other immunosuppressive agents has generally been poor, with relatively few patients demonstrating significant improvement. As a result, interest has shifted away from suppressing the inflammatory response. Clinical investigators now are focusing on identifying and testing agents that suppress fibrosis or interfere with mediators involved in the fibrotic process. Unfortunately, early enthusiasm for treatment with interferon-γ, which inhibits fibrosis, has not been confirmed in controlled trials. In some patients with severe IPF,

---

Prognosis and response to corticosteroid or other immunosuppressive therapy in idiopathic pulmonary fibrosis is generally poor.

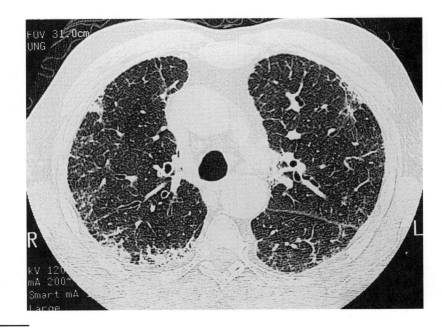

Figure 11-2. High-resolution computed tomographic scan of idiopathic pulmonary fibrosis shows scattered interstitial densities, especially in the subpleural regions.

especially those who are younger, lung transplantation is used as the only therapeutic alternative to progressive respiratory failure and death.

OTHER IDIOPATHIC INTERSTITIAL PNEUMONIAS

Several other disorders besides IPF fall under the category of the idiopathic interstitial pneumonias and have often been confused with IPF. Although these disorders are uncommon, some are briefly described here, largely to clarify how their pathologic features differ from UIP and how their clinical features differ from IPF. They are also mentioned in Chapter 9 as part of the discussion on the pathology of the interstitial pneumonias.

Desquamative interstitial pneumonia (DIP) occurs largely in smokers. It generally has a subacute rather than a chronic onset. Imaging studies with chest radiography and HRCT scanning often show a ground-glass (hazy) pattern. Lung biopsy shows a uniform accumulation of intraalveolar macrophages, with little or no fibrosis. The prognosis is much better than in IPF, and patients often improve after cessation of smoking and respond to corticosteroids.

Nonspecific interstitial pneumonia (NSIP) differs from UIP in its radiographic pattern, histologic appearance, prognosis, and response to treatment. As with DIP, imaging studies often show a ground-glass pattern that reflects inflammation rather than fibrosis. Lung biopsy shows a predominantly inflammatory response in the alveolar walls, with relatively little fibrosis. Although NSIP often is idiopathic and is not associated with any underlying disease or inciting agent, it can represent the histologic appearance of parenchymal lung disease associated with one of the connective tissue diseases or with drug-induced pulmonary toxicity. Based on the prominence of inflammation rather than fibrosis, the prognosis is significantly better than in IPF, and patients often respond to treatment with corticosteroids.

Cryptogenic organizing pneumonia is a disorder characterized by connective tissue plugs in small airways accompanied by mononuclear cell infiltration of the surrounding pulmonary parenchyma. As noted in Chapter 9, the terms *cryptogenic organizing pneumonia* (COP) and *bronchiolitis obliterans with organizing pneumonia* (BOOP) have often been used interchangeably. However, the term BOOP is best reserved for the pathologic picture rather than the clinical syndrome. Although the histologic picture of BOOP can be associated with connective tissue disease, toxic fume inhalation, or infection, the large majority of cases have no identifiable cause and are considered idiopathic. The term COP is most appropriate for patients who have "idiopathic BOOP," that is, the histologic pattern of BOOP but no apparent cause for this pattern

Like chronic eosinophilic pneumonia (see section on chronic eosinophilic pneumonia), COP often has a subacute presentation (over weeks to months) with systemic (constitutional) as well as respiratory symptoms. The chest radiograph shows patchy infiltrates, generally with an alveolar rather than an interstitial pattern, often mimicking a community-acquired pneumonia (Fig. 11-3). Like chronic eosinophilic pneumonia, the response to corticosteroids often is dramatic and occurs over days to weeks. Therapy usually is prolonged for months to prevent relapse.

Acute interstitial pneumonia (AIP) is a more acute or fulminant type of pulmonary parenchymal disease that begins with the clinical picture of acute respiratory distress syndrome (ARDS; see Chapter 28), but without any of the usual inciting events associated with development of ARDS. Imaging studies of AIP typically show features of ARDS, including areas of ground-glass opacification and alveolar filling (as opposed to a purely interstitial pattern). The histologic pattern is that of diffuse alveolar damage, often showing some organization and fibrosis. Although mortality is high overall, some patients do well, with clinical resolution of the disease and no long-term sequelae.

On chest radiograph, bronchiolitis obliterans with organizing pneumonia (BOOP) often mimics a pneumonia, with one or more alveolar infiltrates.

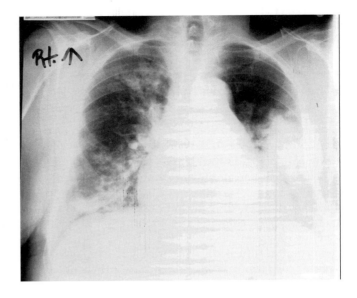

Figure 11-3. Chest radiograph demonstrating patchy alveolar opacities in a patient with bronchiolitis obliterans with organizing pneumonia. The enlarged cardiac silhouette is due to an unrelated cardiomyopathy.

One confusing aspect of the nomenclature of the idiopathic interstitial pneumonias is the relationship underlying AIP, UIP (or IPF), and a disorder called *Hamman-Rich syndrome*. More than 65 years ago, Hamman and Rich described a number of cases of parenchymal lung disease that subsequently were thought to represent the first-described cases of IPF, and for many years the term *Hamman-Rich syndrome* was used synonymously with IPF. However, the cases described by Hamman and Rich now are believed to be cases of AIP rather than IPF, and it is more appropriate that Hamman-Rich syndrome be considered synonymous with AIP rather than either UIP or IPF.

PULMONARY PARENCHYMAL INVOLVEMENT COMPLICATING CONNECTIVE TISSUE DISEASE

The connective tissue diseases, also commonly called *collagen vascular diseases* or *systemic rheumatic diseases,* include rheumatoid arthritis, systemic lupus erythematosus, progressive systemic sclerosis (scleroderma), polymyositis-dermatomyositis, Sjögren's syndrome, and some overlap syndromes that have features of more than one of these disorders. Although they form a diverse group, all are multisystem inflammatory diseases that are mediated immunologically. The organ systems that likely are involved vary with each disease and are mentioned briefly in the following discussion of each entity.

Each disease is complicated and has been the focus of extensive research into etiology and pathogenesis. However, because none of them primarily affects the lung, they are not considered in detail here. Rather, a brief discussion notes how they affect the respiratory system, particularly with regard to development of parenchymal lung disease. Some clinicians include additional disorders among connective tissue diseases, but this discussion is limited to those in the preceding paragraph, each of which has the potential for pulmonary involvement.

Four assertions are true about each of these disorders. First, although patients generally have evidence of the underlying connective tissue disease before pulmonary manifestations develop, some patients have lung disease as the presenting problem, occasionally predating other manifestations of their illness by several years. Second, detailed histologic, physiologic, or autopsy evaluation of patients with these diseases shows that pulmonary involvement is much more common than clinically suspected. Third, the histopathology of interstitial lung disease associated with connective tissue disorders often is that of UIP and therefore is indistinguishable from the pattern seen in IPF. However, in many cases the histopathology demonstrates NSIP rather than UIP. Fourth, the interstitial lung disease that may develop with each of these entities preferentially affects the lower rather than the upper lung zones. This fact usually is apparent on examination of the chest radiograph.

Histologic and physiologic changes suggest that pulmonary involvement in most connective tissue diseases is common, often with a histologic pattern of usual interstitial pneumonia or nonspecific interstitial pneumonia.

Rheumatoid arthritis is a disorder with primary manifestations consisting of inflammatory joint disease. The most common site of involvement within the thorax is the pleura. Involvement takes the form of pleurisy, pleural effusions, or both. The lung parenchyma may become involved, with one or multiple nodules or with development of interstitial lung disease. The latter usually is relatively mild, although severe cases are sometimes seen. Occasionally, patients with rheumatoid arthritis develop airway complications in the form of bronchiolitis (an inflammatory process involving small airways) or bronchiectasis.

In rheumatoid arthritis and lupus, pleural disease is more common than is clinically evident interstitial lung disease.

Systemic lupus erythematosus is a multisystem disease that primarily affects joints and skin but often has more serious involvement of several organ systems, including kidneys, lungs, nervous system, and heart. Its most frequent presentation within the chest takes the form of pleural disease, specifically pleuritic chest pain, pleural effusion, or both. The lung parenchyma may be involved by an acute pneumonitis, in which infiltrates often involve the alveolar spaces as well as the alveolar walls, or less frequently by chronic interstitial lung disease. In the latter, extensive fibrosis usually is not a prominent feature of the histology.

Progressive systemic sclerosis or *scleroderma* is a disease with most obvious manifestations located in the skin and small blood vessels. Other organ systems, including the gastrointestinal tract, lungs, kidneys, and heart, are involved relatively frequently. Of all the connective tissue diseases, scleroderma is the one in which pulmonary involvement tends to be most severe and most likely associated with significant scarring of the pulmonary parenchyma. Pulmonary fibrosis complicating scleroderma appears to be strongly associated with the presence of a particular serologic marker, an autoantibody to topoisomerase I (antitopoisomerase I, also called Scl70). Another potential pulmonary manifestation of scleroderma is disease of the small pulmonary blood vessels producing pulmonary arterial hypertension, which is discussed in Chapter 14. This involvement appears to be independent of the fibrotic process affecting the alveolar walls.

Scleroderma lung disease is notable for interstitial fibrosis. Disease of the small pulmonary vessels may be independent of the interstitial process.

In *polymyositis-dermatomyositis,* muscles and skin are the primary sites of the inflammatory process. The interstitial lung disease of polymyositis-dermatomyositis is relatively infrequent and has no particular distinguishing features. Patients may have respiratory problems as a result of muscle disease, with weakness of the diaphragm or other inspiratory muscles. Involvement of striated muscle in the proximal esophagus may lead to difficulty in swallowing and recurrent episodes of aspiration pneumonia.

In *Sjögren's syndrome,* a lymphocytic infiltration affects salivary and lacrimal glands and is associated with dry mouth and dry eyes (keratoconjunctivitis sicca). When patients with Sjögren's syndrome have pulmonary parenchymal involvement, the histologic appearance is most commonly that of a lymphocytic infiltrate within the alveolar walls (called *lymphocytic interstitial pneumonia*) rather than UIP or NSIP. Other lymphocytic complications of the lung can develop in patients with Sjögren's syndrome, specifically either a localized, masslike lesion called a *pseudolymphoma* or an actual lymphoma.

Finally, a number of overlap syndromes, often called *undifferentiated connective tissue disease,* have features of several of these disorders, particularly scleroderma, lupus, and polymyositis. Patients may develop any of the complications noted with the more classic individual disorders, including interstitial lung disease, pleural disease, and pulmonary vascular disease.

SARCOIDOSIS

Sarcoidosis is defined as a systemic disorder in which granulomas, typically described as noncaseating, can be found in affected tissues or organ systems. An important qualification is that these granulomas occur in the absence of any exogenous (infectious or environmental) agents known to be associated with granulomatous inflammation. The lung is the most frequently involved organ, with potential manifestations including parenchymal lung disease, enlargement of hilar and mediastinal lymph nodes, or both.

Sarcoidosis is a relatively common disorder that particularly affects young adults between the ages of 20 and 40 years. It is slightly more common in women than in men. In the United States it is more common in African-Americans than in whites. However, this racial predilection is not seen throughout the world, as the disease is notably prevalent in the white population of Scandinavia. Although a common stereotype in the United States is that the disease is primarily one of young, African-American women, a substantial number of men and individuals of other ethnic and age groups also are affected. Of all the disorders of unknown cause affecting the alveolar wall, sarcoidosis is clearly the most prevalent.

Despite increasing knowledge about the cells involved in the inflammatory and granulomatous response in sarcoidosis and the identification of multiple cytokines and chemokines that appear to be involved in the pathogenesis of disease, the fundamental etiology of sarcoidosis remains as mysterious as it was when the disease was first described more than a century ago. It has been hypothesized that sarcoidosis represents an immunologic response to an exogenous agent in a genetically susceptible individual. Multiple exogenous antigens and a number of human leukocyte antigens and other candidate genes have been associated with susceptibility to sarcoidosis. However, neither a particular exogenous agent nor a specific genetic susceptibility has been consistently demonstrated. Interest in potential exogenous inciting agents has often focused on microorganisms such as viruses, mycobacteria, and other bacteria (e.g., *Propionibacterium acnes*). However, the identity of an infectious agent as a trigger for sarcoidosis remains elusive, and whether such an infectious agent even exists is not known. At present, it seems most likely that sarcoidosis represents a complex interaction among a number of antigens and the effects of multiple genes.

On the other hand, substantial information is available about cells and mediators that appear to be important in the inflammatory and granulomatous tissue reaction in sarcoidosis (Fig. 11-4). The critical cells are macrophages and T lymphocytes. The presumption is that processing of the responsible antigen by alveolar macrophages results in recruitment of helper T lymphocytes ($CD4^+$ cells) with a T_H1 profile. A host of proinflammatory cytokines and chemokines, such as interleukin-2, interferon-γ, tumor necrosis factor-α (TNF–α), and interleukin-12, appear to be important in recruiting and activating inflammatory cells, perpetuating the inflammatory response, and inducing the formation of granulomas. Profibrotic cytokines, such as TGF–β, PDGF, and insulinlike growth factor-I, subsequently may result in fibrosis as a complication of the initial inflammatory reaction.

Accumulation of $CD4^+$ lymphocytes at sites of active disease appears to result in secondary immunologic phenomena that are well recognized in sarcoidosis. First, presumably because of this concentration of activated lymphocytes in affected tissues, there is a relative depletion of $CD4^+$ cells in peripheral blood. The depletion leads to an apparent depression of cell-mediated immunity, at least as measured by cutaneous

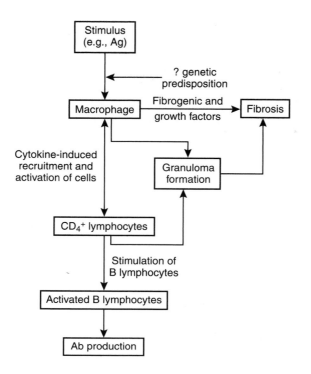

Figure 11-4. Simplified proposed pathogenetic sequence in sarcoidosis.

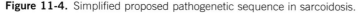

delayed hypersensitivity (skin testing). However, patients with sarcoidosis are not unduly susceptible to opportunistic infections that characteristically affect the immunosuppressed host with impaired cellular immunity. Second, T lymphocytes in sarcoidosis nonspecifically activate B lymphocytes and the humoral immune system, leading to production of a variety of immunoglobulins and the common finding of polyclonal hyperglobulinemia.

The characteristic histopathologic feature of sarcoidosis is the noncaseating granuloma (see Fig. 9-2). These typically well-formed granulomas show a collection of tissue macrophages (also called *epithelioid histiocytes*), multinucleated giant cells, and T lymphocytes, particularly toward the periphery or at the rim of the granuloma. The discrete accumulation of tissue macrophages composing the granuloma does not show evidence of frank necrosis or caseation, as would appear in disorders such as tuberculosis and histoplasmosis. In addition to granulomas in the lung parenchyma or intrathoracic lymph nodes, an alveolitis often occurs. The alveolitis is composed of mononuclear cells, including macrophages and lymphocytes, with the latter presumed to be of particular importance in the pathogenesis of disease.

Patients with sarcoidosis seek consultation most frequently either as a result of abnormalities detected on an incidental chest radiograph or because of respiratory symptoms, mainly dyspnea or a nonproductive cough. Because many other organ systems may be involved with noncaseating granulomas, other manifestations occur but are less common. Eye involvement (e.g., anterior uveitis [inflammation in the anterior chamber of the eye]) and skin involvement (e.g., skin papules or plaques) are particularly common extrathoracic manifestations of sarcoidosis, but cardiac, neurologic, hematologic, hepatic, endocrine, and peripheral lymph node findings also may be seen. Although symptoms often are insidious in onset, some patients with sarcoidosis have a more acute presentation called *Löfgren's syndrome,* in which the chest radiographic finding of bilateral hilar lymphadenopathy is accompanied by erythema nodosum (painful red

The characteristic pathologic feature of sarcoidosis is the noncaseating granuloma. An alveolitis composed primarily of mononuclear cells may occur.

nodules, typically on the anterior surface of the lower legs) and often fever and arthralgias. For unknown reasons, patients who present with Löfgren's syndrome typically have an excellent prognosis with a spontaneous remission rate greater than 80%.

The chest radiograph in sarcoidosis generally shows one of the following patterns: (1) enlargement of lymph nodes, most commonly bilateral hilar lymphadenopathy, with or without paratracheal node enlargement (Fig. 11-5); (2) parenchymal lung disease (in the form of interstitial disease, nodules, or alveolar infiltrates); or (3) both adenopathy and parenchymal disease (Fig. 11-6). HRCT scanning, although not generally necessary, is more sensitive than plain chest radiography in detecting parenchymal lung disease. It may show a particularly characteristic pattern of small nodules preferentially distributed along bronchovascular bundles (Fig. 11-7). In addition, HRCT often demonstrates mediastinal lymphadenopathy that cannot be seen on plain chest radiography.

The course of the radiographic findings in sarcoidosis is quite variable. Over time, both the adenopathy and the interstitial lung disease may regress spontaneously. At the other extreme, the interstitial disease may progress to a condition of extensive scarring and end-stage lung disease, at which time the patient has severe respiratory compromise.

Patients often display immune system abnormalities. Clinically, these patients may have anergy, that is, failure to respond to skin tests requiring intact delayed hypersensitivity. They also may have hyperglobulinemia, which is evidence of a hyperactive humoral immune system. Calcium metabolism may be abnormal in sarcoidosis, occurring as a result of increased formation of the active form of vitamin D (1,25-dihydroxy-D_3) by activated macrophages in granulomas. Increased amounts of the active form of

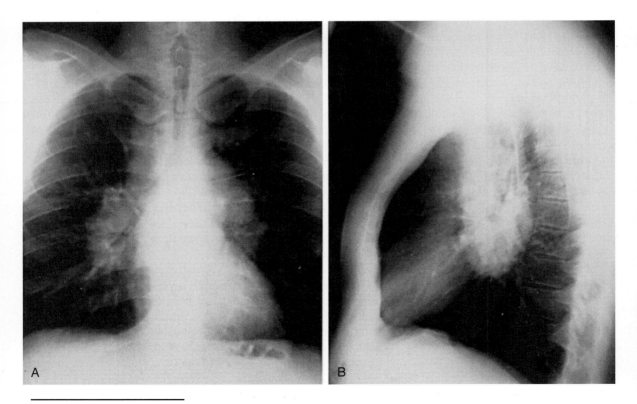

Figure 11-5. Radiographic appearance of stage I sarcoidosis shows bilateral hilar and paratracheal adenopathy. Enlarged nodes can be seen on posteroanterior *(A)* and lateral *(B)* views.

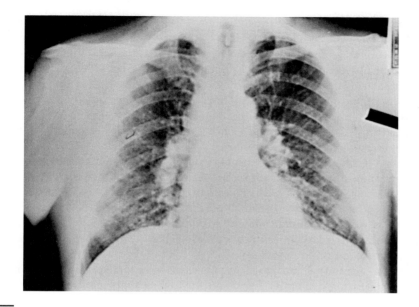

Figure 11-6. Chest radiograph shows characteristic features of stage II sarcoidosis: bilateral hilar adenopathy and diffuse interstitial lung disease. In stage III sarcoidosis (not shown), patients have diffuse interstitial lung disease without hilar adenopathy.

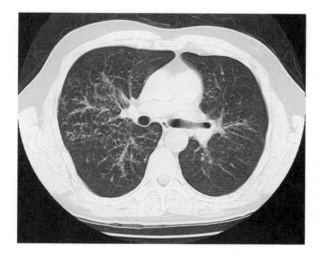

Figure 11-7. Chest computed tomographic scan demonstrates a micronodular pattern in a patient with sarcoidosis.

vitamin D lead to enhanced calcium absorption from the gastrointestinal tract, potentially causing hypercalciuria or, less frequently, hypercalcemia.

The diagnosis of sarcoidosis can be established in several ways. When the clinical diagnosis strongly suggests sarcoidosis, tissue confirmation is sometimes unnecessary. An example of such a presentation is bilateral hilar lymphadenopathy found on an incidental chest radiograph in a symptom-free young African-American woman. On the other hand, when the patient has symptoms or when there is a question about the diagnosis, tissue sampling usually is undertaken to look for noncaseating granulomas and to rule out other causes. The lung is generally the most appropriate source of tissue. Samples of lung tissue are frequently obtained by transbronchial biopsy through a flexible bronchoscope. Interestingly, even when the chest radiograph shows only hilar adenopathy without obvious parenchymal lung disease, the alveolar walls usually are studded with granulomas that may be seen on transbronchial lung biopsy. Other ways of obtaining tissue include performing a biopsy of a lymph node in the mediastinum (via mediastinoscopy) or a thoracoscopic lung biopsy. In addition, biopsy specimens can be obtained easily from involved areas of skin (when skin involvement is suspected on physical examination). Occasionally they are obtained from a variety of other involved tissues or organs, such as peripheral lymph nodes, conjunctiva, minor salivary glands, or liver.

> In sarcoidosis, transbronchial lung biopsy through a fiberoptic bronchoscope usually demonstrates granulomas in the lung parenchyma, even when the chest radiograph does not show interstitial lung disease.

Elevated serum levels of angiotensin-converting enzyme (ACE) have been found in a large percentage of patients with sarcoidosis. This enzyme, which normally is synthesized by vascular endothelial cells, appears to be produced in the granulomas of sarcoidosis, suggesting it may be useful for diagnosing or following the disease. However, because it is not specific for sarcoidosis and often is normal in the presence of relatively inactive disease, ACE levels are not considered reliable in either diagnosing sarcoidosis or assessing its response to treatment.

The natural history of sarcoidosis is quite variable. In some patients, all clinical and radiographic manifestations resolve within 1 to 2 years. Other patients have persistent radiographic changes, either with or without persisting symptoms. In general, nearly two thirds of patients have spontaneous remissions. A minority of patients (10%–30%) show continued progression of radiographic abnormalities, with or without additional extrathoracic disease, and may have debilitating respiratory symptoms. Clinical factors associated with a worse prognosis include age at onset greater than 40 years, African descent, chronic uveitis, chronic hypercalcemia, progressive pulmonary parenchymal fibrosis, and the presence of lupus pernio, a skin lesion affecting the face.

Pulmonary function tests are most useful for quantitating functional impairment. Spirometry, lung volumes, and diffusing capacity all are measured. Techniques for assessing the alveolitis, such as gallium scanning and bronchoalveolar lavage, have been investigated but presently are not thought to provide clinically useful information regarding the "activity" of the disease. Therefore, these techniques are not widely accepted for clinical use in evaluating sarcoidosis.

> The variable natural history of sarcoidosis often makes decisions about use of corticosteroids difficult.

The initial treatment decision confronting the clinician is whether or not to institute therapy for the patient with sarcoidosis. Many patients do not require treatment, especially when the disease is causing neither significant symptoms nor significant functional organ involvement. The fact that the disease may improve or resolve spontaneously also complicates decisions about instituting therapy. When treatment is indicated because of symptoms and significant tissue involvement affecting organ function, the drug of choice usually is systemic corticosteroids. In patients with refractory disease, a variety of other agents, especially immunosuppressive drugs such as methotrexate and cyclophosphamide, have been used, either with or instead of corticosteroids. More recently, there has been interest in using infliximab, an antagonist of TNF-α, in selected cases, but its ultimate potential role in treating sarcoidosis is uncertain.

MISCELLANEOUS DISORDERS INVOLVING THE PULMONARY PARENCHYMA

An exhaustive description of all the remaining diseases of unknown etiology affecting the pulmonary parenchyma cannot be presented here. Instead, a brief description of several additional diseases will acquaint the reader with their major features. They include (1) pulmonary Langerhans cell histiocytosis, (2) lymphangioleiomyomatosis, (3) Goodpasture's syndrome, (4) Wegener's granulomatosis, (5) chronic eosinophilic pneumonia, and (6) pulmonary alveolar proteinosis. For each of these relatively uncommon disorders, certain pathologic, clinical, or radiographic features distinguish them from the diffuse parenchymal lung diseases described earlier in this chapter. However, the defining feature for each of these disorders is a relatively specific pathologic appearance involving various components of the pulmonary parenchyma.

PULMONARY LANGERHANS CELL HISTIOCYTOSIS

Pulmonary Langerhans cell histiocytosis, also called *eosinophilic granuloma of the lung* or *pulmonary histiocytosis X,* is thought to represent part of a spectrum of disorders involving histiocytic infiltration of one or more organ systems. Whereas multisystem involvement in Langerhans cell histiocytosis or histiocytosis X is typically seen with the childhood disorders called *Letterer-Siwe disease* or *Hand-Schüller-Christian disease* (which are not discussed here), isolated or predominant pulmonary involvement in pulmonary Langerhans cell histiocytosis occurs mainly in young to middle-aged adults.

Pulmonary Langerhans cell histiocytosis (also called eosinophilic granuloma of the lung or histiocytosis X) enters into the differential diagnosis of unexplained interstitial disease, particularly in the young or middle-aged adult.

The responsible histiocytic cell appears to be a type of antigen-presenting dendritic or phagocytic cell called a *Langerhans cell.* An interesting ultrastructural feature of these cells is the presence of cytoplasmic rodlike structures called *X bodies* (hence the name histiocytosis X) or Birbeck granules, which can be seen by electron microscopy. Light microscopic examination of the lung, in addition to demonstration of these histiocytes, reveals infiltration by eosinophils, lymphocytes, macrophages, and plasma cells. The process initially involves the lungs in a peribronchiolar distribution and subsequently becomes more diffuse. Although the disease occurs almost exclusively in smokers, the mechanism by which smoking may cause the disease or contribute to its pathogenesis is not well defined.

On chest radiograph, the clinical presentation of pulmonary Langerhans cell histiocytosis typically features a pattern of nodular or reticulonodular disease often accompanied by respiratory symptoms of dyspnea, cough, or both. The radiographic findings tend to be more prominent in the upper lung zones, with HRCT scans showing small cysts in addition to the nodular or reticulonodular changes. The cysts occasionally rupture, leading to a spontaneous pneumothorax, which may be the presenting feature of the disease. In some cases, progression results in a pattern of extensive cystic disease and honeycombing. Unlike the typical restrictive pattern in most of the diffuse parenchymal lung diseases, pulmonary function testing in pulmonary Langerhans cell histiocytosis may show restrictive changes, obstructive changes, or both. The presence of air-filled cysts typically leads to unusually normal or large lung volumes on chest radiography despite the presence of interstitial disease.

The natural history of the disease is variable. In some patients the disease is self-limited, and the radiographic and functional changes may stabilize over time, especially with cessation of smoking. In other patients, extensive disease and significant functional impairment follow. No clearly effective treatment is available, although corticosteroids are often tried if smoking cessation alone is ineffective.

LYMPHANGIOLEIOMYOMATOSIS

Lymphangioleiomyomatosis is a rare pulmonary disease characterized by proliferation of atypical smooth muscle cells around lymphatics, blood vessels, and airways, accompanied by numerous small cysts throughout the pulmonary parenchyma. It occurs almost exclusively in women of childbearing age, suggesting that hormonal influences play a role in the development of disease. An interesting aspect is that the pathologic process in lymphangioleiomyomatosis is essentially identical to that seen in tuberous sclerosis complex (TSC), suggesting a common pathogenetic mechanism. Mutations in the two genes TSC1 and TSC2 are associated with TSC, although in most cases of

Lymphangioleiomyomatosis is characterized by proliferation of atypical smooth muscle cells within the lung.

lymphangioleiomyomatosis the abnormal smooth muscle cells have a mutation in the TSC2 gene.

The normal products of TSC1 and TSC2 are proteins that form a complex that acts as a potent suppressor of cell growth and proliferation. Thus, the abnormal proteins lead to loss of this suppressor activity, resulting in uncontrolled growth. Patients with lymphangioleiomyomatosis appear to have developed an acquired mutation in smooth muscle cells in the lung, whereas patients with TSC appear to have an inborn genetic error. Furthermore, the gene product of TSC2 also interacts directly with intracellular estrogen receptors to cause inhibition of cell growth. This may account for some of the hormonal influences in lymphangioleiomyomatosis.

The clinical manifestations of lymphangioleiomyomatosis result from the presence of cysts and the involvement of lymphatics, blood vessels, and airways. The overall pathologic process in the pulmonary parenchyma may lead to dyspnea and cough. Vascular involvement may result in hemoptysis, lymphatic obstruction may produce chylous (milky appearing) pleural effusions, and airway involvement may produce airflow obstruction. Rupture of subpleural cysts can lead to development of a spontaneous pneumothorax.

The chest radiograph typically shows a reticular pattern, and cystic changes may be seen. HRCT scanning is much better than plain chest radiography for demonstrating cystic disease throughout the pulmonary parenchyma. The mechanism of cyst formation is thought to be a combination of a ball-valve phenomenon resulting from small airway obstruction by the abnormal smooth muscle proliferation and destruction of tissue attributable to elaboration of metalloproteinases by lymphangioleiomyomatosis cells. As is true for pulmonary Langerhans cell histiocytosis, results of pulmonary function testing are not typical of most diffuse parenchymal diseases because patients may demonstrate obstructive disease, restrictive disease, or both. Similarly, lung volumes on chest radiograph appear normal or increased rather than decreased.

Because of the hormonal dependence of the disease, treatment has focused on hormonal manipulation, most commonly with either oophorectomy or administration of progesterone. However, better understanding of the role of the TSC2 gene has led to clinical trials of the drug sirolimus. This drug is an inhibitor of cell growth and proliferation through the same pathway as the TSC1 and TSC2 gene products, and it is hoped that this will act in place of the defective proteins.

GOODPASTURE'S SYNDROME

Goodpasture's syndrome is a disease that has become well known not because of its incidence, which is extremely low, but because of its interesting pathogenetic and immunologic features. Two organ systems are involved in this syndrome: the lungs and the kidneys. In the lungs, patients have episodes of pulmonary hemorrhage, and pulmonary fibrosis may develop, presumably as a consequence of the recurrent episodes of bleeding. In the kidneys, patients have a glomerulonephritis characterized by linear deposits of antibody along the glomerular basement membrane. Studies on peripheral blood have demonstrated that patients have circulating antibodies against a component of type IV collagen in their own glomerular basement membrane (GBM), often abbreviated anti-GBM antibodies. It is believed that these antibodies cross-react with the basement membrane of the alveolar wall and that their deposition in the kidney and lung is responsible for the clinical manifestations of the disease.

In Goodpasture's syndrome, autoantibodies directed against the glomerular basement membrane may cross-react with the basement membrane of alveolar walls.

Why these true autoantibodies develop in patients with Goodpasture's syndrome is not clear. In some patients, onset of disease appears to follow influenza infection or exposure to a toxic hydrocarbon. Presumably, injury to basement membranes and release of previously unexposed antigenic determinants are involved, or incidental formation of antibodies (against an unrelated antigen) may cross-react with alveolar and glomerular basement membranes. The disease is associated with certain human leukocyte antigens (HLA-DRw2 and HLA-B7), indicating an underlying genetic susceptibility.

Unlike many diseases associated with autoantibodies, the anti-GBM antibodies are clearly pathogenetic. Therapy for Goodpasture's syndrome is based on decreasing the burden of anti-GBM antibodies presented to the lung and kidney. Plasmapheresis is capable of directly removing anti-GBM antibodies from the circulation. Immunosuppressive therapy (e.g., prednisone plus cyclophosphamide), aimed at decreasing the formation of anti-GBM antibodies, usually is given in conjunction with plasmapheresis.

WEGENER'S GRANULOMATOSIS

A group of disorders termed the *granulomatous vasculitides* may affect the alveolar wall as part of a more generalized disease. The most well known of these disorders is *Wegener's granulomatosis,* a disease characterized primarily but not exclusively by involvement of the upper respiratory tract, lungs, and kidneys. The pathologic process in the lungs and upper respiratory tract consists of a necrotizing, small-vessel granulomatous vasculitis, whereas a focal glomerulonephritis is present in the kidney. On chest radiograph, patients commonly have one or several nodules (often large) or infiltrates, often with associated cavitation of the lesion(s) (Fig. 11-8). Unlike most of the other disorders of the pulmonary parenchyma discussed in Chapter 10 and this chapter, diffuse interstitial lung disease is not the characteristic radiographic finding in this entity.

Patients with Wegener's granulomatosis typically have antibodies in the serum directed against proteinase 3, a serine protease that is present in the azurophil granules found in the cytoplasm of neutrophils. These antibodies can be detected by immunofluorescent techniques, which demonstrate a coarse, diffuse cytoplasmic pattern of

> Wegener's granulomatosis is characterized pathologically by granulomatous vasculitis of the lung and upper respiratory tract and by glomerulonephritis. The clinical corollary is pulmonary, upper respiratory tract, and renal disease.

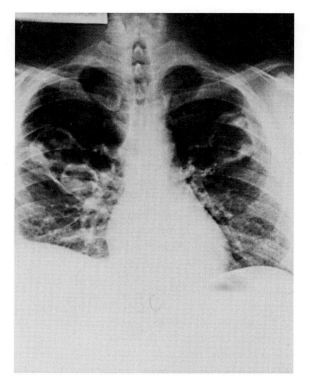

Figure 11-8. Chest radiograph shows multiple cavitary pulmonary nodules in patient with Wegener's granulomatosis.

staining when the patient's serum is incubated with normal neutrophils. The presence of antineutrophil cytoplasmic antibodies (ANCA), specifically with a cytoplasmic staining pattern (c-ANCA), has become an important component of the diagnostic evaluation for Wegener's granulomatosis, although the sensitivity of the test has varied considerably in different series. Antibody levels correlate with disease activity, and these antibodies likely play some role in the pathogenesis of disease. However, other factors probably are involved as well.

Although Wegener's granulomatosis once was considered an aggressive and fatal disease, its prognosis has improved dramatically since cytotoxic agents, specifically cyclophosphamide, have been used in its treatment. Prednisone is also generally added for the initial period of therapy. Whereas the mean survival time without treatment was 5 months, patients are achieving complete and long-term remissions with institution of appropriate therapy. Some data support the use of the combination antibiotic trimethoprim–sulfamethoxazole, either for treatment of selected patients or for prevention of relapse following successful immunosuppressive therapy. The mechanism is uncertain but may involve a reduction in nasal carriage of *Staphylococcus*, which has been associated with flares. The meaning of this finding in terms of pathogenesis of the disease is unclear, as is the place of this less toxic therapy in the overall strategy for management.

CHRONIC EOSINOPHILIC PNEUMONIA

Chronic eosinophilic pneumonia is a disorder in which the pulmonary interstitium and alveolar spaces are infiltrated primarily by eosinophils and, to a lesser extent, by macrophages. The clinical presentation typically occurs over weeks to months, with systemic symptoms such as fever and weight loss accompanying dyspnea and a nonproductive cough. The clues suggesting this diagnosis are often found on the chest radiograph and the routine white blood cell differential count. The radiograph frequently shows pulmonary infiltrates with a peripheral distribution and a pattern more suggestive of alveolar filling than interstitial disease (Fig. 11-9). Because the typical radiographic pattern of pulmonary edema with congestive heart failure has central pulmonary infiltrates with sparing of the lung periphery, the prominent peripheral pattern often seen in chronic eosinophilic pneumonia has been described as the "photographic negative of pulmonary edema." The majority of patients also have increased numbers of eosinophils in peripheral blood, although this finding is not uniformly present and therefore is not critical for the diagnosis. However, bronchoalveolar lavage typically shows a high percentage of eosinophils, reflecting the pathologic process within the pulmonary parenchyma.

> Chronic eosinophilic pneumonia is often suggested on chest radiograph by a pattern of peripheral pulmonary infiltrates.

Treatment is gratifying to patient and physician alike, because chronic eosinophilic pneumonia characteristically shows a dramatic response to corticosteroid therapy. Clinical improvement and radiographic resolution generally occur within days to weeks, although therapy often must be prolonged for months to prevent recurrence.

PULMONARY ALVEOLAR PROTEINOSIS

Pulmonary alveolar proteinosis (PAP) is a parenchymal lung disease in which the primary pathologic process affects the alveolar spaces, not the alveolar walls. Alveolar spaces are filled with a proteinaceous phospholipid material that represents components of pulmonary surfactant. The accumulation of surfactant components is due to either decreased degradation or surfactant dysfunction. PAP is classified as primary, secondary (usually related to hematologic malignancies), or congenital. Primary PAP is by far the most common of the three types and is discussed here.

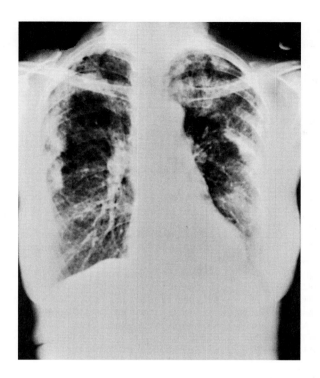

Figure 11-9. Chest radiograph shows pattern of peripheral pulmonary infiltrates characteristic of chronic eosinophilic pneumonia.

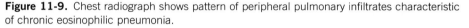

Many aspects of the pathogenesis of primary PAP have been elucidated. In most cases the underlying problem has been identified as the production of an autoantibody to granulocyte-macrophage colony-stimulating factor (GM-CSF). The first clues that GM-CSF was involved came from the discovery that GM-CSF knockout mice (in which both alleles for GM-CSF are disabled) consistently develop a pulmonary process with pathology that is essentially identical to that seen with PAP in humans. GM-CSF, acting through alveolar macrophage-specific transcription factors, regulates a number of essential macrophage functions, including regulation of surfactant degradation, intracellular lipid metabolism, and phagocytosis. Thus, inhibiting the activity of GM-CSF via autoantibodies leads to decreased clearance of surfactant from the alveolar spaces.

An animal model suggests that defective uptake of surfactant by alveolar macrophages, attributable to a decreased amount or effect of GM-CSF, may underlie the pathogenesis of pulmonary alveolar proteinosis.

Patients with alveolar proteinosis present primarily with dyspnea and cough. The chest radiograph is notable for bilateral alveolar infiltrates. HRCT generally shows a distinctive pattern that suggests the diagnosis, called a "crazy paving" pattern (produced by thickening of interlobular septa accompanied by ground-glass alveolar filling). Patients are susceptible to certain types of superimposed respiratory infections that are uncommon in normal hosts, especially with the organism *Nocardia*. The susceptibility to unusual pathogens probably is due to abnormal macrophage function as well as to more recently discovered abnormalities in neutrophil function also mediated by GM-CSF.

Treatment of PAP traditionally has been based on whole-lung lavage, which involves washing out the material filling the alveolar spaces while the patient is under general anesthesia. Preliminary studies suggest that administration of exogenous GM-CSF may be an alternative therapy. The prognosis of the disease is generally relatively good, although patients may require additional treatments with whole-lung lavage. The long-term effects of exogenous GM-CSF in this disease are unknown.

REFERENCES

IDIOPATHIC PULMONARY FIBROSIS

American Thoracic Society and European Respiratory Society: American Thoracic Society/European Respiratory Society international multidisciplinary consensus classification of the idiopathic interstitial pneumonias, *Am J Respir Crit Care Med* 165:277–304, 2002.

American Thoracic Society and European Respiratory Society: Idiopathic pulmonary fibrosis: diagnosis and treatment, *Am J Respir Crit Care Med* 161:646–664, 2000.

British Thoracic Society: The diagnosis, assessment and treatment of diffuse parenchymal lung disease in adults, *Thorax* 54(suppl):S1–S30, 1999.

Costabel U, King TE: International consensus statement on idiopathic pulmonary fibrosis, *Eur Respir J* 17:163–167, 2001.

Daniels CE, Ryu JH: Treatment of idiopathic pulmonary fibrosis, *Semin Respir Crit Care Med* 27:668–676, 2006.

Dempey OJ, Kerr KM, Gomersall L, Rennen H, Currie GP: Idiopathic pulmonary fibrosis: an update, *Q J Med* 99:643–654, 2006.

Gross TJ, Hunninghake GW: Idiopathic pulmonary fibrosis, *N Engl J Med* 345:517–525, 2001.

Lynch JP 3rd, Saggar R, Weigt SS, Zisman DA, White ES: Usual interstitial pneumonia, *Semin Respir Crit Care Med* 27:634–651, 2006.

Maher TM, Wells AV, Laurent GJ: Idiopathic pulmonary fibrosis: multiple causes and multiple mechanisms? *Eur Respir J* 30:835–839, 2007.

Selman M, King TE Jr, Pardo A: Idiopathic pulmonary fibrosis: prevailing and evolving hypotheses about its pathogenesis and implications for therapy, *Ann Intern Med* 134:136–151, 2001.

Selman M, Pardo A: Role of epithelial cells in idiopathic pulmonary fibrosis: from innocent targets to serial killers, *Proc Am Thorac Soc* 3:364–372, 2006.

Walter N, Collard HR, King TE Jr: Current perspectives on the treatment of idiopathic pulmonary fibrosis, *Proc Am Thorac Soc* 3:330–338, 2006.

OTHER IDIOPATHIC INTERSTITIAL PNEUMONIAS

American Thoracic Society and European Respiratory Society: American Thoracic Society/European Respiratory Society international multidisciplinary consensus classification of the idiopathic interstitial pneumonias, *Am J Respir Crit Care Med* 165:277–304, 2002.

Bouros D, Nicholson AC, Polychronopoulos V, du Bois RM: Acute interstitial pneumonia, *Eur Respir J* 15:412–418, 2000.

Caminati A, Harari S: Smoking-related interstitial pneumonias and pulmonary Langerhans cell histiocytosis, *Proc Am Thorac Soc* 3:299–306, 2006.

Collard HR, King TE Jr: Demystifying idiopathic interstitial pneumonia, *Arch Intern Med* 163:17–29, 2003.

Cordier JF: Cryptogenic organizing pneumonia, *Clin Chest Med* 25:727–738, 2004.

Epler GR: Bronchiolitis obliterans organizing pneumonia, *Arch Intern Med* 161:158–164, 2001.

Kinder BW, Collard HR, Koth L, et al: Idiopathic nonspecific interstitial pneumonia: lung manifestation of undifferentiated connective tissue disease? *Am J Respir Crit Care Med* 176:691–697, 2007.

Visscher DW, Myers, JL: Histologic spectrum of idiopathic interstitial pneumonias, *Proc Am Thorac Soc* 3:322–329, 2006.

Young DA, Cherniack RM, King TE, Schwarz MI: Acute interstitial pneumonitis. Case series and review of the literature, *Medicine* 79:369–378, 2000.

PULMONARY PARENCHYMAL INVOLVEMENT COMPLICATING CONNECTIVE TISSUE DISEASE

Gochuico BR: Potential pathogenesis and clinical aspects of pulmonary fibrosis associated with rheumatoid arthritis, *Am J Med Sci* 321:83–88, 2001.

Grutters JC, Wells AU, Wuyts W, et al: Evaluation and treatment of interstitial lung involvement in connective tissue diseases: a clinical update, *Eur Respir Mon* 34:27–49, 2006.

Keane MP, Lynch JP: Pleuropulmonary manifestations of systemic lupus erythematosus, *Thorax* 55:159–166, 2000.

Minai OA, Dweik RA, Arroliga AC: Manifestations of scleroderma pulmonary disease, *Clin Chest Med* 19:713–731, 1998.

Schwarz MI: The lung in polymyositis, *Clin Chest Med* 19:701–712, 1998.

Strange C, Highland KB: Interstitial lung disease in the patient who has connective tissue disease, *Clin Chest Med* 25:549–559, 2004.

Swigris JJ, Fischer A, Gilles J, Meehan RT, Brown KK: Pulmonary and thrombotic manifestations of systemic lupus erythematosus, *Chest* 133:271–280, 2008.

Westhovens R, De Keyser F, van den Hoogen FHJ, et al: The clinical spectrum and pathogenesis of pulmonary manifestations in connective tissue diseases, *Eur Respir Mon* 34:1–26, 2006.

SARCOIDOSIS

American Thoracic Society: Statement on sarcoidosis, *Am J Respir Crit Care Med* 160:736–755, 1999.

Drent M, Costabel U: Sarcoidosis, *Eur Respir Mon* 10(monograph 32):1–341, 2005.

Gibson GJ: Sarcoidosis: old and new treatments, *Thorax* 56:336–339, 2001.

Iannuzzi MC, Rybicki BA, Teirstein AS: Sarcoidosis, *N Engl J Med* 357:2153–2165, 2007.

Johns CJ, Michele TM: The clinical management of sarcoidosis. A 50-year experience at the Johns Hopkins Hospital, *Medicine* 78:65–111, 1999.

Lynch JP 3rd, Ma YL, Koss MN, White ES: Pulmonary sarcoidosis, *Semin Respir Crit Care Med* 28:53–74, 2007.

Mandel J, Weinberger SE: Clinical insights and basic science correlates in sarcoidosis, *Am J Med Sci* 321: 99–107, 2001.

Paramothayan S, Jones PW: Corticosteroid therapy in pulmonary sarcoidosis. A systematic review, *JAMA* 287:1301–1307, 2002.

Weinberger SE: Clinical crossroads: a 47-year-old woman with sarcoidosis, *JAMA* 296:2133–2140, 2006.

Zissel G, Prasse A, Muller-Quernheim J: Sarcoidosis—immunopathogenetic concepts, *Semin Respir Crit Care Med* 28:3–14, 2007.

MISCELLANEOUS DISORDERS INVOLVING THE PULMONARY PARENCHYMA

Ball JA, Young KR: Pulmonary manifestations of Goodpasture's syndrome. Antiglomerular basement membrane disease and related disorders, *Clin Chest Med* 19:777–791, 1998.

Carsillo T, Astrinidis A, Henske EP: Mutations in the tuberous sclerosis complex gene TSC2 are a cause of sporadic pulmonary lymphangioleiomyomatosis, *Proc Natl Acad Sci U S A* 97:6085–6090, 2000.

Collard HR, Schwarz MI: Diffuse alveolar hemorrhage, *Clin Chest Med* 25:583–592, 2004.

Cordier J-F: Organising pneumonia, *Thorax* 55:318–328, 2000.

Costabel U, Guzman J: Alveolar proteinosis, *Eur Respir Mon* 5(monograph 14):194–205, 2000.

Cottin V, Cordier JF: Eosinophilic pneumonias, *Allergy* 60:841–857, 2005.

Doershuk CM: Pulmonary alveolar proteinosis—is host defense awry? *N Engl J Med* 356:547–549, 2007.

Frankel SK, Cosgrove GP, Fischer A, Meehan RT, Brown KK: Update in the diagnosis and management of pulmonary vasculitis, *Chest* 129:452–465, 2006.

Juvet SC, McCormack FX, Kwiatkowski DJ, Downey GP: Molecular pathogenesis of lymphangioleiomyomatosis: lessons learned from orphans, *Am J Respir Cell Mol Biol* 36:398–408, 2007.

Langford CA, Hoffman GS: Wegener's granulomatosis, *Thorax* 54:629–637, 1999.

Langford CA, Sneller MC: Update on the diagnosis and treatment of Wegener's granulomatosis, *Adv Intern Med* 46:177–206, 2001.

Lin FC, Chang GD, Chern MS, Chen YC, Chang SC: Clinical significance of anti-GM-CSF antibodies in idiopathic pulmonary alveolar proteinosis, *Thorax* 61:528–534, 2006.

Marchand E, Cordier JF: Idiopathic chronic eosinophilic pneumonia, *Semin Respir Crit Care Med* 27: 134–141, 2006

Shah PL, Hansell D, Lawson PR, Reid KB, Morgan C: Pulmonary alveolar proteinosis: clinical aspects and current concepts on pathogenesis, *Thorax* 55:67–77, 2000.

Strizheva GD, Carsillo T, Kruger WD, Sullivan EJ, Ryu JH, Henske EP: The spectrum of mutations in TSC1 and TSC2 in women with tuberous sclerosis and lymphangioleiomyomatosis, *Am J Respir Crit Care Med* 163:253–258, 2001.

Sullivan EJ: Lymphangioleiomyomatosis. A review, *Chest* 114:1689–1703, 1998.

Tazi A, Soler P, Hance AJ: Adult pulmonary Langerhans' cell histiocytosis, *Thorax* 55:405–416, 2000.

Vassallo R, Ryu JH, Colby TV, Hartman T, Limper AH: Pulmonary Langerhans'-cell histiocytosis, *N Engl J Med* 342:1969–1978, 2000.

Vassallo R, Schroeder DR, Decker PA, Limper AH: Clinical outcomes of pulmonary Langerhans'-cell histiocytosis in adults, *N Engl J Med* 346:484–490, 2002.

Venkateshiah SB, Yan TD, Bonfield TL, et al: An open-label trial of granulocyte macrophage colony stimulating factor therapy for moderate symptomatic pulmonary alveolar proteinosis, *Chest* 130:227–237, 2006.

12

Anatomic and Physiologic Aspects of the Pulmonary Vasculature

The pulmonary vasculature is responsible for transporting deoxygenated blood to the alveoli and then carrying freshly oxygenated blood back to the left atrium and ventricle for pumping to the peripheral tissues. Although the pulmonary circulation is often called the "lesser circulation," the lungs are the only organ system that receives the entire cardiac output. This extensive system of pulmonary vessels is susceptible to a variety of disease processes, ranging from those that primarily affect the vasculature to those that are either secondary to airway or pulmonary parenchymal disease or due to transport of material that is foreign to the pulmonary vessels, including blood clots.

Before diseases of the pulmonary vasculature are considered in Chapters 13 and 14, this chapter discusses a few of the general anatomic and physiologic aspects of the pulmonary vessels. Included in the discussion on physiology are several topics relating to hemodynamics of the pulmonary circulation as well as a brief consideration of some nonrespiratory, metabolic functions of the pulmonary circulation.

ANATOMY

In contrast to the systemic arteries, which carry blood from the left ventricle to the rest of the body, the pulmonary arteries are relatively thin-walled vessels that normally do not need to withstand particularly high intraluminal pressures. The pulmonary trunk, which carries the outflow from the right ventricle, divides almost immediately into the right and left main pulmonary arteries, which subsequently divide into smaller branches. Throughout these progressive divisions, the pulmonary arteries and their branches travel with companion airways, following closely the course of the progressively dividing bronchial tree. By the time the vessels are considered arterioles, the outer diameter is less than approximately 0.1 mm. An important feature of the smaller pulmonary arteries is the presence of smooth muscle within the walls that is responsible for the vasoconstrictive response to various stimuli, particularly hypoxia.

The pulmonary capillaries form an extensive network of communicating channels coursing through alveolar walls. Rather than being described as a series of separate vessels, the capillary system has been described as a continuous meshwork or sheet bounded by alveolar walls on each side and interrupted by "posts" of connective tissue, akin to the appearance of an underground parking garage. The capillaries are in close proximity to alveolar gas, separated only by alveolar epithelial cells and a small amount of interstitium present in some regions of the alveolar wall (see Figs. 8-1 and 8-2). Overall, the capillary surface area is approximately 125 m^2 and represents approximately 85% of the available alveolar surface area.

The design of this capillary system is extraordinarily well suited to the requirements of gas exchange, inasmuch as it contains an enormous effective surface area of contact between pulmonary capillaries and alveolar gas. The pulmonary veins, which are responsible for transporting oxygenated blood from the pulmonary capillaries to the left atrium, progressively combine into larger vessels until four major pulmonary veins enter the left atrium. Unlike the pulmonary arteries and their branches, the pulmonary venous system does not follow the course of the corresponding bronchial structures until the level of the hilum.

The bronchial arteries, which are part of the systemic circulation, provide nutrient blood flow to a variety of nonalveolar structures, such as the bronchi and the visceral pleural surface. Generally, a single bronchial artery of variable origin (upper right intercostal, right subclavian, or internal mammary artery) supplies the right lung. Two bronchial arteries, usually arising from the thoracic aorta, supply the left lung. Venous blood from the large, extrapulmonary airways drains via bronchial veins into the azygos vein and eventually into the right atrium. In contrast, venous blood from intrapulmonary airways drains into the pulmonary venous system, eventually providing a small amount of anatomic shunting of desaturated blood to the systemic arterial circulation.

An extensive network of lymphatic channels is also located primarily within the connective tissue sheaths around small vessels and airways. Although these channels do not generally course through the interstitial tissue of the alveolar walls, they are in sufficiently close proximity to be effective at removing liquid and some solutes that constantly pass into the interstitium of the alveolar wall.

PHYSIOLOGY

PULMONARY VASCULAR RESISTANCE

Although the pulmonary circulation handles the same cardiac output from the right ventricle as the systemic circulation handles from the left ventricle, the former operates under much lower pressures and has substantially less resistance to flow than does the latter. The systolic and diastolic pressures in the pulmonary artery normally are approximately 25 and 10 mm Hg, respectively, in contrast to 120 and 80 mm Hg in the systemic arteries. The pulmonary vascular resistance (PVR) can be calculated according to Equation 12-1:

$$R = \text{Change in pressure/Flow} \qquad (12\text{-}1)$$

The change or drop in pressure across the pulmonary circuit is the mean pulmonary artery pressure (mPA) minus the mean left atrial pressure (mLA), and the flow is the cardiac output (CO). Thus:

$$PVR = (mPA - mLA)/CO \qquad (12\text{-}2)$$

Left atrial pressure is difficult to measure directly, but a reasonably accurate indirect assessment can be made by measuring the pulmonary artery occlusion pressure or

Pulmonary vascular resistance = (Mean PA pressure − Mean LA pressure)/cardiac output. LA pressure is indirectly determined from occluded PA pressure.

"back" pressure in the pulmonary artery when forward flow has been occluded. A special catheter designed for this purpose, called a *pulmonary artery balloon occlusion catheter,* or *Swan-Ganz catheter,* has been used widely in clinical application for such pressure measurements (Fig. 12-1).

Assuming mean pulmonary artery (PA) and left atrial (LA) pressures of 15 and 6 mm Hg, respectively, along with a CO of 6 L/min, the pulmonary resistance is $(15 − 6)/6$ mm Hg/L/min, or 1.5 mm Hg/L/min. This resistance is approximately one tenth that found in the systemic circulation.

When CO increases (e.g., during exercise), the pulmonary circulation is able to decrease its resistance and handle the extra flow with only a minimal increase in pulmonary artery pressure. Two mechanisms appear to be responsible: recruitment of new vessels and, to a lesser extent, distention of previously perfused vessels. Under normal resting conditions, some pulmonary vessels receive no blood flow but are capable of carrying part of the pulmonary blood flow should the pressure increase. In addition, because pulmonary vessels have relatively thin walls, they are distensible and can enlarge their diameter under increased pressure to accommodate additional blood flow. With a means for increasing the total cross-sectional area of the pulmonary vasculature on demand, the pulmonary circulation is capable of lowering its resistance when the need for increased flow arises.

When cardiac output increases, recruitment and distention of pulmonary vessels prevent a significant increase in pulmonary artery pressure.

Another factor that affects PVR is lung volume. In discussing the nature of this effect, it is useful to distinguish two categories of pulmonary vessels on the basis of their size and location. One category, called *alveolar vessels,* includes the capillary network coursing through alveolar walls. When alveoli are expanded and lung volume is raised, these vessels are compressed within the stretched alveolar walls, and their contribution

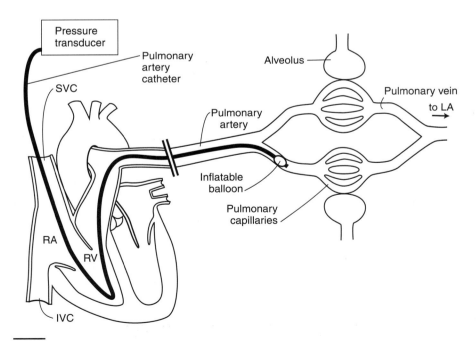

Figure 12-1. Schematic diagram of pulmonary artery (Swan-Ganz) catheter positioned in a pulmonary artery. The catheter is shown with the balloon inflated so that forward flow is occluded and the pressure measured at the catheter tip (pulmonary artery occlusion, or pulmonary capillary wedge pressure) is the pressure transmitted from the left atrium. When the balloon is deflated, the pressure measured at the catheter tip is pulmonary artery pressure. IVC = inferior vena cava; LA = left atrium; RA = right atrium; RV = right ventricle; SVC = superior vena cava.

to PVR is increased. In contrast, when alveoli are emptied and lung volume is lowered, the resistance of these alveolar vessels is diminished. The other category consists of the larger vessels called *extraalveolar vessels*. They are not compressed by air-filled alveoli. The supporting structure that surrounds the walls of these vessels has attachments to alveolar walls, and the elastic recoil of the alveolar walls provides radial traction to keep these vessels open. This concept is similar to the concept discussed in Chapter 6 concerning the effect of alveolar wall attachments on airway diameter (see Fig. 6-6). When lung volume is increased, elastic recoil of the alveolar walls is increased, and the extraalveolar vessels become larger. When lung volume is decreased, the resistance of the extraalveolar vessels increases. This differential effect of lung volume on the resistance of alveolar versus extraalveolar vessels is shown in Figure 12-2. The total PVR is least at the normal resting expiratory position of the lung, that is, at functional residual capacity.

DISTRIBUTION OF PULMONARY BLOOD FLOW

The relatively low pressures in the pulmonary artery have important implications regarding the way blood flow is distributed in the lung. When a person is in the upright position, blood going to the upper zones of the lung is flowing against gravity and must be under sufficient pressure in the pulmonary artery to make this antigravitational journey. Because the top of the lung is approximately 15 cm above the level of the main pulmonary arteries, a pressure of 15 cm H_2O is required to achieve perfusion of the apices. The mPA of 15 mm Hg (approximately 19 cm H_2O) normally is just

The distribution of blood flow within the lung is strongly influenced by gravity.

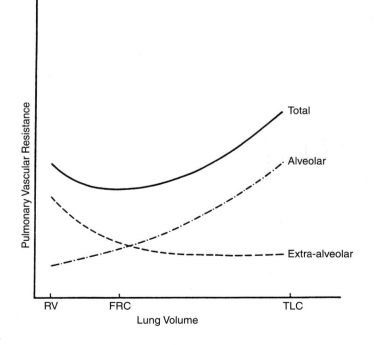

Figure 12-2. Effect of lung volume on total pulmonary vascular resistance (solid line), alveolar vessel resistance (dashed-dotted line), and extraalveolar vessel resistance (dashed line). Note that total resistance is least at functional residual capacity (FRC). RV = Residual volume; TLC = Total lung capacity. (From Taylor AE, Rehder K, Hyatt RE, Parker JC: *Clinical respiratory physiology,* p. 75, Philadelphia, 1989, WB Saunders.)

sufficient to achieve flow to this region. In contrast, flow to the lower lung zones, that is, below the level of the main pulmonary arteries, is assisted by gravity. Therefore, in the upright individual, gravity provides a normal gradient of blood flow from the apex to the base of the lung, with the base receiving substantially greater flow than the apex (see Fig. 1-4). As discussed in Chapter 1, this distribution of blood flow in the lung has major implications regarding the manner in which ventilation and perfusion are matched.

The three-zone model for describing the determinants of pulmonary blood flow discussed in Chapter 1 actually is more complicated now that a zone 4 has been recognized. In this zone, which occupies the base of the lung at low lung volumes, blood flow progressively diminishes as the most dependent region of the lung is approached. In order to explain why a zone 4 exists, we must return to the concept of extraalveolar pulmonary vessels. At the lung bases, the weight of the lung results in decreased alveolar volume, accompanied by distortion and compression of extraalveolar vessels. As a result, the resistance of the extraalveolar vessels increases considerably, the total vascular resistance in this zone increases, and blood flow diminishes.

The distribution of blood flow in the lung can be measured with radioactive isotopes. A *perfusion scan* is a particularly useful technique that involves intravenous injection of radiolabeled particles, specifically macroaggregates of albumin, that are of sufficient size to lodge in the pulmonary capillaries. An external counter over the lung senses the distribution of lodged particles and hence the distribution of blood flow to the lung. This technique, when performed in the upright individual, not only confirms the expected gradient of blood flow in the lung but also detects regions of decreased or absent perfusion in disease states (see Chapter 3).

PULMONARY VASCULAR RESPONSE TO HYPOXIA

An important physiologic feature of the pulmonary circulation is its response to hypoxia. When alveoli in an area of lung contain gas with a low Po_2, generally less than 60 to 70 mm Hg, the vessels supplying that region of lung undergo vasoconstriction. This response occurs primarily at the level of the small arteries or arterioles and serves as a protective mechanism for decreasing perfusion to poorly ventilated alveoli. Hence, ventilation-perfusion mismatch is decreased, and blood flow to areas with a low ventilation-perfusion ratio, which contribute hypoxemic blood, is minimized. When localized regions of lung have a low Po_2, the vasoconstrictive response also is localized. In these circumstances, the overall PVR does not increase significantly. However, with a more generalized decrease in Po_2, as in many forms of lung disease or in persons exposed to high altitude, pulmonary vasoconstriction also is more generalized. In this circumstance, PVR and pulmonary artery pressure both are increased. What would be a protective response in the case of localized disease is thus detrimental in the case of generalized disease and widespread alveolar hypoxia.

There is one setting in which such generalized pulmonary vasoconstriction in response to alveolar hypoxia is most beneficial: the fetus. In utero, the alveoli receive no aeration, making the entire lung hypoxic. The result is marked pulmonary vasoconstriction, accompanied by very high PVR and diversion of blood away from the lung. Blood preferentially flows through the ductus arteriosus from the pulmonary artery to the aorta, and through the foramen ovale from the right to the left atrium. This allows the majority of the blood oxygenated by the placenta to go directly into the systemic circulation of the fetus.

At birth, when the first few breaths are taken, oxygen flows into the alveoli, and the diffuse pulmonary vasoconstriction is reversed. As a result of this pulmonary vasodilation (as well as constriction of the ductus arteriosus), right ventricular output passes

Pulmonary vasoconstriction occurs in response to alveolar hypoxia. This protective mechanism reduces blood flow to poorly ventilated alveoli, minimizing ventilation-perfusion mismatch.

through the lungs, where the blood is oxygenated. Interestingly, the hypoxic vasoconstriction that persists throughout adult life may be directly related to this important fetal response.

The mechanism of hypoxic vasoconstriction is incompletely understood. One theory suggests that alveolar hypoxia acts on pulmonary vascular smooth muscle cells by inhibiting a membrane potassium ion channel, which leads to membrane depolarization and subsequent influx of calcium ions. The increase in intracellular calcium then induces pulmonary vascular smooth muscle cell contraction. Alternatively, hypoxia may alter release of vasoactive mediators; popular candidates are mediators released from vascular endothelial cells, such as the vasodilating factors nitric oxide (previously called endothelial-derived relaxing factor) and endogenously derived carbon monoxide, as well as the constricting factor known as endothelin. Nitric oxide, which is produced by vascular endothelial cells, acts via increasing cyclic guanosine monophosphate to produce vascular smooth muscle relaxation.

OTHER ASPECTS OF PULMONARY VASCULAR PHYSIOLOGY

An additional stimulus for pulmonary vasoconstriction is a low blood pH value. Although this effect is less important than the effect of hypoxia, the two stimuli appear to have a synergistic effect on increasing PVR. Any effect of P_{CO_2} on the pulmonary vasculature appears to be small. Although hypercapnia may increase PVR, the effect apparently is mediated by changes in blood pH.

A variety of other factors that influence pulmonary vascular tone are being increasingly recognized. Autonomic innervation of the pulmonary arterial system is present but not extensive. Sympathetic and parasympathetic stimulation have the expected opposing effects, causing vasoconstriction and vasodilation, respectively. Humoral stimuli altering vascular tone are numerous; examples include histamine and the prostaglandin products of arachidonic acid metabolism. Most recently, interest has focused on two molecules mentioned earlier in the discussion of hypoxic vasoconstriction, each of which is known to have important effects on the pulmonary vasculature: nitric oxide (a potent vasodilator) and endothelin (a potent vasoconstrictor). In addition to the possible role of these compounds in the pathophysiology of disease states involving the pulmonary vasculature are therapeutic benefits in patients with pulmonary arterial hypertension for agents that influence the production or effect of these vasoactive molecules.

Another important aspect of pulmonary vascular physiology relates to fluid movement from pulmonary capillaries into the interstitium of the alveolar wall. Because of the importance of abnormalities in fluid transport across the capillaries in acute respiratory distress syndrome and respiratory failure, this topic is discussed specifically in Chapter 28.

Finally, although transport of blood between the heart and the lungs is the most obvious function of the pulmonary vasculature, these vessels have other nonrespiratory, metabolic functions. The pulmonary circulation has an important role in the inactivation of certain circulating bioactive chemicals. For example, serotonin (5-hydroxytryptamine) and bradykinin are primarily inactivated in the lung, probably at the level of the vascular endothelium. In addition, angiotensin I, an inactive decapeptide derived in the kidney, is converted to the active octapeptide angiotensin II by angiotensin-converting enzyme, which is produced by pulmonary vascular endothelial cells. Although the metabolic functions of the pulmonary vasculature are important in modifying the effects of these substances, whether derangements in these functions are important consequences of diseases affecting the vasculature is not known.

A low pH value in blood is an additional stimulus for pulmonary vasoconstriction.

REFERENCES

Barnes PJ, Liu SF: Regulation of pulmonary vascular tone, *Pharmacol Rev* 47:87–131, 1995.

Brij SO, Peacock AJ: Cellular responses to hypoxia in the pulmonary circulation, *Thorax* 53:1075–1079, 1998.

Fishman AP: A century of pulmonary hemodynamics, *Am J Respir Crit Care Med* 170:109–113, 2004.

Keith IM: The role of endogenous lung neuropeptides in regulation of the pulmonary circulation, *Physiol Rev* 49:519–537, 2000.

Mazza E, Taichman DB. Functions and control of the pulmonary circulation. In Mandel J, Taichman DB, editors: *Pulmonary vascular disease,* Philadelphia, 2006, Saunders Elsevier.

Stenmark KR, Fagan KA, Frid MG: Hypoxia-induced pulmonary vascular remodeling: cellular and molecular mechanisms, *Circ Res* 99:675–691, 2006.

Weibel ER: *The pathway for oxygen: structure and function in the mammalian respiratory system,* Cambridge, MA, 1984, Harvard University Press.

Weir EK, Lopez-Barneo J, Buckler KJ, Archer SL: Acute oxygen-sensing mechanisms, *N Engl J Med* 353: 2042–2055, 2005.

West JB: *Respiratory physiology—the essentials,* ed 7, Baltimore, 2004, Lippincott Williams & Wilkins.

13

Pulmonary Embolism

ETIOLOGY AND PATHOGENESIS	**CLINICAL FEATURES**
PATHOLOGY	**DIAGNOSTIC EVALUATION**
PATHOPHYSIOLOGY	**TREATMENT**

Pulmonary embolism is one of the most important disorders that affect the pulmonary vasculature. Not only is it found in more than 60% of autopsies in which careful search is made, but it is widely misdiagnosed in terms of "overdiagnosis" when not present and "underdiagnosis" when present.

The term *pulmonary embolism* or, more precisely, *pulmonary thromboembolism* refers to movement of a blood clot from a systemic vein through the right side of the heart to the pulmonary circulation, where it lodges in one or more branches of the pulmonary artery. The clinical consequences of this common problem are quite variable, ranging from none to sudden death, depending on the size of the embolus and the underlying medical condition of the patient. Although pulmonary embolism is intimately associated with the development of a thrombus elsewhere in the circulation, this chapter focuses on the pulmonary manifestations of thromboembolic disease, not on the clinical effects or diagnosis of the clot at the site of formation, usually in the deep veins of the lower extremities.

ETIOLOGY AND PATHOGENESIS

A thrombus, that is, a blood clot, is the material that travels to the pulmonary circulation in pulmonary thromboembolic disease. Other material also can travel via the vasculature to the pulmonary arteries, including tumor cells or fragments, fat, amniotic fluid, and a variety of foreign materials that can be introduced into the circulation. This text does not consider these additional, much less common, types of embolism, which have quite different clinical presentations than do thromboemboli.

In the majority of cases, the lower extremities are the source of thrombi that embolize to the lungs. Although these thrombi frequently originate in the veins of the calf, propagation of the clots to the veins of the thigh is necessary to produce sufficiently large thromboemboli that can obstruct major portions of the pulmonary vascular bed and become important clinically. Rarely do pulmonary emboli originate in the arms, pelvis, or right-sided chambers of the heart; combined, these sources probably account for less than 10% of all pulmonary emboli. However, not all thrombi resulting in embolic disease are clinically apparent. In fact, only approximately 50% of patients with pulmonary emboli have previous clinical evidence of venous thrombosis in the lower extremities or elsewhere.

The following three factors are commonly stated to potentially contribute to the genesis of venous thrombosis: (1) alteration in the mechanism of blood coagulation

> Thrombi in the deep veins of the lower extremities are the usual source of pulmonary emboli.

(i.e., hypercoagulability), (2) damage to the endothelium of the vessel wall, and (3) stasis or stagnation of blood flow. In practice, many specific risk factors for thromboemboli have been identified, including immobilization (e.g., bed rest, prolonged sitting during travel, immobilization of an extremity after fracture), the postoperative state, congestive heart failure, obesity, underlying carcinoma, pregnancy and the postpartum state, use of oral contraceptives, and chronic deep venous insufficiency. Patients at particularly high risk are those who had trauma or surgery related to the pelvis or lower extremities, especially hip fracture or hip or knee replacement.

A number of genetic predispositions to hypercoagulability are recognized. They include deficiency or abnormal function of proteins with antithrombotic activity (e.g., antithrombin III, protein C, protein S) or the presence of abnormal variants of some of the clotting factors that are part of the coagulation cascade, especially factor V and prothrombin (factor II). In the genetic defect called factor V Leiden, which usually is due to a single base pair substitution leading to replacement of an arginine residue by glutamine, the factor V protein becomes resistant to the action of activated protein C. Individuals who are heterozygous for factor V Leiden have a threefold to fivefold increased risk for venous thrombosis. The much less common homozygous state confers a significantly higher risk. In the genetic variant of prothrombin often called the *prothrombin gene mutation,* there is also a single base pair deletion that, by an unknown mechanism, leads to increased plasma levels of prothrombin and predisposes to venous thrombosis. Whereas deficiencies of the antithrombotic proteins are rare, factor V Leiden may have a prevalence of up to 5%. The fact that it is found in approximately 20% of patients with a first episode of venous thromboembolism suggests factor V Leiden is an important risk factor. Both factor V Leiden and the prothrombin gene mutation are relatively common in the Caucasian population but rare among African-Americans and Asians in the United States.

PATHOLOGY

The pathologic changes that result from occlusion of a pulmonary artery depend to a large extent on the location of the occlusion and the presence of other disorders that compromise O_2 supply to the pulmonary parenchyma. There are two major consequences of vascular occlusion in the lung parenchyma distal to the site of occlusion. First, if minimal or no other O_2 supply reaches the parenchyma, either from the airways or from the bronchial arterial circulation, then frank necrosis of lung tissue (pulmonary infarction) will result. According to one estimate, only 10% to 15% of all pulmonary emboli result in pulmonary infarction. It is sometimes said that compromise of two of the three O_2 sources to the lung (pulmonary artery, bronchial artery, and alveolar gas) is necessary before infarction results. Second, when the integrity of the parenchyma is maintained and infarction does not result, hemorrhage and edema often occur in lung tissue supplied by the occluded pulmonary artery. The name *congestive atelectasis* has sometimes been applied to this process of parenchymal hemorrhage and edema without infarction.

With either pulmonary infarction or congestive atelectasis, the pathologic process generally extends to the visceral pleural surface, so corresponding radiographic changes often are pleura based. In some cases, pleural effusion also may result. As part of the natural history of infarction, there is generally contraction of the infarcted parenchyma and eventual formation of a scar. With congestive atelectasis but no infarction, resolution of the process and resorption of the blood may leave few or no pathologic sequelae.

In many cases, neither of these pathologic changes occurs, and relatively little alteration of the distal lung parenchyma is found, presumably because of incomplete

Embolic occlusion of a vessel may lead to infarction or congestive atelectasis of the lung parenchyma.

occlusion or sufficient nutrient O_2 from other sources. Frequently, the thrombus quickly fragments or undergoes a process of lysis, with smaller fragments moving progressively distally in the pulmonary arterial circulation. Whether this rapid process of clot dissolution occurs is important in determining the pathologic consequences of pulmonary embolism.

With clots that do not fragment or lyse, generally a slower process of organization in the vessel wall and eventual recanalization are seen. Webs may form within the arterial lumen and sometimes are detected on a pulmonary arteriogram or on postmortem examination as the only evidence for prior embolic disease.

PATHOPHYSIOLOGY

When a thrombus migrates to and lodges within a pulmonary vessel, a variety of consequences ensue. They relate not only to mechanical obstruction of one or more vessels but also to the secondary effects of various mediators released from the thrombus and ischemic tissue. The effects of mechanical occlusion of the vessels are discussed first, followed by a consideration of how chemical mediators contribute to the clinical effects.

When a vessel is occluded by an embolus and forward blood flow through the vessel stops, perfusion of pulmonary capillaries normally supplied by that vessel ceases. If ventilation to the corresponding alveoli continues, then the ventilation is wasted, and the region of lung serves as dead space. As discussed in Chapter 1, assuming that minute ventilation remains constant, increasing the dead space automatically decreases alveolar ventilation and hence CO_2 excretion. However, despite the potential for CO_2 retention in pulmonary embolic disease, hypercapnia is an unusual consequence of pulmonary embolus, mainly because patients routinely increase their minute ventilation after an embolus occurs and more than compensate for the increase in dead space. In fact, the usual consequence of a pulmonary embolus is hyperventilation and hypocapnia, not hypercapnia. However, if minute ventilation is fixed (e.g., in an unconscious or anesthetized patient whose ventilation is controlled by a mechanical ventilator), then a rise in P_{CO_2} may result from the increase in dead space caused by a relatively large pulmonary embolus.

In addition to creating an area of dead space, another potential consequence of mechanical occlusion of one or more vessels is an increase in pulmonary vascular resistance. As discussed in Chapter 12, the pulmonary vascular bed is capable of recruitment and distention of vessels. Not surprisingly, experimental evidence indicates no increase in resistance or pressure in the pulmonary vasculature until approximately 50% to 70% of the vascular bed is occluded. The experimental model is somewhat different from the clinical setting, however, because release of chemical mediators may cause vasoconstriction and additional compromise of the pulmonary vasculature.

With even further limitation of the vascular bed by the combination of mechanical occlusion and the effects of chemical mediators, the pulmonary vascular resistance and pulmonary artery pressure may rise so high that the right ventricle cannot cope with the acute increase in workload. As a result, the forward output of the right ventricle may diminish, blood pressure may fall, and the individual may have a syncopal (fainting) episode or go into cardiogenic shock. In addition, "backward" failure of the right ventricle may occur, which manifests acutely with elevation of systemic venous pressure and appears on physical examination as distention of jugular veins.

The hemodynamic consequences of an acute pulmonary embolus depend to a large extent on the presence of preexisting emboli and whether underlying pulmonary vascular disease or cardiac disease is present. When emboli have occurred previously, the right ventricular wall has already thickened (hypertrophied), and higher pressures can

> Pulmonary emboli typically are associated with hypocapnia, resulting from an increase in overall minute ventilation.

be generated and maintained. On the other hand, an additional embolus in an already compromised pulmonary vascular bed may act as "the straw that broke the camel's back" and induce decompensation of the right ventricle.

In addition to the direct mechanical effects of vessel occlusion, thrombi result in release of chemical mediators that have secondary effects on both airways and blood vessels of the lung. The exact source and nature of the chemical mediators are not entirely clear. Platelets that adhere to the thrombus presumably are an important source of mediators such as histamine, serotonin, and prostaglandins. Bronchoconstriction, largely at the level of small airways, appears to be an important consequence of mediator release and is thought to contribute to the hypoxemia that commonly accompanies pulmonary embolism. In addition, areas of low ventilation and inappropriately high perfusion appear to develop because the process of hypoxic vasoconstriction becomes compromised by mediators related to thromboemboli. However, vasoconstriction of pulmonary arteries and arterioles can occur and add to the likelihood of major cardiovascular compromise.

Three additional features of the pathophysiology of pulmonary embolism are noteworthy. First, as a result of vascular compromise to one or more regions of lung, synthesis of the surface-active material surfactant in the affected alveoli is compromised. Consequently, alveoli may be more likely to collapse, and liquid may more likely leak into alveolar spaces. Second, hypocapnia appears to have the effect of inducing secondary bronchoconstriction of small airways. With the hypocapnia that occurs in pulmonary embolus, and particularly with the low alveolar P_{CO_2} in dead space regions of lung, secondary bronchoconstriction results. Both of these mechanisms, along with the small airway constriction induced by chemical mediators, may contribute to the volume loss or atelectasis that is frequently observed on chest radiographs of patients with pulmonary embolism. Shunt physiology also may contribute to hypoxemia because of either perfusion of atelectatic lung or elevated right heart pressures producing intracardiac shunting across a patent foramen ovale.

A variety of bioactive substances are inactivated in the lung (see Chapter 12). Whether pulmonary embolism disturbs some of these nonrespiratory, metabolic functions of the lung is not clear, and whether clinical consequences might ensue from such a potential disturbance is unknown.

CLINICAL FEATURES

Most frequently, pulmonary embolism develops in the setting of one of the risk factors previously mentioned. Commonly, the embolus does not produce any significant symptoms, and the entire episode goes unnoticed by the patient and the physician. When the patient does have symptoms, acute onset of dyspnea is the most frequent complaint. Less common is pleuritic chest pain or hemoptysis. Syncope is an occasional presentation, particularly in the setting of a massive embolus, defined as the obstruction of two or more lobes (or an equivalent number of segments).

On physical examination, the most common findings are tachycardia and tachypnea. The chest examination may be entirely normal or may reveal a variety of nonspecific findings, such as decreased air entry, localized rales, or wheezing. With pulmonary infarction extending to the pleura, a pleural friction rub may be detected, as may findings of a pleural effusion. Cardiac examination may show evidence of acute right ventricular overload, that is, acute cor pulmonale, in which case the pulmonic component of the second heart sound (P_2) is increased, a right-sided S_4 is heard, and a right ventricular heave may be present. If the right ventricle fails, a right-sided S_3 may be heard, and jugular veins may be distended. Examination of the lower extremities may reveal changes suggesting a thrombus, including tenderness, swelling, or a cord

Common symptoms of pulmonary embolism are the following:
1. Dyspnea
2. Pleuritic chest pain
3. Hemoptysis
4. Syncope

(palpable clot within a vessel). However, only a minority of patients with emboli arising from leg veins have clinical evidence of deep venous thrombosis, so the absence of these findings should not be surprising or overly reassuring.

DIAGNOSTIC EVALUATION

The initial diagnostic evaluation of the patient with suspected pulmonary embolism generally includes a chest radiograph and measurement of arterial blood gases. For patients in whom the diagnosis is considered less likely, the clinician may start with a D-dimer assay (discussed later). The radiographic findings in acute pulmonary embolism are quite variable. Most frequently, the radiographic findings are normal. When they are not, the abnormalities often are nonspecific, including areas of atelectasis or elevation of a hemidiaphragm, indicating volume loss. The volume loss may be related to decreased ventilation to the involved area as a result of small airways constriction and possibly loss of surfactant. If pleuritic chest pain is present, the patient may try to prevent pain by breathing more shallowly, which contributes to atelectasis.

Occasionally, the chest radiograph reveals a localized area of decreased lung vascular markings corresponding to the region in which the vessel has been occluded. This finding is called *Westermark's sign* but often is difficult to read unless prior radiographs are available for comparison. With a large proximal embolus, occasionally enlargement of a pulmonary artery near the hilum occurs as a result of distention of the vessel by the clot itself. An apparent abrupt termination of the vessel may occur, although this usually is difficult to see on a plain chest radiograph.

Both congestive atelectasis and infarction may appear as an opacified region on the radiograph. Classically, the density is shaped like a truncated cone, fanning out toward and reaching the pleural surface. This finding, called a *Hampton's hump*, is relatively infrequent. Pleural effusions may be seen as an accompaniment of pulmonary embolic disease. Pleural effusions associated with pulmonary embolism may be either exudative or transudative and contain a variable number of red blood cells.

Arterial blood gas values show hypoxemia and a respiratory alkalosis, with hypocapnia occurring in more than 80% of cases. Because Pco_2 is decreased, arterial Po_2 is higher than it would be if hyperventilation were not present. However, if the alveolar–arterial O_2 difference in partial pressure of oxygen (PAo_2–Pao_2 [$AaDo_2$]) is calculated, it is increased. Occasionally, Po_2 is normal, so the presence of a normal Po_2 does not exclude the diagnosis of pulmonary embolism.

Traditionally, the major screening test for pulmonary embolism has been the perfusion lung scan (described in Chapter 3). However, the diagnostic evaluation of suspected pulmonary embolism is in a state of transition, as contrast computed tomographic (CT) angiography is increasingly being used either instead of or in addition to perfusion lung scanning. Evaluation of the large veins in the lower extremities, typically using ultrasound techniques, is another commonly used diagnostic strategy. Identification of a clot in a vein above the popliteal fossa warrants the same treatment as a documented pulmonary embolus and often obviates the need for further evaluation.

When blood flow is obstructed by a clot within the pulmonary arterial system, perfusion lung scanning demonstrates absence of perfusion to the region of lung supplied by the occluded vessel (Fig. 13-1). If results of the scan are normal, pulmonary embolism is, for all practical purposes, excluded. However, abnormalities do not automatically indicate the presence of embolic disease. False-positive lung scans are common because local decreases in blood flow may result from primary disease of the parenchyma or the airways. A ventilation scan, which involves inhalation of a xenon radioisotope, is often added because if regions of decreased blood flow are secondary to airway disease, corresponding abnormalities should be seen on the ventilation scan. If a defect in perfusion

Characteristic arterial blood gas values in pulmonary embolic disease are the following:
1. Decreased Po_2
2. Decreased Pco_2
3. Increased pH

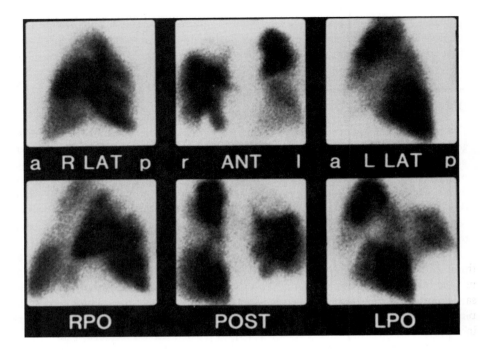

Figure 13-1. Positive results of perfusion scan shows multiple perfusion defects in a patient with pulmonary emboli. Six views of complete scan are shown: right lateral *(R LAT)*, anterior *(ANT)*, left lateral *(L LAT)*, right posterior oblique *(RPO)*, posterior *(POST)*, and left posterior oblique *(LPO)*. Compare with normal scan results in Figure 3-11. a = Anterior; l = left; p = posterior; r = right. (Courtesy Dr. Henry Royal.)

is due to a pulmonary embolism, ventilation still will be present in the area, and the perfusion defect will be "mismatched," that is, will not have a corresponding ventilation defect. If parenchymal disease, such as pneumonia, is the cause of a perfusion defect, then a corresponding abnormality should be seen on the chest radiograph.

Interpretation of the perfusion lung scan is a complicated process that depends on the clinical setting, the results of chest radiograph, and frequently the findings on a ventilation lung scan. Because the perfusion scan often is not definitive, a probability is placed on the likelihood of pulmonary embolism, taking into account the size and number of defects and the presence or absence of corresponding abnormalities on the radiograph and the ventilation lung scan. The scan results are analyzed in conjunction with the *pretest probability* of pulmonary embolism, a term used to represent the clinician's assessment of the likelihood of pulmonary embolism based on the patient's clinical presentation.

When the lung scan is not conclusive, it is critical that additional diagnostic evaluation be performed. Different options for further workup are available, focusing either on the veins of the lower extremities or on the pulmonary vasculature itself. However, because lower extremity studies often are negative even in the presence of documented pulmonary embolism, a negative lower extremity study does not preclude the need for further evaluation of the pulmonary arteries if there is a reasonably high suspicion of pulmonary thromboembolism.

Major techniques for diagnosis of pulmonary emboli include ventilation-perfusion lung scanning, CT angiography, and conventional pulmonary angiography.

The more recent technique of CT angiography (discussed in Chapter 3) is a less invasive, more conveniently performed procedure, although it is not as sensitive as conventional pulmonary angiography in detecting thromboemboli in smaller vessels. Nevertheless, as CT technology continues to improve, CT angiography is rapidly becoming a standard procedure and now is often used in preference to perfusion lung scanning as part of the initial diagnostic evaluation for suspected pulmonary embolism (Fig. 13-2). CT angiography offers the significant advantage of high-quality visualization of the lung parenchyma, which is helpful in considering the likelihood of competing diagnoses.

Direct evaluation of the pulmonary arterial system to identify intraluminal thrombus can be accomplished invasively by advancing a catheter through a jugular or femoral vein into the pulmonary arteries in a more traditional procedure called *conventional pulmonary angiography* (discussed in Chapter 3). Although conventional angiography is generally considered the "gold standard" for diagnosis of thromboembolic disease, it has pitfalls in interpretation and is not entirely without risk. Nevertheless, it frequently is useful, and the finding of a filling defect within a vessel or an abrupt cutoff is considered diagnostic of a pulmonary embolus (Fig. 13-3).

Another test that is increasingly used as part of the diagnostic strategy for venous thromboembolic disease is measurement of plasma levels of D-dimer, which is a degradation product of cross-linked fibrin. Plasma levels of D-dimer increase in the setting of venous thrombosis, but the test is nonspecific, and the results are dependent on the particular assay used. When D-dimer measurement is used in clinical practice, normal levels found using a sensitive assay (e.g., enzyme-linked immunosorbent assay) are considered strong evidence against thromboembolic disease. Thus, a normal D-dimer level is helpful, especially in the patient with a low pretest probability of having a pulmonary embolism, but an elevated level is considered nonspecific and therefore nondiagnostic.

TREATMENT

Standard treatment of a pulmonary embolus involves anticoagulant therapy, initially intravenous unfractionated heparin or subcutaneous low-molecular-weight heparin, and then an oral coumarin derivative (warfarin), the latter usually given for at least

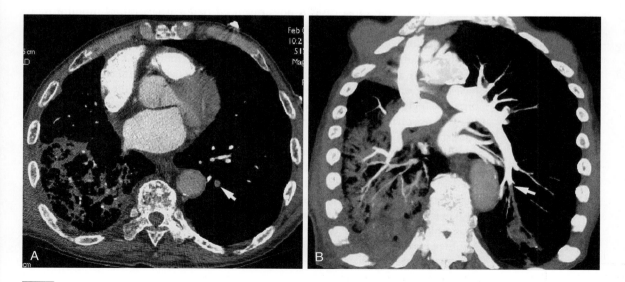

Figure 13-2. Chest computed tomographic angiography shows a pulmonary embolus in a mid-sized vessel in the left lung. **A,** Standard cross-sectional view shows a blood vessel (seen on end) filled by clot rather than radiopaque contrast dye *(arrow).* **B,** Image displayed in a reformatted oblique view shows the same vessel in its longitudinal course. The arrow marks the absence of radiopaque dye in the vessel at the edge of the clot. (Courtesy Dr. Phillip Boiselle.)

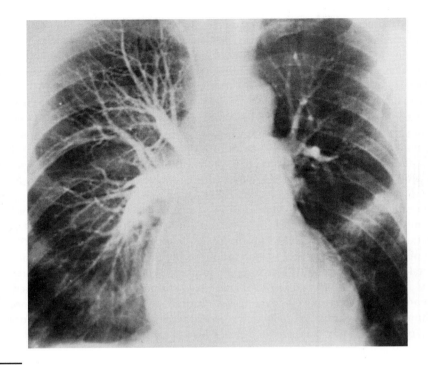

Figure 13-3. Positive results of pulmonary angiogram show occlusion of vessel supplying the left lower lobe. Area of density in left mid-lung probably represents pulmonary infarct. (Courtesy Dr. Morris Simon.)

Options for therapy for pulmonary embolism are the following:
1. Anticoagulation (heparin, warfarin)
2. Thrombolysis (t-PA, streptokinase, urokinase)
3. Inferior vena caval filter

3 to 6 months. Low-molecular–weight heparin has a number of potential advantages over unfractionated heparin, including less risk of heparin-induced thrombocytopenia. In addition, in most cases it does not need frequent laboratory monitoring of coagulation tests to guide dosage adjustment, and it can be given subcutaneously in one or two daily doses, avoiding the need for continuous intravenous infusion.

The most important aspect of treating pulmonary embolism is achieving prompt and adequate anticoagulation. For the most part, after a patient with an embolism that has already entered the pulmonary circulation has sought medical attention, the biggest danger derives from a recurrent embolus that causes hemodynamic instability. For this reason, treatment in high-risk patients can be started before the diagnosis is confirmed.

The rationale for use of anticoagulants is to prevent formation of new thrombi or propagation of old thrombi (in the legs), not to dissolve clots that have already embolized to the lungs. As a result, there has been a great deal of interest in the use of thrombolytic agents such as tissue plasminogen activator (t-PA), streptokinase, and urokinase for treatment of pulmonary emboli. These agents, which may actually lyse recent blood clots, ideally are given within the first several days of the embolic event, but they may be effective even up to 2 weeks after the embolus. Although a difference in mortality rate has not been clearly demonstrated when thrombolytic agents or heparin is used for initial therapy, there may be specific subgroups of patients most likely to benefit from thrombolytic therapy, namely, patients with massive pulmonary embolus and hemodynamic compromise as a result of vascular occlusion. When one of these agents is used, the initial intravenous infusion of the thrombolytic agent is followed by standard anticoagulant therapy.

In some circumstances, treatment of pulmonary embolism involves placement of a filtering device into the inferior vena cava, with the goal of trapping thrombi from the lower extremities en route to the pulmonary circulation. This type of device is used most frequently if there are contraindications to anticoagulant therapy (i.e., bleeding problems), if thromboemboli have recurred despite adequate anticoagulation, or if the patient already has such limited pulmonary vascular reserve that an additional clot to the lungs likely would be fatal.

No discussion of the treatment of pulmonary embolism is complete without a consideration of prophylactic methods used to prevent deep venous thrombosis in the high-risk patient. The most common forms of prophylaxis traditionally have been (1) external compression of the lower extremities with an intermittently inflating pneumatic device and (2) heparin administered subcutaneously in low dosage. Low-molecular–weight heparin is at least as effective and safe as low-dose unfractionated heparin. One or another method of prophylaxis is now generally used in patients about to undergo thoracic or abdominal surgery and in a variety of other high-risk patients who are at bed rest in the hospital. In the highest risk patients (i.e., those with hip fracture or hip or knee replacement surgery), either low-molecular–weight heparin or warfarin is more effective for prophylaxis than is low-dose subcutaneous standard heparin.

REFERENCES

GENERAL REVIEWS

Blann AD, Lip GY: Venous thromboembolism, *BMJ* 332:215–219, 2006.
Goldhaber SZ: Pulmonary embolism, *Lancet* 363:1295–1305, 2004.
Hyers TM: Venous thromboembolism, *Am J Respir Crit Care Med* 159:1–14, 1999.

SPECIFIC ASPECTS

Aguilar D, Goldhaber SZ: Clinical uses of low-molecular-weight heparins, *Chest* 115:1418–1423, 1999.
Arcasoy SM, Kreit JW: Thrombolytic therapy of pulmonary embolism: a comprehensive review of current evidence, *Chest* 115:1695–1707, 1999.
Bell WR, Simon TL, DeMets DL: The clinical features of submassive and massive pulmonary emboli, *Am J Med* 62:355–360, 1977.
Buller HR, Agnelli G, Hull RD, Hyers TM, Prins MH, Raskob GE: Antithrombotic therapy for venous thromboembolic disease: the Seventh ACCP Conference on Antithrombotic and Thrombolytic Therapy, *Chest* 126(3 suppl): 401S–428S, 2004.
Dalen JE: The uncertain role of thrombolytic therapy in the treatment of pulmonary embolism, *Arch Intern Med* 162:2521–2523, 2002.
Dalen JE: Pulmonary embolism: what have we learned since Virchow? Natural history, pathophysiology and diagnosis, *Chest* 122:1440–1456, 2004.
Elliott CG: Pulmonary physiology during pulmonary embolism, *Chest* 101:163S–171S, 1992.
Geerts WH, Pineo GF, Heit JA, et al: Prevention of venous thromboembolism: the Seventh ACCP Conference on Antithrombotic and Thrombolytic Therapy, *Chest* 126(3 suppl):338S–400S, 2004.
Hirsh J, Bates SM: Clinical trials that have influenced the treatment of venous thromboembolism: a historical perspective, *Ann Intern Med* 134:409–417, 2001.
Kanne JP, Lalani TA: Role of computed tomography and magnetic resonance imaging for deep venous thrombosis and pulmonary embolism, *Circulation* 109(12 suppl 1):I15–I21, 2004.
Patel S, Kazerooni EA: Helical CT for the evaluation of acute pulmonary embolism, *AJR Am J Roentgenol* 185:135–149, 2005.
PIOPED Investigators: Value of the ventilation/perfusion scan in acute pulmonary embolism: results of the Prospective Investigation of Pulmonary Embolism Diagnosis (PIOPED), *JAMA* 263:2753–2759, 1990.
Seligsohn U, Lubetsky A: Genetic susceptibility to venous thrombosis, *N Engl J Med* 344:1222–1231, 2001.
Stein PD, Beemath A, Matta F, et al: Clinical characteristics of patients with acute pulmonary embolism: data from PIOPED II, *Am J Med* 120: 871–879, 2007.

Stein PD, Hull RD, Patel KC, et al: D-dimer for the exclusion of acute venous thrombosis and pulmonary embolism: a systematic review, *Ann Intern Med* 140:589–602, 2004.

Stone SE, Morris TA: Pulmonary embolism during and after pregnancy, *Crit Care Med* 33(10 suppl): S294–S300, 2005.

Weichman K, Ansell JE: Inferior vena cava filters in venous thromboembolism, *Prog Cardiovasc Dis* 49: 98–105, 2006.

Pulmonary Hypertension

Elevation of intravascular pressure within the pulmonary circulation is the hallmark of pulmonary hypertension. In this chapter, specific reference is made to elevated pulmonary arterial pressure (defined as mean pulmonary artery pressure greater than 25 mm Hg at rest or 30 mm Hg with exercise), although in some cases an elevation in pulmonary venous pressure is an important forerunner of pulmonary arterial hypertension. Because pulmonary hypertension has a number of causes that presumably act by several different mechanisms, this chapter begins with a consideration of features relevant to pulmonary hypertension in general and follows with a discussion of some important specific causes of pulmonary hypertension.

First, clarification of two points is pertinent. Pulmonary hypertension merely refers to the elevation of pulmonary vascular pressure. Such elevation in pressure may be acute or chronic, depending on the causative factors. In some cases, chronic pulmonary hypertension is punctuated by further acute elevations in pressure, often as a result of exacerbations of the underlying disease. Second, the development of right ventricular hypertrophy is the consequence of pulmonary hypertension, whatever the primary cause of the latter. When pulmonary hypertension is due to disorders of any part of the respiratory apparatus (airways, parenchyma and blood vessels, chest wall, respiratory musculature, or central nervous system controller), the term *cor pulmonale* is used to refer to the resulting right ventricular hypertrophy. This term should not be used to describe the right ventricular changes occurring as a consequence of primary cardiac disease or of increased flow to the pulmonary vascular bed.

PATHOGENESIS

A number of factors contribute to the pathogenesis of pulmonary hypertension, both acutely and chronically. First, occlusion of a sufficient cross-sectional area of the pulmonary arteries by material within the vessels, such as pulmonary emboli, is an important factor (discussed in Chapter 13). In acute embolism, in which massive pulmonary emboli occlude more than half to two thirds of the vasculature, pulmonary arterial pressure is elevated. The right ventricle may dilate in response to its acutely increased workload because of insufficient time for hypertrophy to occur. In contrast, in chronic embolic disease, multiple and recurrent pulmonary emboli may elevate pulmonary arterial pressures during a period sufficient for right ventricular hypertrophy to occur.

Second, diminution of cross-sectional area as a consequence of primary disease of the pulmonary arterial walls is a potential factor. Disorders acting by this mechanism are characterized by intimal and medial changes (see section on pathology) that lead to thickening of the arterial and arteriolar walls and narrowing or obliteration of the lumen. This group of disorders with pulmonary arterial pathology includes *idiopathic pulmonary arterial hypertension* (IPAH; formerly called *primary pulmonary hypertension*). The familial form of this condition, called *familial pulmonary arterial hypertension,* in most cases is related to mutations of the gene on chromosome 2 that encodes the bone morphogenetic protein receptor type 2. Abnormalities in this receptor are believed to lead to dysregulation of proliferative responses in the endothelium and pulmonary arterial smooth muscle cells, producing the well-described pathologic changes in small pulmonary arteries and arterioles (see section on pathology below). Lesions pathologically similar to those seen in IPAH are observed in conditions associated with pulmonary arterial hypertension, such as scleroderma, portal hypertension, and human immunodeficiency virus (HIV) infection, or with exposure to drugs and toxins, such as cocaine, methamphetamine, and certain diet drugs. When compromise of the pulmonary vasculature and increased resistance to flow are sufficiently pronounced in these primary disorders of the vessel wall, the level of pulmonary hypertension can be quite severe, both at rest and with exercise.

Third, the total cross-sectional area of the pulmonary vascular bed is compromised by parenchymal lung disease, with loss of blood vessels from either a scarring or a destructive process affecting the alveolar walls. Interstitial lung disease and emphysema can affect the pulmonary vasculature via this mechanism, although the underlying disorder in the parenchyma appears quite different. With these diseases, pulmonary arterial pressure commonly is relatively normal at rest but is mildly to moderately elevated with exercise because of insufficient recruitment or distention of vessels to handle the increase in cardiac output.

A fourth mechanism of pulmonary hypertension is vasoconstriction in response to hypoxia and, to a lesser extent, to acidosis. The importance of this mechanism is related to its potential reversibility when normal Po_2 and pH value are achieved. In several causes of cor pulmonale, particularly chronic obstructive lung disease with type B physiology, hypoxia is the single most important factor leading to pulmonary hypertension and is potentially the most treatable. Acidosis, either respiratory or metabolic, causes pulmonary vasoconstriction and, although it is less important than hypoxia, may augment the vasoconstrictive response to hypoxia (discussed in Chapter 12).

When flow through the pulmonary vascular bed is increased, as occurs in patients with congenital intracardiac (left-to-right) shunts, the vasculature is initially able to handle the augmented flow without any anatomic changes in the arteries or arterioles. However, over a prolonged period, the vessel walls thicken and pulmonary arterial resistance increases. Eventually, as a result of the high pulmonary vascular resistance, right-sided cardiac pressures may become so elevated that the intracardiac shunt reverses in direction. This conversion to a right-to-left shunt, commonly called *Eisenmenger's syndrome,* is a potentially important consequence of an atrial or ventricular septal defect or a patent ductus arteriosus.

A final and common mechanism of pulmonary arterial hypertension is elevation of pressure distally, in either the left atrium or the left ventricle, and progressive elevation of the "back-pressure," first in the pulmonary veins and capillaries and then in the

Factors contributing to pulmonary arterial hypertension are the following:
1. Occlusion of vessels by emboli
2. Primary thickening of arterial walls
3. Loss of vessels by scarring or destruction of alveolar walls
4. Pulmonary vasoconstriction (from hypoxia, acidosis)
5. Increased pulmonary vascular flow (left-to-right shunt)
6. Elevated left atrial pressure

pulmonary arterioles and arteries. As is the case with pulmonary hypertension eventually induced by increased flow in the pulmonary vasculature, the initial elevation in pressure is not accompanied by anatomic changes in the pulmonary arteries. However, structural changes are seen eventually, and measured pulmonary vascular resistance may be substantially increased. The major disorders that result in pulmonary hypertension by this final mechanism are mitral stenosis and chronic left ventricular failure.

PATHOLOGY

In many ways the pathologic findings in the pulmonary vessels of patients with pulmonary hypertension are similar, regardless of the underlying cause. This section specifically focuses on these general changes.

The most prominent abnormalities are frequently seen in vessels of the pulmonary arterial tree with a diameter of less than 1 mm, namely, the small muscular arteries (0.1–1 mm) and the arterioles (<0.1 mm). The muscular arteries show hypertrophy of the media, composed of smooth muscle, and hyperplasia of the intimal layer lining the vessel lumen. In the arterioles, a significant muscular component to the vessel wall normally is not present, but with pulmonary hypertension these vessels undergo "neomuscularization" of their walls (Fig. 14-1, A). In addition, the arteriolar intima proliferates. As a result of these changes, the luminal diameter is significantly decreased, and the pulmonary vascular resistance is elevated. Ultimately, the lumen may be completely obliterated and the overall number of small vessels greatly diminished. In some cases, particularly when the pulmonary hypertension is due to IPAH or is secondary to congenital intracardiac shunts, the small arterioles may demonstrate so-called *plexiform changes*, appearing as a plexus of small, slitlike vascular channels.

When pulmonary hypertension becomes marked, other changes are commonly seen in the larger (elastic) pulmonary arteries (Fig. 14-1, B). These vessels, which normally have much thinner walls than do vessels of comparable size in the systemic circulation, develop thickening of the wall, particularly in the media. They also develop the types of atherosclerotic plaques that are generally seen only in the higher-pressure systemic circulation.

A secondary problem that may develop in patients with pulmonary hypertension of any cause is in situ thrombosis in the pulmonary vasculature. Presumably, endothelial damage and sluggish flow in some pulmonary arterial vessels can contribute to thrombus formation. Development of in situ thrombosis can worsen the degree of pulmonary hypertension by further compromising the pulmonary vascular bed.

The cardiac consequences of pulmonary hypertension are manifest pathologically as changes in the right ventricular wall. The magnitude of the changes depends primarily on the severity and chronicity of the pulmonary hypertension rather than the nature of the underlying disorder. The major finding is concentric hypertrophy of the right ventricular wall. If the right ventricle fails as a result of the chronic increase in workload, then dilation of the right ventricle is observed.

> Pathologic features of pulmonary hypertension are the following:
> 1. Intimal hyperplasia and medial hypertrophy of small arteries and arterioles
> 2. Eventual obliteration of the lumen of small arteries and arterioles
> 3. Thickening of the wall of larger (elastic) pulmonary arteries
> 4. Right ventricular hypertrophy

PATHOPHYSIOLOGY

The pathophysiologic hallmark of pulmonary hypertension is, by definition, an increase in pressure within the pulmonary circulation. If the primary component of the vascular change occurs at the level of the pulmonary arteries or arterioles, as in the case of cor pulmonale, then pulmonary arterial pressures (both systolic and diastolic) rise, whereas the pressure within pulmonary capillaries remains normal. On the other

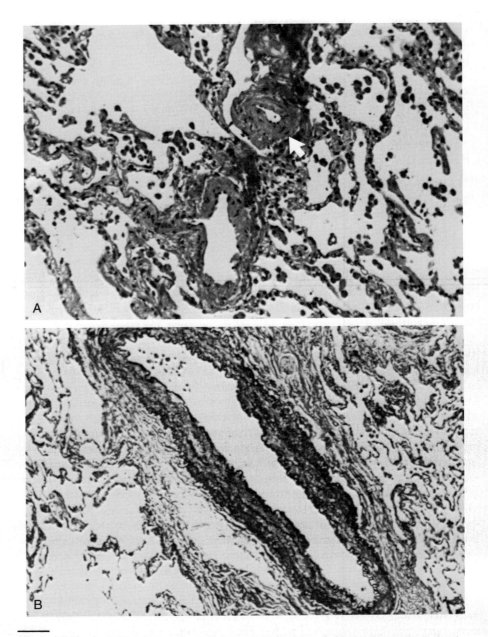

Figure 14-1. Histologic changes in pulmonary hypertension. **A,** Moderate-power photomicrograph shows thickened wall of pulmonary arteriole *(arrow)*. **B,** Low-power photomicrograph (elastic tissue stain) shows thickened wall of branch of pulmonary artery. (Courtesy Dr. Earl Kasdon.)

hand, if pulmonary arterial hypertension is secondary to pulmonary venous and pulmonary capillary hypertension (as in the case of mitral stenosis or left ventricular failure), then pulmonary capillary pressure is elevated above its normal level.

As the architectural changes of pulmonary hypertension progress, both right ventricular and pulmonary arterial pressures rise because of increased pulmonary vascular resistance. Cardiac output usually remains normal early in the course of the process. When the right ventricle fails, right ventricular end-diastolic pressure rises, and cardiac output may decrease as well. Right atrial pressure also rises; this may be apparent on physical examination of the neck veins as elevation in the jugular venous pressure.

CLINICAL FEATURES

Although the overall constellation of symptoms in patients with pulmonary hypertension depends on the underlying disease, certain characteristic complaints can be attributed to the pulmonary hypertension itself. Dyspnea, especially on exertion, is frequently observed in all forms of pulmonary hypertension. However, in patients with pulmonary hypertension related to underlying parenchymal lung disease, it often is difficult to know how much the pulmonary hypertension, as opposed to the underlying lung disease, is responsible for the symptom. Cardiopulmonary exercise testing may be useful in partitioning the relative contributions of each to dyspnea. Patients may have substernal chest pain that is difficult, if not impossible, to distinguish from classic angina pectoris, particularly because the pain is frequently precipitated by exertion. In most instances, the chest pain is presumed to be related to the increased workload of the right ventricle and to right ventricular ischemia, although in some cases an enlarged pulmonary artery can compress the left main coronary artery and produce true left ventricular ischemia. Because of an inability to increase cardiac output with exercise when pulmonary hypertension is severe, patients may experience exertional fatigue or syncope.

Physical examination shows several features that are more related to the cardiac consequences of pulmonary hypertension than to the actual disease of the pulmonary vessels. Pulmonary hypertension itself does not cause any changes that can be noted on examination of the lungs, although patients with underlying lung disease often have findings related to their primary disease. On cardiac examination, patients frequently exhibit an accentuation of the pulmonic component of the second heart sound (P_2) because of earlier and more forceful valve closure attributable to high pressure in the pulmonary artery. Murmurs of tricuspid insufficiency are commonly heard, and a pulmonic insufficiency (Graham-Steell) murmur may be appreciated. With right ventricular hypertrophy, there is often a prominent lift or heave of the region immediately to the left of the lower sternum, corresponding to a prominent right ventricular impulse during systole. As the right atrium contracts and empties its contents into the poorly compliant, hypertrophied right ventricle, a presystolic gallop (S_4) originating from the right ventricle may be heard. When the right ventricle fails, a mid-diastolic gallop (S_3) in the parasternal region is frequently heard, the jugular veins become distended, and peripheral edema may develop.

Clinical features of pulmonary hypertension are the following:
1. Symptoms: dyspnea, substernal chest pain, fatigue, syncope
2. Physical signs: loud P_2, tricuspid insufficiency murmur, prominent parasternal (right ventricular) impulse, right-sided S_4; also, right-sided S_3, jugular venous distention, peripheral edema in case of right ventricular failure

DIAGNOSTIC FEATURES

Pulmonary hypertension usually is provisionally diagnosed by echocardiography. Key findings are right ventricular hypertrophy and elevated right ventricular systolic pressure by Doppler estimates. Detailed description of these echocardiographic techniques is beyond the scope of this chapter but can be found in standard textbooks of cardiology.

Definitive confirmation of pulmonary hypertension and precise quantification of its hemodynamics require cardiac catheterization. Measurements of right ventricular, pulmonary arterial, and pulmonary capillary wedge pressures are important in confirming the diagnosis, determining the severity of disease, and assessing the response to acute vasodilator testing to guide the patient's subsequent management.

Clues to the status of the pulmonary vessels can be provided by chest radiography in some patients. With mild pulmonary hypertension originating at the arterial or arteriolar level, frequently no abnormalities are seen. As pulmonary arterial hypertension becomes more significant, the central (hilar) pulmonary arteries increase in size, and the vessels often rapidly taper off so that the distal vasculature appears attenuated (Fig. 14-2). With hypertrophy of the right ventricle, the cardiac silhouette may enlarge. This feature is most apparent on the lateral radiograph, which shows bulging of the anterior cardiac border.

When pulmonary hypertension is a consequence of either increased flow to the pulmonary vasculature (as in congenital heart disease with initial left-to-right shunting) or increased back pressure from the pulmonary veins and pulmonary capillaries (as in mitral stenosis or left ventricular failure), the findings are significantly different. In the case of congenital heart disease with left-to-right shunting, pulmonary blood flow is prominent until reversal of the left-to-right shunt occurs. When there is elevation of pulmonary venous pressure from mitral stenosis or left ventricular failure, the chest radiograph often shows redistribution of blood flow from lower to upper lung zones, accompanied by evidence of interstitial or alveolar edema.

Perfusion lung scanning is frequently a valuable adjunct in the assessment of patients with pulmonary hypertension. In particular, focal perfusion defects may suggest chronic organized thromboemboli as a likely cause for the elevation in pulmonary arterial pressure. Pulmonary angiography may be useful when perfusion scanning is positive in order to confirm the diagnosis and assess the surgical accessibility of the obstructing lesions.

Pulmonary function tests may demonstrate underlying restrictive or obstructive disease. Tests also may show decreased diffusing capacity from loss of the pulmonary vascular bed.

When evaluating the patient with pulmonary hypertension, pulmonary function tests are useful primarily for detecting underlying airflow obstruction (from chronic obstructive lung disease) or restricted lung volumes (from interstitial lung disease). As a result of the pulmonary hypertension itself and loss of the pulmonary vascular bed, the diffusing capacity may be decreased and often may be the only other abnormality noted.

Arterial blood gas analysis is highly useful for determining whether hypoxemia or acidosis plays a role in the pathogenesis of the pulmonary hypertension. Arterial Po_2

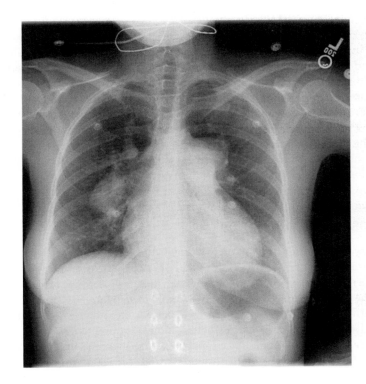

Figure 14-2. Chest radiograph of patient with pulmonary hypertension attributable to recurrent thromboemboli. Central pulmonary arteries are large bilaterally, but rapid tapering of vessels occurs distally.

may be mildly decreased as a result of pulmonary vascular disease, apparently because of nonuniform distribution of disease and ventilation-perfusion mismatch.

SPECIFIC DISORDERS ASSOCIATED WITH PULMONARY HYPERTENSION

Pulmonary hypertension is classified according to the scheme given in Table 14-1. Numerically, pulmonary hypertension most commonly is related to either left heart failure or parenchymal lung disease (most commonly chronic obstructive pulmonary disease). However, treatment directed at pulmonary hypertension in such patients has not been shown to be beneficial. In contrast, patients with IPAH and some other types of pulmonary arterial hypertension now have a variety of medications that can be used for effective treatment.

IDIOPATHIC PULMONARY ARTERIAL HYPERTENSION AND RELATED DISORDERS

Idiopathic pulmonary arterial hypertension (IPAH; formerly called *primary pulmonary hypertension*), is a disease of unknown cause found most commonly in women (female-to-male ratio 1.7:1) from 20 to 45 years old. However, IPAH also occurs in children and

Often, idiopathic pulmonary arterial hypertension occurs in young women, is associated with Raynaud's syndrome, and has a poor prognosis.

Table 14-1
REVISED NOMENCLATURE AND CLASSIFICATION OF PULMONARY HYPERTENSION (2003)

I. PULMONARY ARTERIAL HYPERTENSION
Idiopathic pulmonary arterial hypertension
Familial pulmonary arterial hypertension
Collagen vascular disease
Congenital systemic-to-pulmonary shunts (large, small, repaired or nonrepaired)
Portal hypertension
Human immunodeficiency virus infection
Drugs and toxins
Other (glycogen storage disease, Gaucher's disease, hereditary hemorrhagic telangiectasia, hemoglobinopathies, myeloproliferative disorders, splenectomy)
Associated with significant venous or capillary involvement:
    Pulmonary venoocclusive disease
    Pulmonary capillary hemangiomatosis
II. PULMONARY VENOUS HYPERTENSION
Left-sided atrial or ventricular heart disease
Left-sided valvular heart disease
III. PULMONARY HYPERTENSION ASSOCIATED WITH HYPOXEMIA
Chronic obstructive pulmonary disease
Interstitial lung disease
Sleep-disordered breathing
Alveolar hypoventilation disorders
Chronic exposure to high altitude
IV. PULMONARY HYPERTENSION CAUSED BY CHRONIC THROMBOTIC AND/OR EMBOLIC DISEASE
Thromboembolic obstruction of proximal pulmonary arteries
Thromboembolic obstruction of distal pulmonary arteries
Pulmonary embolism (tumor, parasites, foreign material)
V. MISCELLANEOUS
Sarcoidosis, histiocytosis X, lymphangioleiomyomatosis, compression of pulmonary vessels (adenopathy, tumor, fibrosing mediastinitis)

adults of all ages. In older patients, the disease appears equally in men and women. Other types of pulmonary arterial hypertension have a pathologic appearance and clinical presentation similar to those of IPAH, but with an accompanying process or etiologic agent known to be associated with this disease pattern. Such underlying processes or agents include connective tissue disease (particularly scleroderma), portal hypertension accompanying cirrhosis, HIV infection, and exposure to certain drugs or toxins. In particular, several appetite suppressants have been associated with pulmonary hypertension; they include aminorex (withdrawn from the market many years ago) and the drugs fenfluramine and dexfenfluramine (withdrawn from the market in 1997). The diagnosis of IPAH cannot be made until other causes of pulmonary hypertension have been excluded.

IPAH usually occurs as a sporadic (i.e., nonfamilial) disorder, although the disease has a familial basis in approximately 10% of cases. Information about the genetic basis of familial pulmonary arterial hypertension may have relevance to the pathogenesis of the sporadic, nonfamilial cases of IPAH. In familial pulmonary arterial hypertension, there is a mutation in the gene for the bone morphogenetic protein receptor II (BMPR2), which acts as a receptor in the transforming growth factor-β superfamily. It has been proposed that, under the proper conditions, the presence of the mutant BMPR2 leads to partial loss of an inhibitory effect of BMPR2 on vascular smooth muscle cell growth. The smooth muscle cell changes may lead indirectly to endothelial cell injury and proliferation. Because some patients with IPAH also have been reported to have a mutation in BMPR2, it is reasonable to presume that this and perhaps other genetic factors may play a role in the development of sporadic, nonfamilial IPAH.

The prognosis in IPAH is generally poor; patients frequently die within several years of diagnosis. Treatment has focused on the use of vasodilators and antiremodeling agents in an attempt to reduce pulmonary arterial pressure. Typically, before a particular vasodilator regimen is initiated, patients undergo acute vasodilator testing in the setting of pulmonary artery catheterization so that the effect of one or more short-acting vasodilators on pulmonary arterial pressures, cardiac output, and systemic blood pressure can be evaluated in a controlled setting.

Among the vasodilators that have been used therapeutically are the calcium channel blockers, such as nifedipine or diltiazem, which are given orally. Much more therapeutic success has been achieved with continuous intravenous infusion of prostacyclin derivatives (e.g., epoprostenol, treprostinil), which have been associated with clinical and hemodynamic improvement as well as improved survival. The long-term effect of these drugs indicates that they reverse some of the vascular remodeling and proliferative changes in the pulmonary arterial system separate from their vasodilator effects. However, these drugs are extremely expensive, and the need for continuous infusion makes them inconvenient and logistically more difficult to administer than oral agents. The prostacyclin derivative iloprost can be administered by repetitive inhalation, and oral agents such as the endothelin-1 receptor antagonists bosentan and ambrisentan and the phosphodiesterase-5 inhibitor sildenafil are attractive therapeutic alternatives, particularly in patients with less advanced disease.

Patients with IPAH usually are placed on long-term anticoagulation therapy with warfarin. The rationale is to decrease in situ thrombosis in the pulmonary arterial system. Observational data suggest that anticoagulation may improve survival in these patients.

For some patients with debilitating disease and a poor response to therapy, lung transplantation or combined heart–lung transplantation is indicated. However, this form of therapy has very limited availability and does not offer long-term survival for most patients.

CHRONIC THROMBOEMBOLIC DISEASE

The typical presentation of chronic pulmonary thromboembolism is with symptoms and findings related to pulmonary hypertension rather than with a history suggesting one or more known acute episodes of pulmonary embolism. In some cases the organized thromboemboli are large and proximal and presumably have been occurring over months to years. In these patients, surgical removal of the proximal organized thrombi (pulmonary thromboendarterectomy) may be a feasible and highly effective therapeutic option. Because chronic thrombi are organized and extensively infiltrated with fibroblasts and connective tissue, anticoagulation alone is not effective therapy. In other cases there is extensive thromboembolic occlusion of smaller vessels. Although this type of small vessel occlusion has generally been assumed to result from multiple small pulmonary emboli, primary thrombosis of the microvasculature, perhaps secondary to endothelial damage, has also been suggested to play a role. For the small vessel or microvascular form of chronic pulmonary thromboembolism, therapy involves anticoagulation and agents similar to those used for IPAH.

PULMONARY HYPERTENSION SECONDARY TO AIRWAY OR PARENCHYMAL LUNG DISEASE

The most common causes of cor pulmonale appear to be chronic obstructive lung disease and interstitial lung disease. In the former category, patients with type B physiology, i.e., those with a prominent component of chronic bronchitis who are considered "blue bloaters," are particularly susceptible to development of pulmonary hypertension. Hypoxia is the single most important etiologic factor in these patients. Other contributory factors include respiratory acidosis, which may worsen vasoconstriction; secondary polycythemia, a consequence of chronic hypoxemia, which further increases pulmonary artery pressures as a result of increased blood viscosity; and loss of pulmonary vascular bed caused by coexistent emphysema.

Any of the interstitial lung diseases, when relatively severe, may be associated with cor pulmonale. The major contributing factors appear to be loss of the vascular bed, as a result of the scarring process in the alveolar walls, and hypoxia.

In obstructive and interstitial disease, important therapy can be offered, namely, correction of alveolar hypoxia and hypoxemia by administration of supplemental O_2. The goal is to maintain arterial P_{O_2} at a level greater than approximately 60 mm Hg, above which hypoxic vasoconstriction is largely eliminated. Other forms of therapy aimed more specifically at the underlying disease are discussed in Chapters 6, 10, and 11.

In addition to these two categories of lung disease, other disorders of the respiratory apparatus associated with hypoxemia and hypercapnia may be complicated by development of cor pulmonale. Specifically, disorders of control of breathing, of the chest bellows, and of the neural apparatus controlling the chest bellows may be complicated by cor pulmonale. These disorders are discussed in more detail in Chapters 18 and 19.

> Obstructive disease, interstitial disease, and a variety of neural, muscular, and chest wall diseases may produce pulmonary hypertension and cor pulmonale.

PULMONARY HYPERTENSION ASSOCIATED WITH PULMONARY VENOUS HYPERTENSION

Mitral stenosis and chronic left ventricular failure are the two disorders most frequently associated with pulmonary venous, and subsequently pulmonary arterial, hypertension. The resulting right ventricular hypertrophy is not included in the category of cor pulmonale because the underlying problem resulting in pulmonary hypertension is clearly of cardiac, not pulmonary, origin.

With pulmonary venous hypertension, the pathologic and many of the clinical and diagnostic features are different in a relatively predictable way. Pathologically, dilated and tortuous capillaries and small veins may result from high pressures in the pulmonary veins and capillaries, along with chronic extravasation of red blood cells into the pulmonary parenchyma. During the process of handling the interstitial and alveolar hemoglobin, macrophages may become loaded with hemosiderin, which is a breakdown product of hemoglobin. These macrophages can be detected by appropriate staining of sputum for iron. Not infrequently, the alveolar walls have a fibrotic response, presumably secondary to the long-standing extravasation of blood, so that a component of interstitial lung disease with fibrosis may be seen.

As mentioned in the discussion of radiographic abnormalities, the presence of pulmonary venous hypertension adds several features to the chest radiograph, including redistribution of blood flow to the upper lobes and interstitial and alveolar edema. Another frequent finding is Kerley's B lines, which are small, horizontal lines extending to the pleura at both lung bases that reflect thickening of or fluid in lymphatic vessels in interlobular septa, a consequence of interstitial edema.

Treatment of these disorders revolves around attempts to optimize therapy for the cardiac disease or at least to decrease pulmonary venous and capillary pressures. The potential reversibility of pulmonary arterial hypertension depends on the chronicity of the disease and the degree to which the venous hypertension can be alleviated.

REFERENCES

GENERAL REVIEWS

Chatterjee K, DeMarco T, Alpert JS: Pulmonary hypertension. Hemodynamic diagnosis and treatment, *Arch Intern Med* 162:1925–1933, 2002.

Cool CD, Groshong SD, Oakey J, Voelkel NF: Pulmonary hypertension: cellular and molecular mechanisms, *Chest* 128(6 suppl):565S–571S, 2005.

Fishman AP: A century of pulmonary hemodynamics, *Am J Respir Crit Care Med* 170:109–113, 2004.

Fishman AP, Fishman MC, Freeman BA, et al: Mechanisms of proliferative and obliterative vascular diseases. Insights from the pulmonary and systemic circulations, *Am J Respir Crit Care Med* 158:670–674, 1998.

Gaine S: Pulmonary hypertension, *JAMA* 284:3160–3168, 2000.

Mandel J, Taichman D: *Pulmonary vascular disease,* Philadelphia, 2007, Saunders Elsevier.

Newman JH: Pulmonary hypertension, *Am J Respir Crit Care Med* 172:1072–1077, 2005.

Voelkel NF, Tuder RM: Cellular and molecular mechanisms in the pathogenesis of severe pulmonary hypertension, *Eur Respir J* 8:2129–2138, 1995.

Voelkel NF, Tuder RM: Severe pulmonary hypertensive diseases: a perspective, *Eur Respir J* 14:1246–1250, 1999.

PULMONARY ARTERIAL HYPERTENSION AND RELATED DISORDERS

Abenhaim L, Moride Y, Brenot F, et al: Appetite-suppressant drugs and the risk of primary pulmonary hypertension, *N Engl J Med* 335:609–616, 1996.

Badesch DB, Abman SH, Ahearn GS, et al: American College of Chest Physicians: Medical therapy for pulmonary arterial hypertension: ACCP evidence-based clinical practice guidelines, *Chest* 126(1 suppl):35S–62S, 2004.

Barst RJ, Rubin LJ, Long WA, McGoon MD, et al: A comparison of continuous intravenous epoprostenol (prostacyclin) with conventional therapy for primary pulmonary hypertension, *N Engl J Med* 334:296–301, 1996.

Eddahibi S, Morrell N, d'Ortho MP, Naeije R, Adnot S: Pathobiology of pulmonary arterial hypertension, *Eur Respir J* 20:1559–1572, 2002.

Farber HW, Loscalzo J: Pulmonary arterial hypertension, *N Engl J Med* 351:1655–1665, 2004.

Hoeper MM: Pulmonary hypertension in collagen vascular disease, *Eur Respir J* 19:571–576, 2002.

Humbert M, Sitbon O, Simonneau G: Treatment of pulmonary arterial hypertension, *N Engl J Med* 351:1425–1436, 2004.

Kuo PC, Kuo PC, Plotkin JS, Johnson LB: Distinctive clinical features of portopulmonary hypertension, *Chest* 112:980–986, 1997.

Loscalzo J: Genetic clues to the cause of primary pulmonary hypertension, *N Engl J Med* 345:367–371, 2001.

McGoon M, Gutterman D, Steen V, et al; American College of Chest Physicians: Screening, early detection, and diagnosis of pulmonary arterial hypertension: ACCP evidence-based clinical practice guidelines, *Chest* 126(1 suppl):14S–34S, 2004.

McLaughlin VV, McGoon MD: Pulmonary arterial hypertension, *Circulation* 114:1417–1431, 2006.

Rubin LJ, Badesch DB: Evaluation and management of the patient with pulmonary arterial hypertension, *Ann Intern Med* 143:282–292, 2005.

Rubin LJ, Badesch DB, Barst RJ, et al: Bosentan therapy for pulmonary arterial hypertension, *N Engl J Med* 346:896–903, 2002.

Voelkel NF, Clarke WR, Higenbottam T: Obesity, dexfenfluramine, and pulmonary hypertension, *Am J Respir Crit Care Med* 155:786–788, 1997.

CHRONIC PULMONARY THROMBOEMBOLISM

Fedullo PF, Auger WR, Kerr KM, Rubin LJ: Chronic thromboembolic pulmonary hypertension, *N Engl J Med* 345:1465–1472, 2001.

Hoeper MM, Mayer E, Simonneau G, Rubin LJ: Chronic thromboembolic pulmonary hypertension, *Circulation* 113:2011–2020, 2006.

PULMONARY HYPERTENSION ASSOCIATED WITH CARDIAC DISEASE

Dalen JE, Matloff JM, Evans GL, et al: Early reduction of pulmonary vascular resistance after mitral-valve replacement, *N Engl J Med* 277:387–394, 1967.

Landzberg MJ: Congenital heart disease associated pulmonary arterial hypertension, *Clin Chest Med* 28: 243–253, 2007.

COR PULMONALE

MacNee W: Pathophysiology of cor pulmonale in chronic obstructive pulmonary disease, part one, *Am J Respir Crit Care Med* 150:833–852, 1994.

MacNee W: Pathophysiology of cor pulmonale in chronic obstructive pulmonary disease, part two, *Am J Respir Crit Care Med* 150:1158–1168, 1994.

Ryu JH, Krowka MJ, Pellikka PA, Swanson KL, McGoon MD: Pulmonary hypertension in patients with interstitial lung diseases, *Mayo Clin Proc* 82:342–350, 2007.

Weitzenblum E: Chronic cor pulmonale, *Heart* 89:225–230, 2003.

15

Pleural Disease

In moving from the lung to other structures that are part of the process of respiration, the adjacent pleura is considered next. In clinical medicine, the pleura is important not only because diseases of the lung commonly cause secondary abnormalities in the pleura, but also because the pleura is a major site of disease in its own right. Not infrequently, pleural disease is a manifestation of a multisystem process that is inflammatory, immune, or malignant.

This chapter discusses the anatomy of the pleura, followed by a presentation of several physiologic principles of fluid formation and absorption by the pleura and a discussion of two types of abnormalities that affect the pleura: liquid in the pleural space (pleural effusion) and air in the pleural space (pneumothorax). A comprehensive treatment of all the disorders that affect the pleura is beyond the scope of this text. Rather, this chapter aims to cover the major categories and to give the reader an understanding of how different factors interact in the production of pleural disease. The primary malignancy of the pleura, called *mesothelioma*, is discussed in Chapter 21, which deals with neoplastic disease of the thorax.

ANATOMY

The term *pleura* refers to the thin lining layer on the outer surface of the lung *(visceral pleura)*, the corresponding lining layer on the inner surface of the chest wall *(parietal pleura)*, and the space between them *(pleural space)* (Fig. 15-1). Because the visceral and parietal pleural surfaces normally touch each other, the space between them usually is only a potential space. It contains a thin layer of serous fluid coating the apposing surfaces. When air or a larger amount of fluid accumulates in the pleural space, the visceral and parietal pleural surfaces are separated, and the space between the lung and the chest wall becomes more apparent.

The pleura lines not only the surfaces of the lung that are in direct contact with the chest wall but also the diaphragmatic and mediastinal borders of the lung. These surfaces are called the *diaphragmatic* and *mediastinal pleura*, respectively (see Fig. 15-1).

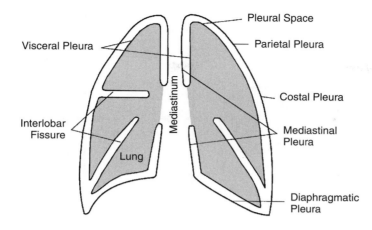

Figure 15-1. Anatomic features of pleura. Pleural space is located between visceral and parietal pleural surfaces. Pleura lines surfaces of lung in contact with chest wall (costal pleura) and mediastinal and diaphragmatic borders (mediastinal and diaphragmatic pleura, respectively). (From Lowell JR: *Pleural effusions: a comprehensive review,* p. 77, Baltimore, 1977, University Park Press.)

Visceral pleura also separates the lobes of the lung from each other; therefore, the major and minor fissures are defined by two apposing visceral pleural surfaces.

Each of the two pleural surfaces, visceral and parietal, is a thin membrane, the surface of which consists of specific lining cells called *mesothelial cells.* Beneath the mesothelial cell layer is a thin layer of connective tissue. Blood vessels and lymphatic vessels course throughout the connective tissue and are important in the dynamics of liquid formation and resorption in the pleural space. On the parietal but not on the visceral pleural surface, openings called *stomata* are located between the mesothelial cells. Each stoma leads to lymphatic channels, allowing a passageway for liquid from the pleural space to the lymphatic system. Sensory nerve endings in the parietal and diaphragmatic pleura apparently are responsible for the characteristic "pleuritic chest pain" arising from the pleura.

The blood vessels supplying the parietal pleural surface originate from the systemic arterial circulation, primarily the intercostal arteries. Venous blood from the parietal pleura drains to the systemic venous system. The visceral pleura is also supplied primarily by systemic arteries, specifically branches of the bronchial arterial circulation. However, unlike the parietal pleura, the visceral pleura has venous drainage into the pulmonary venous system. Depending on their location, the lymphatic vessels that drain the pleural surfaces transport their fluid contents to different lymph nodes. Ultimately, any liquid transported by the lymphatic channels finds its way to the right lymphatic or thoracic ducts, which empty into the systemic venous circulation.

PHYSIOLOGY

The pleural space normally contains only a small quantity of liquid (approximately 10 mL), which lubricates the apposing surfaces of the visceral and parietal pleurae. According to the current concept of pleural fluid formation and resorption, formation of fluid is ongoing primarily from the parietal pleural surface, and fluid is resorbed through the stomata into the lymphatic channels of the parietal pleura (Fig. 15-2). The normal rates of formation and resorption of fluid, which must be equal if the quantity of fluid within the pleural space is not changing, are believed to be approximately 15 to 20 mL/day.

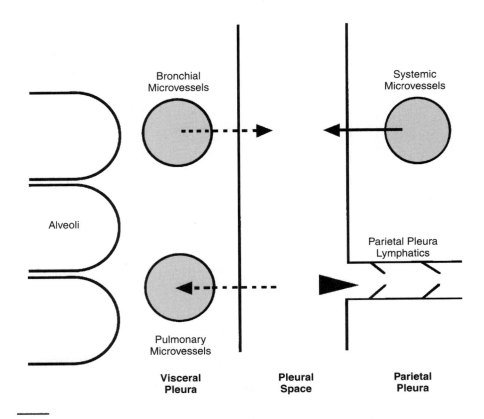

Figure 15-2. Schematic diagram of normal filtration and resorption of fluid in pleural space. Solid arrow shows filtration of fluid from parietal pleural microvessels into pleural space. Arrowhead indicates removal of fluid through stomas and into parietal pleural lymphatics. Dashed arrows indicate a minor role for filtration and resorption of fluid by visceral pleural microvessels. (Adapted from Pistolesi M, Miniati M, Giuntini C: *Am Rev Respir Dis* 140: 825–847, 1989.)

The normally occurring liquid in the pleural space is an ultrafiltrate from the pleural capillaries. Several different forces either promote or oppose fluid filtration. The net movement of fluid from the pleural capillaries to the pleural space depends on the magnitude of these counterbalancing forces. For capillaries adjacent to a pericapillary space, the hydrostatic pressure in the capillary promotes movement of fluid out of the vessel and into the pericapillary space, whereas the colloid osmotic pressure (the osmotic pressure exerted by protein drawing in fluid) hinders movement of liquid out of the capillary. Likewise, hydrostatic and colloid osmotic pressures in the pericapillary space comprise the opposing forces that act on liquid within the pericapillary region.

The effect of these forces is summarized in the Starling equation, which describes the movement of fluid between vascular and extravascular compartments of any part of the body, not just the pleura:

$$\text{Fluid movement} = K[(P_c - P_{is}) - \sigma (COP_c - COP_{is})] \qquad (15\text{-}1)$$

where K = filtration coefficient (a function of the permeability of the pleural surface), P = hydrostatic pressure, COP = colloid osmotic pressure, σ = measure of capillary permeability to protein (called the *reflection coefficient*), and the subscripts "c" and "is" refer to the capillary and the pericapillary interstitial space, respectively. In this case, the pericapillary interstitial space is essentially the pleural space; therefore, P_{is} and

COP_{is} refer to intrapleural pressure and the colloid osmotic pressure of pleural fluid, respectively. The intrapleural pressure, that is, the hydrostatic pressure within the pleural space, is negative, reflecting the outward elastic recoil of the chest wall and the inward elastic recoil of the lung.

When values obtained by direct measurement or by estimation are put into the Starling equation, a net pressure of approximately 9 cm H_2O favors movement of fluid from the parietal pleura to the pleural space. The critical factor responsible for the forces favoring formation of pleural fluid is the difference between the positive hydrostatic pressure in the pleural capillaries and the negative hydrostatic pressure within the pleural space.

Applying the same equation to fluid filtration from the visceral pleura is more difficult. The visceral pleural capillaries are supplied mainly by the systemic arterial circulation but are drained into the pulmonary venous circulation rather than the systemic venous circulation. Although currently unknown, the hydrostatic pressure in the visceral pleural capillaries is estimated to be less than in the parietal pleural capillaries. As a result, the driving pressure for formation of pleural fluid is normally greater at the parietal than at the visceral pleural surface, and most of the small amount of normal pleural fluid is thought to originate from filtration through the systemic capillaries of the parietal pleura.

Resorption of pleural fluid, including protein and cells in the fluid, occurs through the stomata between mesothelial cells on the parietal pleural surface. The fluid enters lymphatic channels, and valves within these channels ensure unidirectional flow. Movement of fluid through the valved lymphatics is believed to be aided by respiratory motion. When pleural fluid formation is increased, as occurs in many of the pathologic states to be discussed, the parietal pleural lymphatics are capable of increasing their flow substantially to accommodate at least some of the excess fluid formed.

> The Starling equation can be applied to the parietal pleura:
> $P_c = 30$ cm H_2O
> P_{is} (mean intrapleural pressure) $= -5$ cm H_2O
> $COP_c = 32$ cm H_2O
> $COP_{is} = 6$ cm H_2O
> $\sigma = 1$, $K = 1$

> Fluid movement at parietal pleura $= [30 - (-5)] - 1(32 - 6) = 9$ cm H_2O.

> Pleural fluid is filtered from the parietal pleura into the pleural space and reabsorbed through stomata into the parietal pleural lymphatics.

PLEURAL EFFUSION

In the normal individual, resorption of pleural fluid maintains pace with pleural fluid formation so that fluid does not accumulate. However, a variety of diseases affect the forces governing pleural fluid filtration and resorption, resulting in fluid formation exceeding fluid removal, that is, development of pleural effusion. The pathogenesis (dynamics) of fluid accumulation is discussed first, followed by a consideration of some of the etiologic factors, clinical features, and diagnostic approaches to pleural effusions.

PATHOGENESIS OF PLEURAL FLUID ACCUMULATION

In theory, a change in the magnitude of any of the factors in the Starling equation can cause sufficient imbalance of pleural fluid dynamics, resulting in pleural fluid accumulation. In practice, it is easiest to divide these changes into the following two categories: (1) alteration of the permeability of the pleural surface, that is, changes in the filtration coefficient (K) and the reflection coefficient (σ) so that the pleura is more permeable to fluid and to larger molecular-weight components of blood, and (2) alteration in the driving pressure, encompassing a change in hydrostatic or colloid osmotic pressures of the parietal or visceral pleura, without any change in pleural permeability.

The most common types of disease causing a change in the filtration and reflection coefficients are inflammatory or neoplastic diseases involving the pleura. In these circumstances the pleural surface becomes more permeable to proteins so that the accumulated fluid has a relatively high protein content. This type of fluid, because of a change in permeability and its association with a relatively high protein content, is termed an *exudate.*

In contrast, an increase in hydrostatic pressure within pleural capillaries (e.g., as might be seen in congestive heart failure) or a decrease in plasma colloid osmotic pressure (as in hypoproteinemia) results in accumulation of fluid with a low protein

> Increased permeability of the pleural surface is associated with exudative pleural fluid. Changes in pleural hydrostatic or colloid osmotic pressures are associated with transudative pleural fluid.

content because the pleural barrier still is relatively impermeable to the movement of proteins. This type of fluid, because of a change in the driving pressure (without increased permeability) and the presence of a low protein content, is termed a *transudate*.

Another general mechanism accounting for some pleural effusions reflects neither altered permeability nor altered driving pressure. Rather, the fluid originates in the peritoneum as ascitic fluid and travels to the pleural space primarily via small diaphragmatic defects and perhaps also by diaphragmatic lymphatics. Considering that intrapleural pressure is more negative than intraperitoneal pressure, it is not surprising that fluid moves from the peritoneum to the pleural space when such defects exist.

Interference with the resorptive process for pleural fluid can contribute to the development of effusions. This is seen primarily with blockage of the lymphatic drainage from the pleural space, as may occur when tumor cells invade the lymphatic channels or the draining lymph nodes.

ETIOLOGY OF PLEURAL EFFUSION

The numerous causes of pleural fluid accumulation are best divided into transudative and exudative categories (Table 15-1). This distinction is generally easy to make and is most important in guiding the physician along the best route for further evaluation. Transudative fluid usually implies that the pathologic process does not primarily involve the pleural surfaces, whereas exudative fluid often suggests that the pleura is affected by the disease process causing the effusion.

Transudative Pleural Fluid

Most frequently, transudative pleural fluid is associated with congestive heart failure. Although traditionally the explanation has been that an elevation of hydrostatic pressure in the pleural capillaries was responsible for increased flux of fluid from these vessels into the pleural space, more recent data suggest an alternative explanation. The source of pleural fluid in congestive heart failure appears primarily to be liquid leaking out of the *pulmonary* capillaries and accumulating in the lung interstitium. This interstitial fluid then leaks across the visceral pleura and into the pleural space, akin to leakage of fluid from the surface of a wet sponge. On the basis of clinical studies, pulmonary venous hypertension (with left-sided heart failure) leading to increased hydrostatic pressure in the pulmonary capillaries appears to be a more important factor contributing to effusions than is systemic venous hypertension (with right-sided failure). Pleural effusion is particularly likely to occur when both ventricles are failing and pulmonary and systemic venous hypertension coexist.

Table	15-1

MAJOR CAUSES OF PLEURAL EFFUSION

TRANSUDATE
Increased hydrostatic pressure; "overflow" of liquid from the lung interstitium
   Congestive heart failure
Decreased plasma oncotic pressure
   Nephrotic syndrome
Movement of transudative ascitic fluid through the diaphragm
   Cirrhosis
EXUDATE
Inflammatory
   Infection (tuberculosis, bacterial pneumonia)
   Pulmonary embolus (infarction)
   Connective tissue disease (lupus, rheumatoid arthritis)
   Adjacent to subdiaphragmatic disease (pancreatitis, subphrenic abscess)
Malignant

Patients with hypoproteinemia have decreased plasma colloid osmotic pressure, and pleural fluid may develop because hydrostatic pressure in pleural capillaries now is less opposed by the osmotic pressure provided by plasma proteins. The most common circumstance resulting in hypoproteinemia and pleural effusion is nephrotic syndrome, with excessive renal losses of protein.

Movement of transudative ascitic fluid through diaphragmatic defects and into the pleural space appears to be the most important mechanism for the pleural effusions sometimes seen in liver disease, especially cirrhosis. Although patients also may have decreased hepatic synthesis of protein, hypoproteinemia has only a minor role in the pathogenesis of these effusions.

Ascitic fluid may travel through diaphragmatic defects into the pleural space.

Exudative Pleural Fluid

Exudative pleural fluid generally implies an increase in the permeability of the pleural surfaces so that protein and fluid more readily enter the pleural space. Although a wide variety of processes can result in exudative pleural effusions, the two main etiologic categories are inflammatory and neoplastic disease. The inflammatory processes often originate within the lung but extend to the visceral pleural surface. Infection (especially bacterial pneumonia and tuberculosis) and pulmonary embolus (often with infarction) are two common examples. In the case of pneumonia extending to the pleural surface, an associated pleural effusion is called a *parapneumonic effusion*. When the effusion itself harbors organisms or has the appearance of pus (as a result of an exuberant inflammatory response with many thousands of neutrophils), then the effusion is called an *empyema* or, more properly, *empyema thoracis*. Although infection within the pleural space is commonly secondary to a pneumonia, empyema also may result from infection introduced through the chest wall, as occurs with trauma or surgery involving the thorax.

In tuberculosis a subpleural focus of infection may rupture into the pleural space, with an ensuing inflammatory response of the pleura (with or without growth of the tubercle bacilli within the pleural space). In some cases the pulmonary focus is not apparent, and pleural involvement is the major manifestation of tuberculosis within the thorax.

Other forms of inflammatory disease affecting the pleura primarily involve the pleural surface as opposed to the lung. Several of the connective tissue diseases, particularly systemic lupus erythematosus and rheumatoid arthritis, are associated with pleural involvement that is independent of changes within the pulmonary parenchyma. Inflammatory processes below the diaphragm, such as pancreatitis and subphrenic abscess, are often accompanied by "sympathetic" pleural inflammation and development of an exudative pleural effusion. With these disorders, inflammation of the diaphragm itself may lead to increased permeability of vessels in the diaphragmatic pleura and leakage of fluid into the pleural space. When ascites is present, as is common in pancreatitis, transport of fluid from the abdomen through defects in the diaphragm may contribute to pleural fluid accumulation.

Malignancy may cause pleural effusion by several mechanisms, but the resulting fluid is generally exudative in nature. Commonly, malignant cells are found on the pleural surface, arriving there either by direct extension from an intrapulmonary malignancy or by hematogenous (bloodstream) dissemination from a distant source. In other cases, lymphatic channels or lymph nodes are blocked by foci of tumor so that the normal lymphatic clearance mechanism for protein and fluid from the pleural space is impaired. In these latter cases, malignant cells are generally not found on examination of the pleural fluid.

A host of other disorders may have pleural effusion as a clinical manifestation. The list includes such varied processes as hypothyroidism, benign ovarian tumors (Meigs' syndrome), asbestos exposure, and primary disorders of the lymphatic channels. Detailed discussion of the various disorders with potential for pleural fluid accumulation can be found in the references.

CLINICAL FEATURES

A patient with pleural fluid may or may not have symptoms caused by the pleural disease. Whether symptoms are present depends on the size of the effusion(s) and the nature of the underlying process. The inflammatory processes affecting the pleura frequently result in pleuritic chest pain, that is, sharp pain aggravated by respiration. When an effusion is large, patients may experience dyspnea resulting from compromise of the underlying lung. With small- or moderate-sized effusions, a patient with otherwise normal lungs generally does not have dyspnea just from the presence of fluid in the pleural space. When the pleural fluid has an inflammatory nature or is frankly infected, fever is commonly present.

On physical examination of the chest, the region overlying the effusion is dull to percussion. Breath sounds usually are decreased in this region as a result of decreased transmission of sound through the fluid medium in the pleura. At the upper level of the effusion, egophony may be heard as a manifestation of increased transmission of sound resulting from compression (atelectasis) of the underlying lung parenchyma. A scratchy, pleural friction rub may be present, particularly with an inflammatory process involving the pleural surfaces.

> Common clinical features with pleural effusion(s) are the following:
> Symptoms: Pleuritic chest pain, dyspnea
> Physical signs: Dullness, decreased breath sounds, egophony at upper level, pleural friction rub

DIAGNOSTIC APPROACH

The posteroanterior and lateral chest radiographs are clearly most important in the initial evaluation of the patient with suspected pleural effusion (Fig. 15-3). With a

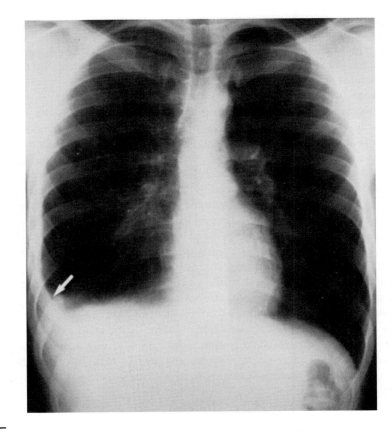

Figure 15-3. Chest radiograph shows small right pleural effusion. Right costophrenic angle is blunted by the effusion *(arrow).* Curvature of lateral rib overlies meniscus of pleural fluid.

small effusion, blunting of the normally sharp angle between the diaphragm and the chest wall (costophrenic angle) is seen. Often this blunting is first apparent on inspection of the posterior costophrenic angle on the lateral radiograph because this is the most dependent area of the pleural space. With a larger effusion, a homogeneous opacity of liquid density appears and is most obvious at the lung base(s) when the patient is upright. The fluid may track along the lateral chest wall, forming a meniscus.

When certain inflammatory effusions persist for a time, fluid may no longer be free-flowing within the pleural space, as fibrous bands of tissue (loculations) form within the pleura. In such circumstances, fluid is not necessarily positioned as expected from the effects of gravity, and atypical appearances may be found. To detect whether fluid is free-flowing or whether small costophrenic angle densities represent pleural fluid, a lateral decubitus chest radiograph may be extremely useful. In this view, the patient lies on a side, and free-flowing fluid shifts position to line the most dependent part of the pleural space (Fig. 15-4).

Ultrasonography is another technique frequently used to evaluate the presence and location of pleural fluid. When pleural fluid is present, a characteristic echo-free space can be detected between the chest wall and the lung. Ultrasonography is particularly useful in locating a small effusion not apparent on physical examination and in guiding the physician to a suitable site for thoracentesis.

When pleural fluid is present and the etiologic diagnosis is uncertain, sampling the fluid by thoracentesis (withdrawal of fluid through a needle or catheter) allows determination of the cellular and chemical characteristics of the fluid. These features define whether the fluid is transudative or exudative and frequently give other clues about the cause. Although different criteria have been used, the most common criteria include

An exudative effusion is defined by one or more of the following:
1. Pleural fluid/serum protein ratio >0.5
2. Pleural fluid/serum LDH ratio >0.6
3. Pleural fluid LDH $>\frac{2}{3} \times$ upper limit of normal serum LDH

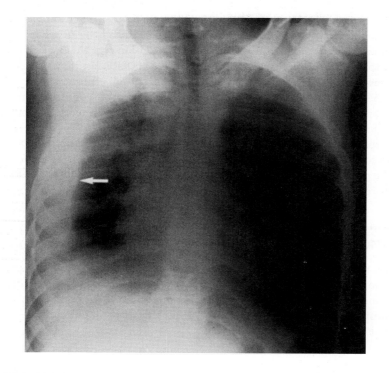

Figure 15-4. Right lateral decubitus chest radiograph of patient shown in Figure 15-3. With the patient lying on right side, pleural fluid *(arrow)* flows freely to the dependent part of pleural space adjacent to right lateral chest wall. Film is shown upright for convenience of comparison with Figure 15-3.

the levels of protein and of the enzyme lactate dehydrogenase (LDH) within the fluid, both in absolute numbers and relative to the corresponding values in serum. Exudative fluid has high levels of protein, LDH, or both, whereas transudative fluid has low levels of protein and LDH.

Pleural fluid obtained by thoracentesis is routinely analyzed for absolute numbers and types of cellular constituents, for bacteria (by stains and cultures), and for glucose level. In many cases, amylase level and pH value of the pleural fluid are measured. Special slides are prepared for cytologic examination, and a search for malignant cells is made. Detailed discussions of the findings in different disorders can be found in the references.

In some cases, pleural tissue is sampled by closed pleural biopsy, generally performed with a relatively large cutting needle inserted through the skin of the chest wall. Histologic examination of this tissue is most useful for demonstrating granulomas of tuberculosis but also can reveal implants of tumor cells from a malignant process in some cases. Pleural tissue also can be obtained under direct vision with the aid of a thoracoscope passed through the chest wall and into the pleural space; this has become the most definitive method for evaluating the pleural space for malignant implants.

Pulmonary function tests are generally not part of the routine evaluation of patients with pleural effusion. However, a significant effusion may impair lung expansion sufficiently to cause a restrictive pattern (with decreased lung volumes) on pulmonary function testing.

TREATMENT

Treatment of pleural effusion depends entirely on the nature of the underlying process and usually is directed at this process rather than the effusion itself. In cases with a high likelihood of the effusion eventuating in extensive fibrosis or loculation of the pleural space, e.g., with an empyema or a hemothorax (blood in the pleural space, often secondary to trauma), the fluid is drained with a catheter or a relatively large-bore tube inserted into the pleural space. If loculation has already occurred, then thoracoscopy or an open surgical approach may be necessary to break up fibrous adhesions and allow effective drainage of the fluid and full reexpansion of the lung.

In other cases with recurrent large effusions, especially those caused by malignancy, the fluid is initially drained with a tube that is passed into the pleural space, and an irritating agent (e.g., talc or a tetracycline derivative) is instilled via the tube into the pleural space to induce inflammation and to cause the visceral and parietal pleural surfaces to become adherent. This process of sclerosis (also called *pleurodesis*) eliminates the pleural space and, if effective, prevents recurrence of pleural effusion on the side where the procedure was performed.

PNEUMOTHORAX

Air is not normally present between the visceral and parietal pleural surfaces. However, air can be introduced into the pleural space by a break in the surface of either pleural membrane, thus creating a *pneumothorax*. Because pressure within the pleural space is subatmospheric, air readily enters the space if there is any communication with air at atmospheric pressure.

ETIOLOGY AND PATHOGENESIS

When a pneumothorax is created by the entry of air through the chest wall and the parietal pleura, the most common causes are (1) trauma (e.g., knife or gunshot wound) and (2) introduction of air via a needle, catheter, or incision through the chest wall and into the pleural space. Alternatively, air may enter the pleura through a break in the visceral pleura, allowing communication between the airways or alveoli and the pleural space. Examples of the latter circumstance include rupture of a subpleural air pocket (e.g., bleb, cyst, or bulla) into the pleural space or necrosis of the lung adjacent to the pleura by a destructive pneumonia or neoplasm.

In some cases a reason for the pneumothorax is apparent, such as an underlying abnormality in the lung, a form of lung disease known to be associated with subpleural air pockets (emphysema or interstitial lung disease with honeycombing and subpleural cysts), or destruction of lung tissue adjacent to the pleural surface (necrotizing pneumonia or neoplasm). Pneumothorax in these clinical settings is said to be secondary to the known lung disease.

In patients with acquired immunodeficiency syndrome, pneumothorax can develop as a complication of pulmonary infection with *Pneumocystis jiroveci* (formerly called *Pneumocystis carinii*), presumably because of necrosis or cyst formation adjacent to the visceral pleura.

In contrast, other patients do not have a defined abnormality of the lung adjacent to the pleura and therefore are said to have a *primary spontaneous pneumothorax*. Even in this latter circumstance, patients frequently have small subpleural pockets of air (blebs), especially at the lung apex, that have gone unrecognized clinically and on routine radiographic examination. If the bleb eventually ruptures, air is released from the lung parenchyma into the pleural space, creating a pneumothorax.

Patients who receive positive pressure to the tracheobronchial tree and alveoli (e.g., with mechanical ventilation) are subject to development of a pneumothorax. In this case, as a result of positive pressure, a preexisting subpleural bleb may rupture, or air may rupture through an alveolar wall into the interstitial space, track through the lung parenchyma to the subpleural surface, and then rupture into the pleural space. Alternatively, and perhaps more commonly, the air following alveolar rupture tracks retrograde to the mediastinum alongside blood vessels and airways and produces a pneumomediastinum (see Chapter 16). A pneumothorax can result when air ruptures through the mediastinal pleura into the pleural space.

> A pneumothorax can result from a break in the parietal pleura (e.g., from trauma, needle or catheter insertion) or in the visceral pleura (e.g., from rupture of a subpleural air pocket, necrosis of lung adjacent to the pleura).

PATHOPHYSIOLOGY

The pathophysiologic consequences of a pneumothorax are variable, ranging from none to the development of acute cardiovascular collapse. The size of the pneumothorax (i.e., the amount of air within the pleural space) is an important determinant of the clinical effects. Because the lung is enclosed within a relatively rigid chest wall, accumulation of a substantial amount of pleural air is accompanied by collapse of the underlying lung parenchyma. In extreme cases, air in the pleural space occupies almost the entire hemithorax, and the lung is totally collapsed and functionless until the air is resorbed or removed.

Air in the pleural space is generally under atmospheric or subatmospheric pressure. In some cases the air may be under positive pressure, creating a *tension pneumothorax*. This tension within the pleural space is believed to occur as a result of a "one-way valve" mechanism, by which air is free to enter the pleural space during inspiration, but the site of entry is closed during expiration. Therefore, only unidirectional movement of air into the pleural space is permitted, the intrapleural pressure increases, and the underlying lung collapses further. When pleural pressure is sufficiently high, the mediastinum and trachea may be shifted away from the side of the pneumothorax. In extreme cases, cardiovascular collapse may result, with a marked fall in cardiac output and blood pressure. These hemodynamic changes are commonly stated to result from inhibition of venous return into the superior and inferior venae cavae as a consequence of positive intrathoracic pressure. However, another explanation is that marked disturbances in

> A tension pneumothorax may be associated with total collapse of the underlying lung, mediastinal shift, and cardiovascular collapse.

gas exchange contribute to the hemodynamic changes. Whatever the mechanism, emergent treatment is necessary to release the air under tension and reverse the cardiovascular collapse. A particularly important risk factor for the development of a tension pneumothorax is positive-pressure ventilation with a mechanical ventilator. When a pneumothorax occurs in this situation, the ventilator may continue to introduce air under high pressure through the site of rupture in the visceral pleura.

For most cases of pneumothorax, after the site of entry into the pleural space is closed, the air is spontaneously resorbed. The reason is that the partial pressure of air in a pneumothorax is higher than the partial pressure of gas in surrounding venous or capillary blood. For example, air within the pleural space might have a pressure a few millimeters of mercury below atmospheric pressure, or approximately 755 to 758 mm Hg. In contrast, gas pressures in mixed venous blood are approximately as follows: $Po_2 = 40$ mm Hg, $Pco_2 = 46$ mm Hg, $Pn_2 = 573$ mm Hg, and $Ph_2o = 47$ mm Hg. Therefore, the total gas pressure in mixed venous blood is 706 mm Hg, which is approximately 50 mm Hg below that of air in the pleural space. Consequently, there is a gradient for diffusion of gas from the pleural space into mixed venous blood. With continued diffusion of gas in this direction, the size of the pneumothorax is slowly reduced, the gas pressures within the pleural space are maintained, and the gradient favoring absorption of gas continues until all the air is resorbed.

If pure O_2 is administered to the patient with a pneumothorax, the process of resorption can be hastened. In arterial blood, most of the nitrogen is replaced by O_2. As a result, Pn_2 in the capillary blood surrounding the pneumothorax becomes quite low, and the gradient for resorption of nitrogen from the pleural space has been increased considerably. At the same time, although arterial Po_2 is high after inhalation of pure O_2, Po_2 falls substantially in capillary and venous blood because of O_2 consumption by the tissues. Therefore, a large partial pressure gradient from pleural gas to pleural capillary blood remains for O_2 as well. The net result is that O_2 administration favors more rapid resorption of nitrogen (the main component of gas in the pneumothorax) without significantly compromising the gradient promoting resorption of O_2.

When a pneumothorax is causing important clinical problems, the physician need not wait for spontaneous resorption of the air but can actively remove the air with a needle, catheter, or tube inserted into the pleural space.

CLINICAL FEATURES

Clinical features of pneumothorax are the following:
Symptoms: Chest pain, dyspnea
Physical signs: Asymmetric (decreased) breath sounds, hyperresonance, tracheal deviation (tension), ↓ blood pressure (tension)

In many cases the clinical setting is appropriate for the development of a pneumothorax. For example, the patient may have predisposing underlying lung disease or may be receiving positive-pressure ventilation with a mechanical ventilator. Interestingly, the group of patients in whom a primary spontaneous pneumothorax develops shows a striking predominance of males. In addition, the patients are often smokers, young adults, and frequently are tall and thin.

The most common complaint at the time of pneumothorax is the acute onset of chest pain, dyspnea, or both. However, some patients may be totally free of symptoms, particularly if the pneumothorax is small. On physical examination the findings depend to a large extent on the size of the pneumothorax. Because of decreased transmission of sound, breath sounds and tactile fremitus are diminished or absent. With a significant amount of air in the pleural space, increased resonance to percussion over the affected lung may be observed.

When the pneumothorax is under tension, the patient often is in acute distress, and a decrease in blood pressure or even frank cardiovascular collapse may be present. Palpation of the trachea frequently demonstrates deviation away from the side of the pneumothorax.

DIAGNOSTIC APPROACH

The diagnosis of pneumothorax is made or confirmed by chest radiograph. The characteristic finding is a curved line representing the edge of the lung (the visceral pleura) separated from the chest wall. Between the edge of the lung and the chest wall, the pleural space is lucent, and none of the normal vascular markings of the lung are seen in this region (Figs. 15-5 and 15-6). When the pneumothorax is small, separation of the visceral and parietal pleura appears on upright chest films only at the apex of the lung, where the pleural air generally accumulates first. If the pneumothorax is substantial, the lung loses a significant amount of volume and therefore has a greater density than usual.

When both fluid and air are present in the pleural space *(hydropneumothorax),* the fluid no longer appears as a meniscus tracking up along the lateral chest wall. Rather, the fluid falls to the most dependent part of the pleural space and appears as a liquid density with a perfectly horizontal upper border (see Fig. 15-6). Finally, when gas in the pleural space is under tension, evidence is often seen of structures (e.g., trachea and mediastinum) being "pushed" away from the side of the pneumothorax (Fig. 15-7).

TREATMENT

Treatment of a pneumothorax is determined by its size as well as by the ensuing clinical consequences. With a small pneumothorax causing few symptoms, it is best to wait for spontaneous resolution of the pneumothorax. This process can be hastened by administration of 100% O_2, which alters the partial pressures of gases in capillary

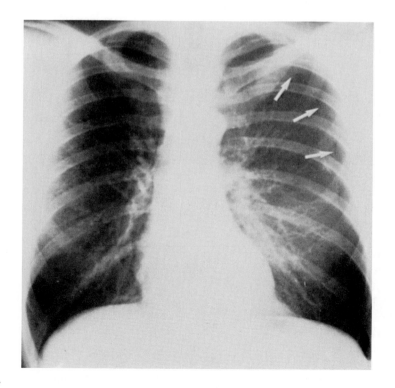

Figure 15-5. Chest radiograph of patient with spontaneous pneumothorax on left. Arrows point to visceral pleural surface of lung. Beyond visceral pleura is air within pleural space. No lung markings can be seen in this region.

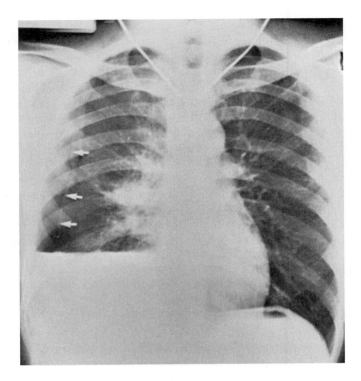

Figure 15-6. Chest radiograph shows right hydropneumothorax. Horizontal line in lower right hemithorax is interface between air and liquid in pleural space. Arrows point to visceral pleura above level of effusion. There is air in pleural space between visceral pleura and chest wall.

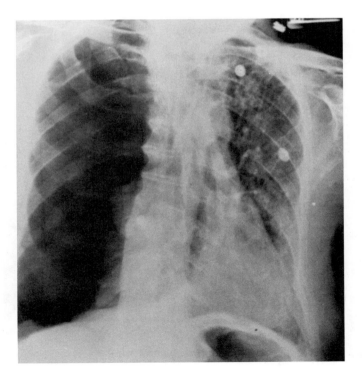

Figure 15-7. Chest radiograph shows right-sided tension pneumothorax. No lung markings are seen in the right hemithorax, and the mediastinum is shifted to the left.

blood, favoring the resorption of pleural air. When the pneumothorax is large (i.e., involves >20% of the hemithorax) or the patient has significant clinical sequelae, the air is best removed, usually by a needle, catheter, or chest tube inserted into the pleural space. Occasionally, patients have recurrent spontaneous pneumothoraces that require obliteration of the pleural space by instilling agents, such as talc, into the pleura to promote pleural inflammation and sclerosis. Concomitant thoracoscopic resection of subpleural apical blebs is frequently performed.

If a patient has hemodynamic compromise because of a tension pneumothorax, a needle, catheter, or tube must be inserted immediately to relieve the pressure. When this technique is performed, the sound of air under pressure escaping from the pleural space can readily be heard. The most important results of decompression are improvements in gas exchange, venous return to the thorax, cardiac output, and arterial blood pressure.

REFERENCES

GENERAL REVIEWS

Colt HG: Thoracoscopy. Window to the pleural space, *Chest* 116:1409–1415, 1999.

Light RW: *Pleural diseases,* ed 5, Philadelphia, 2007, Lippincott Williams & Wilkins.

Loddenkemper R, Antony VB: Pleural diseases, *Eur Respir Mon* 7(monograph 22):1–326, 2002.

Pistolesi M, Miniati M, Giuntini C: Pleural liquid and solute exchange, *Am Rev Respir Dis* 140:825–847, 1989.

Sahn SA: The pleura, *Am Rev Respir Dis* 138:184–234, 1988.

Sahn SA, editor: Pleural disease, *Clin Chest Med* 27:157–394, 2006.

Wiener-Kronish JP, Broaddus VC: Interrelationship of pleural and pulmonary interstitial liquid, *Annu Rev Physiol* 55:209–226, 1993.

Zocchi L: Physiology and pathophysiology of pleural fluid turnover, *Eur Respir J* 20:1545–1558, 2002.

PLEURAL EFFUSION

American Thoracic Society: Management of malignant pleural effusions, *Am J Respir Crit Care Med* 162:1987–2001, 2000.

Bartter T, Santarelli R, Akers SM, Pratter MR: The evaluation of pleural effusion, *Chest* 106:1209–1214, 1994.

Colice GL: Medical and surgical treatment of parapneumonic effusions. An evidence-based guideline, *Chest* 18:1158–1171, 2000.

Light RW: Pleural effusion, *N Engl J Med* 346:1971–1977, 2002.

Light RW: Parapneumonic effusions and empyema, *Proc Am Thorac Soc* 3:75–80, 2006.

Light RW, MacGregor MI, Luchsinger PC, Ball WC Jr: Pleural effusions: the diagnostic separation of transudates and exudates, *Ann Intern Med* 77:507–513, 1972.

Rodriguez-Panadero F, Janssen JP, Astoul P: Thoracoscopy: general overview and place in the diagnosis and management of pleural effusion, *Eur Respir J* 28:409–422, 2006.

Thomsen TW, DeLaPena J, Setnik GS: Videos in clinical medicine: Thoracentesis, *N Engl J Med* 355:e16, 2006.

PNEUMOTHORAX

Baumann MH: Management of spontaneous pneumothorax, *Clin Chest Med* 27:369–381, 2006.

Baumann MH, Strange C, Heffner JE, et al: Management of spontaneous pneumothorax. An American College of Chest Physicians Delphi consensus statement, *Chest* 119:590–602, 2001.

O'Connor AR, Morgan WE: Radiological review of pneumothorax, *BMJ* 330:1493–1497, 2005.

Sahn SA, Heffner JE: Spontaneous pneumothorax, *N Engl J Med* 342:868–874, 2000.

Tschopp JM, Rami-Porta R, Noppen M, Astoul P: Management of spontaneous pneumothorax: state of the art, *Eur Respir J* 28:637–650, 2006.

Wakai A, O'Sullivan RG, McCabe G: Simple aspiration versus intercostal tube drainage for primary spontaneous pneumothorax in adults, *Cochrane Database Syst Rev* 1:CD004479, 2007.

Weissberg D, Refaely Y: Pneumothorax. Experience with 1,199 patients, *Chest* 117:1279–1285, 2000.

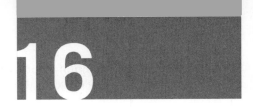

Mediastinal Disease

ANATOMIC FEATURES	PNEUMOMEDIASTINUM
MEDIASTINAL MASSES	Etiology and Pathogenesis
Etiology	Pathophysiology
Clinical Features	Clinical Features
Diagnostic Approach	Diagnostic Approach
Treatment	Treatment

The mediastinum is the region of the thoracic cavity located between the two lungs. Included within the mediastinum are numerous structures, ranging from the heart and the great vessels (aorta, superior and inferior venae cavae) to lymph nodes and nerves. The physician dealing with diseases of the lung is confronted with mediastinal disease in two main ways: (1) an imaging study (chest radiograph or computed tomogram [CT]) shows an abnormal mediastinum or (2) the patient has symptoms similar to those originating from primary pulmonary disease. This chapter describes some of the anatomic features of the mediastinum and discusses two of its most common clinical problems: mediastinal masses and pneumomediastinum.

ANATOMIC FEATURES

The mediastinum is bounded superiorly by bony structures of the thoracic inlet and inferiorly by the diaphragm. Laterally, the mediastinal pleura on each side serves as a membrane separating the medial aspect of the lung (with its visceral pleura) from the structures contained within the mediastinum. The mediastinum most frequently is divided into three anatomic compartments: anterior, middle, and posterior (Table 16-1). This division is particularly useful for characterizing mediastinal masses because specific etiologic factors often have a predilection for a particular compartment. Normal structures located within or coursing through each of the compartments may serve as the origin of a mediastinal mass. Consequently, knowledge of the structures contained in each of the three compartments is important for the clinician in evaluating a patient with a mediastinal mass.

The borders of the three mediastinal compartments are visualized most easily on a lateral chest radiograph (Fig. 16-1). Several descriptions exist for the limits defining each compartment. According to the scheme used here, the anterior mediastinum extends from the sternum to the anterior border of the pericardium. Included within this region are the thymus, lymph nodes, and loose connective tissue.

The borders of the middle mediastinum are the anterior and posterior pericardium. This region includes the heart, pericardium, great vessels, trachea, lymph nodes, and phrenic nerves. The upper portion of the vagus nerve also courses through the middle mediastinum.

Table 16-1

MEDIASTINAL COMPARTMENTS: ANATOMY AND PATHOLOGY

Compartment	Borders	Normal Structures	Masses
Anterior	Anterior: Sternum Posterior: Pericardium, ascending aorta, brachiocephalic vessels	Lymph nodes Connective tissue Thymus (remnant in adults)	Thymoma Germ cell neoplasm Lymphoma Thyroid enlargement (intrathoracic goiter) Other tumors
Middle	Anterior: Anterior pericardium, ascending aorta, brachiocephalic vessels Posterior: Posterior pericardium	Pericardium Heart Vessels: Ascending aorta, venae cavae, main pulmonary arteries Trachea Lymph nodes Nerves: Phrenic, upper vagus	Carcinoma Lymphoma Pericardial cyst Bronchogenic cyst Benign lymph node enlargement (granulomatous disease)
Posterior	Anterior: Posterior pericardium Posterior: Posterior chest wall	Vessels: Descending aorta Esophagus Vertebral column Nerves: Sympathetic chain, lower vagus Lymph nodes Connective tissue	Neurogenic tumor Diaphragmatic hernia

The posterior mediastinum extends from the posterior pericardium to the posterior chest wall. This compartment normally includes the vertebral column, neural structures (including the chain of sympathetic nerves and the lower portion of the vagus nerves), esophagus, and descending aorta. Some lymph nodes and loose connective tissue may be found in the posterior mediastinum.

MEDIASTINAL MASSES

ETIOLOGY

Because of the predilection for certain types of masses to occur in specific mediastinal compartments, it is easiest to consider separately masses occurring in each of the three anatomic regions. However, a fair amount of overlap occurs; that is, many types of mediastinal masses are not exclusively limited to the compartment in which they most frequently appear. A summary of the types of mediastinal masses, arranged by anatomic compartment, is given in Table 16-1.

Anterior Mediastinal Masses

The major types of anterior mediastinal mass are thymoma, germ cell tumor, lymphoma, thyroid gland enlargement, and miscellaneous other tumors.

Thymomas, or tumors of the epithelium of the thymus gland, are the most common type of neoplasm originating in the anterior compartment. They may be benign or malignant in behavior, depending more on whether they are locally invasive than on any

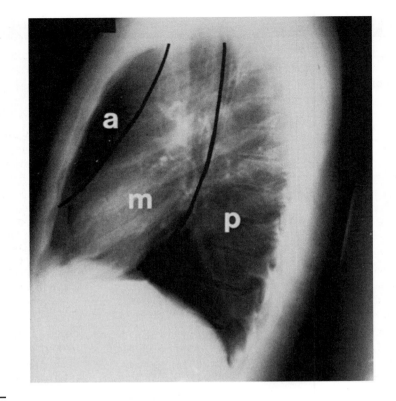

Figure 16-1. Lateral chest radiograph shows borders of three mediastinal compartments. a = Anterior; m = middle; p = posterior.

Myasthenia gravis occurs frequently in patients with thymoma.

particular morphologic features. Thymomas are diagnosed most commonly in patients between the ages of 40 and 60 years and are found equally in men and woman. These tumors are notable for their association with a variety of systemic paraneoplastic syndromes. The best known and most common of these is myasthenia gravis, which is found in 10% to 50% of patients with thymic tumors. Myasthenia gravis is characterized clinically by muscle fatigue and weakness and pathophysiologically by a decreased number of acetylcholine receptors at neuromuscular junctions. The latter is due to antibodies against the acetylcholine receptor. Other systemic syndromes associated with thymoma include pure red blood cell aplasia, hypogammaglobulinemia, and several conditions that appear to have an autoimmune origin, such as systemic lupus erythematosus and polymyositis.

Germ cell tumors are believed to originate from primitive germ cells that probably underwent abnormal migration during an early developmental period. Several types of germ cell tumors have been described. The most common is the teratoma, a tumor composed of ectodermal, mesodermal, and endodermal derivatives. The types of tissue seen are clearly foreign to the area from which the tumor arose and may include elements such as skin, hair, cartilage, and bone. Like thymomas, these tumors may be benign or malignant, with approximately 80% described as benign. Other, less common, germ cell tumors include seminomas and choriocarcinomas.

Lymphoma and carcinoma commonly affect anterior or middle compartments. Mediastinal disease may be isolated or part of more widespread involvement.

Lymphomas may involve the mediastinum, either as part of a disseminated process, in which the mediastinum is only one locus of the disease, or as primary mediastinal masses without other clinically apparent areas of involvement. Hodgkin's disease, particularly the nodular sclerosis subtype, is well described as manifesting solely as a mediastinal mass, although non-Hodgkin's lymphoma may have a similar presentation. Like carcinoma, lymphoma involving the mediastinum is most common in the anterior or the middle mediastinal compartment.

The thyroid gland may be the origin of a mediastinal mass as a result of extension of thyroid tissue from the neck into the mediastinum. Because these masses are generally not functional, patients do not have clinical or laboratory evidence of hyperthyroidism. Only rarely do these masses of thyroid origin prove to be malignant.

Other tumors, including carcinomas, may produce a mediastinal mass. In many cases mediastinal involvement is secondary to a primary neoplasm found elsewhere, particularly in the lung. In occasional cases, no other tumor is apparent, and patients are believed to have a primary carcinoma originating in the mediastinum. Carcinomatous involvement of the mediastinum is not limited to the anterior mediastinum but is also common in the middle mediastinal compartment.

A variety of less common neoplasms may occur in the anterior mediastinum, including parathyroid tumors and tumors of fatty or connective tissue origin. Given the infrequency of these tumors, they are not discussed in this book.

Middle Mediastinal Masses

Carcinomas and lymphomas may be found in the middle mediastinum, as mentioned in the discussion of anterior mediastinal masses. In addition, the middle mediastinum is frequently the location of benign cysts originating from structures found within this region. For example, fluid-filled pericardial and bronchogenic cysts originate from the pericardium and the tracheobronchial tree, respectively. However, these cysts are generally self-contained and usually do not directly communicate with either the pericardium or the airways. Benign enlargement of lymph nodes in the middle mediastinum, often associated with enlarged hilar nodes, is commonly found in granulomatous diseases, particularly sarcoidosis, histoplasmosis, and tuberculosis.

Posterior Mediastinal Masses

The posterior mediastinum is characteristically the location of tumors of neurogenic origin. These tumors may arise from a variety of nerve elements found in the peripheral nerves, the sympathetic nervous system chain, or the paraganglionic tissue. Examples include neurilemomas (arising from Schwann's sheath), ganglioneuromas and neuroblastomas (benign and malignant lesions arising from the sympathetic nervous system, respectively), and pheochromocytomas. Diaphragmatic hernias, either congenital or acquired, frequently are posterior, with the herniated intraabdominal organ appearing as a mediastinal mass.

CLINICAL FEATURES

Almost half of patients with a mediastinal mass have no symptoms, and the mass is first detected on incidentally performed chest imaging. In patients with symptoms, the most common are chest pain, cough, and dyspnea. Occasionally evidence is seen of esophageal or superior vena caval compression, leading to difficulty swallowing (dysphagia) or to facial and upper extremity edema attributable to impairment of venous return (superior vena cava syndrome). Thymic tumors may manifest with one of the associated systemic syndromes, such as muscle weakness (from myasthenia gravis) or anemia (from pure red cell aplasia). A variety of systemic symptoms may be related to the presence of a lymphoma or other malignancy or to hormone production by hormonally active mediastinal tumors.

DIAGNOSTIC APPROACH

In almost all cases the initial diagnostic test is the chest radiograph, which generally shows the mass and allows determination of its location within the mediastinum (Fig. 16-2). The mass can be further characterized by a variety of other techniques, but

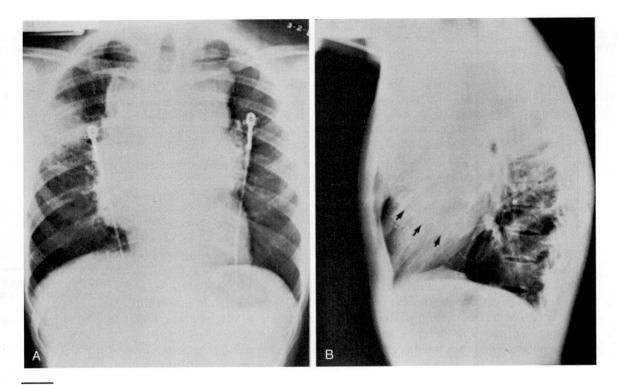

Figure 16-2. Chest radiographs of a patient with a large mediastinal mass shown in the posteroanterior *(A)* and lateral *(B)* views. The mass, proved at surgery to be a germ cell tumor (seminoma), involves anterior and middle mediastinal compartments. Arrows outline inferior border of mass on lateral view.

CT is useful in the evaluation of mediastinal masses.

CT is generally the most valuable. The CT scan is particularly useful for defining the cross-sectional appearance of the lesion, its density, and its relationship to other structures within the mediastinum. With magnetic resonance imaging (MRI), blood vessels appear as hollow rather than solid structures so that vessels can be distinguished from other mediastinal structures without the use of radiographic contrast. Unlike the traditional presentation of CT images as cross-sectional views, MRI can display images in coronal and sagittal planes as well as cross-sectional views. ^{18}F-Fluorodeoxyglucose positron emission tomography yields information on tissue metabolism, which is generally increased in active neoplastic or infectious processes.

The definitive diagnosis of the type of mediastinal mass generally depends on examination of tissue by histopathologic techniques. Tissue frequently is obtained either by mediastinoscopy, in which a rigid scope is inserted into the mediastinum via an incision at the suprasternal notch, or by exploration of the mediastinum by a surgical approach that is anterior and adjacent to the sternum (parasternal mediastinotomy). The technique of video-assisted thoracic surgery also has been used to obtain tissue from the mediastinum. In some patients, aspiration or biopsy of the mass by a needle inserted percutaneously may provide sufficient tissue to make a diagnosis. In many cases, the patient undergoes a more extensive procedure that allows biopsy and removal of the mass at the same time.

Techniques for biopsy of a mediastinal mass are the following:
1. Mediastinoscopy
2. Parasternal mediastinotomy
3. Video-assisted thoracic surgery
4. Percutaneous needle aspiration or biopsy

TREATMENT

Treatment of the various mediastinal masses depends to a large extent on the nature of the lesion. In many cases, complete removal of the mass by surgery is the preferred procedure if technically feasible. Because benign lesions may enlarge and compress vital mediastinal structures, excision of the mass is frequently indicated. In addition, there may be complicating hemorrhage or infection of a benign lesion and eventually even malignant transformation of an initially benign tumor; these factors also favor removal, if possible, following initial diagnosis.

Treatment of malignant tumors depends on the type of tumor and the presence or absence of invasion of other mediastinal structures. Because surgical removal of malignant lesions often is neither indicated nor possible, chemotherapy and radiotherapy are frequently the primary forms of treatment.

PNEUMOMEDIASTINUM

Normally, free air is not present within the mediastinum. When air enters the mediastinum for any number of reasons, a *pneumomediastinum* is said to be present.

ETIOLOGY AND PATHOGENESIS

The three major sources of air entry to the mediastinum are (1) through the skin and chest wall, as commonly seen in the setting of penetrating trauma; (2) from a tear or defect in the esophagus or the trachea, allowing air to enter the mediastinum directly; and (3) from the alveoli. In the last circumstance, an increase in intraalveolar pressure may induce air entry into interstitial tissues of the alveolar wall. This interstitial air may dissect alongside the wall of blood vessels coursing through the interstitium. After air tracks back proximally, it eventually may enter the mediastinum at the site of origin of the vessels in the mediastinum.

Proximal dissection of extraalveolar air probably is the most common cause of a pneumomediastinum. In some cases the reason for the increase in intraalveolar pressure is obvious, for example, severe coughing, vomiting, or straining. In patients receiving mechanical ventilation, the positive pressure produced by the ventilator may initiate alveolar rupture and a pneumomediastinum. A pneumomediastinum may develop in asthmatic persons, presumably because of the development of high intraalveolar pressure in a lung unit behind an obstructed bronchus. In other circumstances, the immediate cause of the pneumomediastinum is not apparent, and the patient truly has a "spontaneous pneumomediastinum."

> Sources of air entry in a pneumomediastinum are the following:
> 1. External (penetrating trauma)
> 2. Tracheal or esophageal tear
> 3. Alveolar rupture and tracking of air proximally

PATHOPHYSIOLOGY

With the accumulation of air in the mediastinum, an increase in pressure would be expected to cause a decrease in venous return to the great veins, with resulting cardiovascular compromise. However, when pressure builds up within the mediastinum, air usually dissects further along fascial planes into the neck, allowing release of the pressure and preventing disastrous cardiovascular complications. In addition, an increase in mediastinal pressure sometimes results in rupture of the mediastinal pleura and escape of air into the pleural space, with consequent development of a pneumothorax (see Chapter 15).

After air has entered the soft tissues of the neck, the patient is said to have *subcutaneous emphysema*. With continued entry of air from the mediastinum into the neck, the air dissects further over soft tissues of the chest and abdominal walls, producing more extensive subcutaneous emphysema.

> Mediastinal air often results in subcutaneous emphysema.

Because of the escape route available for mediastinal air and the opportunity for decompression, major cardiovascular complications are quite uncommon. The development of subcutaneous emphysema, although unsightly and frequently uncomfortable, usually is not associated with major clinical sequelae.

CLINICAL FEATURES

At the onset, patients with a pneumomediastinum often experience relatively sudden substernal chest pain. They may have dyspnea and, rarely, cardiovascular compromise and hypotension. In some cases, the pneumomediastinum causes no symptoms, and the problem is detected on chest radiograph, for example, on a film obtained during the course of an asthmatic attack.

Physical examination may reveal a crunching or clicking sound synchronous with the heartbeat on cardiac auscultation (Hamman's sign). If the patient has subcutaneous emphysema associated with the pneumomediastinum, popping and crackling sounds (crepitations) may be heard and felt on palpation of the affected skin and subcutaneous tissue.

DIAGNOSTIC APPROACH

The chest radiograph and chest CT scan are the most important studies for documenting a pneumomediastinum. Gas may be seen within the mediastinal tissues and usually is visible as one or more radiolucent stripes alongside and parallel to the heart border or the aorta (Fig. 16-3).

TREATMENT

Generally, no treatment is necessary for a pneumomediastinum, even when accompanied by subcutaneous emphysema. The air usually is resorbed spontaneously over time. When a pneumomediastinum is a consequence of tracheobronchial or esophageal rupture, surgery may be necessary to repair the underlying tear. In the rare circumstance when pressure builds up within the mediastinum, an incision or placement of a catheter or chest tube may be necessary to allow escape of air from the mediastinum and release of the pressure.

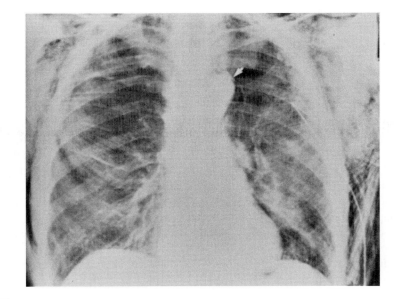

Figure 16-3. Chest radiograph shows pneumomediastinum and air in subcutaneous tissues (subcutaneous emphysema). Note numerous radiolucent stripes outlining mediastinal structures; these stripes represent air within mediastinum. Arrow points to air around aortic arch.

REFERENCES

Detterbeck FC, Parsons AM: Thymic tumors, *Ann Thorac Surg* 77:1860–1869, 2004.

Duwe BV, Sterman DH, Musani AI: Tumors of the mediastinum, *Chest* 128:2893–2909, 2005.

Laurent F, et al: Mediastinal masses: diagnostic approach, *Eur Radiol* 8:1148–1159, 1998.

Lin JC, Hazelrigg SR, Landreneau RJ: Video-assisted thoracic surgery for disease within the mediastinum, *Surg Clin North Am* 80:1511–1533, 2000.

Maunder RJ, Pierson DJ, Hudson LD: Subcutaneous and mediastinal emphysema: pathophysiology, diagnosis, and management, *Arch Intern Med* 144:1447–1453, 1984.

Ribet ME, Cardot GR: Neurogenic tumors of the thorax, *Ann Thorac Surg* 58:1091–1095, 1994.

Ribet ME, Copin MC, Gosselin B: Bronchogenic cysts of the mediastinum, *J Thorac Cardiovasc Surg* 109:1003–1010, 1995.

Strollo DC, Rosado de Christenson ML, Jett JR: Primary mediastinal tumors. Part 1. Tumors of the anterior mediastinum, *Chest* 112:511–522, 1997.

Strollo DC, Rosado de Christenson ML, Jett JR: Primary mediastinal tumors. Part 2. Tumors of the middle and posterior mediastinum, *Chest* 112:1344–1357, 1997.

17

Anatomic and Physiologic Aspects of Neural, Muscular, and Chest Wall Interactions with the Lungs

RESPIRATORY CONTROL
  Organization of Respiratory Control
  Ventilatory Response to
    Hypercapnia and Hypoxia

  Ventilatory Response to Other
    Stimuli
RESPIRATORY MUSCLES

The movement of gas into and out of the lungs requires the action of a pump that is capable of creating negative intrathoracic pressure, expanding the lungs, and initiating airflow with each inspiration. This pumplike action is provided by the respiratory muscles, including the diaphragm, working in conjunction with the chest wall. However, the muscles themselves do not have any rhythmic activity in the way that cardiac muscle does; they must be driven by rhythmic impulses provided by a "controller."

This chapter centers on a discussion of anatomic and physiologic features of the controlling system and the respiratory muscles to provide background for the discussion in Chapters 18 and 19. Those chapters discuss disorders affecting respiratory control, respiratory musculature, and the chest wall. Although much of the physiology and many of the clinical problems discussed here and in the next two chapters do not directly involve the lungs, they are so closely intertwined with respiratory function and dysfunction that they are appropriately considered in a textbook of pulmonary disease.

RESPIRATORY CONTROL

Although the process of breathing is a normal rhythmic activity that occurs without conscious effort, it involves an intricate controlling mechanism at the level of the central nervous system. The central nervous system transmits signals to the respiratory muscles, initiating inspiration approximately 12 to 20 times per minute. Remarkably, this controlling system normally is able to respond to varied needs of the individual, appropriately increasing ventilation during exercise and maintaining arterial blood gases within a narrow range.

This section begins with a description of the structural organization of neural control of ventilation and proceeds to a consideration of how various stimuli may interact with and adjust the output of the respiratory controller. The ways in which the output of the controller can be quantified and how these techniques have proved useful in the evaluation of patients with a variety of clinical disorders are briefly discussed.

ORGANIZATION OF RESPIRATORY CONTROL

The basic organization of the respiratory control system is shown in Figure 17-1. Crucial to this system is the central nervous system "generator." Signals that originate from the generator travel down the spinal cord to the various respiratory muscles. The inspiratory muscles, the most important of which is the diaphragm, respond to the signals by contracting and initiating inspiration. This process is described in more detail in the section on respiratory muscles.

As a result of inspiratory muscular contraction, the diaphragm descends, the chest wall expands, and air flows from the mouth through the tracheobronchial tree to the alveolar spaces. Gas exchange in the distal parenchyma allows movement of O_2 into the blood and a corresponding release of CO_2 from the blood to the alveoli.

Although this sequence of events sounds relatively straightforward, it is complicated by an intricate feedback system that adjusts the output of the generator to achieve the desired effect. If the response of the respiratory muscles to the generator's signal is inadequate, as judged by a variety of respiratory "reflexes," the generator increases its output to compensate for the lack of expected effect. If the arterial blood gases deviate from the desired level, chemosensors for O_2 and CO_2 alter their input to the respiratory generator, ultimately affecting its output. In addition, input from other regions of the central nervous system, particularly the cerebral cortex and the pons, can adjust the net output of the generator.

The Respiratory Generator

Considering the importance of the respiratory generator in this scheme of respiratory control, its anatomy and mode of action are described here. Much of the work clarifying the location of the respiratory generator involved animal experiments with

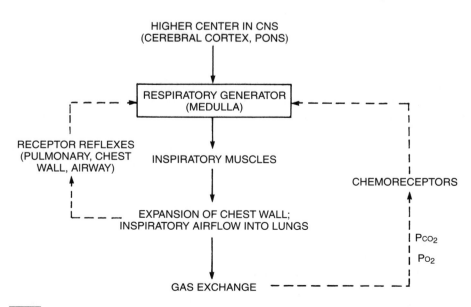

Figure 17-1. Schematic diagram shows organization of respiratory control system. Dashed lines show feedback loops affecting respiratory generator.

transections at various levels of the central nervous system and assessment of the effects on ventilation. Because transection between the brain and the brainstem does not significantly alter ventilation, the generator apparently resides somewhere at the level of the brainstem or lower and does not require interaction with higher cortical centers. When transections are made at various points within the brainstem, the breathing pattern is substantially altered but ventilation is not eliminated. Only when a transection is made between the medulla and the spinal cord does ventilation cease, indicating that the respiratory generator resides within the medulla.

> A central respiratory generator within the medulla controls activity of the respiratory muscles.

Although the respiratory center (or the generator) has been referred to as a single region, it appears that more than one network of neurons within the medulla is involved in initiating and coordinating respiratory activity. According to a popular model, one group of neurons is responsible for initiating inspiration and regulating its speed as a result of the intensity of neuronal activity; another group of neurons controls the "switching off" of inspiration and hence determines the onset of expiration.

Therefore, there are two aspects of ventilatory control: (1) the degree of inspiratory drive or central inspiratory activity (which regulates the inspiratory flow rate), and (2) the timing mechanism (which controls the termination of inspiration). These two determining factors act in concert to set the respiratory rate and tidal volume and thus the minute ventilation and the specific pattern of breathing.

Input from Other Regions of the Central Nervous System

Even though the medullary respiratory center does not require additional input to drive ventilation, it does receive other information that contributes to a regular pattern of breathing and to more precise ventilatory control. For example, input from the pons appears to be necessary for a normal, coordinated breathing pattern. When the influence of the pons is lost, irregularities in the breathing pattern ensue.

In addition to pathways involved in the "automatic" or involuntary control of ventilation, the cerebral cortex exerts a conscious or voluntary control over ventilation. Cortical overriding of automatic control can be seen with either voluntary breathholding or hyperventilation. Its usefulness is readily apparent in a person's need for voluntary control of breathing during such activities as speaking, eating, and swimming. Interestingly, the automatic control of ventilation may be disturbed while conscious control remains intact. In these cases, during wakefulness the cerebral cortex exerts sufficient voluntary control over ventilation to maintain normal arterial blood gas values. During periods when the patient is dependent on automatic ventilatory control (e.g., during sleep), marked hypoventilation or apnea may occur. This rare condition was known as *Ondine's curse*, after a mythologic tale in which the suitor of Neptune's daughter was cursed to lose automatic control over all bodily functions when he fell asleep. The disorder now is called congenital central hypoventilation syndrome. Defects in the *PHOX2b* gene mapped to chromosome 4p12 have been identified in most cases. *PHOX2b* encodes a highly conserved domain for transcription factors important in neural development. Further research into the pathogenesis of this condition undoubtedly will lead to better understanding of the mechanisms of normal ventilatory control.

Chemoreceptors

Maintenance of arterial blood gases is the ultimate goal of ventilatory control, and an important feedback loop adjusts respiratory center output if blood gases are not maintained at the appropriate level (see Fig. 17-1). Elevation of P_{CO_2} (hypercapnia) and depression of P_{O_2} (hypoxemia) both are capable of stimulating ventilation. In each case, one or more chemoreceptors "sense" alterations in P_{CO_2} or P_{O_2} and accordingly vary their input to the medullary respiratory center.

> Changes in P_{CO_2} are sensed primarily at a central chemoreceptor in the medulla.

The primary sensor for CO_2 is located near the ventrolateral surface of the medulla and is called the *central chemoreceptor*. Even though it is located in the medulla, the central chemoreceptor is clearly separate from the medullary respiratory center and should not be confused with it. The central chemoreceptor does not appear to respond directly to blood Pco_2 but rather to the pH of the extracellular fluid (ECF) surrounding the chemoreceptor. The pH level, in turn, is determined by the level of hydrogen (H^+) and bicarbonate (HCO_3^-) ions as well as Pco_2 (see Appendix C for further discussion). The blood–brain barrier, the permeability properties of which govern the composition of cerebrospinal fluid (CSF) and brain ECF, prevents the free movement of either H^+ or HCO_3^- from blood to brain ECF, whereas CO_2 passes freely. The feedback loop for changes in Pco_2 can be summarized as follows:

Increased arterial blood Pco_2 → Increased brain ECF Pco_2 → Decreased brain ECF pH → Decreased pH at central chemoreceptor → Stimulation of central chemoreceptor → Stimulation of medullary respiratory center → Increased ventilation → Decreased arterial blood Pco_2.

The primary sensors for O_2 are not located in the central nervous system but in two *peripheral chemoreceptors* called the *carotid body* and *aortic body chemoreceptors*. The carotid chemoreceptors, which are quantitatively much more important than the aortic chemoreceptors, are located just beyond the bifurcation of each common carotid artery into the internal and external carotid branches. The aortic chemoreceptor is found between the pulmonary artery and the arch of the aorta. These chemoreceptors are sensitive to changes in Po_2, with hypoxia stimulating chemoreceptor discharge. In adults, the peripheral carotid body chemoreceptors also have a role in sensing Pco_2. Under normoxic conditions, the peripheral chemoreceptors are much less important for this purpose than are the central chemoreceptors. However, arterial hypoxemia increases the sensitivity of the peripheral Pco_2 receptors. Therefore, if hypoxemia and hypercarbia both are present, the carotid body chemoreceptor will be maximally stimulated to increase ventilation. Peripheral chemoreceptor discharge is transmitted back to the central nervous system by cranial nerves: the glossopharyngeal nerve in the case of the carotid bodies and the vagus nerve for the aortic bodies. The information ultimately is transmitted to the medullary respiratory center so that its output is augmented.

The major sensors for Po_2 are the peripheral (carotid and aortic body) chemoreceptors.

Input from Other Receptors

In addition to chemoreceptor effects, input that originates from receptors in the lung (including the airways) and is carried via the vagus nerve to the central nervous system must be considered. Stretch receptors, located within the smooth muscle of airway walls, respond to changes in lung inflation. As the lung is inflated, receptor discharge increases. In animals, this stretch receptor reflex (the Hering-Breuer reflex) is responsible for apnea that occurs as a result of lung inflation. In contrast, conscious human adults do not readily demonstrate the Hering-Breuer reflex, and the role of the stretch receptors in ventilatory control is not entirely clear. Presumably, stretch receptors contribute to the "switching off" of inspiration and initiation of expiration after a critical level of inspiratory inflation has been reached.

Irritant receptors, located superficially along the lining of airways, may initiate tachypnea, usually in response to some noxious stimulus, such as a chemical or irritating dust. Juxtacapillary (or J) receptors are found within the pulmonary interstitium, adjacent to capillaries. One of their effects is to cause tachypnea, and they may be responsible for the respiratory stimulation caused by inflammatory processes or accumulation of fluid within the pulmonary interstitium.

Receptors in the chest wall, particularly in the intercostal muscles, appear to play a role in the fine-tuning of ventilation. The muscle spindles are part of a reflex arc that adjusts the output of respiratory muscles if the desired degree of muscular work has not been achieved. When a mismatch occurs between the output from the central nervous system controller and the amount of "stretch" that is sensed by these receptors, feedback from the receptors is involved in causing dyspnea. For example, for the patient with severe emphysema and lung hyperinflation, the increased output from the brain is not matched by an "appropriate" change in lung inflation. That is, the output does not match the result, so feedback is transmitted through the stretch receptors in the chest wall to the brain, and the patient experiences dyspnea. The precise mechanisms of this pathway are incompletely understood.

VENTILATORY RESPONSE TO HYPERCAPNIA AND HYPOXIA

Two of the stimuli for ventilation that have been best studied are well-defined chemical stimuli, hypercapnia and hypoxia. Hypercapnia is sensed primarily, but not exclusively, by the central chemoreceptor, and the stimulus appears to be the pH level of brain ECF. In contrast, hypoxia stimulates ventilation by acting on peripheral chemoreceptors, carotid much more than aortic.

When arterial Po_2 is held constant, ventilation increases by approximately 3 L/min for each millimeter of mercury rise in arterial Pco_2 in adults. This relatively linear response, the magnitude of which varies considerably among individuals, is shown in Figure 17-2. Furthermore, Figure 17-2 shows that the response to increments in Pco_2 also depends on Po_2. At a lower Po_2, the response to hypercapnia is heightened.

With chronic hypercapnia, the ventilatory response to further increases in Pco_2 is diminished. The reason for the blunted CO_2 responsiveness is relatively straightforward. When CO_2 retention persists for days, the kidneys compensate for the more acidic pH by excreting less bicarbonate, and the levels of bicarbonate rise in both plasma and brain ECF. The elevated bicarbonate level can buffer more successfully any acute changes in Pco_2 so that the brain ECF pH value changes less for any given increment in Pco_2.

With hypoxemia, the same linear relationship does not exist between alterations in partial pressure and ventilation. Rather, the ventilatory response is relatively small until Po_2 falls to approximately 60 mm Hg, below which the rise in ventilation is much more dramatic (Fig. 17-3). The curvilinear relationship between Po_2 and ventilation

> Ventilatory responsiveness to CO_2 is blunted in patients with chronic hypercapnia.

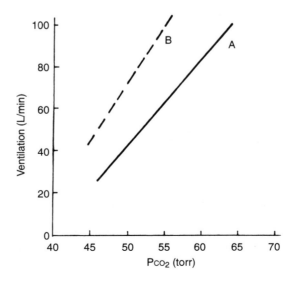

Figure 17-2. Ventilatory response to progressive elevation of Pco_2 in normal individual. Solid line *(A)* shows response when simultaneous Po_2 is high (hyperoxic conditions). Dashed line *(B)* shows heightened response when simultaneous Po_2 is low (hypoxic conditions).

can be made linear if ventilation is plotted against O_2 saturation instead of partial pressure (Fig. 17-4). However, despite the linear relationship between ventilation and O_2 saturation, it is the partial pressure of O_2, not the content or saturation, that is sensed by the chemoreceptor.

Pco_2 also has an effect on a patient's response to hypoxia. The sensitivity to hypoxia is increased as Pco_2 is raised and is decreased as Pco_2 is lowered (see Fig. 17-4). This feature is important to consider when testing for responsiveness to hypoxia. As the patient hyperventilates in response to a low Po_2, Pco_2 drops, and ventilation is stimulated less than it would be if Pco_2 were unchanged. Therefore, Pco_2 should be kept constant so that the condition for testing actually is "isocapnic" hypoxia.

When the clinician suspects a disorder of ventilatory control, quantitation of the ventilatory response to hypercapnia or hypoxia can be performed. However, the responses to these stimuli vary widely even in seemingly normal individuals. This fact must be taken into account in the interpretation of ventilatory response data.

VENTILATORY RESPONSE TO OTHER STIMULI

One of the most important times for a rapid and appropriate increase in ventilation is in response to a change in metabolic requirements. For example, with the metabolic needs of exercise, a normal individual can increase ventilation from a resting value of 5 L/min to 60 L/min or more, without any demonstrable change in arterial blood gas values. According to one popular theory, the initial rapid increase in ventilation at the onset of exercise is due to a neural stimulus, although the origin is not clear. After the initial rapid augmentation in ventilation there occurs a later and slower rise that probably is due to a bloodborne chemical stimulus. However, many questions about the remarkably appropriate way that ventilation is capable of responding to the demands of exercise remain unanswered.

Another important ventilatory response occurs to alterations in acid-base status. With excess metabolic acid production (i.e., metabolic acidosis), ventilation increases as pH is lowered, and elimination of additional CO_2 aids in returning the pH toward normal. The peripheral chemoreceptors appear to be primarily responsible for sensing acute metabolic acidosis and stimulating the increase in ventilation. However, how much the central chemoreceptors modify or contribute to this response is not entirely settled.

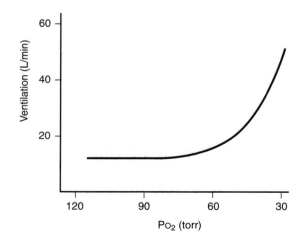

Figure 17-3. Ventilatory response to progressively decreasing Po_2 with Pco_2 kept constant in a normal individual. Ventilation does not rise significantly until Po_2 falls to approximately 60 mm Hg.

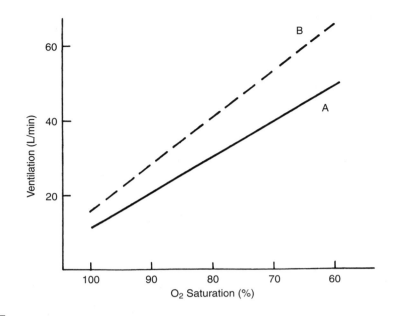

Figure 17-4. Ventilatory response to hypoxia, plotted using O_2 saturation rather than Po_2. The relationship between ventilation and O_2 saturation during progressive hypoxia is linear. Solid line *(A)* shows response when measured at normal Pco_2. Dashed line *(B)* shows augmented response at elevated Pco_2.

RESPIRATORY MUSCLES

The purpose of signals emanating from the respiratory generator is to initiate inspiratory muscle activity. Although the primary inspiratory muscle is the diaphragm, other muscle groups contribute to optimal movement of the chest wall under a variety of conditions and needs. Notable among these other inspiratory muscle groups are the scalene and the parasternal intercostal muscles, which display inspiratory activity even during normal quiet breathing. The so-called *accessory muscles of inspiration* (e.g., sternocleidomastoid and trapezius muscles) are not normally used during quiet inspiration but can be recruited when necessary, either when diaphragm function is impaired or when ventilation is significantly increased. Another set of intercostal muscles, the external intercostal muscles, are also inspiratory muscles, but their overall importance during inspiration is less clear. Finally, additional muscles coordinate upper airway activity during inspiration. Proper functioning of these muscles maintains patency of the upper airway, whereas dysfunction may be important in the pathogenesis of certain clinical disorders associated with upper airway obstruction, such as obstructive sleep apnea (see Chapter 18).

> The diaphragm is the major muscle of inspiration. The less important inspiratory and accessory muscles may increase their role in disease states.

During inspiration, the diaphragm contracts and its muscle fibers shorten. To understand the effect of this contraction, consider the configuration of the diaphragm within the chest. At its lateral aspect, the diaphragm is adjacent to the inner part of the lower rib cage. This portion of the chest wall and the diaphragm is known as the *zone of apposition* (Fig. 17-5). In this region, the muscle fibers of the diaphragm are oriented vertically. When the diaphragm contracts, shortening of these vertically oriented fibers diminishes the zone of apposition and causes the more medial dome of the diaphragm to descend. At the same time, by pushing abdominal contents downward, diaphragmatic contraction increases not only intraabdominal pressure but also the lateral pressure on the lower rib cage transmitted through the apposed diaphragm. The effect of

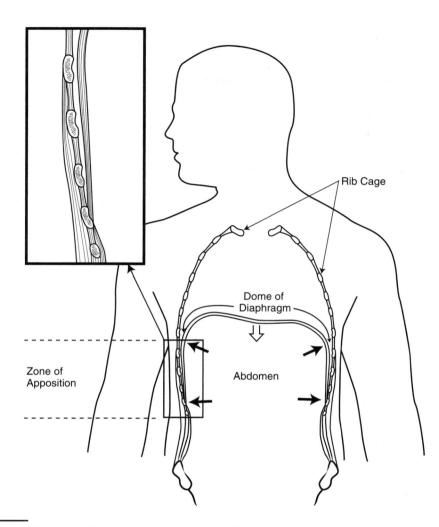

Figure 17-5. Functional anatomy and action of diaphragm during breathing. At the zone of apposition, fibers of the diaphragm are oriented vertically alongside the inner aspect of lower rib cage. During inspiration, descent of diaphragm *(open arrow)* causes increase in abdominal pressure that is transmitted through apposed diaphragm to expand lower rib cage *(solid arrows).* (Adapted from De Troyer A, Estenne M: *Clin Chest Med* 9:175–193, 1988.)

diaphragmatic contraction is thus to lift the lower ribs and expand the lower chest wall at the same time the abdominal wall moves outward. The external intercostal muscles, located between the ribs, also contract during inspiration, contributing as well to the lower rib cage being lifted and rotated outward.

   As the reader can now appreciate, the act of inspiration is more complex than it initially seemed. While the diaphragm acts on the abdomen and the lower chest wall, the scalene muscles and the parasternal intercostals (perhaps along with the external intercostals) act to expand the upper chest wall. The net effect is that abdominal contents are pushed downward, intraabdominal pressure is increased, the chest wall expands, intrathoracic pressure is lowered, and air flows into the lungs. With normal resting breathing, the most apparent inspiratory motion is the outward movement of the abdomen, which results from diaphragmatic descent and increased abdominal pressure. In the face of high workloads, increased ventilation, or certain disease states, the accessory muscles are additionally recruited to assist the primary inspiratory muscles.

An important determinant of the efficacy of diaphragmatic contraction is the initial shape and length of the diaphragm. For any muscle, the strength of contraction is decreased when its initial length is less. The diaphragm is no exception. Therefore, at high lung volumes, the diaphragm is lower and foreshortened before its active contraction, so the strength of contraction is diminished. At the same time, the lower, flatter diaphragm means that the zone of apposition is decreased, with less downward movement of the diaphragm and outward movement of the lower chest wall associated with inspiration. At the extreme, the diaphragm is oriented horizontally, there is no zone of apposition, and contraction results in an indrawing of the lower rib cage but no useful inspiratory function. The importance of these factors will become apparent in the discussion of diaphragmatic function in obstructive lung disease, in which resting lung volume may be abnormally high and, even before contraction, the diaphragm is in a flatter, more horizontal position.

> The effectiveness of diaphragmatic contraction is decreased at high resting lung volumes, when the diaphragm is flatter and shorter.

In contrast to inspiration, expiration is a relatively passive process whereby the lung and chest wall return to the resting position. However, when breathing is deep and forceful, when airways resistance is increased during expiration, or when a person coughs, the action of expiratory muscles may be important in aiding expiratory airflow. In particular, abdominal muscles (transverse abdominis, internal and external obliques) and internal intercostals are important in this role.

In summary, the normal operation of the respiratory apparatus depends on a signal generated by the respiratory center and eventually translated into an efficient pattern of respiratory muscle contraction. Although feedback and control systems ensure optimal functioning of this system, this finely coordinated mechanism may fail in numerous ways. Chapters 18 and 19 examine clinically important dysfunction occurring at various levels of this complex system.

REFERENCES

RESPIRATORY CONTROL

Bianchi AL, Denavit-Saubié M, Champagnat J: Central control of breathing in mammals: neuronal circuitry, membrane properties, and neurotransmitters, Physiol Rev 75:1–45, 1995.

Burton MD, Kazemi H: Neurotransmitters in central respiratory control, Respir Physiol 122:111–121, 2000.

Calverley PMA: Control of breathing. In Hughes JMB, Pride NB, editors: Lung function tests: physiological principles and clinical applications, London, 2000, WB Saunders, pp. 107–120.

Caruana-Montaldo B, Gleeson K, Zwillich CW: The control of breathing in clinical practice, Chest 117: 205–225, 2000.

Duffin J, Hung S: Respiratory rhythm generation, Can Anaesth Soc J 32:124–137, 1985.

Hedemark LL, Kronenberg RS: Chemical regulation of respiration, Chest 82:488–494, 1982.

Schwartzstein RM, Parker MJ: The controller: directing the orchestra. In Schwartzstein RM, Parker MJ, editors: Respiratory physiology: a clinical approach, Philadelphia, 2006, Lippincott Williams & Wilkins, pp. 126–148.

von Euler C: Neural organization and rhythm generation. In Crystal RG, West JB, Weibel ER, Barnes PJ, editors: The lung: scientific foundations, ed 2, Philadelphia, 1997, Lippincott-Raven, pp. 1711–1724.

West JB: Respiratory physiology—the essentials, ed 8, Philadelphia, 2008, Lippincott Williams & Wilkins.

RESPIRATORY MUSCLES

American Thoracic Society and European Respiratory Society: ATS/ERS statement on respiratory muscle testing, Am J Respir Crit Care Med 166:518–624, 2002.

Derenne J-P, Macklem PT, Roussos C: The respiratory muscles: mechanics, control, and pathophysiology, Am Rev Respir Dis 118:119–133, 1978.

Derenne J-P, Macklem PT, Roussos C: The respiratory muscles: mechanics, control, and pathophysiology, part 2, Am Rev Respir Dis 118:373–390, 1978.

Derenne J-P, Macklem PT, Roussos C: The respiratory muscles: mechanics, control, and pathophysiology, part 3, Am Rev Respir Dis 118:581–601, 1978.

De Troyer A: The mechanism of inspiratory expansion of the rib cage, J Lab Clin Med 114:97–104, 1989.

De Troyer A, Estenne M: Functional anatomy of the respiratory muscles, *Clin Chest Med* 9:175–193, 1988.

Epstein SK: An overview of respiratory muscle function, *Clin Chest Med* 15:619–639, 1994.

Guenter CA, Whitelaw WA: The role of diaphragm function in disease, *Arch Intern Med* 139:806–808, 1979.

Macklem PT: Respiratory muscles: the vital pump, *Chest* 78:753–758, 1980.

Moxham J: Respiratory muscle testing, *Monaldi Arch Chest Dis* 51:483–488, 1996.

Polkey MI, Moxham J: Terminology and testing of respiratory muscle dysfunction, *Monaldi Arch Chest Dis* 54:514–519, 1999.

Roussos C, Macklem PT: The respiratory muscles, *N Engl J Med* 307:786–797, 1982.

Schwartzstein RM, Parker MJ: Statics: snapshots of the ventilatory pump. In Schwartzstein RM, Parker MJ, editors: *Respiratory physiology: a clinical approach,* Philadelphia, 2006, Lippincott Williams and Wilkins, pp. 34–60.

18

Disorders of Ventilatory Control

PRIMARY NEUROLOGIC DISEASE	SLEEP APNEA SYNDROME
Presentation with Hyperventilation	Types
Presentation with Hypoventilation	Clinical Features
Abnormal Patterns of Breathing	Pathophysiology
CHEYNE-STOKES BREATHING	Treatment
CONTROL ABNORMALITIES	
SECONDARY TO LUNG DISEASE	

The finely tuned system of ventilatory control described in Chapter 17 is altered in a variety of clinical circumstances. In some cases a primary disorder of the nervous system affects the neurologic network involved in ventilatory control and therefore may either diminish or increase the "drive" to breathe. In other instances the controlling system undergoes a process of adaptation in response to primary lung disease, so any alteration in function is a secondary phenomenon.

This chapter considers primary and secondary disturbances in ventilatory control. Of the secondary disorders, the most commonly seen is that associated with chronic obstructive pulmonary disease; therefore, the discussion of secondary disorders of ventilatory control focuses on this particular disorder. A common disturbance in the pattern of breathing, termed *Cheyne-Stokes breathing*, is covered, with a brief discussion of its pathogenesis. The final topic is ventilatory disorders associated with sleep, because alteration of ventilatory control may be an important component of the pathogenesis of sleep-related respiratory dysfunction.

PRIMARY NEUROLOGIC DISEASE

Several diseases of the nervous system alter ventilation, apparently by affecting regions involved in ventilatory control. However, the results are variable, depending on the type of disorder and the region involved. In some cases hyperventilation is prominent, whereas in others hypoventilation is significant. In a third category the most apparent change occurs in the pattern of breathing.

PRESENTATION WITH HYPERVENTILATION

With certain acute disorders of the central nervous system, hyperventilation (i.e., decreased Pco_2 and respiratory alkalosis) is relatively common. Acute infections (meningitis, encephalitis), strokes, and trauma affecting the central nervous system

Many acute disorders of the central nervous system are associated with hyperventilation.

are notable examples. The exact mechanism of hyperventilation in these situations is not known with certainty. Patients with hyperthyroidism frequently present with hyperventilation that resolves after treatment. Increased sensitivity of the chemoreceptors in the brain during hyperthyroidism appears to account for the effect. Hyperventilation frequently complicates severe hepatic disease, presumably because of increased blood levels of substances stimulating ventilation that normally are metabolized by the healthy liver. Some proposed substances causing central stimulation of respiration in patients with hepatic disease include progesterone, ammonia, and glutamate.

PRESENTATION WITH HYPOVENTILATION

A presentation with hypoventilation presumably results from a primary insult to the nervous system that affects centers involved with control of breathing. In such circumstances, patients have an elevated Pco_2, but because the clinical problems are generally not acute, the pH level has returned toward normal as a result of renal compensation with retention of bicarbonate. When no specific etiologic factor or prior event can be found to explain the hypoventilation, the patient is said to have *idiopathic hypoventilation* or *primary alveolar hypoventilation.* Other patients have suffered a significant insult to the nervous system at some time in the past, such as encephalitis, and chronic hypoventilation presumably is a sequela of the past event.

Patients with these syndromes of hypoventilation are characterized by depressed ventilatory responses to the chemical stimuli of hypercapnia and hypoxia. Measurement of arterial blood gases generally reveals an elevation in arterial Pco_2 accompanied by a decrease in Po_2, the latter primarily attributable to hypoventilation. As in other disorders associated with these blood gas abnormalities, cor pulmonale may result and be the presenting problem in these syndromes. The term *congenital central hypoventilation syndrome* or *Ondine's curse* (see Chapter 17) has been applied to a rare subset of patients with congenital alveolar hypoventilation. However, an element of decreased ventilatory response to hypercapnia and hypoxia is much more commonly seen in clinical practice and probably represents a spectrum of abnormalities in ventilatory response.

In the past, treatment of alveolar hypoventilation generally centered around two modalities: drugs (most commonly the hormone progesterone) and electrical stimulation of the phrenic nerve. Progesterone is well known to be a respiratory stimulant and in some cases may improve respiratory drive and decrease CO_2 retention. In the second approach, the diaphragm can be induced to contract by repetitive electrical stimulation of the phrenic nerve, which can be achieved by intermittent current applied to an implanted electrode. Although both of these modalities are still used, the most common current therapy for patients with clinically significant hypoventilation is noninvasive positive-pressure (i.e., assisted) ventilation. This topic is discussed in Chapter 29.

Treatment of alveolar hypoventilation due to depressed central respiratory drive consists of the following:
1. Pharmacologic (e.g., progesterone)
2. Electrical stimulation of phrenic nerve
3. Assisted ventilation

ABNORMAL PATTERNS OF BREATHING

In addition to disturbances in overall alveolar ventilation, patients with neurologic disease may demonstrate abnormal patterns of breathing. The term *ataxic breathing* is applied to a grossly irregular breathing pattern observed with some types of lesions in the medulla. In contrast, certain lesions in the pons result in a breathing pattern characterized by a prolonged inspiratory pause; this pattern is called *apneustic breathing.*

Another type of abnormal breathing pattern is termed *Cheyne-Stokes breathing.* Unlike the other patterns, Cheyne-Stokes breathing is common and warrants a special section to describe it and discuss what is known about its pathogenesis.

CHEYNE-STOKES BREATHING

Cheyne-Stokes breathing is a cyclic pattern in which periods of gradually increasing ventilation alternate with periods of gradually decreasing ventilation (even to the point of apnea). This type of ventilation is shown schematically in Figure 18-1. It has been known for many years that two main types of disorders are associated with this type of breathing: heart failure and some forms of central nervous system disease. Cheyne-Stokes breathing can also be seen under certain physiologic situations even in the absence of underlying disease. Examples include the onset of sleep and exposure to high altitude.

Common causes of Cheyne-Stokes ventilation are heart failure and some forms of central nervous system disease.

Central to the pathogenesis of Cheyne-Stokes ventilation is a problem with the feedback system of ventilatory control. Normally, the controlling system can adjust its output to compensate for arterial blood gas values that differ from the ideal or desired state. For example, with an elevated arterial P_{CO_2}, the central chemoreceptor signals the medullary respiratory center to increase its output in order to augment ventilation and restore P_{CO_2} to normal. Similarly, the peripheral chemoreceptor responds to hypoxemia by increasing its output, signaling the medullary respiratory center to augment ventilation and restore P_{O_2} to normal.

At times, this feedback system may fail, especially if there is a delayed response to the signal or if the system responds more than necessary and overshoots the mark. Such defects in the feedback process appear to be at work in Cheyne-Stokes breathing. This section touches on a few aspects of theories proposed to explain Cheyne-Stokes ventilation. For further discussion the interested reader is referred to the references.

A prolongation in circulation time, which is one mechanism postulated to play a role in heart failure, results in an abnormal delay between events in the lung and sensing of P_{CO_2} changes by the central chemoreceptor. Hence, medullary respiratory output is out of phase with gas exchange at the lungs, and oscillations in ventilation occur as the central chemoreceptor and the medullary respiratory center make belated attempts to maintain a stable P_{CO_2} (see Fig. 18-1).

An alternative explanation for Cheyne-Stokes breathing that occurs with heart failure is an accentuated ventilatory response to hypercapnia. This type of heightened responsiveness of the feedback system produces "instability" of respiratory control and a cyclical overshooting and undershooting of ventilation. Such increased responsiveness of the ventilatory control system may also play a role in patients with central nervous system disease who exhibit periods of Cheyne-Stokes respiration.

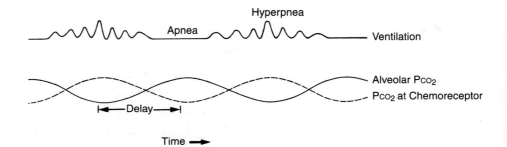

Figure 18-1. Cheyne-Stokes breathing shows cyclic pattern of ventilation. In patients with prolonged circulation time, delay between signal to chemoreceptor (P_{CO_2} at chemoreceptor) and ventilatory output (reflected by alveolar P_{CO_2}) is shown.

A similar type of instability of ventilatory control occurs when hypoxia is driving the feedback system, as is seen on exposure to high altitude. The ventilatory response to hypoxia is alinear. For the same drop in P_{O_2}, the increment in ventilation is larger at a lower absolute P_{O_2} (see Fig. 17-3). This means that at a relatively high initial P_{O_2}, the system is less likely to respond to small changes in P_{O_2} but then is apt to overshoot as P_{O_2} falls further. This instability of the respiratory control system results in a widely oscillating output from the respiratory center and thus a cyclic pattern of ventilation.

CONTROL ABNORMALITIES SECONDARY TO LUNG DISEASE

Ventilatory control mechanisms often respond to various forms of primary lung disease by altering respiratory center output. Either stimulation of peripheral chemoreceptors by hypoxemia or stimulation of receptors by diseases affecting the airways or the pulmonary interstitium can induce the respiratory center to increase its output, resulting in a respiratory alkalosis. For example, patients with asthma commonly demonstrate increased respiratory drive and hyperventilation during acute attacks as a consequence of stimulation of airway receptors. Similarly, patients with acute pulmonary embolism, pneumonia, or chronic interstitial lung disease often hyperventilate, presumably as a result of stimulation of one or more types of intrathoracic receptors, with or without the additional ventilatory stimulus contributed by hypoxemia.

In contrast, patients with chronic obstructive pulmonary disease (COPD) have variable levels of P_{CO_2}. Some patients with COPD (type A pathophysiology) do not generally demonstrate CO_2 retention, whereas the condition of others (type B) is often characterized by hypercapnia (see Chapter 6). In the latter group, the ventilatory control mechanism appears to be reset to operate at a higher setpoint for P_{CO_2}. When responsiveness to increased levels of P_{CO_2} is measured in hypercapnic patients, it is apparent that their ventilatory response is diminished. However, these patients with chronic, compensated respiratory acidosis have higher levels of plasma (as well as cerebrospinal fluid) bicarbonate because of bicarbonate retention by the kidneys. Therefore, for any increment in P_{CO_2}, the effect on pH at the medullary chemoreceptor is attenuated by the increased buffering capacity available. A "chicken and egg" question then becomes important: Is CO_2 retention secondary to an underlying ventilatory control abnormality in these patients, or is the diminution in ventilatory sensitivity merely secondary to chronic CO_2 retention? Although this question remains unanswered, some evidence suggests that familial factors may be important and that CO_2 retention is more likely to develop in patients with a genetically lower respiratory sensitivity.

Whatever the answer to this question, there is a clinically important corollary to this depression in CO_2 sensitivity, irrespective of the cause of CO_2 retention. When O_2 is administered to the chronically hypoxemic and hypercapnic patient, P_{CO_2} may rise even further. At the extreme, if very high levels of inspired O_2 are administered, even life-threatening CO_2 retention may occasionally be seen. In the past, this phenomenon has been ascribed to loss of sensitivity to CO_2 as a ventilatory stimulus, resulting from chronic CO_2 retention. Such patients were thought to be primarily dependent on hypoxic drive as a ventilatory stimulus. Removal of the hypoxic stimulus by the administration of supplemental oxygen was thought to be the cause of the observed increase in P_{CO_2}.

However, it now is known that hypoxic drive plays only a limited role in the frequently observed increase in P_{CO_2} occurring in patients with underlying hypoventilation who are given supplemental oxygen. Three factors account for this well-recognized clinical event: changes in minute ventilation, changes in ventilation-perfusion matching, and the Haldane effect. To grasp this complicated phenomenon, each of these factors should be understood. The easiest factor to understand is the change in minute ventilation. If a patient is hypoxemic, low Pa_{O_2} is sensed by the peripheral chemoreceptors, causing

Administration of O_2 to the chronically hypoxemic and hypercapnic patient may elevate P_{CO_2}.

stimulation of the respiratory center. When supplemental oxygen is given and the patient is no longer hypoxemic, this stimulation abates. As discussed, this was previously thought to be the primary explanation for the rise in Pco_2 seen in hypoxic, hypercapnic patients who were given supplemental oxygen. However, it now is known from a number of studies that the decrease in ventilation accounts for only a small proportion of the rise in Pco_2. More important is a worsening of ventilation-perfusion matching. Recall that alveolar hypoxia results in decreased perfusion to the hypoxic lung segments, an effect that is mediated through hypoxic vasoconstriction of the pulmonary arterioles leading to hypoxic alveoli. However, administration of supplemental O_2 may alleviate alveolar hypoxia in these poorly ventilated regions, thus aborting the compensatory localized vasoconstriction. Ventilation-perfusion mismatch becomes more marked in the absence of hypoxic vasoconstriction, leading to less efficient elimination of CO_2 and increased levels of Pco_2. The third factor contributing to the rise in Pco_2 is the Haldane effect, in which deoxygenated hemoglobin has a higher affinity for CO_2 (see Chapter 1). When supplemental oxygen is given, the more oxygenated hemoglobin has a lower affinity for CO_2, leading to enhanced release of CO_2 from hemoglobin and a higher Pco_2.

Significant elevations in Pco_2 upon administration of supplemental O_2 to the chronically hypercapnic patient can generally be prevented by avoiding excessive concentrations of supplemental O_2 beyond those needed to raise oxygen saturation to approximately 90%. The clinician should not withhold supplemental O_2 from hypoxemic patients who have chronic hypercapnia because significant hypoxemia poses more of a risk than does a further increase in Pco_2. Nevertheless, such patients usually are given relatively limited amounts of supplemental O_2 (often called "low-flow O_2" because of the low flow rate of O_2 given via nasal prongs) in order to minimize the degree of further hypercapnia.

SLEEP APNEA SYNDROME

Sleep apnea syndrome is a comparatively recently recognized disorder of respiration during sleep. Although a number of factors contribute to its pathogenesis, sleep-related changes in ventilatory control, specifically control of upper airway muscles, constitute an important component.

In this syndrome, patients have repetitive periods of apnea (i.e., cessation of breathing) that occur during sleep. A period of more than 10 seconds without airflow is generally considered to constitute an apneic episode, and patients with this syndrome often have hundreds of such episodes during the course of a night's sleep. The term *hypopnea* is used to describe a reduction in airflow of 50% or more but without the complete cessation of airflow implied by the term *apnea*. Because episodes of apnea and hypopnea commonly coexist, the broader term *sleep apnea–hypopnea syndrome* is sometimes used. Sleep apnea syndrome is surprisingly common; estimates suggest a prevalence of 2% to 4% in middle-aged adults. Men are affected more commonly than women, and affected women are typically postmenopausal.

TYPES

Sleep apnea syndrome is commonly divided into several types (obstructive, central, and mixed) depending on the nature of the episodes. In obstructive apnea the drive to breathe still is present during the apneic episode, but transient obstruction of the upper airway prevents inspiratory airflow. Inspiratory muscles are active during obstructive apnea; however, their attempts at initiating airflow are unsuccessful. In central apnea, there is no drive to breathe during the apneic period, that is, there is no signal from the respiratory center to initiate inspiration. Hence, no respiratory muscle activity can be observed when airflow ceases. Frequently, patients may have episodes of apnea that have features of both central and obstructive apnea, a condition called *mixed apnea*. Typically, such episodes start without ventilatory effort (central apnea), but upper airway obstruction is present when ventilatory effort resumes (obstructive apnea). Because clinically significant episodes of obstructive apnea are more frequent than those of central apnea, the focus here is on the clinical features, pathophysiology, and treatment of obstructive apnea.

Categories of sleep apnea syndrome are the following:
1. Obstructive
2. Central
3. Mixed

CLINICAL FEATURES

Patients with sleep apnea syndrome may seek medical consultation because of (1) symptoms or signs that they or their partner have noticed during a night's sleep, (2) daytime symptoms, or (3) complications that arise from the repetitive apneic episodes. During sleep, patients with episodes of obstructive apnea are often noted to have a markedly deranged sleep pattern. Loud snoring is particularly prominent, and patients may have obvious snorting and agitation as a result of trying to breathe against the obstructed airway. They also may have violent movements during periods of obstruction. Not uncommonly the sleep partner complains of being hit or injured as a result of these violent movements. On waking, patients often complain of a severe headache, presumably related to cerebral vasodilation associated with derangements in gas exchange that occur during the apneic episodes. It is important to note, however, that many patients, especially those with milder cases, will not report any problems to their physician. Symptoms may be noted only when the physician specifically inquires about sleep issues.

With such a disordered pattern of sleep, patients are effectively sleep deprived, and not surprisingly they may be overly somnolent during the normal waking hours. Even though the patient is in bed and "asleep," only the lightest phases of sleep are entered, and adequate amounts of the deeper phases of sleep are not achieved because of repeated "microarousals." The degree of somnolence can be debilitating and even dangerous. Patients may fall asleep while driving, eating, or working or during a variety of other usual daytime activities. Patients are often considered to have a personality disorder, partially because of their extreme hypersomnolence and partially because of psychologic changes that have presumably resulted from their disease. Inability to concentrate and depression are also seen.

Clinical features of sleep apnea syndrome are the following:
1. Disordered respiration during sleep
2. Daytime hypersomnolence
3. Cardiovascular complications

Secondary cardiovascular complications of obstructive sleep apnea are believed to be mediated in part by increased sympathetic nervous system activity. During the episodes of apnea, patients may have a variety of cardiac arrhythmias or conduction disturbances, although they rarely are life threatening. As a result of episodes of prolonged hypoxemia at night, pulmonary hypertension can result, and unexplained cor pulmonale may be the presenting clinical problem. Systemic hypertension appears to be associated with and perhaps is a consequence of obstructive sleep apnea.

PATHOPHYSIOLOGY

During the last 2 decades, a great deal has been learned about the pathogenesis and the risk factors leading to obstructive sleep apnea syndrome. Normally, inspiration is characterized not only by contraction of the diaphragm, resulting in negative airway pressure, but also by increased activity of a number of upper airway muscles acting to keep the pharynx patent. The genioglossus muscle is particularly important in this regard because it prevents the tongue from falling against the posterior pharyngeal wall and occluding the pharynx.

In patients with obstructive sleep apnea, structural and functional factors often work together to allow the upper airway to close during inspiration. In most patients, an excess of soft tissue in the upper airway, often as a consequence of obesity, compromises the size of the pharyngeal opening. During sleep, particularly rapid eye movement sleep, loss of activity of the upper airway muscles allows inspiratory collapse of the soft tissues and obstruction of the upper airway. Airflow eventually resumes after each episode of obstruction as the patient arouses (although these "microarousals" often are not evident to the patient), when activity of the upper airway muscles is restored, and when the airway temporarily becomes patent. However, as the patient falls asleep again, inspiratory muscle activity is again lost, and the cycle repeats itself. Because of the importance of structural factors contributing to a small upper airway, patients who are obese (with short, fat necks) or who have a small jaw (micrognathia), a large tongue, or large tonsils are at particular risk for obstructive sleep apnea.

During an episode of central apnea, monitoring of chest wall motion reveals no movement, corresponding to cessation of airflow and a fall in O_2 saturation (Fig. 18-2, A). With obstructive apnea, chest wall and abdominal movement can be detected during a fruitless attempt to move air through the obstructed airway. Airflow

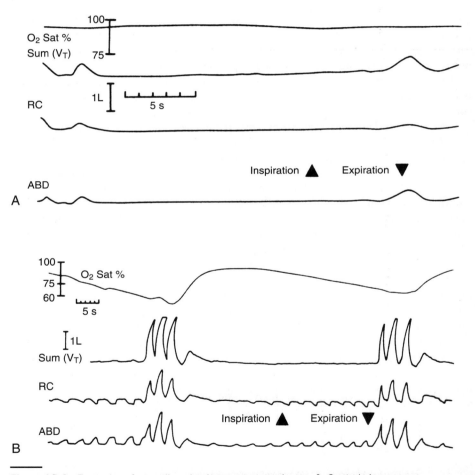

Figure 18-2. Examples of recordings in sleep apnea syndrome. **A,** Central sleep apnea. Absence of abdominal, rib cage, and sum movements are associated with a small fall in arterial oxygen saturation. **B,** Obstructive sleep apnea. Apneas at the beginning and midportion of the recording are marked by absence of sum movements (V_T) despite respiratory efforts. When the diaphragm contracts and the upper airway is obstructed during attempted inspiration, the abdomen moves out (upward on tracing) while rib cage moves inward (downward). Each apnea shown is associated with marked fall in O_2 saturation and is terminated by three deep breaths. ABD = Abdominal movement; O_2 Sat = O_2 saturation; RC = rib cage; V_T = tidal volume (monitored as sum of rib cage and abdominal movements). (From Tobin MJ, Cohn MA, Sackner MA: *Arch Intern Med* 143:1221–1228, 1983. Copyright 1983, American Medical Association.)

measured simultaneously is found to be absent (tidal volume $= 0$) and O_2 saturation drops, often to profoundly low levels (Fig. 18-2, *B*). When O_2 saturation drops significantly during sleep, disturbances in cardiac rhythm occur, and elevation of pulmonary artery pressure may be seen as a consequence of hypoxia-induced pulmonary vasoconstriction.

TREATMENT

In patients with central apnea, treatment generally consists of the use of respiratory stimulants, an electrical, implanted phrenic nerve pacemaker to stimulate the diaphragm or mechanical ventilation, either invasive via a tracheostomy tube or noninvasive via a face mask. In obstructive apnea, a variety of forms of therapy have been used. With patients who are markedly obese, an attempt at significant weight loss is often made. Although weight loss can sometimes dramatically improve the number and severity of the apneic episodes, long-term weight reduction is difficult for most patients to maintain, making other forms of therapy necessary. In all patients, respiratory depressants, including alcohol and sedative–hypnotic drugs, should be avoided because they may worsen obstructive sleep apnea.

The first-line therapy used in most patients with obstructive sleep apnea syndrome is nasal continuous positive airway pressure, commonly called *nasal CPAP*. A mask connected to an air compressor is placed over the nose of the patient at bedtime. The compressor maintains positive pressure in the upper airway throughout the respiratory cycle, thus providing a pneumatic splint to keep the airway open.

An alternative but less common form of therapy involves nocturnal use of an oral appliance to maintain the tongue and/or the jaw in a relatively anterior position. This mechanical form of therapy facilitates airway patency by keeping the tongue away from the posterior pharyngeal wall.

Because nasal CPAP and oral appliances are so often effective, other forms of therapy now are used less frequently. Nevertheless, surgical modes of therapy may be beneficial in selected patients. For example, some patients are treated by a surgical procedure called *uvulopalatopharyngoplasty,* which involves removal of redundant soft tissue in the upper airway. However, the procedure is not without a risk of complications. Patients with particularly severe obstructive apnea whose disease is refractory to other forms of therapy can be treated with a tracheostomy, which involves placement of a tube in the trachea to allow air to bypass the site of upper airway obstruction. Despite the apparently drastic nature of tracheostomy as a form of treatment, the therapeutic response often is quite gratifying. Patients may have a dramatic reversal of symptoms and a striking improvement in their lifestyle, which previously was limited by intractable daytime sleepiness.

Nasal continuous positive airway pressure (CPAP) is often applied at night to patients with obstructive sleep apnea to prevent "upper airway closure.

REFERENCES

PRIMARY NEUROLOGIC DISEASE

Burton MD, Kazemi H: Neurotransmitters in central respiratory control, *Respir Physiol* 122:111–121, 2000.

Garay SM, Turino GM, Goldring RM: Sustained reversal of chronic hypercapnia in patients with alveolar hypoventilation syndromes: long-term maintenance with noninvasive nocturnal mechanical ventilation, *Am J Med* 70:269–274, 1981.

Krachman S, Criner GJ: Hypoventilation syndromes, *Clin Chest Med* 19:139–155, 1998.

Lustik SJ , Chhibber AK, Kolano JW, et al: The hyperventilation of cirrhosis: progesterone and estradiol effects, *Hepatology* 25:55–58, 1997.

Mellins RB, Balfour HH, Turino GM, Winters RW: Failure of automatic control of ventilation (Ondine's curse), *Medicine* 49:487–504, 1970.

Pino-Garcia JM, García-Río F, Díez JJ, et al: Regulation of breathing in hyperthyroidism: relationship to hormonal and metabolic changes, *Eur Respir J* 12:400–407, 1998.

Reichel J: Primary alveolar hypoventilation, *Clin Chest Med* 1:119–124, 1980.

CHEYNE-STOKES BREATHING

Cherniack NS, Longobardo GS: Cheyne-Stokes breathing: an instability in physiologic control, *N Engl J Med* 288:952–957, 1973.

Cherniack NS, Longobardo GS: Abnormalities in respiratory rhythm. In Fishman AP, Cherniack NS, Widdicombe JG, Geiger SR, editors: *Handbook of physiology. Section 3: the respiratory system, vol. II. Control of breathing, part 2,* Bethesda, MD, 1986, American Physiological Society, pp. 729–749.

Cherniack NS, Longobardo G, Evangelista CJ: Causes of Cheyne-Stokes respiration, *Neurocrit Care* 3: 271–279, 2005.

Naughton MT: Pathophysiology and treatment of Cheyne-Stokes respiration, *Thorax* 53:514–518, 1998.

CONTROL ABNORMALITIES SECONDARY TO LUNG DISEASE

Aubier M, Murciano D, Milic-Emili J, et al: Effects of the administration of O₂ on ventilation and blood gases in patients with chronic obstructive pulmonary disease during acute respiratory failure, *Am Rev Respir Dis* 122:747–754, 1980.

Caruana-Montaldo B, Gleeson K, Zwillich CW: The control of breathing in clinical practice, *Chest* 117:205–225, 2000.

Dunn WF, Nelson SB, Hubmayr RD: Oxygen-induced hypercarbia in obstructive pulmonary disease, *Am Rev Respir Dis* 144:526–530, 1991.

Epstein SK, Singh N: Respiratory acidosis, *Respir Care* 46:366–383, 2001.

Kutty K: Sleep and chronic obstructive pulmonary disease, *Curr Opin Pulm Med* 10:104–112, 2004.

Milic-Emili J, Aubier M: Some recent advances in the study of the control of breathing in patients with chronic obstructive lung disease, *Anesth Analg* 59:865–873, 1980.

Mountain R, Zwillich C, Weil J: Hypoventilation in obstructive lung disease: the role of familial factors, *N Engl J Med* 298:521–525, 1978.

Park SS: Respiratory control in chronic obstructive pulmonary diseases, *Clin Chest Med* 1:73–84, 1980.

Weinberger SE, Schwartzstein RM, Weiss JW: Hypercapnia, *N Engl J Med* 321:1223–1231, 1989.

SLEEP APNEA SYNDROME

American Academy of Sleep Medicine Task Force: Sleep-related breathing disorders in adults: recommendations for syndrome definition and measurement techniques in clinical research, *Sleep* 22:667–689, 1999.

Caples SM, Garcia-Touchard A, Somers VK: Sleep-disordered breathing and cardiovascular risk, *Sleep* 30:291–303, 2007.

Cartwright R: Obstructive sleep apnea: a sleep disorder with major effects on health, *Dis Mon* 47:109–147, 2001.

Chan AS, Lee RW, Cistulli PA: Dental appliance treatment for sleep apnea, *Chest* 132:693–699, 2007.

Eckert DJ, Jordan AS, Merchia P, Malhotra A: Central sleep apnea pathophysiology and treatment, *Chest* 131:595–607, 2007.

Flemons WW: Obstructive sleep apnea, *N Engl J Med* 347:498–504, 2002.

Gozal D, Kheirandish-Gozal L: Cardiovascular morbidity in obstructive sleep apnea: oxidative stress, inflammation and much more, *Am J Respir Crit Care Med* 177:369–375, 2008.

Horner RL, Bradley TD: Update in sleep and control of ventilation 2006, *Am J Respir Crit Care Med* 175:426–431, 2006.

Netzer N, Eliasson AH, Netzer C, Kristo DA: Overnight pulse oximetry for sleep-disordered breathing in adults: a review, *Chest* 120:625–633, 2001.

Roldan G, Ang RC: Overview of sleep disorders, *Respir Care Clin North Am* 12:31–54, 2006.

Simonds AK: New developments in the treatment of obstructive sleep apnea, *Thorax* 55(suppl 1):S45–S50, 2000.

Skomro RP, Kryger MH: Clinical presentations of obstructive sleep apnea syndrome, *Prog Cardiovasc Dis* 41:331–340, 1999.

Teran-Santos J, Jimenez-Gomez A, Cordero-Guevera J: The association between sleep apnea and the risk of traffic accidents, *N Engl J Med* 340:847–851, 1999.

Veasey SC, Guilleminault C, Strohl KP, Sanders MH, Ballard RD, Magalang UJ: Medical therapy for obstructive sleep apnea: a review by the Medical Therapy for Obstructive Sleep Apnea Task Force of the Standards of Practice Committee of the American Academy of Sleep Medicine, *Sleep* 29:1036–1044, 2006.

White DP: Pathogenesis of obstructive and central sleep apnea, *Am J Respir Crit Care Med* 172:1363–1370, 2005.

Disorders of the Respiratory Pump

NEUROMUSCULAR DISEASE AFFECTING THE MUSCLES OF RESPIRATION	Diaphragmatic Fatigue
	Unilateral Diaphragmatic Paralysis
	Bilateral Diaphragmatic Paralysis
Specific Diseases	**DISEASES AFFECTING THE CHEST WALL**
Pathophysiology and Clinical Consequences	
DIAPHRAGMATIC DISEASE	Kyphoscoliosis
	Obesity

The chest wall, diaphragm, and related neuromuscular apparatus moving the chest wall act in concert to translate signals from the ventilatory controller into expansion of the thorax. Together, these structures constitute the respiratory pump, an important system that may fail as a result of diseases affecting any of its parts. Because disorders of the respiratory pump include a variety of problems, this discussion is limited to those disorders that are most common and most important clinically: (1) neuromuscular disease affecting the muscles of respiration (Guillain-Barré syndrome, myasthenia gravis, poliomyelitis, and amyotrophic lateral sclerosis); (2) diaphragmatic fatigue; (3) diaphragmatic paralysis; and (4) diseases affecting the chest wall (kyphoscoliosis, obesity).

NEUROMUSCULAR DISEASE AFFECTING THE MUSCLES OF RESPIRATION

A number of neuromuscular diseases have the potential for affecting the muscles of respiration. In some cases the underlying process is acute and generally reversible (e.g., Guillain-Barré syndrome), and the muscles of respiration are transiently affected for a variable amount of time. In other cases the neuromuscular damage is permanent, and any consequences that affect the muscles of respiration are chronic and irreversible. This chapter provides brief definitions of some specific neurologic disorders with respiratory sequelae, followed by a discussion of the pathophysiology and clinical consequences of these diseases as they relate to the respiratory system.

SPECIFIC DISEASES

The major neuromuscular diseases that can affect the muscles of respiration are listed in Table 19-1; several are discussed here.

Guillain-Barré syndrome is a disorder characterized by demyelination of peripheral nerves. It is thought to be triggered by exposure to an antigen (typically an infectious

Table	19-1

DISORDERS OF THE RESPIRATORY PUMP

Neuromuscular Diseases	Chest Wall Diseases
Guillain-Barré syndrome	Kyphoscoliosis
Myasthenia gravis	Obesity
Poliomyelitis	Ankylosing spondylitis
Postpolio syndrome	
Amyotrophic lateral sclerosis	
Quadriplegia	
Polymyositis	
Muscular dystrophy	

agent). The resulting immune response is misdirected to similar antigenic determinants (epitopes) on neural tissue. Patients frequently have a history of a recent viral or bacterial illness, followed by development of an ascending paralysis and variable sensory symptoms. Classically, weakness or paralysis starts symmetrically in the lower extremities and progresses or ascends proximally to the upper extremities and trunk. In up to one third of cases, the disease is more severe, with respiratory muscle weakness or paralysis accompanying the more usual limb and trunk symptoms. When respiratory muscles are affected, respiratory failure often supervenes but usually is reversible over the course of weeks to months. Generally, the natural history of the disease leads to recovery, although 3% to 8% of patients die, and up to 10% of survivors have permanent sequelae.

In *myasthenia gravis,* patients experience weakness and fatigue of voluntary muscles, most frequently those innervated by cranial nerves, but peripheral (limb) and, potentially, respiratory muscles also are affected. The primary abnormality is found at the neuromuscular junction, where transmission of impulses from nerve to muscle is impaired by a decreased number of receptors on the muscle for the neurotransmitter acetylcholine and by the presence of antibodies against these receptors. Although myasthenia gravis is a chronic illness, the manifestations often can be controlled by appropriate therapy, and individual episodes of respiratory failure are potentially reversible.

Poliomyelitis is a viral disease in which the poliovirus attacks motor nerve cells of the spinal cord and brainstem. Both the diaphragm and intercostal muscles can be affected, with resulting weakness or paralysis and respiratory failure. Surviving patients generally recover respiratory muscle function, although some patients have chronic respiratory insufficiency from prior disease. New cases are quite rare as the result of mass vaccination of the population.

In *postpolio syndrome,* patients develop new or progressive symptoms of weakness that occur decades after the initial episode of poliomyelitis. Involvement occurs in muscles originally affected by the disease; therefore, respiratory muscle involvement is more likely in patients who had respiratory failure with their initial disease.

Amyotrophic lateral sclerosis is a degenerative disease of the nervous system that involves both upper and lower motor neurons. Commonly, muscles innervated by either cranial nerves or spinal nerves are affected. Clinically, progressive muscle weakness and wasting develop, eventually leading to profound weakness of respiratory muscles and death. Although the time course of the disease is variable among patients, the natural history is one of irreversibility and progressive deterioration. As a result, patients and families must confront the difficult decision of whether to use mechanical ventilation either noninvasively or through a tracheostomy tube when the patient is in respiratory failure, knowing that no treatment will arrest the progressive neurologic deterioration.

PATHOPHYSIOLOGY AND CLINICAL CONSEQUENCES

Weakness of respiratory muscles is the hallmark of respiratory involvement in the neuromuscular diseases. Depending on the specific disease, chest wall (intercostal) muscles, diaphragm, and expiratory muscles of the abdominal wall are affected to variable extents.

Because of the impairment of inspiratory muscle strength, patients may be unable to maintain sufficient minute ventilation for adequate CO_2 elimination. In addition, patients often alter their pattern of breathing, taking shallower and more frequent breaths. Although this pattern of breathing may be easier and more comfortable, it also is less efficient because a greater proportion of each breath is wasted on ventilating the anatomic dead space (see Chapter 1). Therefore, even if total minute ventilation is maintained, alveolar ventilation (and thus CO_2 elimination) is impaired by the altered pattern of breathing.

The respiratory difficulty that develops in patients with neuromuscular disease is complicated by weakness of expiratory muscles and by an ineffective cough. Recurrent respiratory tract infections, accumulation of secretions, and areas of collapse or atelectasis contribute to the clinical problems seen in these patients.

Symptoms include dyspnea and anxiety. Patients also may have a feeling of suffocation. Often, the presence of generalized muscle weakness severely limits patients' activity and lessens the degree of dyspnea that would be present if they were capable of more exertion.

With severe neuromuscular disease, pulmonary function tests show a restrictive pattern of impairment. Although muscle weakness is the primary cause of the restriction, the compliance of the lung and the chest wall may be secondarily affected, further contributing to the restrictive pattern. The decrease in pulmonary compliance presumably is due to microatelectasis, that is, alveolar collapse, resulting from the shallow tidal volumes. At the same time, stiffening of various components of the chest wall (e.g., tendons, ligaments, and joints) over time is thought to be responsible for decreased distensibility of the chest wall. Functional residual capacity (FRC) is normal or decreased, depending on how much respiratory system compliance is altered. Total lung capacity is decreased primarily as a result of inspiratory muscle weakness, but changes in respiratory system compliance may contribute as well. Residual volume (RV) frequently is increased as a result of expiratory muscle weakness (Fig. 19-1). The degree of muscle weakness can be quantitated by measuring the maximal inspiratory and expiratory pressures that the patient is able to generate with maximal inspiratory and expiratory efforts against a closed mouthpiece. Both maximal inspiratory pressure (MIP) and maximal expiratory pressure may be significantly depressed.

In the setting of severe muscle weakness, arterial blood gases are most notable for the presence of alveolar hypoventilation, that is, hypercapnia. Hypoxemia also occurs as a result of alveolar hypoventilation and the associated depression in alveolar P_{O_2}. When hypoventilation is the sole cause of hypoxemia, the alveolar–arterial oxygen difference ($A a D_{O_2}$) is normal. However, complications of atelectasis, respiratory tract infections, and inadequately cleared secretions may add a component of ventilation-perfusion mismatch or shunt that further depresses P_{O_2} and increases $A a D_{O_2}$.

Features of neuromuscular disease are the following:
1. Altered pattern of breathing (↑ rate, ↓ tidal volume)
2. Ineffective cough
3. Restrictive pattern on pulmonary function tests
4. Decreased maximal inspiratory/expiratory pressures
5. ↑ P_{CO_2}, often with ↓ P_{O_2}

DIAPHRAGMATIC DISEASE

Although diaphragmatic involvement is a significant component of many of the neuromuscular diseases that affect the muscles of respiration, additional etiologic and clinical considerations justify a separate discussion of diaphragmatic disease. First we consider diaphragmatic fatigue, a potential consequence of disorders affecting other parts of the respiratory system that significantly increase the workload placed on the

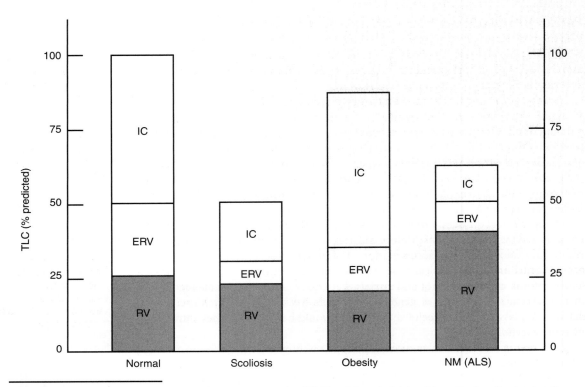

Figure 19-1. Examples of lung volumes (total lung capacity *[TLC]* and its subdivisions) in patients with chest wall and neuromuscular *(NM)* disease compared with values in a normal subject. Clear area represents vital capacity a nd its subdivisions. ALS = Amyotrophic lateral sclerosis; ERV = expiratory reserve volume; IC = inspiratory capacity; RV = residual volume. (Adapted from Bergofsky EH: *Am Rev Respir Dis* 119:643–669, 1979.)

diaphragm. We then discuss diaphragmatic paralysis, with separate considerations of unilateral and bilateral paralysis because the causes and the clinical manifestations are often quite different.

DIAPHRAGMATIC FATIGUE

Excluding cardiac muscle, the diaphragm is the single muscle used most consistently and repetitively throughout the course of a person's lifetime. It is well suited for sustained activity and for aerobic metabolism, and under normal circumstances the diaphragm does not become fatigued.

However, if the diaphragm is required to perform an excessive amount of work or if its energy supplies are limited, fatigue may develop and may contribute to respiratory dysfunction in certain clinical settings. For example, if a healthy individual repetitively uses the diaphragm to generate 40% or more of its maximal force, fatigue develops and prevents this degree of effort from being sustained indefinitely. For patients with diseases that increase the work of breathing, particularly obstructive lung disease and diseases of the chest wall (described in the section on diseases affecting the chest wall), the diaphragm works at a level much closer to the point of fatigue. When a superimposed acute illness further increases the work of breathing or when an intercurrent problem (e.g., depressed cardiac output, anemia, or hypoxemia) decreases the energy supply available to the diaphragm, then diaphragmatic fatigue may contribute to the development of hypoventilation and respiratory failure.

Inefficient diaphragmatic contraction is another factor that may contribute to diaphragmatic fatigue, especially in patients with obstructive lung disease. When the diaphragm is flattened and its fibers are shortened as a result of hyperinflated lungs, the force or pressure developed during contraction is less for any given level of diaphragmatic excitation (see Chapter 17). Therefore, a higher degree of stimulation is necessary to generate comparable pressure by the diaphragm, and increased energy consumption results.

Diaphragmatic fatigue often is difficult to detect because the force generated by the diaphragm cannot be measured conveniently. Ideally, diaphragmatic fatigue is documented by measuring the pressure across the diaphragm (i.e., the difference between abdominal and pleural pressure, called the *transdiaphragmatic pressure*) during diaphragmatic stimulation or contraction. As an alternative to measurement of transdiaphragmatic pressure, the strength of the inspiratory muscles in general can be assessed by measuring the pressure that a patient can generate with a maximal inspiratory effort against a closed mouthpiece, i.e., the maximal inspiratory pressure (MIP). A useful finding on physical examination is the pattern of motion of the abdomen during breathing when the patient is supine. If diaphragmatic contraction is especially weak or absent, pleural pressure falls, mainly as a result of contraction of other inspiratory muscles. The negative pleural pressure is transmitted across the relatively flaccid diaphragm to the abdomen, which then moves paradoxically inward during inspiration.

Along with investigation of the role of diaphragmatic fatigue in respiratory failure have been attempts to improve or reverse fatigue. Use of assisted ventilation with a mechanical ventilator to rest the diaphragm is one potential method for reversing fatigue. Alternatively, use of theophylline has been shown experimentally to increase the strength of diaphragmatic contraction. However, whether this type of pharmacologic therapy produces a clinically beneficial effect has yet to be proven.

UNILATERAL DIAPHRAGMATIC PARALYSIS

Paralysis of the diaphragm on one side of the thorax (also called a *hemidiaphragm*) typically results from disease affecting the ipsilateral phrenic nerve. A particularly common cause of unilateral diaphragmatic paralysis is invasion of the phrenic nerve by malignancy. The underlying tumor frequently is lung cancer that has invaded or metastasized to the mediastinum, and either the primary tumor itself or mediastinal lymph nodes affected by tumor invade the phrenic nerve somewhere along its course through the mediastinum. With treatment, some diaphragmatic function may return, but frequently diaphragmatic paralysis resulting from malignancy is irreversible.

Paralysis of the left hemidiaphragm may be seen following cardiac surgery attributable to either a stretch injury or a cooling injury to the phrenic nerve. In these cases, a cold solution is instilled in the pericardium during the procedure to stop cardiac contraction (cold cardioplegia) and allow surgery on a nonbeating heart while circulation is maintained by cardiopulmonary bypass. However, the cold solution causes temporary paralysis of the left phrenic nerve, leading to diaphragmatic paralysis of variable duration. With changes in surgical techniques, phrenic nerve injury is becoming less common following cardiac surgery. When it does occur, function usually recovers within 1 year.

In some patients with unilateral diaphragmatic paralysis, no underlying reason for the paralysis can be identified, and the problem is considered *idiopathic*. A viral infection affecting the phrenic nerve may be responsible in such cases. Many but not all of these patients recover some function over time.

Factors contributing to diaphragmatic fatigue are the following:
1. Increased work of breathing
2. Decreased energy supply to diaphragm
3. Inefficient diaphragmatic contraction

Diaphragmatic weakness can be demonstrated in the supine position by inward motion of the abdomen during inspiration.

The possibility of unilateral diaphragmatic paralysis usually is first suggested by a characteristic appearance on the chest radiograph (Fig. 19-2). The affected hemidiaphragm is elevated above its usual position, in the absence of any associated lobar atelectasis or other reason for volume loss on the affected side. Standard chest radiographs taken during a full inspiration (to total lung capacity) reveal that the normal hemidiaphragm descends during inspiration whereas the paralyzed hemidiaphragm cannot. Patients may or may not be symptomatic with dyspnea as a result of the paralyzed hemidiaphragm, often depending on the presence or absence of additional underlying lung disease.

Because an elevated diaphragm may result from causes other than diaphragmatic paralysis (e.g., processes below the diaphragm, such as a subphrenic abscess), it is generally useful to confirm objectively that diaphragmatic paralysis is the cause of diaphragmatic elevation. This can be achieved relatively easily by real-time observation of diaphragmatic movement during a "sniff test." With this technique, the radiologist observes diaphragmatic motion under fluoroscopy while the patient sniffs. During the act of sniffing, which is a rapid inspiratory activity, the normal diaphragm contracts and therefore descends, while the paralyzed diaphragm moves passively (and paradoxically) upward as a result of rapid development of negative intrathoracic pressure during the sniff.

For appropriate patients who are dyspneic because of the hemidiaphragmatic paralysis, a treatment option is diaphragmatic plication. In this surgical procedure, the hemidiaphragm is fixed in a flattened position; although the hemidiaphragm does not move, the lung is maintained at a higher volume and the hemidiaphragm can no longer move paradoxically upward during inspiration.

BILATERAL DIAPHRAGMATIC PARALYSIS

Paralysis of both diaphragms has much more serious clinical implications than does unilateral paralysis because the patient must depend on the accessory muscles of inspiration to maintain minute ventilation. The causes of bilateral diaphragmatic paralysis are the neuromuscular diseases listed in Table 19-1, with bilateral diaphragmatic paralysis being the most severe consequence of respiratory involvement by these disorders.

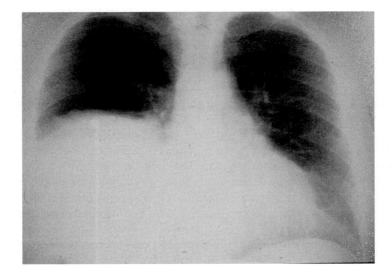

Figure 19-2. Chest radiograph shows elevation of the right hemidiaphragm resulting from unilateral (right) phrenic nerve paralysis.

A characteristic clinical manifestation of bilateral diaphragmatic paralysis is dyspnea that is significantly exacerbated when the patient assumes the recumbent position, i.e., severe orthopnea. When the patient is supine, the abdominal contents push on the flaccid diaphragm, as the beneficial effects of gravity on abdominal contents and on lowering the position of the diaphragm are lost. On physical examination, patients typically demonstrate paradoxical inward motion of the abdomen during inspiration while they are supine, as described in the discussion on diaphragmatic fatigue. The deleterious effect of assuming the recumbent position is also seen with pulmonary function testing, in that the vital capacity measured in the supine position is significantly lower than that measured in the upright position.

DISEASES AFFECTING THE CHEST WALL

With certain diseases of the chest wall, difficulty in expanding the chest may impede normal inspiration (see Table 19-1). This section focuses on two specific disorders that pose the greatest clinical problems: kyphoscoliosis and obesity.

KYPHOSCOLIOSIS

Kyphoscoliosis is an abnormal curvature of the spine in both the anterior (kyphosis) and lateral (scoliosis) directions (Fig. 19-3). As a result of this deformity, the rib cage becomes stiffer and more difficult to expand, i.e., chest wall compliance is decreased. Respiratory difficulties are common in patients with significant kyphoscoliosis. In particularly severe cases, chronic respiratory failure is the consequence. Although some cases of kyphoscoliosis actually are secondary to neuromuscular disease such as poliomyelitis, the majority of severe cases associated with respiratory impairment are idiopathic.

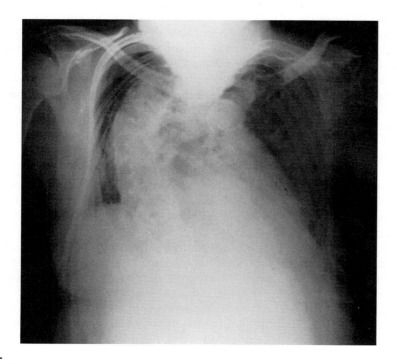

Figure 19-3. Chest radiograph of patient with severe kyphoscoliosis. Note marked spinal curvature and chest wall distortion.

Several pathophysiologic features contribute to respiratory dysfunction in patients with kyphoscoliosis. A crucial underlying problem is the increased work of breathing resulting from the poorly compliant chest wall. To maintain even a normal minute ventilation, the work expenditure of the respiratory muscles is greatly increased. In addition, patients decrease their tidal volume and increase respiratory frequency because of difficulty expanding the abnormally stiff chest wall. Consequently, the proportion of wasted ventilation rises, and alveolar ventilation falls unless total ventilation undergoes a compensatory increase. Hence, the increased work of breathing acts together with the altered pattern of breathing to decrease alveolar ventilation and to increase PCO_2. Chest wall compliance further decreases with age, and respiratory complications of uncorrected kyphoscoliosis become increasingly prevalent as the patient ages.

The marked distortion of the chest wall causes underventilation of some regions of the lung, microatelectasis, ventilation-perfusion mismatch, and hypoxemia. Therefore, two frequent causes of hypoxemia in kyphoscoliosis are hypoventilation and ventilation-perfusion mismatch.

A common complication of severe kyphoscoliosis is pulmonary hypertension and cor pulmonale. Hypoxemia and, to a lesser extent, hypercapnia are important for the development of pulmonary hypertension. However, increased resistance of the pulmonary vessels also results from compression and possibly from impaired development in regions in which the chest wall is especially distorted. Long-standing pulmonary hypertension itself also causes structural changes in the vessels, with thickening of the walls of pulmonary arteries. This thickening is not acutely reversible, even with correction of the hypoxemia.

Exertional dyspnea probably is the most common symptom experienced by patients with severe kyphoscoliosis and respiratory impairment. Unlike patients with neuromuscular disease, those with a chest wall deformity such as kyphoscoliosis have normal muscle strength and therefore are capable of normal levels of exertion. Patients with kyphoscoliosis also are not subject to the same difficulty in generating an effective cough as are patients with neuromuscular disease. Expiratory muscle function is preserved, an effective cough is maintained, and problems with secretions and recurrent respiratory tract infections are not prominent clinical features.

Pulmonary function tests in patients with kyphoscoliosis are notable for a restrictive pattern of impairment, with a decrease in the total lung capacity. Vital capacity is significantly decreased, whereas RV tends to be relatively preserved. Functional residual capacity, determined by the outward recoil of the chest wall balanced by the inward recoil of the lung, is decreased because the poorly compliant chest wall has a diminished propensity to recoil outward (see Fig. 19-1).

Severe cases of kyphoscoliosis are generally characterized by hypercapnia and hypoxemia. The latter usually is due to both hypoventilation and ventilation-perfusion mismatch. Chronic respiratory insufficiency and cor pulmonale are the end results of severe kyphoscoliosis, and the level of respiratory difficulty appears to correlate with the severity of chest wall deformity.

Surgical therapy aimed at improving or correcting the spinal deformity may be useful in children or adolescents, but rarely is it effective in adults. Supportive therapy that may be beneficial includes a variety of measures that provide ventilatory assistance to the patient. Treatments with an intermittent positive-pressure breathing machine augment tidal volume by delivering positive pressure to the patient during inspiration. The increase in tidal volume improves microatelectasis and lung compliance, affording the patient several hours with decreased work of breathing after each treatment. At night, ventilatory assistance with either inspiratory positive pressure delivered via a mask or through a tracheostomy tube or negative pressure around the chest wall allows the respiratory muscles to rest. Nocturnal ventilatory support may provide sufficient rest for

Features of severe kyphoscoliosis are the following:
1. Increased work of breathing
2. Altered pattern of breathing (↑ rate, ↓ tidal volume)
3. Exertional dyspnea
4. Ventilation-perfusion mismatch
5. ↑ PCO_2, often with ↓ PO_2
6. Pulmonary hypertension, cor pulmonale
7. Restrictive pattern on pulmonary function tests

the inspiratory muscles to diminish daytime respiratory muscle fatigue. These types of ventilatory support are discussed further in Chapter 29.

OBESITY

Obesity has many consequences for health, and respiratory symptoms are one aspect. Obesity can produce a wide spectrum in severity of respiratory impairment, ranging from no symptoms to marked limitation in function. Surprisingly, the degree of obesity does not appear to correlate with the presence or severity of respiratory dysfunction. Some patients who are massively obese have no difficulty in comparison with much less obese patients who may be severely limited. This may be partially explained by the distribution of body fat: central distribution of fat is more associated with decreased lung function as measured by pulmonary function testing. A full explanation of the discrepancies in symptoms among different patients is based on several factors, including smoking history, underlying lung disease, effects of obesity on the cardiovascular system, and underlying physical deconditioning.

The problem of respiratory impairment in obesity was popularly known for years as the *pickwickian syndrome* or *obesity-hypoventilation syndrome.* The term "pickwickian" was applied because of the description of the fat boy, Joe, in Dickens' *Pickwick Papers,* who had many of the characteristics described in this syndrome. Specifically, Joe had features of massive obesity, somnolence, and peripheral edema, the latter presumably related to cor pulmonale and right ventricular failure. With the accumulation of knowledge about the pathogenesis of respiratory impairment in obesity, the term pickwickian syndrome has become less meaningful.

Obesity appears to exert two mechanical effects on the respiratory system. As a result of excess soft tissue, the chest wall becomes stiffer or less compliant, so more work is necessary for expansion of the thorax. In addition, the massive accumulation of soft tissue in the abdominal wall exerts pressure on abdominal contents, forcing the diaphragm up to a higher resting position.

In a fashion similar to that of kyphoscoliosis, the stiff chest wall results in lower tidal volumes and increased wasted or dead space ventilation. Therefore, in order to maintain adequate alveolar ventilation, overall minute ventilation must increase in the face of increased work of breathing. Some patients are able to compensate appropriately by increasing their overall minute ventilation, and Pco_2 remains normal. Other patients do not compensate fully, and hypercapnia is the necessary consequence.

Exactly what distinguishes these two types of patients is not really known. Perhaps patients in the latter group, for whom the term obesity-hypoventilation syndrome can be applied, started out with a central nervous system respiratory controller that was relatively hyporesponsive. Output of the controller might not have responded sufficiently to keep pace with increased ventilatory requirements, and CO_2 retention resulted. After hypercapnia actually develops, it is much more difficult to assess the innate responsiveness of the patient's ventilatory controller because chronic hypercapnia (i.e., chronic respiratory acidosis with a compensatory metabolic alkalosis) blunts the responsiveness of the central chemoreceptor.

Another distinguishing feature between normocapnic and hypercapnic obese patients may relate to inspiratory muscle strength. Whereas inspiratory muscle strength is normal in obese patients with normal Pco_2, it is reduced by approximately 30% in patients with the obesity-hypoventilation syndrome, perhaps as a result of respiratory muscle fatigue.

The high resting position of the diaphragm in obesity, occurring as a result of pressure from the obese abdomen, is associated with decreased expansion of the lung and closure of small airways and alveoli at the bases. Thus, the dependent regions are hypoventilated relative to their perfusion, and this ventilation-perfusion mismatch results in arterial hypoxemia.

Features of obesity are the following:
1. Decreased chest wall compliance
2. High diaphragm (low functional residual capacity)
3. Altered pattern of breathing (↑ rate, ↓ tidal volume)
4. Ventilation-perfusion mismatch
5. Variable ↑ Pco_2, ↓ Po_2
6. Obstructive apnea (common)

Another factor that contributes to the overall clinical picture in many massively obese patients is upper airway obstruction during sleep, i.e., the obstructive form of sleep apnea syndrome. Soft tissue deposition in the neck and tissues surrounding the upper airway presumably predisposes the person to episodes of complete upper airway obstruction during sleep (see Chapter 18). In a large percentage of cases, somnolence that occurs in patients who supposedly have the obesity-hypoventilation syndrome is related to the presence of obstructive sleep apnea.

Although obesity, depressed respiratory drive, respiratory muscle weakness, and sleep apnea syndrome contribute to respiratory dysfunction, exactly how they interact in individual patients often is difficult to assess. Because sleep apnea syndrome and depressed respiratory drive also occur in patients who are not obese, it is reasonable to view some of the contributing pathophysiologic factors in terms of a Venn diagram (Fig. 19-4). Probably the most marked symptoms and respiratory dysfunction are seen in patients who are represented at the intersection of the three circles.

The symptoms that may occur in obese patients can be associated with the increased work of breathing (e.g., dyspnea) or with the sleep apnea syndrome (e.g., daytime somnolence and disordered sleep with profound snoring). Patients may have clinical manifestations related to the complications of pulmonary hypertension, cor pulmonale, and right ventricular failure. These complications are largely related to arterial hypoxemia both during the day and at night, particularly if patients have sleep apnea syndrome.

Pulmonary function tests frequently demonstrate a restrictive pattern of dysfunction, with a decrease in total lung capacity. The diaphragm is pushed up in massively obese patients, reducing FRC, which in these patients is much closer to RV; thus, spirometric examination shows the expiratory reserve volume is greatly reduced. This pattern of functional impairment is shown in Figure 19-1.

In most obese patients, arterial blood gases show a decrease in the Po_2 and an increase in the $AaDo_2$ as a consequence of high diaphragms, airway and alveolar closure, and ventilation-perfusion mismatch. If Pco_2 is not elevated, these patients are sometimes said to have "simple obesity." When Pco_2 is elevated, the term *obesity-hypoventilation syndrome* is often used, and in these cases superimposed hypoventilation is another

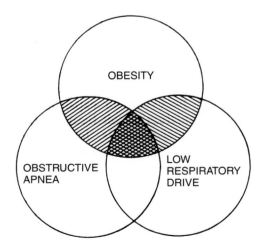

Figure 19-4. Venn diagram shows hypothetical indication of the way obesity interacts with obstructive apnea and low respiratory drive. Overlap on left indicates obese, normocapnic patients with obstructive apnea. Overlap on right indicates hypercapnic obese patients without obstructive apnea. Overlap at center indicates obese, hypercapnic patients with obstructive apnea.

factor contributing to hypoxemia. If patients have sleep apnea syndrome, arterial blood gas values become even more deranged at night during episodes of apnea.

Weight loss is crucial in the treatment of obese patients with respiratory dysfunction. If weight loss is successful, many of the clinical problems may resolve. Unfortunately, attempts at significant and sustained weight loss often are futile, and other modes of therapy must be instituted. In patients who hypoventilate, respiratory stimulants, especially progesterone (a centrally acting respiratory stimulant), have been used with some success. If the patient has obstructive sleep apnea syndrome, therapy aimed at eliminating the episodes of nocturnal upper airway obstruction is crucial (see Chapter 18).

REFERENCES

NEUROMUSCULAR DISEASE AFFECTING THE MUSCLES OF RESPIRATION

Bach JR: Management of post-polio respiratory sequelae, *Ann N Y Acad Sci* 753:96–102, 1995.

Benditt JO: Management of pulmonary complications in neuromuscular disease, *Phys Med Rehabil Clin North Am* 9:167–185, 1998.

Derenne J-P, Macklem PT, Roussos C: The respiratory muscles: mechanics, control, and pathophysiology, *Am Rev Respir Dis* 118:581–601, 1978.

Dhand UK: Clinical approach to the weak patient in the intensive care unit, *Respir Care* 51:1024–1040, 2006.

Kaplan LM, Hollander D: Respiratory dysfunction in amyotrophic lateral sclerosis, *Clin Chest Med* 15:675–681, 1994.

Lacomis D: Myasthenic crisis, *Neurocrit Care* 3:189–194, 2005.

Mansel JK, Norman JR: Respiratory complications and management of spinal cord injuries, *Chest* 97:1446–1452, 1990.

Mehta S: Neuromuscular disease causing acute respiratory failure, *Respir Care* 51:1016–1021, 2006.

Orlikowski D, Prigent H, Sharshar T, Lofaso F, Raphael JC: Respiratory dysfunction in Guillain-Barré syndrome, *Neurocrit Care* 1:415–422, 2004.

Piepers S, van den Berg JP, Kalmijn S, et al: Effect of non-invasive ventilation on survival, quality of life, respiratory function and cognition: a review of the literature, *Amyotroph Lateral Scler* 7:195–200, 2006.

Roussos C, Macklem PT: The respiratory muscles, *N Engl J Med* 307:786–797, 1982.

Smith PEM, Calverley PM, Edwards RH, Evans GA, Campbell EJ: Practical problems in the respiratory care of patients with muscular dystrophy, *N Engl J Med* 316:1197–1205, 1987.

Seneviratne J, Mandrekar J, Wijdicks EF, Rabenstein AA: Non-invasive ventilation in myasthenia crisis, *Arch Neurol* 65:54–58, 2008.

Sunderrajan EV, Davenport J: The Guillain-Barré syndrome: pulmonary-neurologic correlations, *Medicine* 64:333–341, 1985.

DIAPHRAGMATIC DISEASE

Aldrich TK: Respiratory muscle fatigue, *Clin Chest Med* 9:225–236, 1988.

Aubier M, De Troyer A, Sampson M, Macklem PT, Roussos C: Aminophylline improves diaphragmatic contractility, *N Engl J Med* 305:249–252, 1981.

Belman MJ, Sieck GC: The ventilatory muscles: fatigue, endurance and training, *Chest* 82:761–766, 1982.

Celli B: The diaphragm and respiratory muscles, *Chest Surg Clin North Am* 8:207–224, 1998.

Cohen CA, Zagelbaum G, Gross D, Roussos C, Macklem PT: Clinical manifestations of inspiratory muscle fatigue, *Am J Med* 73:308–316, 1982.

Mador MJ: Respiratory muscle fatigue and breathing patterns, *Chest* 100:1430–1435, 1991.

Pacia EB, Aldrich TK: Assessment of diaphragm function, *Chest Surg Clin North Am* 8:225–236, 1998.

Roussos C, Macklem PT: The respiratory muscles, *N Engl J Med* 307:786–797, 1982.

Tripp HF, Bolton JW: Phrenic nerve injury following cardiac surgery: a review, *J Card Surg* 13:218–223, 1998.

DISEASES AFFECTING THE CHEST WALL

Baydur A, Milic-Emili J: Respiratory mechanics in kyphoscoliosis, *Monaldi Arch Chest Dis* 48:69–79, 1993.

Berger KI, Ayappa I, Chatr-Amontri B, et al: Obesity hypoventilation syndrome as a spectrum of respiratory disturbances during sleep, *Chest* 120:1231–1238, 2001.

Bergofsky EH: Respiratory failure in disorders of the thoracic cage, *Am Rev Respir Dis* 119:643–669, 1979.

Chen Y, Rennie D, Cormier YF, Dosman J: Waist circumference is associated with pulmonary function in normal-weight, overweight, and obese subjects, *Am J Clin Nutr* 85:35–39, 2007.

Kafer ER: Respiratory and cardiovascular functions in scoliosis, *Bull Eur Physiopathol Respir* 13:299–321, 1977.

Koenig SM: Pulmonary complications of obesity, *Am J Med Sci* 321:249–279, 2001.

Luce JM: Respiratory complications of obesity, *Chest* 78:626–631, 1980.

McMaster MJ, Glasby MA, Singh H, Cunningham S: Lung function in congenital kypnosis and kypnoscoliosis, *J Spinal Disord Tech* 20:203–208, 2007.

Piper A, Grunstein RR: Current perspectives on the obesity hypoventilation syndrome, *Curr Opin Pulm Med* 13:490–496, 2007.

Sutton FD Jr, Zwillich CW, Creagh CE, Pierson DJ, Weil JV: Progesterone for outpatient treatment of pickwickian syndrome, *Ann Intern Med* 83:476–479, 1975.

Lung Cancer: Etiologic and Pathologic Aspects

Carcinoma of the lung is a public health problem of immense proportions. It has been a source of great frustration to individual physicians and to the medical profession in general. Several decades ago, the primary cause of carcinoma of the lung—cigarette smoking—was identified without a shadow of a doubt. Fortunately, the prevalence of smoking in developed countries has been falling gradually after peaking in the mid-1970s. Unfortunately, any optimism is tempered by the following concerns: (1) approximately 20% of all American adults still smoke; (2) although smoking prevalence declined substantially in the years before 1990, it has changed only slowly since then; and (3) tobacco use is continuing to increase in developing countries, where the tobacco industry is focusing its marketing efforts.

A few statistics put the magnitude of the problem of lung cancer into perspective. In the United States, nearly 213,000 new cases of lung cancer are diagnosed annually, and more than 160,000 individuals each year die as a result of the disease. For many years, carcinoma of the lung has been the leading cause of cancer deaths among men, and in 1987 lung cancer surpassed breast cancer as the leading cause of death among women. Lung cancer is responsible for 25% to 30% of all deaths attributable to cancer and approximately 5% of all deaths from any cause. It is sobering to realize that during the last 5 years more Americans were killed by lung cancer than were killed in all the wars in U.S. history.

The number of cases and the number of deaths related to lung cancer have increased dramatically over the last several decades. For no other form of cancer has the increase approached that of lung cancer. For men, the death rate appears to have reached a peak in 1990 and fortunately has been decreasing since then. In women the death rate increased fivefold in the 30 years from 1960 to 1990 but more recently appears to be reaching a plateau. Despite the magnitude of the problem, our ability to treat carcinoma of the lung has improved only minimally. Five-year survival has increased from approximately 7% to 14% during the last several decades, making the prognosis of this disease still dismal in the vast majority of cases.

The discussion of carcinoma of the lung is presented in two parts. This chapter considers what is known about the etiology and pathogenesis of lung cancer, followed by a description of the pathologic aspects and classification of the different types of tumors. Chapter 21 continues with a discussion of the clinical aspects of the disease, including diagnostic and therapeutic considerations. Chapter 21 concludes with a brief discussion of two additional types of neoplastic disease affecting the respiratory system, bronchial carcinoid tumor (bronchial adenoma) and mesothelioma, along with a consideration of the common problem of the patient with a solitary pulmonary nodule.

ETIOLOGY AND PATHOGENESIS

For no other common cancer affecting humans have the causative factors been worked out so well as for lung cancer. Cigarette smoking clearly is responsible for the vast majority of cases (>85%, according to some estimates), and additional risk factors associated with occupational exposure have been identified. This chapter begins with a discussion of these two major risk factors of cigarette smoking and occupational exposure, followed by consideration of genetic factors as a potential contributor to lung cancer risk. Next is a brief description of the importance of previous scarring within the pulmonary parenchyma, which has been implicated in the development of "scar carcinomas," and several miscellaneous proposed risk factors are mentioned. Finally, the role of oncogenes and tumor suppressor genes in the pathogenesis of lung cancer is discussed.

SMOKING

Cigarette smoking is the single most important risk factor for the development of carcinoma of the lung. As might be expected, the duration of the smoking history, the number of cigarettes smoked each day, the depth of inhalation, and the amount of each cigarette smoked all correlate with the risk for development of lung cancer. As a rough but easy way to quantitate prior cigarette exposure, the number of years of smoking can be multiplied by the average number of packs smoked per day, giving the number of "pack years."

Although the evidence incriminating smoking with lung cancer is incontrovertible, the responsible component of cigarette smoke has not been identified with certainty. Cigarette smoke consists of a gaseous phase and a particulate phase, and potential carcinogens have been found in both phases, ranging from nitrosamines to benzo[a]pyrene and other polycyclic hydrocarbons. Filters appear to decrease but certainly do not eliminate the potential carcinogenic effects of cigarettes. A substantially lower risk for lung cancer is associated with cigar and pipe smoking, presumably related to the fact that cigar and pipe smoke is generally not inhaled deeply into the lungs in the same manner as cigarette smoke. The smoking of marijuana and cocaine also has been associated with lung cancer.

The actual development of lung cancer as a result of smoking requires many years of exposure. However, histologic abnormalities before the development of a frank carcinoma are well documented in the bronchial epithelium of smokers. These changes, including loss of bronchial cilia, hyperplasia of bronchial epithelial cells, and nuclear abnormalities, may be the histologic forerunners of a true carcinoma. If a person stops smoking, many of these precancerous changes appear to be reversible. Epidemiologic studies have suggested that the risk for developing lung cancer decreases progressively after cessation of smoking but probably never returns to the level in nonsmokers, even after more than 10 to 15 years. In many cases, the initial cellular changes leading to or predisposing to malignant transformation have already developed by the time the

> Histologic abnormalities in the bronchial epithelium induced by smoking precede the development of carcinoma.

patient stops smoking, and it is merely a matter of time before the carcinoma develops or becomes clinically apparent.

Data indicate that the risk of lung cancer is increased for nonsmoking spouses because of their exposure to sidestream or "secondhand" smoke. Although the risk attributable to "passive smoking" is relatively small compared with the risk of active smoking, involuntary exposure to cigarette smoke likely is responsible for some cases of lung cancer occurring in nonsmokers. The comparably small but apparent risk of lung cancer from passive smoking has been a major justification for legislation prohibiting smoking in shared spaces such as commercial aircraft, restaurants, and offices.

OCCUPATIONAL FACTORS

A number of potential environmental risk factors have been identified, most of which occur with occupational exposure. Perhaps the most widely studied of the environmental or occupationally related carcinogens is asbestos, a fibrous silicate formerly in wide use because of its properties of fire resistance and thermal insulation. Shipbuilders, construction workers, and those who work with insulation and brake linings are among those who may be exposed to asbestos.

Carcinoma of the lung is the most likely malignancy to result from asbestos exposure, although other tumors, especially mesothelioma (see Chapter 21), are also strongly associated with prior asbestos contact. The risk for development of lung cancer is particularly high among smokers exposed to asbestos, in which case these two risk factors probably have a multiplicative effect. Specifically, asbestos alone appears to confer a twofold to fivefold increased risk for lung cancer, whereas smoking alone is associated with an approximately 10-fold increased risk. Together, the two risk factors make the person who smokes and has an asbestos exposure 20 to 50 times more likely to have carcinoma of the lung than a nonsmoking, nonexposed counterpart. Like other forms of asbestos-related disease, a long time elapses before complications develop. In the case of lung cancer, the tumor generally becomes apparent more than 2 decades after exposure.

> The risk of lung cancer is markedly increased by the combined risk factors of asbestos exposure and smoking.

A number of other types of occupational exposure have been implicated. Examples include exposure to arsenic (in workers making pesticides, glass, pigments, and paints), ionizing radiation (especially in uranium miners), halo ethers (bis-chloromethyl ether and chloromethyl methyl ether in chemical industry workers), and polycyclic aromatic hydrocarbons (in petroleum, coal tar, and foundry workers). As is the case with asbestos, there is generally a long latent period of at least 2 decades from the time of exposure until presentation of the tumor.

GENETIC FACTORS

Why lung cancer develops in some heavy smokers and not in others is a question of great importance but with no definite answer at present. The assumption is that genetic factors must place some individuals at higher risk for lung cancer after exposure to carcinogens. The finding of an increased risk of lung cancer among first-degree relatives of lung cancer patients, even after confounding factors have been taken into account, supports this hypothesis. Candidate genetic factors have primarily included specific enzymes of the cytochrome P-450 system. These enzymes may have a role in metabolizing products of cigarette smoke to potent carcinogens so that genetically determined increased activity or expression of the enzymes is associated with a greater risk of developing lung cancer following exposure to cigarette smoke.

One example is the enzyme aryl hydrocarbon hydroxylase, which can convert hydrocarbons to carcinogenic metabolites. This enzyme is induced by smoking, and genetically determined inducibility of this enzyme by smoking may correlate with the risk for lung cancer. Another enzyme of the cytochrome P-450 system can be identified by its ability to metabolize the antihypertensive drug debrisoquine. Some data suggest an association between extensive metabolism of debrisoquine and the development of lung cancer. Presumably, the action of this enzyme on a potentially carcinogenic substrate from cigarette smoke affects an individual's risk for developing lung cancer. However, the available data for both of these cytochrome P-450 enzymes are inconsistent, and a role for these enzymes is not universally accepted.

Other as yet unidentified genetic factors potentially affect the susceptibility to environmental carcinogens and may include the activity of tumor suppressor genes. If such factors eventually are recognized, then preventing susceptible individuals from being exposed to the known environmental carcinogens or targeting more aggressive screening techniques toward the populations at greatest risk may be possible.

PARENCHYMAL SCARRING

Scar tissue within the lung can be a locus for the subsequent occurrence of lung cancer, called a *scar carcinoma*. The scarring may be either localized (e.g., resulting from an old focus of tuberculosis or another infection) or diffuse (e.g., from pulmonary fibrosis, whether idiopathic or associated with a specific cause). Most frequently, scar carcinoma of the lung is an adenocarcinoma and often a specific subtype called *bronchioloalveolar carcinoma*. These cell types are discussed in the section on adenocarcinoma.

Although it is easy to consider carcinomas occurring within or adjacent to scar tissue to be scar carcinomas, adenocarcinomas of the lung also may develop fibrotic areas within the tumor. Therefore, in some cases it may be impossible to know whether the scar preceded or followed development of the carcinoma.

MISCELLANEOUS FACTORS

The lay press has expressed a great deal of interest and publicized the risk of lung cancer from exposure to radon, a gas that is a decay product of radium-226 (itself a decay product of uranium). Exposure to this known carcinogen may occur indoors in homes built on soil that has a high radium content and is releasing radon into the surrounding environment. Although the finding of unacceptably high levels of radon in some home environments has sparked concern about the risk of lung cancer and interest in widespread testing of houses, uncertainty remains about the overall risk posed by exposure to radon. At the extreme, it has been suggested that radon is the second most important factor contributing to lung cancer and potentially is responsible for 20,000 lung cancer deaths per year in the United States. However, this magnitude of risk is not universally accepted.

Some evidence suggests that at least one dietary factor may affect the risk of lung cancer. Some studies have reported an association between low intake and serum levels of β-carotene, the provitamin form of vitamin A, with an increased risk of lung cancer. However, the data relating to this issue are controversial. An increased risk associated with low dietary intake of β-carotene, if it exists, is relatively minor compared with the risk posed by cigarette smoking. Three large randomized trials have failed to demonstrate a protective effect of β-carotene, α-tocopherol, or retinoid supplementation on lung cancer risk. The issue is further complicated by data suggesting a slight increase in the incidence of lung cancer in some trials of individuals given supplements.

CONCEPTS IN THE PATHOGENESIS OF LUNG CANCER

There has been a great deal of interest in identifying the cell(s) of origin, that is, the histogenesis, of the various types of lung cancer and in elucidating the genetic changes involved in the malignant transformation of these cells. For many years, it was assumed that the different histopathologic types of lung cancer (described in the section on pathology) were each associated with a different cell of origin. It was thought that previously well-differentiated normal cells underwent a process of dedifferentiation and unrestricted growth when exposed to a carcinogenic stimulus. However, based in part on the common finding of cellular heterogeneity, that is, more than one cell type within a single tumor, it is currently believed that many, if not all, types of lung cancer arise from an undifferentiated precursor or stem cell. During this cell's malignant transformation, it differentiates along one or more particular pathways that determine its ultimate histologic appearance, that is, its cell type(s).

Alterations in genes that code for proteins controlling or regulating cell growth have been found in a high proportion of patients with lung cancer. These molecular changes may play a central role in the pathogenesis of lung cancer. Two types of oncogenes have been identified: proto-oncogenes (which code for growth-promoting factors) and tumor suppressor genes (which code for factors having a negative regulatory effect on cell proliferation). A mutation in one of the paired alleles of a proto-oncogene can result in production of a protein with a growth-promoting effect so that a "dominant" behavior or effect would be observed. In contrast, both alleles of a tumor suppressor gene must be altered before the absence of the gene product would be clinically manifest as increased cell growth or malignant transformation. This requirement produces a "recessive" pattern of clinical expression.

> Alterations in proto-oncogenes and tumor suppressor genes have been found in many patients with lung cancer.

Specific common alterations in proto-oncogenes that have been identified in lung cancer include mutations in the ras, EGFR, HER2, and Bcl-2 families of dominant oncogenes. A variety of mutations in recessive tumor suppressor genes also have been identified, including the retinoblastoma *(rb)* and *p53* genes. In addition, deletion of genetic material from chromosome 3p (the short arm of chromosome 3) has been recognized in lung cancer, and it is thought that deletion may involve loss of one or more tumor suppressor genes. Particularly interesting experimental data link a carcinogenic metabolite of benzo[a]pyrene, which is found in cigarette smoke, to those mutations of the *p53* gene that are most commonly seen in lung cancer.

PATHOLOGY

The term *bronchogenic carcinoma* is often used interchangeably with the term *lung cancer,* implying that lung cancers arise from bronchi or bronchial structures. Many, if not most, lung cancers do originate within airways, but other tumors arise in the periphery of the lung and may not necessarily originate in an airway. This section focuses on the currently accepted classification of lung cancer and summarizes what is known about the behavior patterns of the various types of tumors.

Almost all lung cancers fall within one of four histologic categories: (1) squamous cell carcinoma, (2) small cell carcinoma, (3) adenocarcinoma, and (4) large cell carcinoma. Within each category are several subcategories that, for our purposes, are less important. However, two of these subcategories are discussed—bronchioloalveolar carcinoma (a type of adenocarcinoma) and oat cell carcinoma (a type of small cell carcinoma)—because they are frequent diagnoses and are often used terms in the clinical setting.

> Major histologic categories of lung cancer are the following:
> 1. Squamous cell carcinoma
> 2. Small cell carcinoma
> 3. Adenocarcinoma
> 4. Large cell carcinoma

One of the most important distinctions to make is between small cell carcinoma and all the other cell types, which are grouped together as *non–small cell carcinoma.* The importance of this distinction relates to the propensity of small cell carcinoma for early clinical and subclinical metastasis, which affects the approaches to staging and treatment of this tumor compared with those of all the other cell types.

Each of the four major categories of lung cancer is associated with cigarette smoking. However, the statistical association between smoking and the individual cell types is greatest for squamous cell carcinoma and small cell carcinomas, which are seen almost exclusively in smokers. Even though smoking also increases the risk for adenocarcinoma and large cell carcinoma, these cell types also occur with some regularity in nonsmokers.

SQUAMOUS CELL CARCINOMA

Approximately 28% of all bronchogenic carcinomas are of the squamous cell type. These tumors originate within the epithelial layer of the bronchial wall, in which a series of progressive histologic abnormalities result from chronic or repetitive cigarette smoke–induced injury.

Initially, there is metaplasia of the normal bronchial columnar epithelial cells, which are replaced by squamous epithelial cells. Over time these squamous cells become more and more atypical in appearance until there is development of a well-localized carcinoma, that is, carcinoma in situ. Eventually, the carcinoma extends beyond the bronchial mucosa and becomes frankly invasive. After the tumor reaches this stage, it generally comes to eventual clinical attention by producing either symptoms or radiographic changes. In some cases, detection of the carcinoma is made at the earlier in situ stage, usually by recognition of the malignant cells in a specimen of sputum obtained for cytologic examination or by biopsy of grossly abnormal-appearing bronchial mucosa during bronchoscopic evaluation undertaken for other reasons.

Specific histologic features of squamous cell carcinoma allow the pathologist to establish this diagnosis. These tumors are characterized by the presence of keratin, "squamous pearls," and intercellular bridges (Fig. 20-1).

Squamous cell carcinomas tend to be located in relatively large or proximal airways, most commonly at the subsegmental, segmental, or lobar level. With growth of the tumor into the bronchial lumen, the airway may become obstructed. The lung distal to

Features of squamous cell carcinomas are the following:
1. Generally arise in proximal airways
2. May cause airway obstruction, leading to distal atelectasis or pneumonia
3. May cavitate
4. Intrathoracic spread rather than distant metastases

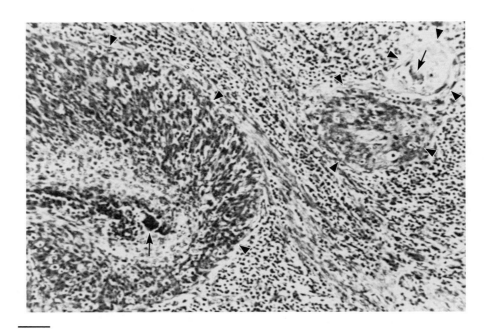

Figure 20-1. Low-power photomicrograph of squamous cell carcinoma. Note three foci of tumor, each highlighted by arrowheads. Intervening regions show connective tissue and inflammatory cells. Arrows point to two areas of keratin formation by the tumor. (Courtesy Dr. Earl Kasdon.)

the obstruction frequently collapses (becomes atelectatic), and a postobstructive pneumonia may develop. Sometimes a cavity develops within the tumor mass; this finding of cavitation is much more common with squamous cell than with other types of bronchogenic carcinoma.

Spread of squamous cell carcinoma beyond the airway usually involves (1) direct extension to the pulmonary parenchyma or to other neighboring structures or (2) invasion of lymphatic vessels, with spread to local lymph nodes in the hilum or mediastinum. These tumors have a general tendency to remain within the thorax and to cause problems by intrathoracic complications rather than by distant metastasis. The overall prognosis in terms of 5-year survival is better for patients with squamous cell carcinoma than for patients with any of the other cell types.

SMALL CELL CARCINOMA

Small cell carcinoma, which comprises 14% of all lung cancers, previously was considered to have several subtypes, of which *oat cell carcinoma* was the most important. The most recent (1999) classification of lung cancer simplifies the classification and no longer includes oat cell carcinoma as a separate subtype. Like squamous cell carcinoma, small cell carcinomas generally originate within the bronchial wall, most commonly at a proximal level. The cell of origin of small cell carcinoma is disputed. An older theory proposed that these tumors arise from a neurosecretory type of epithelial cell termed the *Kulchitsky cell* or *K cell.* These cells have the capacity for polypeptide production and are considered a type of APUD cell (i.e., capable of *a*mine *p*recursor *u*ptake and *d*ecarboxylation). A more recent theory suggests that small cell carcinomas, like other lung cancers, have their origin from a pluripotent stem cell. The eventual cell type then depends on the pattern and degree of differentiation from this precursor cell. Molecular and chromosomal studies have shown that more than 90% of small cell carcinomas demonstrate deletions on the short arm of chromosome 3 (3p).

In small cell carcinoma, the malignant cells appear as small, darkly stained cells with sparse cytoplasm (Fig. 20-2). Local growth of the tumor often follows a submucosal pattern, but the tumor quickly invades lymphatics and submucosal blood vessels. Hilar and mediastinal nodes are involved and enlarged early in the course of the disease and frequently are the most prominent aspect of the radiographic presentation.

Because of rapid dissemination of small cell carcinoma, metastatic spread to distant sites is a common early complication. Distant disease, which may be clinically occult at the time of presentation, often affects the brain, liver, bone (and bone marrow), and adrenal glands. It is this propensity for early metastatic involvement that gives small cell carcinoma the worst prognosis among the four major categories of bronchogenic carcinoma.

Features of small cell carcinomas are the following:
1. Generally arise in proximal airways
2. Commonly produce polypeptide hormones
3. Hilar and mediastinal node involvement
4. Early, distant metastatic disease

ADENOCARCINOMA

Adenocarcinoma has surpassed squamous cell carcinoma as the most frequent cell type, accounting for approximately 37% of all lung tumors. Because the majority of adenocarcinomas occur in the periphery of the lung, it is much harder to relate their origin to the bronchial wall. At present, these tumors are believed to arise at the level of bronchioles or the alveolar walls. Adenocarcinomas sometimes appear at a site of parenchymal scarring that is either localized or part of a diffuse fibrotic process.

Adenocarcinoma is the most common type of lung cancer to develop among nonsmokers. Nearly 18% of lung adenocarcinomas are diagnosed in nonsmokers versus less than 2% of squamous cell carcinomas and less than 1% of small cell carcinomas. A link between human papillomavirus and adenocarcinoma of the lung has been hypothesized but is not definitively established.

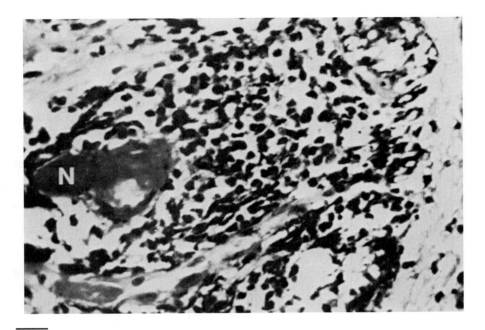

Figure 20-2. High-power photomicrograph of small cell carcinoma. Malignant cells have irregular, darkly stained nuclei and sparse cytoplasm. Note small area of necrosis *(N)* within tumor. (Courtesy Dr. Earl Kasdon.)

The characteristic appearance defining adenocarcinoma is the tendency to form glands and in many cases to produce mucus (Fig. 20-3). In the bronchioloalveolar subcategory of adenocarcinoma, the malignant cells seem to grow and spread along the preexisting alveolar walls, almost as though they were using the alveolar wall as scaffolding for their growth (Fig. 20-4).

The usual presenting pattern of adenocarcinoma is a peripheral lung nodule or mass. Occasionally, the tumors arise within a relatively large bronchus and therefore may be observed clinically because of complications of localized bronchial obstruction, as seen with squamous cell carcinoma. The bronchioloalveolar subcategory can manifest in several ways: as a nodule or mass lesion, as a localized infiltrate simulating a pneumonia, or as widespread parenchymal disease.

Although adenocarcinoma may spread locally to adjacent regions of lung or to pleura, it also has a propensity for nodal involvement (hilar and mediastinal) and for distant metastatic spread. Like small cell carcinoma, it spreads to liver, bone, central nervous system, and adrenal glands. In comparison with small cell carcinoma, however, adenocarcinoma is more likely to be localized at the time of presentation, particularly when it manifests as a solitary peripheral lung nodule. The overall prognosis for adenocarcinoma is not surprising given this behavior; its natural history and survival rates are intermediate between those of squamous cell and small cell carcinomas.

Features of adenocarcinomas are the following:
1. Often manifest as a solitary, peripheral pulmonary nodule
2. May arise in an old parenchymal scar
3. Generally localized when manifest as a peripheral lung nodule
4. Spread to hilar and mediastinal nodes and to distant sites

LARGE CELL CARCINOMA
Large cell carcinoma accounts for approximately 15% to 20% of all lung cancers. It is the most difficult carcinoma to define well because the tumors often are defined by the characteristics they lack, that is, the specific features that would otherwise classify them as one of the other three cell types.

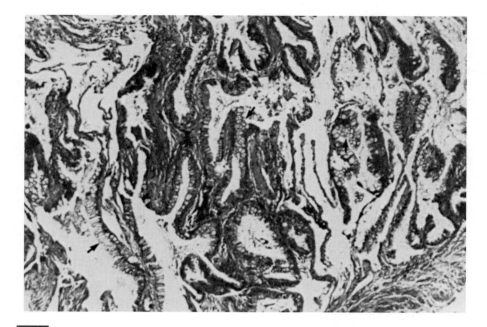

Figure 20-3. Low-power photomicrograph of adenocarcinoma of lung. Malignant cells form glandlike structures and produce mucus *(arrows)*. (Courtesy Dr. Earl Kasdon.)

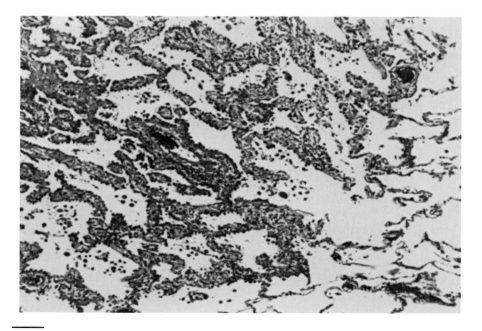

Figure 20-4. Low-power photomicrograph of bronchioloalveolar carcinoma. Tumor cells appear to be growing along preexisting alveolar walls. Lower right corner of photograph shows normal alveolar walls, which can be contrasted with areas of tumor. (Courtesy Dr. Earl Kasdon.)

The behavior of these tumors is relatively similar to that of adenocarcinoma. They often appear in the periphery of the lung as mass lesions, although they tend to be somewhat larger than adenocarcinomas. Their natural history is also similar to that of adenocarcinoma in terms of both propensity for spread and overall prognosis.

Table 21-1 (see Chapter 21) summarizes the distinguishing features of each cell type and reiterates many of the points discussed here.

REFERENCES

ETIOLOGY AND PATHOGENESIS

Alberg AJ, Ford JG, Samet JM: Epidemiology of lung cancer. ACCP evidence-based clinical practice guidelines, 2nd ed, *Chest* 132:29S–55S, 2007.

Denissenko MF, Pao A, Tang M, Pfeifer GP: Preferential formation of benzo[a]pyrene adducts at lung cancer mutational hotspots in p53, *Science* 274:430–432, 1996.

Dhala A, Pinsker K, Prezant DJ: Respiratory health consequences of environmental tobacco smoke, *Med Clin North Am* 88:1535–1552, 2004.

Field RW, Krewski D, Lubin JH, et al: An overview of the North American residential radon and lung cancer case-control studies, *J Toxicol Environ Health A* 69:599–631, 2006.

Goodman GE: Prevention of lung cancer, *Thorax* 57:994–999, 2002.

Miller YE: Pathogenesis of lung cancer. 100 year report, *Am J Respir Cell Mol Biol* 33:216–223, 2005.

Rom WN, Hay JG, Lee TC, Jiang Y, Tchou-Wong KM: Molecular and genetic aspects of lung cancer, *Am J Respir Crit Care Med* 161:1355–1367, 2000.

Sato M, Shames DS, Gazdar AF, Minna JD: A translational view of the molecular pathogenesis of lung cancer, *J Thorac Oncol* 2:327–343, 2007.

Spiro SG, Silvestri GA: One hundred years of lung cancer, *Am J Respir Crit Care Med* 172:523–529, 2005.

Subramanian J, Govindan R: Lung cancer in never smokers: a review, *J Clin Oncol* 25:561–570, 2007.

Whitesell PL, Drage CW: Occupational lung cancer, *Mayo Clin Proc* 68:183–188, 1993.

PATHOLOGY

Brambilla E, Travis WD, Colby TV, Corrin B, Shimosato Y: The new World Health Organization classification of lung tumors, *Eur Respir J* 18:1059–1068, 2001.

Franklin WA: Diagnosis of lung cancer: pathology of invasive and preinvasive neoplasia, *Chest* 117(suppl):80S–89S, 2000.

Müller K-M: Lung cancer: morphology, *Eur Respir Mon* 17:34–47, 2001.

Schwartz AM, Henson DE: Diagnostic surgical pathology in lung cancer. ACCP evidence-based clinical practice guidelines, 2nd ed, *Chest* 132:78S–93S, 2007.

Travis WD: Pathology of lung cancer, *Clin Chest Med* 23:65–81, 2002.

Verbeken EK, Brambilla E: WHO classification of lung and pleural tumours. The WHO/IASLC 1999 revision, *Eur Respir Rev* 12 (review 84):172–176, 2002.

21

Lung Cancer: Clinical Aspects

CLINICAL FEATURES	Functional Assessment
Symptoms Relating to Primary Lung Lesion	Diagnostic Screening for Lung Cancer
Symptoms Relating to Nodal and Distant Metastasis	**PRINCIPLES OF THERAPY**
	BRONCHIAL CARCINOID
Paraneoplastic Syndromes	**TUMORS**
DIAGNOSTIC APPROACH	**MALIGNANT MESOTHELIOMA**
Macroscopic Evaluation	**SOLITARY PULMONARY**
Microscopic Evaluation	**NODULE**

The goal of this chapter is to extend the discussion of lung cancer into the clinical realm and to relate how the pathologic processes considered in Chapter 20 are encountered in a clinical setting. An outline of the major clinical features of lung cancer is followed by a discussion of the diagnostic approach and general principles of management. The chapter concludes with a brief discussion of bronchial carcinoid tumors, malignant mesothelioma, and the clinical problem of the solitary pulmonary nodule.

CLINICAL FEATURES

Because lung cancer presumably starts with a single malignant cell, a long period of repetitive divisions and doubling of cell number must occur before the tumor becomes clinically apparent. During this preclinical period, an estimated 30 divisions take place before the tumor reaches a diameter of 1 cm. This process most likely requires a number of years, during which time the patient and the physician are unaware of the tumor.

In general, the possibility of lung cancer is raised because of findings on imaging studies (chest radiography or computed tomographic [CT] scan) or because of an assortment of symptoms that may ensue. This section focuses primarily on symptoms; imaging studies and diagnostic sampling are discussed in the section on diagnostic approach. The symptoms at the time of presentation may relate to the primary lung lesion, to metastatic disease (either in intrathoracic lymph nodes or at distant sites), or to what are commonly called "paraneoplastic syndromes."

Potential clinical problems with lung cancer are the following:

1. Symptoms of endobronchial tumor: cough, hemoptysis
2. Problems of bronchial obstruction: postobstructive pneumonia, dyspnea
3. Pleural involvement: chest pain, pleural effusion, dyspnea
4. Involvement of adjacent structures: heart, esophagus
5. Complications of mediastinal involvement: phrenic or recurrent laryngeal nerve paralysis, superior vena cava obstruction
6. Distant metastases: brain, bone or bone marrow, liver, adrenals
7. Ectopic hormone production: ACTH, ADH, parathyroid hormone-related peptide
8. Other paraneoplastic syndromes: neurologic, clubbing, hypertrophic osteoarthropathy
9. Nonspecific systemic effects: anorexia, weight loss

SYMPTOMS RELATING TO PRIMARY LUNG LESION

Perhaps the most common symptoms associated with lung cancer are cough and hemoptysis. Because bronchogenic carcinoma generally develops in smokers, these patients often dismiss their symptoms (particularly cough) as routine complications of smoking and chronic bronchitis. With tumors originating in large airways, such as squamous cell carcinoma or small cell carcinoma, patients may also have problems related to bronchial obstruction, such as pneumonia behind the obstruction or shortness of breath secondary to occlusion of a major bronchus. In contrast, with tumors that arise in the periphery of the lung, including many adenocarcinomas and large cell carcinomas, patients tend not to have symptoms related to bronchial involvement, and their lesions are often found on a chest radiograph obtained for unrelated purposes.

When tumors involve the pleural surface, either by direct extension or by metastatic spread, patients may have chest pain, often pleuritic in nature, or dyspnea resulting from substantial accumulation of pleural fluid. Other adjacent structures, particularly the heart and esophagus, can be involved by direct invasion or extrinsic compression by the tumor. Resulting complications include pericardial effusion, cardiac dysrhythmias, and dysphagia.

Tumors originating in the most apical portion of the lung, which are called *superior sulcus* or *Pancoast tumors*, often produce a characteristic constellation of symptoms and physical findings caused by direct extension to adjacent structures. Involvement of the nerves composing the brachial plexus can result in pain and weakness of the shoulder and arm. Involvement of the cervical sympathetic chain produces the typical features of Horner's syndrome—ptosis (drooping upper eyelid), miosis (constricted pupil), and anhidrosis (loss of sweat) over the forehead and face—all occurring on the same side as the lung mass. Invasion of neighboring bony structures (e.g., ribs and vertebrae) is a common complication.

SYMPTOMS RELATING TO NODAL AND DISTANT METASTASIS

When the mediastinum has metastatic lymph nodes from a primary lung cancer, symptoms often arise from invasion or compression of important structures within the mediastinum, such as the phrenic nerve, recurrent laryngeal nerve, and superior vena cava. As a consequence, the following conditions, respectively, may develop: diaphragmatic paralysis (often with accompanying dyspnea), vocal cord paralysis (with hoarseness), and superior vena cava obstruction (with edema of the face and upper extremities resulting from obstruction to venous return).

Distant metastases, most commonly to the brain, bone or bone marrow, liver, and adrenal gland(s), frequently are asymptomatic. In other cases, symptoms depend on the particular organ system involved. Small cell carcinoma is the cell type most likely to generate distant metastases (see Chapter 20). Squamous cell carcinoma is least likely, and both adenocarcinoma and large cell carcinoma occupy an intermediate position.

PARANEOPLASTIC SYNDROMES

Many lung tumors are capable of producing clinical syndromes that are not readily attributable to the space-occupying nature of the tumor or to direct invasion of other structures or organs. These syndromes are sometimes called the "paraneoplastic" manifestations of malignancy and frequently are due to production of a hormone or a hormonelike substance by the tumor. When a detectable hormone is produced by the lung tumor (or, for that matter, by any type of tumor), the patient is said to have "ectopic" hormone production. Sometimes clinical symptoms result from high circulating levels of the hormone; in other cases, only sensitive techniques of measurement are capable of demonstrating production of the hormone.

Why some tumors are capable of hormone production is not clear. It has been hypothesized that genetic information coding for the particular hormone is present but not expressed in the normal, nonmalignant cell. In the course of becoming malignant, the cell undergoes a process of gene dysregulation, during which it regains the ability to express this normally silent genetic material coding for hormone production.

The cell type most frequently associated with ectopic production of humoral substances is small cell carcinoma, presumably because of its similarity or relationship to a type of neuroendocrine cell in the airway (the Kulchitsky cell), with secretory granules and the potential for peptide synthesis. Adrenocorticotropic hormone (ACTH) and antidiuretic hormone (ADH) are the best described hormones produced by small cell carcinoma, potentially giving rise to the ectopic ACTH syndrome or to the syndrome of inappropriate ADH (SIADH), respectively. Squamous cell carcinoma is capable of causing hypercalcemia, which results from production of parathyroid hormone-related peptide, a peptide with parathyroid hormonelike activity. Production of other hormones, such as calcitonin and human chorionic gonadotropin, also are well described with bronchogenic carcinoma.

Some of the other paraneoplastic syndromes cannot be attributed to a known hormone, and our understanding of their mechanisms varies. Examples range from a wide variety of neurologic syndromes (some of which appear to be due to autoimmune antibody production) to the soft tissue and bony manifestations of clubbing and hypertrophic osteoarthropathy (see Chapter 3). The nonspecific systemic effects of malignancy, such as anorexia, weight loss, and fatigue, are potential consequences of lung cancer, and it has been hypothesized that production of various mediators, such as tumor necrosis factor, may mediate these systemic effects.

DIAGNOSTIC APPROACH

A wide variety of diagnostic methods are used in evaluating cases of known or suspected lung cancer. Some of these techniques also have been proposed for screening of asymptomatic individuals with risk factors for lung cancer, in an attempt to detect early, preclinical lesions. However, a beneficial effect of any method of lung cancer screening on mortality has not been objectively demonstrated.

Many of the studies assessing the lung on a macroscopic level aim to demonstrate the presence, location, and probability of spread of a bronchogenic carcinoma. Evaluation on a microscopic level is essential for defining the histologic type of lung cancer, which is an important factor in determining what modalities of therapy are most appropriate. Functional assessment of the patient with lung cancer plays a role primarily in quantitating the severity of underlying lung disease, particularly chronic obstructive lung disease resulting from prior heavy smoking. Knowledge of a patient's functional limitation from lung disease is essential before the clinician can decide whether operative removal of a lung cancer even is feasible without precipitating disabling respiratory insufficiency.

MACROSCOPIC EVALUATION

The initial test for detection and macroscopic evaluation of bronchogenic carcinoma is generally the chest radiograph. The presence of a nodule or mass within the lung on chest radiograph always raises the question of lung cancer, especially when the patient has a history of heavy smoking. The location of the lesion may give an indirect clue about its histology: peripheral lesions are more likely to be large cell carcinoma or adenocarcinoma, whereas central lesions are statistically more likely to be squamous cell carcinoma or small cell carcinoma (Figs. 21-1 and 21-2). The chest radiograph is

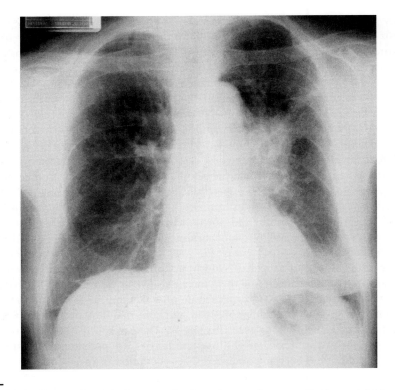

Figure 21-1. Chest radiograph shows small cell carcinoma of lung manifesting as left hilar mass.

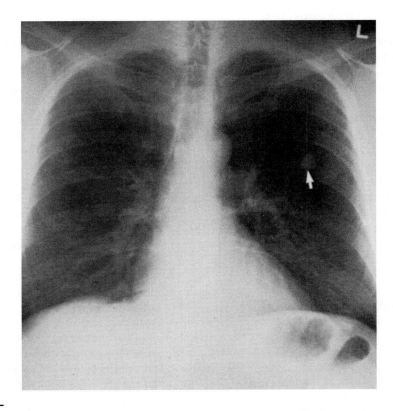

Figure 21-2. Chest radiograph shows adenocarcinoma of lung manifesting as solitary pulmonary nodule *(arrow).*

also useful for determining the presence of additional suspicious lesions, such as a second primary tumor or metastatic spread from the original carcinoma. Involvement of hilar or mediastinal nodes or the pleura (with resulting pleural effusion) may be detected on the chest radiograph, and such a finding will substantially affect the overall approach to therapy.

CT has become a standard part of the diagnostic evaluation of patients with lung cancer. Besides helping to define the location, extent, and spread of tumor within the chest, this technique has been particularly useful for the detection of enlarged, potentially malignant, lymph nodes within the mediastinum, which are often not seen with conventional radiography. However, even though CT effectively identifies enlarged mediastinal nodes, it cannot determine whether such nodes simply are hyperplastic or are enlarged because of tumor involvement. Consequently, histologic sampling of enlarged mediastinal nodes still is necessary to confirm tumor involvement of the nodes.

A relatively new technique that has gained increasing popularity in the evaluation of patients with known or suspected lung cancer is positron emission tomographic (PET) scanning (see Chapter 3). Because of their high metabolic activity, malignant lesions typically exhibit high uptake of the tracer ^{18}F-fluorodeoxyglucose (FDG). Focal uptake in the region of a parenchymal nodule or mass suggests that the lesion is malignant, and uptake in the mediastinum or at distant sites often reflects spread of the tumor to those sites. However, other metabolically active lesions, such as focal areas of infection, also may show FDG uptake. Thus, a positive PET scan in the appropriate clinical scenario is very suggestive but is not diagnostic of malignancy.

The best way to directly examine the airways of a patient with presumed or known bronchogenic carcinoma is by bronchoscopy with either a rigid or, much more frequently, a flexible bronchoscope (see Chapter 3). The location and intrabronchial extent of many tumors can be directly observed, and samples can be obtained from the lesion, either for cytologic or histopathologic examination. Diagnostic specimens can be obtained in many cases even when the lesion is beyond direct visualization with the bronchoscope. In addition, the bronchoscopist can assess whether an intrabronchial carcinoma is impinging significantly on the bronchial lumen and causing either partial or complete airway occlusion.

Staging of Lung Cancer

After a tumor has been documented, evaluation of the extent and spread of the malignancy often is formally achieved by staging. In the case of non–small cell carcinoma of the lung (i.e., all cell types other than small cell carcinoma), staging is based on (1) the primary intrathoracic tumor—its size, location, and local complications, such as direct extension to adjacent structures or obstruction of the airway lumen; (2) the presence or absence of tumor within hilar and mediastinal lymph nodes; and (3) the distant spread of tumor beyond the thorax to other tissues or organ systems. In the case of small cell carcinoma, the disease is classified as either limited (localized within one hemithorax) or extensive (beyond the limits of one hemithorax).

The first component of staging, taking into account characteristics of the primary tumor itself, is generally accomplished with a combination of chest radiography and bronchoscopy, sometimes with additional information obtained from CT.

The second component, based on involvement of mediastinal lymph nodes by tumor, often is initially assessed by CT, sometimes complemented by PET scanning. Definitive evaluation has generally been based on direct examination (and biopsy) of the nodes by either mediastinoscopy or mediastinotomy. In *suprasternal mediastinoscopy,* the mediastinum is visualized with a scope placed through an incision made just above the sternal notch. Biopsy specimens can be obtained by this technique if there is any suspicion that abnormal nodes are present. In *parasternal mediastinotomy,* the mediastinum is examined through a small incision made adjacent to the sternum, and samples of suspicious

Basis for staging of non–small cell lung cancer includes the following:
1. Size, location, and local complications of the primary tumor
2. Hilar and mediastinal lymph node involvement
3. Distant metastasis

nodes can be taken. In selected cases, *transbronchial needle aspiration* is an option for needle sampling of cellular material from lymph nodes adjacent to major airways. This technique, which is performed as part of flexible bronchoscopy, is especially useful for sampling nodes in the subcarinal region. The development of real-time ultrasound and CT guidance for transbronchoscopic needle aspiration is making this approach more useful for sampling lymph nodes in other areas of the thorax as well. Ultrasound-guided biopsy of certain mediastinal lymph nodes can be performed via an endoscope introduced into the esophagus rather than the tracheobronchial tree.

The third component involves determining whether the tumor has disseminated to distant sites. Spread of a lung tumor to other organs is often documented with either radioisotope or CT scanning. If available, a total body PET scan often will indicate sites of distant metastasis in the bones, liver, and adrenal glands. If a PET scan is not available, metastatic disease in bone can be well demonstrated with radioisotope bone scanning. CT is particularly suitable for detection of metastases to the liver, brain, and adrenal glands. Importantly, PET scanning is not very useful for assessing intracranial metastasis because brain tissue is so metabolically active at baseline that distinguishing between a metastasis and surrounding normal brain tissue is difficult. A CT scan or magnetic resonance imaging is best for detecting intracranial metastasis.

MICROSCOPIC EVALUATION

Evaluation of lung cancer on a microscopic level is crucial for establishing the specific cell type of the tumor. Some of the techniques used were mentioned briefly in Chapter 3. Specimens are obtained either for cytologic examination of abnormal cells shed from the tumor or for histologic examination of a biopsy specimen obtained directly from the lesion. Cytologic examination can be performed on sputum, on washings or brushings obtained through a bronchoscope, or on material aspirated from the tumor with a small-gauge needle. Biopsy material can be obtained by passing a biopsy forceps through a bronchoscope, by using a cutting needle passed through the chest wall directly into the tumor, or by directly sampling tissue at the time of a surgical procedure. The staining techniques for processing these materials are discussed in Chapter 3.

FUNCTIONAL ASSESSMENT

Functional assessment of the patient with lung cancer provides important information that can guide the clinician in the choice of treatment. As discussed in the section on principles of therapy, surgery usually is the procedure of choice if staging techniques have shown that the disease is limited and approachable surgically. However, when surgery is performed, usually a lobe and sometimes an entire lung must be removed. Because patients are generally smokers, they are at high risk for having significant underlying chronic obstructive pulmonary disease, and they may not tolerate removal of a substantial amount of lung tissue. Helpful studies for the clinician to use in evaluating patients are spirometry and sometimes other tests to determine exercise tolerance or the relative amount of function contributed by the area of lung to be removed. Further specification of guidelines precluding surgery is beyond the scope of this chapter but may be found in the references.

Assessment of pulmonary function helps to determine whether surgical resection can be tolerated by the functionally compromised patient.

DIAGNOSTIC SCREENING FOR LUNG CANCER

Given that the likelihood of "curing" lung cancer through surgical resection is greatest when the lesion has not yet metastasized to lymph nodes or distant sites, it seems logical that screening high-risk individuals for early, small lesions that have not yet caused symptoms would improve overall survival. Nevertheless, controlled studies of sputum cytology and chest radiography in a high-risk population of smokers have not been able to demonstrate improved mortality from lung cancer with use of these screening techniques. As a result and despite some methodologic problems with these studies, routine screening of high-risk current or former smokers by sputum cytology or chest radiography currently is not recommended.

More recently, low-dose fast helical chest CT has been shown to be more sensitive than chest radiography for detecting small lung cancers. However, whether screening with chest CT will improve mortality from lung cancer is unknown. In addition, such scans detect many benign lesions, which may result in unnecessary diagnostic procedures with some associated morbidity. At present, this important public health issue of screening for lung cancer has generated great interest as well as controversy, and it remains a subject of active investigation. The overall benefit of CT screening for lung cancer is expected to be defined by the National Lung Screening Trial, which has randomized approximately 50,000 current or former smokers to receive either chest CT scan or chest x-ray screening for 3 years. The trial is powered to detect a 20% reduction in lung cancer mortality related to differences in screening methods.

PRINCIPLES OF THERAPY

Although many advances in the treatment of a variety of malignancies have been made over the last three decades, patients with lung cancer have seen only a minor improvement in their prognosis during the same time. The 5-year survival of all patients with lung cancer is approximately 14%, certainly a dismal overall outlook.

The three major forms of treatment available for lung cancer are surgery, radiation therapy, and chemotherapy. During the past 10 to 15 years, somewhat more radical approaches have been used, particularly combination modalities of therapy. General guidelines for the clinician suggest when and how to use these modalities, but what therapy or combination of therapies will prove most beneficial for a given patient often is not known with certainty. Two primary factors appear to determine how a particular tumor should be treated: its staging (i.e., size, location, and extent of spread) and its cell type.

According to current practice for treatment of bronchogenic carcinoma, surgery is the treatment of choice for localized tumors. When the tumor has extended directly to the pleura (with malignant cells found in the pleural fluid) or to the adjacent mediastinum, the tumor usually is considered unresectable, and alternative therapy is used. Similarly, when contralateral mediastinal nodes are involved, the tumor is generally considered to have spread sufficiently so that it has become unresectable. At present, there is great interest in trying to determine the best modes of therapy for patients in whom the benefit of surgery is debatable, such as patients with ipsilateral mediastinal node involvement or chest wall involvement. Combining surgery with another modality, either chemotherapy or radiation therapy, has been a promising approach to this subcategory of patients. Finally, if metastases to distant tissues or organs have occurred, then surgery almost invariably is not an appropriate form of therapy.

The cell type is an important consideration in making decisions about management because small cell carcinoma has a high likelihood of having already metastasized by the time it is detected. Because of the early spread of small cell carcinoma, surgery is not considered the treatment of choice unless the particular small cell tumor is a solitary peripheral nodule without any evidence of mediastinal or distant spread. In the more usual presentation of small cell carcinoma as a central mass, unresectable disease is virtually ensured, and chemotherapy (with or without radiotherapy) is considered the primary mode of therapy.

When one of the non–small cell tumors is unresectable on the basis of any criteria, the clinician is faced with a choice of no treatment, radiotherapy, or chemotherapy. The final choice often is highly individual, depending not only on the particular tumor but also on the physician's and patient's preferences. In some cases, radiation therapy treatments are instituted early in an attempt to shrink the tumor and delay local complications. In other circumstances, therapy is withheld until a complication ensues, such as bleeding or airway obstruction. Radiation treatments then are given with the goal of palliation or tumor size reduction for temporary alleviation of the acute problem. Unfortunately, by definition palliation is not curative therapy, and further problems with the tumor are certain to develop.

Other palliative forms of therapy are being used to establish patency of an airway that has been partially or completely occluded or compressed by tumor. The treatment typically is accomplished with either flexible or rigid bronchoscopy, using techniques such as laser, argon plasma coagulation, photodynamic therapy, cryotherapy, or electrocautery to diminish the size of the endobronchial tumor and reestablish an effective lumen. Alternatively or as a combined approach used in addition to the above techniques, an endobronchial stent (i.e., a hollow and relatively rigid plastic or metal sheath) can be positioned within the airway lumen to maintain airway patency.

The overall 5-year survival in patients with carcinoma of the lung is less than 15%. Patients who survive had localized disease at presentation and were amenable to surgical therapy. In this latter group, 5-year survival approaches 50%.

Table 21-1 summarizes many of the specific features of lung cancer discussed in this chapter and in Chapter 20. Each of the major cell types is considered separately, with emphasis on clinical, radiographic, and therapeutic aspects of each category of tumor.

BRONCHIAL CARCINOID TUMORS

Bronchial carcinoid tumors have often been called *bronchial adenomas* because they were thought to represent a benign or adenomatous form of neoplasm involving the bronchial tree. In fact, although many patients with these tumors have an excellent prognosis and are cured by surgical removal, it is more accurate to view these tumors as low-grade malignancies, and they are currently classified as such. They constitute approximately 5% of primary lung tumors.

Bronchial carcinoid tumors arise most commonly in relatively central airways of the tracheobronchial tree. Although the cell of origin is not known with certainty, these tumors have been postulated to arise from the neurosecretory Kulchitsky cells (K cells). Alternatively, they may arise from undifferentiated stem cells within the airway wall. Bronchial carcinoid tumors also have been suggested to represent a more benign variant of small cell carcinoma, which some pathologists consider to arise also from K cells. In some carcinoid tumors, the histology has atypical features more suggestive of frank malignancy; these tumors have a poorer overall prognosis than those without such features.

Two important epidemiologic features distinguish bronchial carcinoid tumors from the other pulmonary neoplasms discussed here. First, smoking does not appear to be a risk factor. Second, as a group, patients with bronchial carcinoid tumors are younger than those with other pulmonary malignancies; frequently, young adults are affected.

Bronchial carcinoid tumors are often discovered on either an abnormal chest radiograph or during episodes of hemoptysis or pneumonia distal to an obstructing airway tumor. Ectopic hormone production may be found, probably relating to the presumed neurosecretory origin of the neoplastic cells. The carcinoid syndrome, generally involving episodic flushing, diarrhea, and wheezing that results from the effects of serotonin produced by the tumor, is uncommon, being found in less than 5% of all cases of bronchial carcinoid tumors.

Treatment of these tumors is surgical resection if at all possible. For many patients the prognosis is excellent, and recurrent or distant disease does not occur after surgical removal. However, metastatic disease is found more commonly in patients whose tumors have atypical histology, and the prognosis is worse for these patients.

Common features of bronchial carcinoid tumors are the following:
1. Often found in young adults
2. Hemoptysis
3. Pneumonia distal to an obstructing endobronchial mass

Table 21-1

LUNG CANCER: COMPARATIVE FEATURES

Cell Type	Frequency (%)[a]	Location[b]	Radiographic Appearance[c]	Spread	Treatment	Relative Prognosis[d]	Miscellaneous
Squamous cell	30–35	Proximal, endobronchial	1. Central mass 2. Obstructive atelectasis 3. Postobstructive pneumonia	Contiguous intrathoracic spread; nodal metastasis	Surgery, combined modality therapy, or palliative therapy	Best	Hypercalcemia (occasional)
Small cell (including oat cell)	20	Proximal, endobronchial (submucosal)	1. Central mass 2. Hilar, mediastinal adenopathy	Hilar, mediastinal nodes; distant metastasis	Chemotherapy (± radiation therapy)	Worst	Ectopic hormone production (ADH, ACTH) relatively common
Adenocarcinoma (including bronchoalveolar cell)	35	Peripheral	Solitary peripheral nodule or mass	Contiguous intrathoracic spread; nodal and distant metastasis	Surgery, combined modality therapy, or palliative therapy	Intermediate	
Large cell	15–20	Variable	Variable; often large peripheral mass	Contiguous intrathoracic spread; nodal and distant metastasis	Surgery, combined modality therapy, or palliative therapy	Intermediate	

[a]Approximate percent of all lung cancers.
[b]Most common location; for all cell types, variable locations are seen.
[c]Common presentations on chest radiograph.
[d]For all cell types, the overall prognosis is generally poor.
ACTH = Adrenocorticotropic hormone; ADH = antidiuretic hormone.

MALIGNANT MESOTHELIOMA

Unlike the other tumors discussed, *malignant mesothelioma* primarily involves the pleura rather than the airways or the pulmonary parenchyma. Like bronchial carcinoid tumors, smoking is not a risk factor. Malignant mesothelioma is relatively uncommon but is important at least partially because in many of the cases a specific etiologic factor can be identified.

The primary risk factor for development of malignant mesothelioma is a history of exposure to asbestos, generally in the range of 30 to 40 years earlier. Individuals who have worked in the types of jobs that expose them to asbestos (see Chapter 20) are the persons at highest risk, but a heavy exposure is not necessary for predisposing a person to malignant mesothelioma. In fact, mesothelioma develops even in spouses of asbestos workers, presumably because of inhalation of asbestos dust while exposed to their partners' clothes.

In patients with malignant mesothelioma, the main symptoms are chest pain, dyspnea, and possibly cough. The chest radiograph usually is most notable for the presence of pleural fluid and often irregular or lobulated thickening of the pleura (Fig. 21-3). Diagnosis requires biopsy of the pleura and histologic demonstration of the malignancy. Because the tumor originates in the pleura and does not directly communicate with airways, malignant cells are not shed into the tracheobronchial tree and cannot be found on cytologic examination of sputum or bronchoscopy specimens.

The prognosis for malignant mesothelioma is poor. The tumor eventually entraps the lung and spreads to mediastinal structures. Death generally results from respiratory failure. No clearly effective form of therapy is available, and fewer than 10% of patients survive 3 years. A radical surgical approach, extrapleural pneumonectomy, has been used in conjunction with chemotherapy and/or radiotherapy. This procedure involves removal of the entire ipsilateral lung along with both the visceral and parietal pleura. Alternatively, obliteration of the pleural space (pleurodesis) with a sclerosing

> Mesothelioma is suggested by pleural fluid, irregular or lobulated pleural thickening, and a distant history of asbestos exposure.

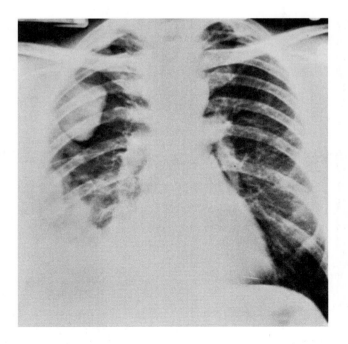

Figure 21-3. Chest radiograph of patient with mesothelioma. Note several lobulated, pleural-based masses in right hemithorax accompanied by right pleural effusion.

agent can be performed in an attempt to prevent reaccumulation of large amounts of pleural fluid. Because of the poor prognosis, mesothelioma has become a target for a variety of new types of investigational therapy, including immunotherapy, use of biologic response modifiers (e.g., interferons and interleukin-2), and gene therapy.

SOLITARY PULMONARY NODULE

Although the solitary pulmonary nodule on chest radiograph (defined as a single, rounded lesion 3 cm or less in diameter) is a common presentation of lung cancer, there is actually a broad differential diagnosis for this radiographic abnormality. The physician is faced with judging the likelihood that a nodule is malignant and choosing the appropriate pathway for diagnosis and management. Because lung cancer that manifests as a pulmonary nodule may be curable by surgical resection, management of such a lesion should not be neglected until the lesion is no longer curable. On the other hand, to subject a patient to thoracotomy, which is a major surgical procedure, for removal of a benign lesion requiring no therapy is likewise undesirable.

The diagnostic possibilities for the solitary pulmonary nodule are listed in Table 21-2. Besides primary lung cancer, the major alternative diagnoses are benign pulmonary neoplasms, solitary metastases to the lung from a distant primary carcinoma, and infections (especially healed granulomatous lesions from tuberculosis or fungal disease). Estimating the likelihood of a malignant versus a benign lesion from its radiographic appearance is based on three major factors:

1. *Growth.* Perhaps the most helpful piece of information a physician can have is a prior chest radiograph. Comparison of old and new films shows whether a lesion is stable and gives an approximation of the rate of growth. Although it is difficult to say with certainty whether a lesion is benign or malignant based on the rate of growth, the absence of any increase in size for at least 2 years is an extremely good (but not infallible) indication that a lesion is benign.

2. *Calcification.* The presence of calcification within a pulmonary nodule, best demonstrated on CT scan, may favor the diagnosis of a benign lesion, especially a granuloma or hamartoma. If certain patterns of calcification are found—diffuse speckling, dense calcification, laminated (onion-skin) calcification, or "popcorn" calcification—then the lesion almost assuredly is benign. On the other hand, calcification at the periphery of a lesion or amorphous calcification within the lesion may be suggestive of malignancy. For example, a peripheral area of calcification

> Criteria for assessing the likelihood that a solitary pulmonary nodule is malignant are the following:
> 1. Stability or change in size of the lesion
> 2. Presence or absence of calcification; pattern of calcification
> 3. Smooth versus irregular appearance of the border

Table	21-2

DIFFERENTIAL DIAGNOSIS OF THE SOLITARY PULMONARY NODULE

Neoplasms	**Infection**
Malignant	Infectious granuloma
Primary lung cancer	Tuberculosis ("tuberculoma")
Solitary pulmonary metastasis	Histoplasmosis ("histoplasmoma")
from distant carcinoma	
Bronchial carcinoid (bronchial adenoma)	Bacterial abscess
	Miscellaneous (e.g., hydatid cyst, canine
Benign	heartworm)
Hamartoma	
Miscellaneous (e.g., fibroma, lipoma)	**Miscellaneous**
	Rounded atelectasis
Vascular Abnormality	Hematoma
Arteriovenous malformation	Pseudotumor (fluid loculated in a fissure)

is entirely consistent with a scar carcinoma arising in the region of an old, calcified parenchymal scar (e.g., an old calcified granuloma).

3. *Border Appearance.* An irregular or spiculated margin is suggestive of a malignant lesion, whereas a benign lesion commonly has a smooth and discrete border.

Additional clinical features may be more suggestive of a benign versus a malignant lesion but are somewhat less reliable. In individuals younger than 35 years, primary lung cancer is an unlikely but certainly not impossible diagnosis. A history of heavy smoking (and/or exposure to asbestos) indicates a high risk for a malignant lesion; however, the absence of a smoking history does not rule out the diagnosis of lung cancer, particularly a peripheral adenocarcinoma. The size of a lesion may be helpful because those larger than 3 cm in diameter (usually called masses rather than nodules when they exceed 3 cm) are much more likely to be malignant than are nodules less than 2 cm in diameter. Finally, the presence of a previously diagnosed distant carcinoma obviously raises the possibility that a lung nodule is a metastatic focus of tumor.

The practical question of how to evaluate and manage these cases often is difficult, and the decision-making process must be individualized for each patient. A simple noninvasive test such as sputum cytologic examination is most helpful if results are positive; however, the yield is low, even with peripheral nodules that eventually are proven to be carcinoma. Unless the lesion has been stable on chest radiograph for more than 2 years, chest CT scanning is performed routinely to look at border characteristics, assess the presence and pattern of calcification, and identify other abnormalities, especially lymph nodes within the mediastinum. PET scanning (see Chapter 3), when available, is being performed increasingly when the diagnosis is uncertain after evaluation of the clinical information and other imaging studies. Uptake of labeled FDG suggests that the lesion has high metabolic activity and could be malignant, whereas lack of uptake suggests a metabolically inactive, benign lesion.

More invasive procedures, such as percutaneous needle aspiration or biopsy and transbronchial biopsy (through a flexible bronchoscope), may be used in an attempt to make a histologic diagnosis. However, in many cases biopsy findings that are negative for malignancy do not obviate the need for surgery because malignant cells may be missed by the limited sampling of a needle or biopsy forceps. Hence, a commonly used approach with a lesion suspicious for carcinoma is to proceed directly with resection, assuming no contraindications to surgery and no clinical evidence that the lesion has spread elsewhere or has metastasized from a distant primary malignancy. With the increasing availability since the early 1990s of video-assisted thoracic surgery using a thoracoscope, this procedure is commonly used as a less invasive means of removing and therefore diagnosing small, peripheral lung nodules. A more definitive resection, such as a lobectomy performed by thoracotomy, then is performed if the nodule is found to be malignant.

When lung cancer manifests as a solitary peripheral nodule, the prognosis is much better than for the general group of patients with lung cancer. As a result of frequently curative surgical resection, more than 50% of patients with an initial solitary peripheral lung cancer survive 5 years, compared with less than 15% of all lung cancer patients.

REFERENCES

LUNG CANCER: GENERAL REVIEWS AND CLINICAL ASPECTS

American College of Chest Physicians: Diagnosis and management of lung cancer: ACCP evidence-based clinical practice guidelines, 2nd ed, *Chest* 132(suppl):1S–422S, 2007.

Ginsberg MS, Grewal RK, Heelan RT: Lung cancer, *Radiol Clin North Am* 45:21–43, 2007.

Matthay RM, editor: Lung cancer, *Clin Chest Med* 23:1–277, 2002.

Spiro SG, editor: Lung cancer, *Eur Respir Mon* 17:1–329, 2001.

Spiro SG, Silvestri GA: One hundred years of lung cancer, *Am J Respir Crit Care Med* 172: 523–529, 2005.

LUNG CANCER: DIAGNOSTIC APPROACHES

Alberts WM: Diagnosis and management of lung cancer executive summary: ACCP evidence-based clinical practice guidelines, 2nd ed, *Chest* 132: 1S–19S, 2007.

Bach PB, Silvestri GA, Hanger M, Jett JR: Screening for lung cancer: ACCP evidence-based clinical practice guidelines, 2nd ed, *Chest* 132: 69S–77S, 2007.

Birim O, Kappetein AP, Stijnen T, Bogers AJ: Meta-analysis of positron emission tomographic and computed tomographic imaging in detecting mediastinal lymph node metastases in nonsmall cell lung cancer, *Ann Thorac Surg* 79:375–382, 2005.

Boiselle PM, Ernst A, Karp DD: Lung cancer detection in the 21st century: potential contributions and challenges of emerging technologies, *AJR Am J Roentgenol* 175:1215–1221, 2000.

Hollings N, Shaw P: Diagnostic imaging of lung cancer, *Eur Respir J* 19:722–742, 2002.

Hyer JD, Silvestri G: Diagnosis and staging of lung cancer, *Clin Chest Med* 21:95–106, 2000.

Mulshine JL, Sullivan DC: Clinical practice. Lung cancer screening, *N Engl J Med* 352:2714–2720, 2005.

Petty TL: The early diagnosis of lung cancer, *Dis Mon* 47:204–264, 2001.

Pieterman RM, van Putten JW, Meuzelaar JJ, et al: Preoperative staging of non-small-cell lung cancer with positron-emission tomography, *N Engl J Med* 343:254–261, 2000.

Silvestri GA, Gould MK, Margolis ML, et al: Noninvasive staging of small cell lung cancer: ACCP evidence-based clinical practice guidelines, 2nd ed, *Chest* 132: 178S–201S, 2007.

LUNG CANCER: TREATMENT

Ernst A, Feller-Kopman D, Becker HD, Mehta AC: Central airway obstruction, *Am J Respir Crit Care Med* 169:1278–1297, 2004.

Krupnick AS, Kreisel D, Hope A, Bradley J, Govindan R, Meyers B: Recent advances and future perspectives in the management of lung cancer, *Curr Probl Surg* 42:540–610, 2005.

Mazzone PJ, Arroliga AC: Lung cancer: preoperative pulmonary evaluation of the lung resection candidate, *Am J Med* 118:578–583, 2005.

Spira A, Ettinger DS: Multidisciplinary management of lung cancer, *N Engl J Med* 350:379–392, 2004.

Spiro SG, Porter JC: Lung cancer—where are we today? Current advances in staging and nonsurgical treatment, *Am J Respir Crit Care Med* 166:1166–1196, 2002.

Visbal AL, Leighl NB, Feld R, Shepherd FA: Adjuvant chemotherapy for early-stage non-small cell lung cancer, *Chest* 128:2933–2943, 2005.

BRONCHIAL CARCINOIDS

Fink G, Krelbaum T, Yellin A, et al: Pulmonary carcinoid: presentation, diagnosis, and outcome in 142 cases in Israel and review of 640 cases from the literature, *Chest* 119:1647–1651, 2001.

Hasleton PS: Histopathology and prognostic factors in bronchial carcinoid tumors, *Thorax* 49:S56–S62, 1994.

Kulke MH, Mayer RJ: Carcinoid tumors, *N Engl J Med* 340:858–868, 1999.

MALIGNANT MESOTHELIOMA

Boutin C, Schlesser M, Frenay C, Astoul PH: Malignant pleural mesothelioma, *Eur Respir J* 12:972–981, 1998.

British Thoracic Society Standards of Care Committee: Statement on malignant mesothelioma in the United Kingdom, *Thorax* 56:250–265, 2001.

Robinson BW, Lake RA: Advances in malignant mesothelioma, *N Engl J Med* 353:1591–1603, 2005.

Robinson BW, Musk AW, Lake RA: Malignant mesothelioma, *Lancet* 366:397–408, 2005.

SOLITARY PULMONARY NODULE

Jeong YJ, Yi CA, Lee KS: Solitary pulmonary nodules: detection, characterization, and guidance for further diagnostic workup and treatment, *AJR Am J Roentgenol* 188:57–68, 2007.

Ost D, Fein AM, Feinsilver SH: Clinical practice. The solitary pulmonary nodule, *N Engl J Med* 348:2535–2542, 2003.

Swensen SJ, Silverstein MD, Ilstrup DM, Schleck CD, Edell ES: The probability of malignancy in solitary pulmonary nodules, *Arch Intern Med* 157:849–855, 1997.

Winer-Muram HT: The solitary pulmonary nodule, *Radiology* 239:34–49, 2006.

22

Lung Defense Mechanisms

PHYSICAL OR ANATOMIC
  FACTORS
ANTIMICROBIAL PEPTIDES
PHAGOCYTIC AND
  INFLAMMATORY CELLS
  Pulmonary Alveolar
    Macrophages
  Dendritic Cells
  Polymorphonuclear
    Leukocytes
  Natural Killer Cells
ADAPTIVE IMMUNE
  RESPONSES
  Humoral Immune Mechanisms
  Cellular Immune Mechanisms

FAILURE OF RESPIRATORY
  DEFENSE MECHANISMS
  Impairment of Physical Clearance
  Impairment of Antimicrobial
    Peptides
  Impairment of Phagocytic
    and Inflammatory Cells
  Defects in the Adaptive Immune
    System
IMMUNOSUPPRESSED PATIENT
  WITH PULMONARY
  INFILTRATES
AUGMENTATION OF
  RESPIRATORY DEFENSE
  MECHANISMS

In the process of exchanging thousands of liters of air each day for O_2 uptake and CO_2 elimination, the lung is exposed to a multitude of foreign substances transported with the inhaled air. Some of these are potentially injurious; others are relatively harmless. Inhaled air is not the only source of foreign material. Secretions from the mouth and pharynx frequently are aspirated into the tracheobronchial tree, especially during sleep, even in healthy individuals. This myriad of foreign substances is perhaps best classified into three major categories: small particulate material, noxious gases, and microorganisms. Because the oropharynx is rich with bacteria, aspirated secretions are particularly important as a source of unwanted bacteria entering the airways.

To protect itself against potentially toxic inhaled material, the respiratory system has evolved complex protective mechanisms that can be dissected into different components. Each component appears to have a distinct role, but a tremendous degree of redundancy and interaction exists among different components. That the distal lung parenchyma is normally sterile (and is not in a state of constant inflammation) serves as testimony to the effectiveness of the defense system. However, the protective mechanisms can break down, resulting in respiratory infection. Such a breakdown in defense can occur as a result of certain diseases, a large inoculum of microorganisms that overwhelms a normal host, an especially virulent organism, or frequently as a consequence of medical treatment that impairs the immune system.

Before the discussion of infectious disorders of the respiratory system in Chapters 23, 24, and 25 it is appropriate to first consider how the lung protects itself against the infectious agents to which it is exposed. Although this chapter focuses on protective mechanisms against infection, defenses against noninfectious substances, especially inhaled particulate material, also are addressed. The major categories of defense mechanisms to be discussed include (1) physical or anatomic factors relating to deposition and clearance of inhaled material, (2) antimicrobial peptides, (3) phagocytic and inflammatory cells that interact with the inhaled material, and (4) adaptive immune responses, which depend on prior exposure to, and recognition of, the foreign material. The chapter concentrates on the aspects of the host defense system that are specific to the lung and then proceeds with a discussion of several ways that the system breaks down, resulting in an inability to handle microorganisms and an increased risk for certain types of respiratory tract infection. The chapter concludes by briefly considering how we can activate or augment specific immune responses through vaccination, thus enhancing our defenses against selected respiratory pathogens.

PHYSICAL OR ANATOMIC FACTORS

The pathway from the mouth or nose down to the lung parenchyma requires that inhaled air traverse a series of progressively branching airways. The laminar flow of air through the airways is disrupted at the branch points (subcarinae), thus enhancing deposition of particulate material at these locations. Hence, inhaled particulates frequently are deposited at various points in the airway, never reaching the most distal region of lung, the alveolar spaces. Particle size is an important determinant of deposition along the airway and thus affects the likelihood of a particle's reaching the distal parenchyma. When an inhaled particle is greater than 10 μm in diameter, it is likely to settle high in the upper airway, for example, in the nose. For particles 5 to 10 μm in diameter, settling tends to occur somewhat lower, in the trachea or the conducting airways but not down to the level of the small airways and alveoli. The particles most likely to reach the distal lung parenchyma range in size from 0.5 to 5 μm. Many bacteria fall within this size range, so deposition along the airways is not very effective for excluding bacteria from the lower respiratory tract. However, large particles of dust and other inhaled material are effectively excluded from the distal lung parenchyma by virtue of their size. Of note, the target size for particles of inhaled medications is less than 5 μm so that the medication can bypass the conducting airways and reach the more distal lung.

When particles are deposited in the trachea or bronchi, two major processes, cough and mucociliary transport, are responsible for physical removal of these particles from the airways. Cough is an important protective mechanism, frequently triggered by stimulation of airway irritant receptors, which are most prominent in the proximal airways and are activated by inhaled or aspirated foreign material. Rapid acceleration and high flow rates of air achieved by a cough often are effective in clearing irritating foreign material from the airways.

The term *mucociliary transport* or *mucociliary clearance* refers to a process of waves of beating cilia moving a blanket of mucus (and any material trapped within the mucus) progressively upward along the tracheobronchial tree. From the trachea down to the respiratory bronchioles, the most superficial layer of epithelial cells lining the airway has cilia projecting into the airway lumen. These cilia have a structure identical to that of cilia found elsewhere in the body, consisting of longitudinal microtubules with a characteristic architecture. Specifically, a cross-sectional view of cilia shows two central microtubules surrounded by nine pairs of microtubules arranged around the periphery (Fig. 22-1). Small, projecting sidearms from each doublet, called *dynein arms,* are crucial to the contractile function of the microtubules and hence to the beating of the cilia.

Strikingly, the movement of cilia on a particular cell and the movement between cells are quite coordinated, producing actual "waves" of ciliary motion. How such a pattern of ciliary motion is coordinated from cell to cell or even within the same cell

Factors affecting deposition and physical clearance of particles are the following:
1. Particle size
2. Cough
3. Mucociliary transport

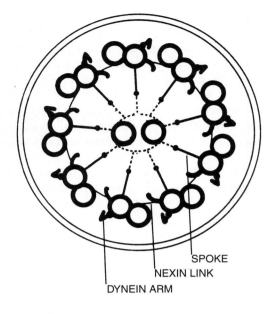

Figure 22-1. Schematic diagram of cross-section of cilium. Two central microtubules and nine pairs of peripheral microtubules are shown. Dynein arm projects from each peripheral doublet, and nexin links and radial spokes provide connections within microtubular structure. (From Eliasson R, Mossberg B, Camner P, Afzelius BA: *N Engl J Med* 297:1–6, 1977. Copyright 1977 Massachusetts Medical Society. All rights reserved.)

is not known. What this wavelike motion accomplishes is movement of the overlying mucous layer in a cephalad direction (i.e., from distal to more proximal parts of the tracheobronchial tree), at an estimated speed of 6 to 20 mm/min in the trachea. If inhaled particles are trapped in the mucous layer, they too are transported upward and eventually are either expectorated or swallowed.

Two layers compose the mucous blanket bathing the epithelial cells. Directly adjacent to the cells is the *sol layer*, within which the cilia are located. The aqueous sol layer contains a number of molecules in solution that are part of the innate immune system (discussed in antimicrobial peptides section). Superficial to the sol layer is the more viscous *gel layer*, which is produced by both submucosal mucous glands and goblet cells. Picture the viscous gel layer floating on top of the sol layer and being propelled upward as the cilia are able to beat more freely within the less viscous sol layer.

ANTIMICROBIAL PEPTIDES

The sol layer contains a number of substances that are important in innate immunity. The innate immune system can be thought of as a fast-acting system that is ready to quickly protect the lungs and ideally to prevent activation of the adaptive immune system (discussed in adaptive immune responses section). In addition to mucociliary clearance, the innate immune system is composed of small molecules, proteins, and cells that are able to respond to inhaled particles in a way that does not require any previous exposure to the particle. These molecules are generally highly conserved in evolution and are present in many invertebrate species as well as in humans. They are able to immediately interact with microorganisms through recognition of conserved structures on the microbes, and they can act directly to kill the invader and stimulate a further host immune response. They provide a fast, energy-efficient, effective front-line defense, with broad overlap in actions. There are many components of innate immunity in the lung, and a full description is beyond the scope of this chapter. The interested reader is referred to the in-depth reviews listed in the references. In order for the reader to get a sense of this system, this chapter focuses on a few of the best described of these molecules: lysozyme, lactoferrin, defensins, and collectins (surfactant protein A [SP-A] and surfactant protein D [SP-D]).

Lysozyme is present throughout the respiratory tract but is most prominent in the proximal airways. It is synthesized by respiratory epithelial cells, serous glandular cells, and macrophages. As the name implies, lysozyme causes bacterial cell death by inducing lysis. It is most active against gram-positive organisms. Decreased levels of lysozyme have been correlated with increased susceptibility to acute bronchitis.

Lactoferrin is present in airway fluid. It is produced by serous cells and neutrophils. Lactoferrin acts to agglutinate and kill bacteria, to enhance neutrophil adherence, and to prime neutrophil superoxide production. Its name derives from the fact that lactoferrin also functions to block iron from bacterial metabolism. Lactoferrin binds to bacteria through recognition of highly conserved carbohydrate moieties on the microbial cell surface.

Defensins are a family of small proteins with intrinsic antimicrobial activity that are found in the lung and on other mucosal surfaces, including the gastrointestinal and reproductive tracts. The two most important types of defensins in the lung are α-defensins and β-defensins. α-Defensins are synthesized by resident neutrophils; β-defensins are made by respiratory epithelial cells. Defensins have broad antimicrobial activity against both gram-positive and gram-negative organisms. They act by making the microbial cell wall permeable, thus causing release of microbial cell contents and destruction of the membrane potential. Defensins are highly sensitive to salt concentrations, and they are inactivated in the abnormal milieu in the lungs of patients with cystic fibrosis.

SP-A and SP-D are members of the collectin family of proteins. They function by binding and aggregating microbes and by facilitating interaction with other immune cells. They also appear to be important in regulation of pulmonary macrophage activity. Animal models indicate that defects in either of these proteins increase the susceptibility to respiratory infection; however, human disease related to a genetic mutation or deletion has not been identified.

Respiratory immunoglobulin A (IgA) can be considered part of the innate immune system because it is also constitutively produced by the respiratory epithelium and does not require prior exposure. IgA is further discussed in the section on humoral immune mechanisms.

Airway innate immunity substances are the following:
1. Lysozyme
2. Lactoferrin
3. Defensins
4. Collectins (surfactant proteins A and D)
5. IgA

PHAGOCYTIC AND INFLAMMATORY CELLS

PULMONARY ALVEOLAR MACROPHAGES

In the airways and at the level of the alveoli, particles and bacteria can be scavenged by mononuclear phagocytic cells called *pulmonary alveolar macrophages*. These cells constitute a major form of defense against material that has escaped deposition in the upper airway and has reached the intrathoracic airways or the alveolar structures.

Pulmonary alveolar macrophages are large, mobile cells approximately 15 to 50 μm in diameter. They are descendants of circulating monocytes derived from the bone marrow. These cells adhere to the alveolar epithelium. Their cytoplasm contains a variety of granules of various shapes and sizes, many of which are packages of digestive enzymes that can dispose of ingested foreign material. Alveolar macrophages have a major role in killing microorganisms that have reached the lower respiratory tract. They also release chemoattractant cytokines (chemokines) that recruit other inflammatory cells.

When an alveolar macrophage is exposed to inhaled particles or bacteria, attachment of the foreign material to the surface of the macrophage is the first step in the processing sequence. The particles or bacteria are engulfed within the plasma membrane, which invaginates and pinches off within the cell to form a cytoplasmic phagosome containing the now isolated foreign material. In some circumstances, this sequence of attachment and phagocytosis is facilitated by opsonins, which coat the foreign material. Opsonins are proteins that bind to extracellular materials and make them more adherent to phagocytic cells and more amenable to engulfment or ingestion. Opsonins can be specific for the particular foreign substance, such as antibodies directed against antigenic material, or they may demonstrate nonspecific binding to a variety of substances. Particularly important specific opsonins are antibodies of the IgG class directed against antigenic foreign material, either bacteria or other antigenic particles. Nonspecific opsonins in the lung include secretory IgA, complement, and fibronectin. All these opsonins greatly promote attachment to and ingestion by macrophages.

After bacteria or other foreign material is isolated within phagosomes, a process of intracellular digestion occurs within the macrophage. Often the phagosomes combine with lysosomes to form phagolysosomes, in which proteolytic enzymes supplied by the lysosome digest, detoxify, or destroy the phagosomal contents. In addition to lysosomal enzymes, a variety of oxidation products, such as hydrogen peroxide and other intermediate products of oxidative metabolism, are toxic to bacteria and may play a role in the ability of the macrophage to kill ingested microorganisms.

After they are activated, the resident pulmonary macrophages participate in orchestrating further immune responses. Macrophages release inflammatory mediators, such as tumor necrosis factor-α and interleukin-1β, as well as other cytokines and chemokines that are active in recruiting additional inflammatory cells.

The macrophage does not always kill or totally eliminate inhaled foreign material to which it is exposed. In some cases, such as with inhaled silica particles, the ingested material is toxic to the macrophage and eventually may kill the cell. In other cases, ingested material is inert but essentially indigestible and may persist indefinitely in the form of an indigestible residue. Organisms that are especially capable of persistent infection of macrophages without being killed or deactivated include *Mycobacterium tuberculosis* and the human immunodeficiency virus (HIV).

An increasingly appreciated role of the alveolar macrophage is to *suppress* inflammation in the lung. The lung is unique in that it is constantly exposed to inhaled foreign substances but at the same time must maintain an exquisitely delicate gas-exchange apparatus. Even a small amount of inflammation within the alveolar wall would have a negative effect on gas exchange, and a fine balance keeps the distal airways sterile but not in a state of constant, harmful inflammation. Alveolar macrophages are able to process a large amount of inhaled substances without inciting an immune response external to the macrophage itself. It is estimated that the normal pool of alveolar macrophages can handle up to 10^9 inhaled bacteria before the bacteria overwhelm the macrophages and cause infection in the alveoli. In addition, alveolar macrophages, through complex signaling mechanisms, function to keep dendritic cell and T-cell activation in check. The detailed working of this fine equilibrium between inflammation and quiescence in the lung is an area of active research.

Major phagocytic and resident inflammatory cells are the following:
1. Dendritic cells (airway and parenchymal)
2. Pulmonary alveolar macrophages
3. Polymorphonuclear leukocytes
4. Natural killer lymphocytes

DENDRITIC CELLS

Dendritic cells are present throughout the body in various forms. They are bone marrow–derived cells that, in the lung, are located in the airway epithelium as well as in alveolar walls and peribronchial connective tissue. These cells have long and irregular cytoplasmic extensions that form a contiguous network. The primary function of dendritic cells is to sample the airway microenvironment, phagocytose and process antigens, and then migrate to regional lymph nodes. In the lymph nodes, dendritic cells present antigen to T cells, a critical step for the later immunologic defense provided by lymphocytes. *Langerhans cells,* a type of dendritic cell with a particular ultrastructural appearance, are the cells with abnormal proliferation that appear to be responsible for Langerhans cell histiocytosis of the lung (also called *eosinophilic granuloma;* see Chapter 11).

POLYMORPHONUCLEAR LEUKOCYTES

Another important cell involved in pulmonary defense is the polymorphonuclear leukocyte (PMN). The PMN is a particularly important component of the defense mechanism for an established bacterial infection of the lower respiratory tract. Normally, few PMNs reside in the small airways and alveoli. When bacteria overwhelm the initial defense mechanisms already discussed, they may replicate within alveolar spaces, causing a bacterial pneumonia. Examination of the histologic features of a bacterial pneumonia reveals that a prominent component of the inflammatory response is an outpouring of PMNs into the alveolar spaces. These cells probably are attracted to the lung by a variety of stimuli, particularly products of complement activation and chemotactic factors released by alveolar macrophages.

The eventual movement of PMNs out of the vasculature and into the lung parenchyma depends on the initial adherence of PMNs to the vascular endothelium. A variety of factors mediate this process of adhesion, including integrins (on the surface of the PMNs) and adhesion molecules (on the surface of the vascular endothelial cells).

When PMNs are involved, they play a crucial role in phagocytosis and killing of the population of invading and proliferating bacteria. Neutrophil granules contain several antimicrobial substances, including defensins, lysozyme, and lactoferrin. In addition, neutrophils are capable of generating products of oxidative metabolism that are toxic to microbes.

NATURAL KILLER CELLS

Natural killer (NK) cells are part of the rapid initial response and are capable of killing microorganisms without prior sensitization. These cells lack surface markers characteristic of either T or B lymphocyte (discussed in the section on cellular immune mechanisms). NK cells are important in rapid protection against viral infections. They act by recognizing and killing virus-infected cells that have been transformed and no longer express certain markers on the cell surface. NK cells also are important in surveillance for neoplasms, and they use the same methods to detect and kill malignantly transformed cells.

ADAPTIVE IMMUNE RESPONSES

The final category of defense mechanisms for the respiratory system is the adaptive immune response, which involves recognizing and responding to specific antigenic material after prior sensitization. Bacteria, viruses, and other microorganisms are perhaps the most important antigens to which the respiratory tract is repetitively exposed. Presumably, immune defense mechanisms are particularly important in protecting the individual against these agents. The processes of the adaptive immune response are not unique to the lung, and only a superficial discussion of general principles is provided here as a basis for understanding the adaptive immune responses in the lung. For more detailed information, the reader is referred to specialized texts and review articles on immunology.

The two major components of the adaptive immune system are humoral (or B-lymphocyte related) and cellular (or T-lymphocyte related). Humoral immunity involves activation of B lymphocytes (which do not require the thymus for differentiation) and production of antibodies by plasma cells (which are derived from B lymphocytes). *Cellular immunity* refers to activation of T lymphocytes (which depend on the thymus for differentiation) and execution of certain specific T-lymphocyte functions, including the production of soluble mediators or cytokines. The two lymphocyte systems are not independent of each other. In particular, T lymphocytes appear to have an important role in regulating immunoglobulin or antibody synthesis by the humoral immune system.

Both humoral and cellular immunity are important in protection of the respiratory system against microorganisms. For certain infectious agents, humoral immunity is the primary mode of protection. For other agents, cellular immunity appears to be paramount. In the lung and in the blood, T lymphocytes are more numerous than are B lymphocytes, but both systems are essential for effective defense against the spectrum of potentially harmful microorganisms.

Lymphocytes can be found in many locations within the respiratory tract, extending from the nasopharynx down to distal regions of the lung parenchyma. True lymph nodes are present around the trachea, the carina, and at the hilum of each lung, in the region of the mainstem bronchi. These lymph nodes receive the lymphatic drainage from most of the airways and lung parenchyma. Lymphoid tissue is present in the nasopharynx, and collections of lymphocytes arranged in nodules are found along medium to large bronchi. These latter collections are called *bronchus-associated lymphoid tissue* and may be responsible for intercepting and handling antigens deposited along the conducting airways. Smaller aggregates of lymphocytes can be found in more distal airways and even scattered throughout the pulmonary parenchyma.

Major components of the adaptive immune system operative in the respiratory tract are the following:
1. T lymphocytes
2. B lymphocytes
3. IgG

HUMORAL IMMUNE MECHANISMS

Humoral immunity in the respiratory tract appears in the form of two major classes of immunoglobulins: IgA and IgG. Antibodies of the IgA class are particularly important in the nasopharynx and upper airways, where they constitute the primary antibody type. The form of IgA present in these areas is secretory IgA, which includes a pair of IgA molecules (joined by a polypeptide) plus an extra glycoprotein component termed the *secretory component*. Secretory IgA appears to be synthesized locally, and the quantities of IgA are much greater in the respiratory tract than in the serum.

Evidence suggests that secretory IgA plays a role in as the respiratory defense system. By virtue of its ability to bind to antigens, IgA may bind to viruses and bacteria, preventing their attachment to epithelial cells. In addition, IgA is efficient in agglutinating microorganisms; the agglutinated microbes are more easily cleared by the mucociliary transport system. Finally, IgA appears to have the ability to neutralize a variety of respiratory viruses as well as some bacteria.

In contrast to IgA, IgG is particularly abundant in the lower respiratory tract. It is synthesized locally to a large extent, although a fraction also originates from serum IgG. It has a number of biologic properties, such as agglutinating particles, neutralizing viruses and bacterial toxins, serving as an opsonin for macrophage handling of bacteria, activating complement, and causing lysis of gram-negative bacteria in the presence of complement.

The overall role of the humoral immune system in respiratory defenses includes protecting the lung against a variety of bacterial and, to some extent, viral infections. The clinical implications of this role and the consequences of impairment in the humoral immune system are discussed in the section on defects in the adaptive immune system.

CELLULAR IMMUNE MECHANISMS

Cellular immune mechanisms, those mediated by thymus-dependent (T) lymphocytes, also operate as part of the overall defense system of the lungs. Sensitized T lymphocytes produce a variety of soluble, biologically active mediators called *cytokines,* some of which (e.g., interferon-γ) have the ability to attract or activate other protective cell types, particularly macrophages. T lymphocytes also are capable of interacting with the humoral immune system and modifying antibody production.

Two important types of T lymphocytes have been well characterized on the basis of specific cell surface markers and functional characteristics. One type consists of cells that are positive for the CD4 surface marker, commonly called CD4$^+$ or helper T cells. CD4$^+$ cells, in turn, are divided into T_H1 and T_H2 subsets, which mediate cellular immune defense and allergic inflammation, respectively. The other major type of T lymphocyte consists of cells that are positive for the CD8 surface marker. These CD8$^+$ cells include suppressor and cytotoxic T cells. On exposure to specific antigens, both CD4$^+$ and CD8$^+$ cells produce a variety of cytokines that interact with other components of the immune system, particularly B lymphocytes and macrophages.

One important role for the cellular immune system is to protect against bacteria that have a pattern of intracellular growth, especially *M. tuberculosis* (see discussion of tuberculosis in Chapter 24). In addition, the cellular immune system has a critical role in the handling of many viruses, fungi, and protozoa.

Although separating the immune protection of the lung into different categories is important for discussion purposes, all of these limbs are deeply intertwined, and dysfunction in one aspect likely will cause problems in other parts of the system. The development of a respiratory infection generally indicates that a number of defense mechanisms have been overcome by the infecting organism.

FAILURE OF RESPIRATORY DEFENSE MECHANISMS

Clinically important deficiencies have been recognized for each of the major categories of respiratory defense mechanisms. As a result, respiratory infections may ensue, and analysis of the specific types of infections associated with each type of defect is both extremely informative and clinically useful.

IMPAIRMENT OF PHYSICAL CLEARANCE

The simplest impairment of physical clearance to understand is the inability to cough effectively. Three factors are required to generate the high velocities of an effective cough: (1) a large inspiration, (2) an increase in intrathoracic pressure against a closed glottis, and (3) a coordinated expiratory blast during which the glottis opens. Considering each of these steps, it becomes easier to appreciate why certain patients have difficulty with clearing inhaled particles and respiratory secretions. The patient with a weakened or paralyzed diaphragm will not be able to take a deep breath. The patient with weak expiratory muscles, such as the person with quadriplegia, will not be able to generate the large increase in intrathoracic pressure. The patient with a chronic tracheostomy or paralyzed vocal cord will not be able to effectively close the glottis in order to increase intrathoracic pressure. All these patients are prone to respiratory tract infections, even if the underlying immune systems are normal.

Other physical or anatomic factors that influence deposition and clearance of particles include genetic abnormalities and environmental factors affecting the mucociliary transport system. Especially interesting information has been provided by a genetic abnormality termed the *dyskinetic cilia syndrome,* also sometimes called the *immotile cilia syndrome.* In this disorder, a defect in ciliary structure and function leads to absent or impaired ciliary motility and hence to ineffective mucociliary clearance. More than 20 types of defects are recognized, but the most common is absence of dynein arms on the microtubules. Clinically, the impairment in mucociliary clearance is associated with chronic sinusitis, chronic bronchitis, and bronchiectasis. In males, the sperm tail, which has a structure similar to that of cilia, is abnormal, resulting in poor sperm motility and infertility. The disorder called *Kartagener's syndrome,* which consists of the triad of chronic sinusitis, bronchiectasis, and situs inversus, is a variant of the dyskinetic cilia syndrome (see Chapter 7). Normal ciliary motion in a specific direction is believed to be responsible for the proper rotation of the heart and positioning of intraabdominal organs during embryogenesis. When ciliary function is significantly disturbed, the positioning of the heart and the intraabdominal organs becomes random, thus accounting for the situs inversus found in approximately 50% of patients with dyskinetic cilia syndrome.

Viral respiratory tract infections frequently cause temporary structural damage to the tracheobronchial mucosa. Functionally, alteration of the mucosa is associated with impaired mucociliary clearance, which may retard the transport of invading bacteria out of the tracheobronchial tree. This is only one of the mechanisms by which viral respiratory tract infections predispose the individual to complicating bacterial superinfections.

Environmental factors also may cause impairment of mucociliary clearance. Exposure to cigarette smoke is the most important clinically and probably contributes to the predisposition of heavy smokers to recurrent respiratory tract infections. Some atmospheric pollutants, such as sulfur dioxide (SO_2), nitrogen dioxide (NO_2), and ozone (O_3), appear to depress mucociliary clearance, but the clinical consequences are not entirely clear. High concentrations of O_2, such as 90% to 100% inhaled for more than several hours, appear to be associated with impaired mucociliary function. Here the consequences are relevant to patients with respiratory failure who require these extremely high concentrations. In addition, general anesthesia with inhalational drugs administered during surgery is associated with short-term cilia dysfunction and contributes to the increased risk of pneumonia in patients during the postoperative period.

Management of patients with respiratory failure often involves insertion of a tube into the trachea (an endotracheal tube) and support of gas exchange with a mechanical ventilator (see Chapter 29). Endotracheal tubes pose a significant risk for bacterial infection of the lower respiratory tract, often called *ventilator-associated pneumonia,* in part by preventing glottic closure, a critical component of the sequence of events leading to an effective cough. In addition, the endotracheal tube provides a direct conduit into the trachea for any bacteria that have colonized or contaminated the ventilator tubing or the endotracheal tube itself.

Causes of impaired mucociliary clearance are the following:
1. Dyskinetic (immotile) cilia syndrome
2. Viral respiratory tract infection
3. Cigarette smoking
4. High concentrations of O_2 for prolonged periods
5. General anesthesia

IMPAIRMENT OF ANTIMICROBIAL PEPTIDES

There is tremendous overlap in function of the antimicrobial substances present in the sol layer. Thus, an isolated defect in any one component is unlikely to cause catastrophic consequences. Deficiencies of lysozyme have been associated with an increased risk of acute bacterial bronchitis. In patients with cystic fibrosis, the high salt content in their respiratory secretions appears to inactivate defensins and contributes to the severe respiratory infections that commonly occur. In animals, defects in SP-A or SP-D are associated with an increase in respiratory infections, but analogous problems in humans have not yet been identified.

IMPAIRMENT OF PHAGOCYTIC AND INFLAMMATORY CELLS

Clinical problems result from deficiencies in the number or function of the two major phagocytic and inflammatory cell types: alveolar macrophages and PMNs. One of the more important ways in which macrophage function can be impaired is by viral respiratory tract infections. These infections may paralyze the ability of the macrophage to kill bacteria, another reason why patients with viral infections are more susceptible to superimposed bacterial bronchitis or pneumonia.

Cigarette smoking depresses the ability of alveolar macrophages to take up and kill bacteria. Hypoxia, starvation, alcoholism, and cold exposure similarly appear to be conditions in which impaired bacterial killing is at least partly due to depressed macrophage function. Treatment with corticosteroids, given for a myriad of diseases, seems to alter migration and function of macrophages, and this may compound additional adverse effects of steroids on lymphocytes and the immune system. Some data suggest that macrophage migration is impaired in the acquired immunodeficiency syndrome (AIDS), possibly complicating the other host defense defects recognized in the disease (see Chapter 26).

PMNs are depressed in number in several clinical circumstances, generally as a result of an underlying disease of the bone marrow, such as leukemia, or as a result of treatment administered. Chemotherapeutic agents used to treat malignancy commonly destroy rapidly proliferating cells of the bone marrow, resulting in temporary loss of PMN precursors and marked depression in the number of circulating PMNs. When PMNs are present at a concentration less than $1000/mm^3$ of blood, the risk of bacterial infection begins to rise, becoming particularly marked when the count drops below $500/mm^3$. Although opportunistic fungal infections are generally associated with impairment of cellular immunity rather than with neutropenia, the fungus *Aspergillus* is an important respiratory pathogen in the neutropenic patient.

DEFECTS IN THE ADAPTIVE IMMUNE SYSTEM

The adaptive immune system is subject to defects in function that affect its humoral and cellular components. In comparison with innate immunity, there is much less redundancy in the adaptive immune system, and, as a general principle, defects in adaptive immunity result in a much greater risk of infection. Deficiencies in the humoral immune system, such as decreased or absent immunoglobulin production (i.e., hypogammaglobulinemia or agammaglobulinemia), are associated with recurrent bacterial respiratory infections, often leading to bronchiectasis. The risk of infection is best defined for individuals with IgG or global immunoglobulin deficiency. Although some individuals with selective IgA deficiency seem to have an increased risk of respiratory infections, either viral or bacterial, this risk may be at least partly related to a coexisting deficiency of one of the four recognized IgG subclasses.

Cellular immunity is disturbed most frequently by treatment with corticosteroids, cytotoxic agents, or other immunosuppressive drugs and in some well-defined disease states, such as Hodgkin's disease and AIDS. Unlike most other deficits in respiratory defenses, problems with cell-mediated immunity may lead to infection with a special group of microorganisms, including intracellular bacteria (especially mycobacteria), fungi, *Pneumocystis,* and certain viruses, particularly cytomegalovirus. Some of these organisms, such as *Pneumocystis* and several of the fungi, rarely affect individuals with normal cellular immunity, whereas other organisms, such as *M. tuberculosis,* can affect individuals without any defined defects in cellular immunity.

In summary, the defense mechanisms available to protect the respiratory tract from invading microorganisms are varied and complex. People are capable of thwarting these defenses by exposing themselves to damaging influences such as cigarette smoke and ethanol. Just as important, physicians often manage patients with pharmacologic agents or other modalities that disrupt host defense mechanisms, making it essential that physicians be aware of the potential infectious complications of therapy.

In the clinical setting, deficiencies in immunoglobulins and PMNs are strongly associated with an increased risk of bacterial infections. Although problems with mucociliary clearance and macrophage function are somewhat less well defined in terms of

---

Causes of problems with macrophage function are the following:
1. Viral respiratory tract infections
2. Cigarette smoking
3. Alcoholism
4. Starvation
5. Cold exposure
6. Hypoxia
7. Corticosteroid therapy
8. HIV/AIDS

Causes of decreased numbers of PMNs are the following:
1. Bone marrow replacement by tumor
2. Cancer chemotherapeutic agents

Causes of adaptive immune deficiency are the following:
1. Humoral: decreased or absent immunoglobulins
2. Cellular: corticosteroids, cytotoxic drugs, Hodgkin's disease and other lymphomas, HIV/AIDS

the specific infectious risk, bacterial infections also appear to be prominent in these settings. In contrast, disturbances in cellular immunity are characterized by an increased risk of a different subset of infections, especially infections caused by mycobacteria, *Pneumocystis,* fungi, and certain viruses.

Because of the frequency and serious nature of respiratory infections in immunosuppressed patients, this chapter briefly considers the problems posed by the immunocompromised patient with pulmonary infiltrates. More detailed discussions can be found in several articles listed in the references.

IMMUNOSUPPRESSED PATIENT WITH PULMONARY INFILTRATES

During the last several decades, physicians have been faced with increasing numbers of patients who have impaired host defense mechanisms, particularly neutropenia (decreased PMNs) and depressed cellular immunity. These conditions occur frequently as a result of chemotherapy given for malignancy or immunosuppressive agents administered for inflammatory diseases or following organ transplantation. Individuals infected with the virus causing HIV/AIDS are another major category of immunosuppressed patients. Because of the importance of AIDS, Chapter 26 is devoted to the respiratory complications associated with this particular form of immunodeficiency.

Immunocompromised patients are extremely susceptible to the development of respiratory tract infections with a variety of organisms, some of which rarely cause disease in the immunocompetent host. When the immunosuppressed patient has fever and new pulmonary infiltrates, the possibility of an "opportunistic" infection comes immediately to mind. However, patients with malignancy also are susceptible to noninfectious complications of their tumor or its treatment, so such complications must be seriously considered in the differential diagnosis.

The spectrum of infectious and noninfectious causes of pulmonary infiltrates in the immunosuppressed host is given in Table 22-1. Although fungi and other relatively unusual types of organisms are commonly thought to be the major causes of infiltrates in patients receiving treatment for malignancy, bacterial pneumonia actually is the most frequent problem in this setting. Neutropenia is the primary predisposing factor for bacterial pneumonias, which frequently are due to gram-negative rods or to *Staphylococcus.*

Table 22-1
CAUSES OF PULMONARY INFILTRATES IN THE IMMUNOCOMPROMISED HOST

Infections	Infections *(Continued)*
Bacteria	*Pneumocystis jiroveci*
Gram-positive cocci, especially	Protozoa
Staphylococcus	*Toxoplasma gondii* (rare)
Gram-negative bacilli	Pulmonary effects of therapy
Mycobacterium tuberculosis	Chemotherapeutic agents
Nontuberculous mycobacteria	Radiation therapy
Nocardia	Pulmonary hemorrhage
Viruses	Congestive heart failure
Cytomegalovirus	Disseminated malignancy
Herpesvirus	Nonspecific interstitial pneumonitis
Fungi	(no defined etiology)
Aspergillus	
Cryptococcus	
Candida	
Mucor	

Other bacteria, namely mycobacteria (either *M. tuberculosis* or nontuberculous mycobacteria) and *Nocardia,* cause problems mainly in the patient with impaired cellular immunity. Defective cellular immunity also predisposes the individual to infections with *Pneumocystis jiroveci,* fungi, and viruses. The fungus *Aspergillus,* which causes an invasive pneumonia in the immunosuppressed patient, seems to be most commonly found in the patient who is neutropenic (and also has impaired cellular immunity) from cytotoxic chemotherapy.

Common noninfectious diagnoses are the interstitial lung diseases resulting as a side effect of radiation therapy or a variety of chemotherapeutic agents (see Chapter 10). However, heart failure (often secondary to cardiac toxicity from chemotherapeutic agents), pulmonary dissemination of the underlying malignancy, and hemorrhage into the pulmonary parenchyma are other causes of infiltrates that can closely mimic infectious etiologies. In many circumstances, an interstitial inflammatory process can be proved histologically, but no definite cause can be identified. These cases often are diagnosed as nonspecific interstitial pneumonitis, with the realization that neither the pathology nor the clinical history provides a specific etiologic diagnosis.

The approach to treatment of the immunocompromised patient with pulmonary infiltrates revolves around the attempt to identify an infectious agent or a noninfectious etiology. Traditional methods have included examination of sputum and specimens obtained by bronchoscopy or thoracoscopic lung biopsy. There has been great interest in the use of newer, more rapid, more sensitive techniques for identifying a variety of opportunistic pathogens. Improved methods of culture, molecular probes, and polymerase chain reaction technology are being investigated and sometimes used clinically in the diagnosis of specific opportunists. The particular procedure chosen is based on specific clinical features relevant to each patient, such as the nature of the underlying disease, the suspected cause of the pulmonary infiltrate, the presence or absence of other predisposing factors, and the potential risks of a diagnostic procedure. However, in some immunocompromised patients with pulmonary infiltrates, empiric treatment is given without a definitive diagnosis, particularly when the patients are at high risk for invasive procedures.

AUGMENTATION OF RESPIRATORY DEFENSE MECHANISMS

In contrast to disease and the actions of physicians in treating patients that can lead to impairment of normal lung defense mechanisms, there are important opportunities to augment defense mechanisms and protect against some forms of respiratory tract infection. Immunization against certain respiratory pathogens has induced production of antibodies against the organisms and has conferred either relative or complete protection against infection by these microbes. Perhaps the most notable examples are immunization against the bacteria that cause pertussis (whooping cough) and immunization against influenza viruses and many subtypes of the common bacterium *Streptococcus pneumoniae* (pneumococcus). Universal immunization against pertussis is recommended during childhood, and, as of 2006, the U.S. Centers for Disease Control recommend a booster vaccine for all adults. Immunization with influenza and pneumococcal vaccines is generally targeted to individuals believed to be at relatively high risk for contracting or developing complications from these infections. Influenza vaccine is also recommended for individuals who come in contact with high-risk persons, such as health care providers and family members of susceptible individuals. We look to the future for other vaccines that will enhance immunity against other respiratory pathogens and allow us to approach these infections more from a preventive standpoint.

REFERENCES

PULMONARY HOST DEFENSES

Bals R: Epithelial antimicrobial peptides in host defects against infection, *Respir Res* 1:141–150, 2000.

Boyton RJ, Openshaw PJ: Pulmonary defences to acute respiratory infection, *Br Med Bull* 61:1–12, 2002.

Curtis JL: Cell-mediated adaptive immune defense of the lungs, *Proc Am Thorac Soc* 2:412–416, 2005.

Fraser RS, Müller NL, Colman N, Paré PD: Pulmonary defense and other nonrespiratory functions. In *Diagnosis of diseases of the chest,* ed 4, Philadelphia, 1999, WB Saunders, pp. 126–135.

Hance AJ: Pulmonary immune cells in health and disease: dendritic cells and Langerhans' cells, *Eur Respir J* 6:1213–1220, 1993.

Hiemstra PS: The role of epithelial beta-defensins and cathelicidins in host defense of the lung, *Exp Lung Res* 33:537–542, 2007.

Holt PG: Pulmonary dendritic cells in local immunity to inert and pathogenic antigens in the respiratory tract, *Proc Am Thorac Soc* 2:116–120, 2005.

Kim S, Shao MXG, Nadel JA: Mucous production, secretion and clearance. In Mason RJ, Broaddus VC, Murray JF, Nadel JA, editors: *Textbook of pulmonary medicine,* ed 4, Philadelphia, 2005, Elsevier Saunders, pp. 330–354.

Kingma PS, Whitsett JA: In defense of the lung: surfactant protein A and surfactant protein D, *Curr Opin Pharmacol* 6:277–283, 2006.

Lambrecht BN: Alveolar macrophage in the driver's seat, *Immunity* 24:366–368, 2006.

Lambrecht BN, Prins J-B, Hoogsteden HC: Lung dendritic cells and host immunity to infection, *Eur Respir J* 18:692–704, 2001.

Lipscomb MF: Lung defenses against opportunistic infections, *Chest* 96:1393–1399, 1989.

Martin TR, Frevert CW: Innate immunity in the lungs, *Proc Am Thorac Soc* 2:403–411, 2005.

Mason CM, Nelson S: Pulmonary host defenses. Implications for therapy, *Clin Chest Med* 20:475–488, 1999.

Moore BB, Moore TA, Toews GB: Role of T- and B-lymphocytes in pulmonary host defences, *Eur Respir J* 18:846–856, 2001.

Pilette C, Ouadrhiri Y, Godding V, Vaerman JP, Sibille Y: Lung mucosal immunity: immunoglobulin-A revisited, *Eur Respir J* 18:571–588, 2001.

Riches DW, Fenton MJ: Monocytes, macrophages and dendritic cells of the lung. In Mason RJ, Broaddus VC, Murray JF, Nadel JA, editors: *Textbook of pulmonary medicine,* ed 4, Philadelphia, 2005, Elsevier Saunders, pp. 355–376

Zhang P, Summer WR, Bagby GJ, Nelson S: Innate immunity and pulmonary host defense, *Immunol Rev* 173:39–51, 2000.

PULMONARY DISEASE ASSOCIATED WITH IMPAIRED DEFENSE MECHANISMS

Dukes RJ, Rosenow EC III, Hermans PE: Pulmonary manifestations of hypogammaglobulinemia, *Thorax* 33:603–607, 1978.

Eliasson R, Mossberg B, Camner P, Afzelius BA: The immotile cilia syndrome, *N Engl J Med* 297:1–6, 1977.

Fishman JA, Rubin RH: Infection in organ-transplant recipients, *N Engl J Med* 338:1741–1751, 1998.

Mayaud C, Cadranel J: A persistent challenge: the diagnosis of respiratory disease in the non-AIDS immunocompromised host, *Thorax* 55:511–517, 2000.

Rañó A, Agusti C, Sibila O, Torres A: Pulmonary infections in non-HIV-immunocompromised patients, *Curr Opin Pulm Med* 11:213–217, 2005.

Rosenow EC III, Wilson WR, Cockerill FR III: Pulmonary disease in the immunocompromised host: I, *Mayo Clin Proc* 60:473–487, 1985.

Shelhamer JH, Gill VJ, Quinn TC, et al: The laboratory evaluation of opportunistic pulmonary infections, *Ann Intern Med* 124:585–599, 1996.

Talbot EA, Hicks CB: Opportunistic thoracic infections. Bacteria, viruses, and protozoa, *Chest Surg Clin North Am* 9:167–192, 1999.

Walsh FW, Rolfe MW, Rumbak MJ: The initial pulmonary evaluation of the immunocompromised patient, *Chest Surg Clin North Am* 9:19–38, 1999.

Wilson WR, Cockerill FR III, Rosenow EC III: Pulmonary disease in the immunocompromised host. II, *Mayo Clin Proc* 60:610–631, 1985.

AUGMENTATION OF RESPIRATORY DEFENSE MECHANISMS

Ahmed F, Singleton JA, Franks AL: Influenza vaccination for healthy young adults, *N Engl J Med* 345:1543–1547, 2001.

Couch RB: Influenza: prospects for control, *Ann Intern Med* 133:992–998, 2000.

Couch RB: Prevention and treatment of influenza, *N Engl J Med* 343:1778–1787, 2000.

Örtqvist A: Pneumococcal vaccination: current and future issues, *Eur Respir J* 18:184–195, 2001.

Pneumonia

By any of several criteria, pneumonia (infection of the pulmonary parenchyma) must be considered one of the most important categories of disease affecting the respiratory system. First, pneumonia is extraordinarily common, accounting for nearly 10% of admissions to many large general hospitals. Overall, it has been estimated that more than 5 million cases of pneumonia occur each year in the United States. Second, pneumonia is a significant cause of death. More than 80,000 Americans die of bacterial pneumonia each year, making it the sixth most common cause of death in the nation. It is no wonder that Sir William Osler referred to pneumonia as "the captain of the men of death," particularly as he spoke before the era of effective antibiotic therapy. For many types of pneumonia, medical therapy with antibiotics (along with supportive care) has great impact on the duration and outcome of the illness. Because of the effectiveness of treatment, the diseases discussed in this chapter typically are gratifying to treat for all involved medical personnel. Unfortunately, the emerging trend during the past 15 years has been the acquisition of antibiotic resistance by some of the organisms causing pneumonia. Therefore, it has been necessary for the treatment of pneumonia to evolve in order to keep pace with patterns of antibiotic resistance.

Although many of the specific agents causing pneumonia are considered here, this chapter is organized primarily as a general discussion of the problem of pneumonia. As appropriate, the focus on individual etiologic agents highlights some characteristic features of each that are particularly useful to the physician. Also covered is a commonly used categorization of pneumonia based on the clinical setting: community-acquired versus nosocomial (hospital-acquired) pneumonia. According to current clinical practice, the approach to evaluation and management of these two types of pneumonia often is quite different.

The chapter concludes with a brief discussion of several infections that were uncommon or primarily of historical interest until September 11, 2001. After the terrorist attacks on the World Trade Center and the Pentagon, the threat of bioterrorism became a reality when spores of *Bacillus anthracis* sent through the mail resulted in cases of cutaneous and inhalational anthrax. In addition to reviewing inhalational anthrax, the chapter briefly describes two other organisms considered to be of concern as potential weapons of bioterrorism: *Yersinia pestis* (the cause of plague) and *Francisella tularensis* (the cause of tularemia).

ETIOLOGY AND PATHOGENESIS

The host defenses of the lung are constantly challenged by a variety of organisms, both viruses and bacteria (see Chapter 22). Viruses in particular are likely to avoid or to overwhelm some of the defenses of the upper respiratory tract, causing a transient, relatively mild clinical illness with symptoms limited to the upper respiratory tract. When host defense mechanisms of the upper and lower respiratory tracts are overwhelmed, microorganisms may establish residence, proliferate, and cause a frank infectious process within the pulmonary parenchyma. With particularly virulent organisms, no major impairment of host defense mechanisms is needed; pneumonia may occur even in normal and otherwise healthy individuals. At the other extreme, if host defense mechanisms are quite impaired, microorganisms that are not particularly virulent, that is, unlikely to cause disease in a healthy host, may produce a life-threatening pneumonia.

In practice, several factors frequently cause enough impairment of host defenses to contribute to the development of pneumonia, even though individuals with such impairment are not considered "immunosuppressed." Viral upper respiratory tract infections, ethanol abuse, cigarette smoking, heart failure, and preexisting chronic obstructive pulmonary disease are a few of the contributing factors. More severe impairment of host defenses is caused by diseases associated with immunosuppression (e.g., acquired immunodeficiency syndrome), by various underlying malignancies (particularly leukemia and lymphoma), and by use of corticosteroids and other immunosuppressive or cytotoxic drugs. In these cases associated with impairment of host defenses, individuals are susceptible to both bacterial and more unusual nonbacterial infections (see Chapters 24–26).

Microorganisms, especially bacteria, find their way to the lower respiratory tract in two major ways. The first is by inhalation, whereby organisms usually are carried in small droplet particles that are inhaled into the tracheobronchial tree. The second is by aspiration, whereby secretions from the oropharynx pass through the larynx and into the tracheobronchial tree. Aspiration usually is thought of as a process occurring in individuals unable to protect their airways from secretions by glottic closure and coughing. Although clinically significant aspiration is more likely to occur in such individuals, everyone is subject to aspirating small amounts of oropharyngeal secretions, particularly during sleep. Defense mechanisms seem able to cope with this nightly onslaught of bacteria, and frequent bouts of aspiration pneumonia are not experienced.

Less commonly, bacteria reach the pulmonary parenchyma through the bloodstream rather than by the airways. This route is important for the spread of certain organisms, particularly *Staphylococcus*. When pneumonia results in this way from bacteremia, the implication is that a distant, primary source of bacterial infection is present or that bacteria were introduced directly into the bloodstream, for example, as a consequence of intravenous drug abuse.

Contributing factors for pneumonia in the immunocompetent host are the following:
1. Viral upper respiratory tract infection
2. Ethanol abuse
3. Cigarette smoking
4. Heart failure
5. Chronic obstructive pulmonary disease

Many individual infectious agents are associated with the development of pneumonia. The frequency with which each agent is involved is difficult to assess and depends to a large extent on the specific population studied. The largest single category of agents probably is bacteria. The other two major categories are viruses and mycoplasma. Of the bacteria, the organism most frequently associated with pneumonia is *Streptococcus pneumoniae,* in common parlance often called the pneumococcus. It has been estimated that in adults approximately half of all pneumonias serious enough to require hospitalization are pneumococcal in origin.

BACTERIA

S. pneumoniae, a normal inhabitant of the oropharynx in a large proportion of adults, is a gram-positive coccus seen in pairs or diplococci. Pneumococcal pneumonia is commonly acquired in the community (i.e., in nonhospitalized patients) and frequently occurs after a viral upper respiratory tract infection. The organism has a polysaccharide capsule that protects the bacteria from phagocytosis and therefore is an important factor in its virulence. There are many antigenic types of capsular polysaccharide, and in order for host defense cells to phagocytize the organism, antibody against the particular capsular type must be present. Antibodies contributing in this way to the phagocytic process are called *opsonins* (see Chapter 22).

Staphylococcus aureus is another gram-positive coccus but usually appears in clusters when examined microscopically. Three major settings in which this organism is seen as a cause of pneumonia are (1) as a secondary complication of respiratory tract infection with the influenza virus; (2) in the hospitalized patient, who often has some impairment of host defense mechanisms and whose oropharynx has been colonized by *Staphylococcus;* and (3) as a complication of widespread dissemination of staphylococcal organisms through the bloodstream.

A variety of gram-negative organisms are potential causes of pneumonia, but only a few of the most important examples from this group of organisms are mentioned here. *Haemophilus influenzae,* which is a small coccobacillary gram-negative organism, is often found in the nasopharynx of normal individuals and in the lower airways of patients with chronic obstructive lung disease. It can cause pneumonia in children and adults, the latter often with underlying chronic obstructive lung disease as a predisposing factor. *Klebsiella pneumoniae,* a relatively large gram-negative rod that normally is found in the gastrointestinal tract, has been best described as a cause of pneumonia in the setting of underlying alcoholism. *Pseudomonas aeruginosa,* which may be found in a variety of environmental sources (especially in the hospital environment), is seen primarily in patients who are debilitated, hospitalized, and, often, previously treated with antibiotics.

The bacterial flora normally present in the mouth are potential etiologic agents in the development of pneumonia. A multitude of organisms (both gram-positive and gram-negative) that favor or require anaerobic conditions for growth are the major organisms composing mouth flora. The most common predisposing factor for anaerobic pneumonia is aspiration of secretions from the oropharynx into the tracheobronchial tree. Patients with impaired consciousness (e.g., as a result of coma, alcohol ingestion, or seizures) and those with difficulty swallowing (e.g., as a result of diseases causing muscle weakness) are prone to aspirate and are at risk for pneumonia caused by anaerobic mouth organisms. In addition, patients with poor dentition or gum disease are more likely to develop aspiration pneumonia because of the larger burden of organisms in their oral cavity.

In some settings, such as prolonged hospitalization or recent use of antibiotics, the type of bacteria residing in the oropharynx may change. Specifically, aerobic

Streptococcus pneumoniae (pneumococcus) is the most common cause of bacterial pneumonia. The polysaccharide capsule is an important factor in its virulence.

Factors predisposing to oropharyngeal colonization and pneumonia with gram-negative organisms are the following:
1. Hospitalization or residence in a chronic care facility
2. Underlying disease and compromised host defenses
3. Recent antibiotic therapy

Anaerobes normally found in the oropharynx are the usual cause of aspiration pneumonia.

gram-negative bacilli and *S. aureus* are more likely to colonize the oropharynx, and any subsequent pneumonia resulting from aspiration of oropharyngeal contents may include these aerobic organisms as part of the process.

The two final types of bacteria mentioned here are more recent additions to the list of etiologic agents. The first of these organisms, *Legionella pneumophila,* was identified as the cause of a mysterious outbreak of pneumonia in 1976 affecting American Legion members at a convention in Philadelphia. Since then it has been recognized as an important cause of pneumonia occurring in epidemics as well as in isolated, sporadic cases. In addition, it seems to affect both previously healthy individuals and those with prior impairment of respiratory defense mechanisms. In retrospect, several prior outbreaks of unexplained pneumonia have been shown to be due to this organism. Although the organism is a gram-negative bacillus, it stains very poorly and is generally not seen by conventional staining methods.

The other organism, *Chlamydophila pneumoniae,* has been recognized in epidemiologic studies as the cause of approximately 5% to 10% of cases of pneumonia. It is an obligate intracellular parasite that appears more related to gram-negative bacteria than to viruses, the category in which it previously had been placed. Diagnosis is rarely made clinically because of the lack of distinguishing clinical and radiographic features, and the organism is not readily cultured. As a result, serologic studies, which are not readily available, serve as the primary means of diagnosis.

Many other types of bacteria can cause pneumonia. Because all of them cannot be covered in this chapter, the interested reader should consult some of the more detailed publications listed in the references.

VIRUSES

Although viruses are extremely common causes of upper respiratory tract infections, they are diagnosed relatively infrequently as a cause of frank pneumonia, except in children. In adults, influenza virus is the most commonly diagnosed agent. Outbreaks of pneumonia caused by adenovirus also are well recognized, particularly in military recruits. A relatively rare cause of a fulminant and often lethal pneumonia was described in the southwest United States, but cases in other locations have also been recognized. The virus responsible for this pneumonia, called *hantavirus,* is found in rodents and previously was described as a cause of fever, hemorrhage, and acute renal failure in other parts of the world.

An outbreak of highly contagious and highly lethal pneumonia was reported in 2003 in East Asia and Canada. Termed *severe acute respiratory syndrome* (SARS), the outbreak was attributed to a novel coronavirus that may have evolved from a type normally found in the civet (a weasel-like mammal found in Chinese markets).

MYCOPLASMA

Mycoplasma appears to be a class of organisms intermediate between viruses and bacteria. Unlike bacteria, they have no rigid cell wall. Unlike viruses, they do not require the intracellular machinery of a host cell to replicate and are capable of free-living growth. Similar in size to large viruses, mycoplasmas are the smallest free-living organisms that have yet been identified. These organisms now are recognized as a common cause of pneumonia, perhaps responsible for a minimum of 10% to 20% of all cases of pneumonia. Mycoplasmal pneumonia occurs most frequently in young adults but is not limited to this age group. The pneumonia is generally acquired in the community, that is, by previously healthy, nonhospitalized individuals, and may occur either in isolated cases or in localized outbreaks.

Mycoplasma, the smallest known free-living organism, is a frequent cause of pneumonia in young adults.

PATHOLOGY

The pathologic process common to all pneumonias is infection and inflammation of the distal pulmonary parenchyma. An influx of polymorphonuclear leukocytes (PMNs), edema fluid, erythrocytes, mononuclear cells, and fibrin is seen to a variable extent in all cases. The bacterial pneumonias, in particular, are characterized by an exuberant outpouring of PMNs into alveolar spaces as they attempt to limit proliferation of the invading bacteria.

The individual types of pneumonia may differ in the exact location and mode of spread of the infection. In the past, a distinction was often made between pneumonias that follow a "lobar" distribution, those that behave more like a "bronchopneumonia," and those with the pattern of an "interstitial pneumonia." However, these distinctions often are difficult to make because individual cases of pneumonia frequently do not adhere to any one particular pattern but have mixtures of the three patterns in varying proportions. Given this limitation, a brief mention of the three major types follows.

> *Lobar Pneumonia.* Lobar pneumonia has classically been described as a process not limited to segmental boundaries but rather tending to spread throughout an entire lobe of the lung. Spread of the infection is believed to occur from alveolus to alveolus and from acinus to acinus through interalveolar pores, known as the *pores of Kohn.* The classic example of a lobar pneumonia is that due to *S. pneumoniae,* although many cases of pneumonia recognized as being due to pneumococcus do not necessarily follow this typical pattern.
>
> *Bronchopneumonia.* In bronchopneumonia, distal airway inflammation is prominent along with alveolar disease, and spread of the infection and the inflammatory process tends to occur through airways rather than through adjacent alveoli and acini. Whereas lobar pneumonias appear as dense consolidations involving part or all of a lobe, bronchopneumonias are more patchy in distribution, depending on where spread by airways has occurred. Many of the other bacteria, such as staphylococci and a variety of gram-negative bacilli, may produce this patchy pattern.
>
> *Interstitial Pneumonia.* Interstitial pneumonias are characterized by an inflammatory process within the interstitial walls rather than the alveolar spaces. Although viral pneumonias classically start as interstitial pneumonias, severe cases generally show extension of the inflammatory process to alveolar spaces as well.

In some cases of pneumonia, the organisms are not highly destructive to lung tissue, even though an exuberant inflammatory process may be seen. Pneumococcal pneumonia classically (although not always) behaves in this way, and the healing process is associated with restoration of relatively normal parenchymal architecture. In other cases, when the organisms are more destructive, tissue necrosis may occur, with resulting cavity formation or scarring of the parenchyma. Many cases of staphylococcal and anaerobic pneumonias follow this more destructive course.

PATHOPHYSIOLOGY

Infections of the pulmonary parenchyma produce their clinical sequelae not only by altering the normal functioning of the lung parenchyma but also by inducing a more generalized, systemic response to the invading microorganisms. The major pathophysiologic consequence of inflammation and infection involving the distal air spaces is a decrease in ventilation to the affected areas. If perfusion is relatively maintained, as it often is, ventilation-perfusion mismatch results, with low ventilation-perfusion ratios in the diseased regions. When alveoli are totally filled with inflammatory exudate, there may be no ventilation to these regions, and extreme ventilation-perfusion inequality (i.e., shunt) results.

Ventilation-perfusion inequality generally manifests as hypoxemia. Although frank shunting may explain part of the hypoxemia, ventilation-perfusion mismatch with areas of low ventilation-perfusion ratio usually is a more important factor. Carbon dioxide retention is not a feature of pneumonia unless the patient already has an extremely limited reserve, especially from underlying chronic obstructive lung disease. In fact, patients with pneumonia frequently hyperventilate and have a Pco_2 less than 40 mm Hg.

The systemic response to pneumonia is not unique but rather is a reflection of the body's response to serious infection. Perhaps the most apparent aspects of this response are fever, an outpouring of PMNs into the circulation (particularly with bacterial pneumonia), and often a "toxic" appearance of the patient. These indirect systemic responses can be clues that an infectious process is the cause of a new pulmonary infiltrate.

> Pneumonia commonly results in ventilation-perfusion mismatch (with or without shunting) and hypoxemia.

CLINICAL FEATURES

In many ways the clinical manifestations of pneumonia are similar, even when different infectious agents are involved. In other ways the presentations and manifestations are quite different. Although recognition of subtle clinical differences sometimes allows the astute clinician to suggest an etiologic diagnosis, methods for identifying a specific infectious agent play an equally if not more important role in the final diagnosis. However, in many cases, a specific agent cannot be clearly identified, and patients often are managed in an empiric way based on the setting in which they present.

Perhaps the most important constellation of symptoms in almost any type of pneumonia consists of fever, cough, and, often, shortness of breath. The cough is nonproductive in some cases, particularly in those pneumonias caused by viruses or mycoplasma; in others, especially bacterial pneumonias, sputum production is a prominent feature. When the inflammatory process in the pulmonary parenchyma extends out to the pleural surface, the patient often reports pleuritic chest pain. If the fever is high and "spiking," patients frequently experience shaking chills associated with the rapid rise in body temperature.

> Frequent clinical features in patients with pneumonia are the following:
> 1. Fever (with or without chills)
> 2. Cough (with or without sputum)
> 3. Dyspnea
> 4. Pleuritic chest pain
> 5. Crackles overlying affected region
> 6. Dullness and bronchial breath sounds with frank consolidation
> 7. Polymorphonuclear leukocytosis

Physical examination reflects the systemic response to infection and the ongoing inflammatory process in the lung. Patients often have tachycardia, tachypnea, and fever. Examination of the chest typically reveals crackles or rales overlying the region of the pneumonia. If dense consolidation is present and the bronchus supplying the area is patent, then sound transmission is greatly increased through the consolidated, pneumonic area. As a result, breath sounds may be bronchial in quality, fremitus is increased, and egophony is present. The consolidated area is characteristically dull to percussion of the overlying chest wall. Examination of the peripheral blood generally shows an increase in the white blood count (leukocytosis). Especially in patients with bacterial pneumonia, the leukocytosis is composed primarily of PMNs, and a shift toward immature, younger neutrophils (i.e., bands) may be seen.

In pneumococcal pneumonia, the onset of the clinical illness often is relatively abrupt, with shaking chills and high fever. Cough may be productive of yellow, green, or blood-tinged (rusty-colored) sputum. Before the development of pneumonia, patients often experience a viral upper respiratory tract infection, which presumably is an important predisposing feature.

Mycoplasmal pneumonia, in contrast to pneumococcal pneumonia, characteristically has a somewhat slower, more insidious onset. Cough is a particularly prominent symptom, but it often is nonproductive. Fever is not as high, and shaking chills are uncommon. Young adults are the individuals most likely to have mycoplasmal pneumonia, although the disease is not limited to this age group.

Patients with either staphylococcal or gram-negative bacillary pneumonias are often quite ill. Frequently, these patients have complex underlying medical problems and have already been hospitalized. Many have impaired defense mechanisms or have recently received antibiotics. Staphylococcal pneumonia may be seen as a secondary complication of influenza infection or as a result of dissemination of the organism through the bloodstream.

Pneumonia with anaerobic organisms generally occurs in patients with impaired consciousness or difficulty swallowing who cannot adequately protect the airway from aspiration of oropharyngeal secretions. Dentition often is poor, and patients frequently have gingivitis or periodontal abscesses. Clinical onset of the pneumonia tends to be gradual, and sputum may have a foul odor, suggesting anaerobic infection. Because the organisms are likely to cause substantial tissue destruction, necrosis of affected tissue and abscess formation are relatively common sequelae.

Pneumonia caused by *L. pneumophila,* commonly called legionnaires' disease, can be seen as isolated cases or localized outbreaks. Otherwise healthy hosts may be affected, but patients with impaired respiratory defense mechanisms appear to be predisposed. Patients often are extremely ill, not only with respiratory compromise and even respiratory failure but also with nonrespiratory manifestations; specifically, gastrointestinal, central nervous system, hepatic, and renal abnormalities may accompany the pneumonia.

DIAGNOSTIC APPROACH

As with other disorders affecting the pulmonary parenchyma, the single most useful tool for assessing pneumonia at the macroscopic level is the chest radiograph. The radiograph not only confirms the presence of a pneumonia; it also shows the distribution and extent of disease and sometimes gives clues about the nature of the etiologic agent. The classic pattern for *S. pneumoniae* (pneumococcus) and *K. pneumoniae* is a lobar pneumonia (Fig. 23-1). Staphylococcal and many of the gram-negative pneumonias may be localized or extensive and often follow a patchy distribution (Fig. 23-2). *Mycoplasma* organisms can produce a variety of radiographic presentations, classically described as being more impressive than the clinical picture would suggest. Pneumonias caused by aspiration of oropharyngeal secretions characteristically involve the dependent regions of lung: the lower lobe in the upright patient or the posterior segment of the upper lobe or superior segment of the lower lobe in the supine patient (Fig. 23-3).

The chest radiograph is useful for demonstrating pleural fluid, which frequently accompanies pneumonia, particularly of bacterial origin. The pleural fluid can be either thin and serous or thick and purulent; in the latter case the term *empyema* is used (discussed later in the Empyema section).

Microscopic examination of the sputum may play an important role in the evaluation of patients with pneumonia. However, the importance of obtaining a sputum specimen and using it as a guide to treatment, as opposed to treating the patient empirically without a sputum specimen, is an issue of substantial controversy. Most authorities now recommend basing initial treatment on clinical presentation. In cases in which a sputum specimen is obtained, it is important to evaluate the quality of the specimen because a poor-quality specimen may provide inadequate or

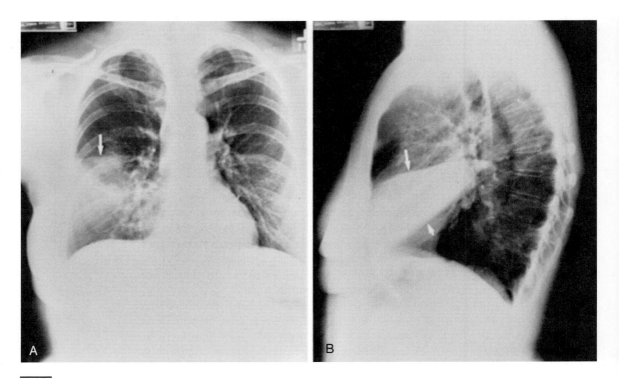

Figure 23-1. Posteroanterior *(A)* and lateral *(B)* chest radiographs show lobar pneumonia (probably caused by *Streptococcus pneumoniae)* affecting the right middle lobe. In **A,** arrow points to the minor fissure, which defines the upper border of the middle lobe. In **B,** long arrow points to the minor fissure, and short arrow points to the major fissure.

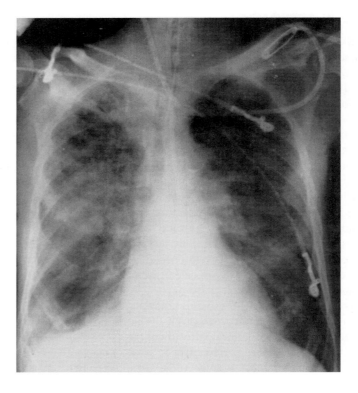

Figure 23-2. Chest radiograph of a patient with extensive gram-negative pneumonia. Note patchy infiltrates throughout both lungs, more prominent on the right.

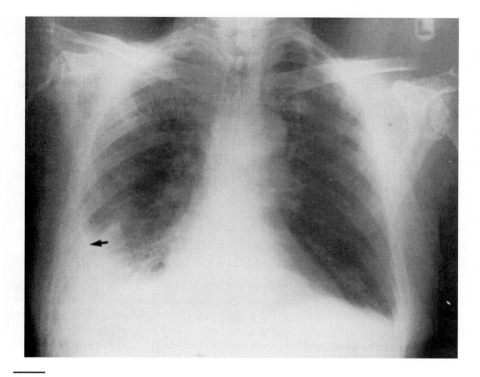

Figure 23-3. Chest radiograph of right lower lobe aspiration pneumonia. In addition to infiltrate at right base, note loculated pleural effusion, which represents empyema complicating pneumonia. Arrow points to edge of loculated effusion. (Courtesy Dr. T. Scott Johnson.)

inaccurate information. In a good sputum specimen (i.e., one that contains few squamous epithelial cells picked up in transit through the upper respiratory tract), inflammatory cells and bacteria can be seen.

In most bacterial pneumonias, large numbers of PMNs are seen in the sputum. In contrast, mycoplasmal and viral pneumonias have fewer PMNs and more mononuclear inflammatory cells. Pneumococcal, staphylococcal, and gram-negative bacillary pneumonias commonly demonstrate a relatively homogeneous population of the infecting bacteria. Anaerobic aspiration pneumonias, caused by a mixture of organisms from the oropharynx, show a mixed population of bacteria of many different morphologies. In legionnaires' disease, the bacterium does not stain well with the usual Gram stain reagent and therefore is not seen with conventional staining techniques. In mycoplasmal and viral pneumonia, the infecting agent is not visualized by light microscopy, and only the predominantly mononuclear cell inflammatory response is seen.

In conjunction with the initial Gram stain and microscopic examination of sputum, the specimen is cultured for bacteria. However, some bacteria are relatively difficult to grow, and in many, if not most, cases the initial Gram stain is just as important in making the etiologic diagnosis. Special culture media are available to facilitate the growth of *Legionella* species.

When sputum is not spontaneously expectorated by the patient, other methods for obtaining respiratory secretions (or even material directly from the lung parenchyma) may be necessary. The techniques that have been used, including flexible bronchoscopy, needle aspiration of the lung, and occasionally surgical lung biopsy, are described in greater detail in Chapter 3.

Routine stains and cultures of sputum are not useful for three of the important causes of pneumonia: *Mycoplasma*, *Chlamydophila*, and *Legionella*. Sometimes the diagnosis can be confirmed by a variety of serologic techniques that demonstrate a rise in antibody titer against the organism, but these techniques provide a retrospective diagnosis and are not useful clinically. Several newer methods are seeing increasing clinical usefulness over time. For example, direct fluorescent antibody staining can be performed for *Legionella*, especially on tissue specimens, but more recent methods include culture on special supplemented media and a commonly used urinary antigen radioimmunoassay (only for certain *L. pneumophila* serotypes). Polymerase chain reaction methods are being investigated for all three organisms and may have an important role in the future.

The functional assessment of patients with acute infectious pneumonia usually is limited to evaluation of gas exchange. Arterial blood gas values characteristically demonstrate hypoxemia, accompanied by a normal or decreased P_{CO_2}. Pulmonary function tests have little usefulness in this setting.

THERAPEUTIC APPROACH: GENERAL PRINCIPLES AND ANTIBIOTIC SUSCEPTIBILITY

The cornerstone of treatment of bacterial pneumonia is antibiotic therapy directed at the infecting organism. However, because the causative organism often is not known when the pneumonia is first diagnosed and, in fact, frequently is not identified at any point during the clinical course, initial treatment strategies have been developed on the basis of the clinical setting (e.g., community-acquired vs hospital-acquired pneumonia). These initial treatment strategies are outlined in the section on initial management strategies based on clinical setting of pneumonia. If and when an organism is identified, the regimen may be changed to allow for more focused or more effective antibiotic coverage. Because knowledge of antibiotic susceptibility of specific organisms helps with understanding the rationale behind initial treatment strategies, this section first considers some of the general patterns of antibiotic susceptibility for the major organisms causing pneumonia.

In the case of pneumococcal pneumonia, penicillin traditionally has been the most appropriate agent, assuming the patient is not allergic to penicillin, although cases with various degrees of resistance to penicillin are now being encountered with increasing frequency. In addition, because penicillin is not effective against some of the other common causes of community-acquired pneumonia, such as *Mycoplasma pneumoniae* and *C. pneumoniae*, other classes of antibiotics with a broader spectrum against agents causing community-acquired pneumonia typically are used when antibiotics are initiated. They include the macrolides (erythromycin or a derivative, e.g., azithromycin) and quinolones (e.g., levofloxacin). When high-level resistance of pneumococcus to penicillin is found, then either a quinolone or vancomycin typically is necessary. Intermediately resistant strains often can be treated with ceftriaxone.

Staphylococci generally produce penicillinase, which requires use of a penicillinase-resistant derivative of penicillin, such as oxacillin or nafcillin. Some staphylococci are also resistant to these derivatives, in which case vancomycin is the antibiotic of choice. *H. influenzae* may be sensitive to ampicillin, but the high frequency of organisms resistant to this antibiotic generally justifies alternative coverage, such as a second- or third-generation cephalosporin, an extended spectrum macrolide, trimethoprim-sulfamethoxazole, or a quinolone. Many of the other gram-negative bacillary pneumonias often display resistance to a variety of antibiotics. Aminoglycosides (e.g., gentamicin and tobramycin), third- or fourth-generation cephalosporins, quinolones, carbapenems (e.g., meropenem), or an extended spectrum penicillin with a β-lactamase inhibitor (e.g., piperacillin/tazobactam) may be used initially while antibiotic sensitivity testing is performed. Pneumonia caused by anaerobes is treated most commonly with either penicillin or clindamycin.

Frequently used antibiotics for common pneumonias are the following:

1. *S. pneumoniae* (penicillin, macrolide, selected quinolones)
2. *Staphylococcus* (oxacillin, nafcillin, cefazolin, vancomycin)
3. *Haemophilus influenzae* (second- or third-generation cephalosporins, trimethoprim-sulfamethoxazole, quinolone, macrolide)
4. Gram-negative rods (aminoglycosides, third- or fourth generation cephalosporins, carbapenems, extended-spectrum penicillin with β-lactamase inhibitor)
5. Anaerobes (penicillin, clindamycin)
6. *Mycoplasma* organisms (macrolide, quinolone)
7. *Legionella* (macrolide, quinolone)
8. *Chlamydophila pneumoniae* (tetracycline, macrolide)

A macrolide or a quinolone is the antibiotic of choice for pneumonias caused by either *Legionella* or *Mycoplasma*.

No definitive forms of therapy for most viral pneumonias are available, although rapid advances in this field may lead to development of more clinically useful therapeutic agents. Influenza vaccine (see Chapter 22) is effective in preventing influenza in the majority of individuals who receive it, whereas antiviral agents (amantadine or rimantadine for influenza A, a neuraminidase inhibitor such as zanamivir or oseltamivir for influenza A or B) may reduce the duration of the illness if given soon after onset of clinical symptoms.

Other modalities of therapy are mainly supportive. Chest physical therapy and other measures to assist clearance of respiratory secretions are useful for some patients with pneumonia, particularly if neuromuscular disease or other factors impair the effectiveness of the patient's cough. If patients have inadequate gas exchange as demonstrated by significant hypoxemia, administration of supplemental O_2 is beneficial. Occasionally, frank respiratory failure develops, and appropriate supportive measures are instituted (see Chapter 29).

INITIAL MANAGEMENT STRATEGIES BASED ON CLINICAL SETTING OF PNEUMONIA

During the past 2 decades, greater emphasis on the cost-effective use of medical resources has spurred the development of algorithms and guidelines for the clinician approaching common clinical problems. Pneumonia is a particularly good example of an important clinical problem for which such management strategies have been developed, relating to both diagnostic evaluation and initiation of therapy. Separate strategies are being promulgated for two distinct groups of patients with pneumonia, depending on the setting in which the pneumonia developed, that is, *community-acquired pneumonia* and *nosocomial (hospital-acquired) pneumonia*. The patients in these categories to whom the guidelines apply do not have significant underlying impairment of systemic host defense mechanisms, such as patients with acquired immunodeficiency syndrome or those receiving immunosuppressive drugs or cancer chemotherapy.

COMMUNITY-ACQUIRED PNEUMONIA

Community-acquired pneumonia refers to pneumonia that develops in the community setting, that is, in an individual who is not hospitalized. Although this category is not meant to include patients with significant impairment of systemic host defense mechanisms, it can include patients with other coexisting illnesses or risk factors that alter the profile of organisms likely to be responsible for pneumonia.

Surprisingly, the cause of community-acquired pneumonia is never identified in a high proportion of patients, estimated to be up to 50%. The likelihood of particular agents is believed to be influenced by a number of modifying factors: presence of coexisting illness, recent treatment with antibiotics, residence in a nursing home, and severity of illness at initial presentation. One issue that has sparked controversy is whether an attempt should be made to identify a specific etiologic agent, using Gram stain and culture, in patients with community-acquired pneumonia, or whether empiric therapy should be used based on the patient's risk factors and clinical characteristics. If a specific pathogen is identified, then modification of the initial antibiotic regimen often is appropriate, particularly to avoid an overly broad spectrum of coverage.

Four broad subcategories of patients with community-acquired pneumonia have been defined, as summarized in Table 23-1.

The first group comprises patients who do not have coexisting cardiopulmonary disease or other modifying risk factors, who have not used antibiotics in the previous 3 months, and who do not require hospitalization. The most common pathogens in this group of patients include *S. pneumoniae, M. pneumoniae, C. pneumoniae,* respiratory viruses, and, in smokers, *H. influenzae.* The preferred therapeutic regimen is one of the newer (advanced-generation) macrolide antibiotics, such as azithromycin or clarithromycin.

The second group includes patients who have coexisting cardiopulmonary disease or other modifying risk factors but who still can be treated in an outpatient setting. Important comorbidities that place a patient in this category include chronic heart, lung, hepatic, or renal disease, diabetes mellitus, alcoholism, malignancies, asplenia, immunosuppressive conditions or drugs, or use of antibiotics within the prior 3 months (in which case antibiotics from a different class should be used). Local resistance patterns of *S. pneumoniae* should be taken into account, and residence in a nursing home should be considered a factor that increases the risk of pneumonia caused by a gram-negative organism. Poor dentition (leading to an increased burden of anaerobic organisms in the mouth), problems with swallowing, or impaired consciousness increase the risk of an anaerobic aspiration pneumonia. Recommended options for management of this group have included either an oral quinolone (used as a single agent) or a β-lactam antibiotic (e.g., second- or third-generation cephalosporin) given in combination with a macrolide (particularly an advanced-generation macrolide such as azithromycin or clarithromycin).

The third and fourth groups differ from the first two on the basis of the severity of the pneumonia. The third group is defined by a need for hospitalization. The fourth group includes patients with the most severe disease, that which necessitates admission to an intensive care unit. These patients still commonly have pneumonia caused by *S. pneumoniae* or the other organisms found in outpatients but with additional concern for gram-negative bacilli, *Legionella,* and sometimes *Staphylococcus aureus.* Therapy for these patients is adjusted accordingly (see Table 23-1). Antibiotics, such as a quinolone or an advanced-generation macrolide, plus a β-lactam (particularly a third-generation cephalosporin), a carbapenem, or an extended spectrum penicillin with β-lactamase inhibitor, typically are used in these settings, sometimes in combination with vancomycin.

NOSOCOMIAL (HOSPITAL-ACQUIRED) PNEUMONIA

In contrast to community-acquired pneumonia, nosocomial pneumonia is acquired by hospitalized patients, generally after more than 48 hours of hospitalization. Patients in intensive care units, especially those who are receiving mechanical ventilation, are at particularly high risk for developing this form of pneumonia. Perhaps the most common problem leading to nosocomial pneumonia is colonization of the oropharynx by organisms not usually present in this site, which is followed by microaspiration of oropharyngeal secretions into the tracheobronchial tree. Patients at risk often have other underlying medical problems, have been receiving antibiotics, or have an endotracheal tube in their airway that bypasses some of the normal protective mechanisms of the respiratory tract.

Organisms of particular concern in patients who develop hospital-acquired pneumonia are enteric gram-negative bacilli and *S. aureus,* but other organisms such as *Pseudomonas aeruginosa* and *Legionella* can be involved. Diagnostic evaluation is difficult and often complicated by the need to distinguish bacterial colonization of the tracheobronchial tree from true bacterial pneumonia. The clinical issues involved with diagnostic testing and optimal forms of therapy are beyond the scope of this discussion but can be found in the references.

In community-acquired pneumonia, factors influencing the likelihood of certain organisms and therefore the therapeutic approach include age, presence of coexisting illness, and severity of pneumonia at initial presentation.

Organisms of particular concern in nosocomial pneumonia include *Staphylococcus aureus,* gram-negative bacilli, and *Legionella.*

Table 23-1

ETIOLOGY AND INITIAL MANAGEMENT OF COMMUNITY-ACQUIRED PNEUMONIA*

Patient Category	Common Organisms	Other Miscellaneous Organisms	Initial Therapy
Outpatient, no cardiopulmonary disease or other modifying risk factors	S. pneumoniae M. pneumoniae C. pneumoniae Respiratory viruses H. influenzae (in smokers)	Legionella M. tuberculosis Endemic fungi	Advanced generation macrolide (e.g., azithromycin or clarithromycin) or Doxycycline
Outpatient, with cardiopulmonary disease and/or other modifying factors	S. pneumoniae M. pneumoniae H. influenzae Aerobic gram-negative bacilli Respiratory viruses Anaerobes C. pneumoniae	M. catarrhalis Legionella M. tuberculosis Endemic fungi	Oral quinolone (with activity against pneumococcus) or β-Lactam plus macrolide
Hospitalized	S. pneumoniae H. influenzae Polymicrobial (including anaerobes) Aerobic gram-negative bacilli Legionella C. pneumoniae Respiratory viruses	M. pneumoniae M. catarrhalis M. tuberculosis Endemic fungi	Intravenous (IV) β-lactam plus IV or oral macrolide or doxycycline or IV quinolone
Hospitalized, severe pneumonia	S. pneumoniae Legionella H. influenzae Aerobic gram-negative bacilli M. pneumoniae Respiratory viruses S. aureus	M. tuberculosis C. pneumoniae Endemic fungi	IV β-lactam plus either IV macrolide (azithromycin) or IV quinolone†

*Excludes patients with human immunodeficiency virus infection.

†If high risk for *Pseudomonas*, adjust regimen to include two antipseudomonal agents.

C. pneumoniae = *Chlamydophila pneumoniae*; *H. influenzae* = *Haemophilus influenzae*; *M. catarrhalis* = *Moraxella catarrhalis*; *M. pneumoniae* = *Mycoplasma pneumoniae*; *M. tuberculosis* = *Mycobacterium tuberculosis*; *S. aureus* = *Staphylococcus aureus*; *S. pneumoniae* = *Streptococcus pneumoniae*.

Adapted from Mandell LA, Wunderink RG, Anzueto A, et al; Infectious Diseases Society of America; American Thoracic Society: *Clin Infect Dis* 44(Suppl 2):S27–S72, 2007.

INTRATHORACIC COMPLICATIONS OF PNEUMONIA

As part of the discussion of pneumonia, two specific intrathoracic complications of pneumonia—lung abscess and empyema—are briefly considered because they represent important clinical sequelae.

LUNG ABSCESS

A lung abscess, like an abscess elsewhere, represents a localized collection of pus. In the lung, abscesses generally result from tissue destruction complicating a pneumonia. The abscess contents are primarily PMNs, often with collections of bacterial organisms. When antibiotics have been administered, organisms may no longer be obtainable from the abscess cavity.

Etiologic agents associated with formation of a lung abscess are generally those bacteria that cause significant tissue necrosis. Most commonly, anaerobic organisms are responsible, suggesting that aspiration of oropharyngeal contents is the predisposing event. However, aerobic organisms, such as *Staphylococcus* or enteric gram-negative rods, also can cause significant tissue destruction, with excavation of a region of lung parenchyma and abscess formation.

> Anaerobic bacteria are the agents most frequently responsible for lung abscesses.

Treatment of a lung abscess involves antibiotic therapy, often given for a more prolonged duration than for an uncomplicated pneumonia. Although abscesses elsewhere in the body are drained by surgical incision, lung abscesses generally drain through the tracheobronchial tree, and surgical intervention or placement of a drainage catheter is needed only rarely.

EMPYEMA

When a pneumonia extends to the pleural surface, the inflammatory process eventually may lead to empyema, another intrathoracic complication of pneumonia. The term *empyema* refers to pus in the pleural space. In its most florid form, an empyema represents thick, creamy, or yellow fluid within the pleural space. The fluid contains enormous numbers of leukocytes, primarily PMNs, often accompanied by bacterial organisms. With a frank empyema or often even with other grossly inflammatory pleural effusions accompanying pneumonia (parapneumonic effusions), pleural inflammation can result in formation of localized pockets of fluid or substantial scarring and limited mobility of the underlying lung.

Several different bacterial organisms may be associated with development of an empyema. Anaerobes are particularly common, but staphylococci and other aerobic organisms also are potential causes. After an empyema has been demonstrated, usually by thoracentesis and sampling of pleural fluid, drainage of the fluid is required. Most commonly, thoracoscopic surgery is performed to completely drain the pleural space. Alternative techniques are used in some specific clinical situations and can include open surgical procedures or placement of large-bore chest tubes with repeated instillation of fibrinolytic agents (e.g., streptokinase) into the pleural space.

> Adequate drainage of pleural fluid is important in the management of empyema.

RESPIRATORY INFECTIONS ASSOCIATED WITH BiOTERRORISM

The magnitude of society's concerns about bioterrorism changed abruptly after September 11, 2001, following the terrorist attacks on the World Trade Center and the Pentagon. Subsequent recognition of cases of both cutaneous and inhalational anthrax contracted by handling mail containing anthrax spores illustrated all too vividly not only the danger posed by some previously uncommon biologic agents but also the widespread fear elicited by the threat of bioterrorism. This section briefly discusses three biologic agents with life-threatening effects that can be mediated by infection involving the respiratory system: *Bacillus anthracis, Yersinia pestis,* and *Francisella tularensis.*

ANTHRAX

Bacillus anthracis, a gram-positive, spore-forming rod found in the soil, causes infection in farm stock and wild animals. Human cases have occurred as a result of exposure to infected animals, contaminated animal products, and inhalation of aerosolized spores. The virulence and potential lethality of the organism are related to elaboration of a toxin that causes prominent edema, inhibits neutrophil function, and alters the production of a number of cytokines. Whereas cutaneous anthrax results from spores introduced through a break in the skin, inhalational anthrax follows inhalation of spores into alveolar spaces and transport of viable spores via lymphatics to mediastinal lymph nodes. Germination of the spores in the mediastinum is associated with toxin release and with a hemorrhagic lymphadenitis and mediastinitis.

Clinically, patients with inhalational anthrax typically present with a flulike illness, with symptoms of mild fever, myalgias, nonproductive cough, malaise, and chest discomfort. Several days later, patients become acutely and severely ill, with fever, dyspnea, cyanosis, septic shock, and often findings of meningitis. The most prominent abnormality on chest radiograph is mediastinal widening from the hemorrhagic lymphadenitis and mediastinitis. Because viable spores are present in the mediastinum and not in the alveoli, anthrax is generally *not* transmitted from person to person via droplet nuclei. Despite treatment with ciprofloxacin or doxycycline, mortality is extremely high after the onset of clinical illness, and public health guidelines have focused on prophylaxis (with either of these antibiotics) to prevent inhalational anthrax following confirmed or suspected exposure to aerosolized spores. An anthrax vaccine is available but requires a complex administration schedule and annual booster injections.

> Inhalational anthrax characteristically produces a widened mediastinum on chest radiograph.

PLAGUE

Despite its association with epidemics of devastating proportions, such as the Black Death of the fourteenth century, plague is now an uncommon disease in the United States, although it is endemic in some parts of the world. However, plague is one of the conditions thought to be of major concern as a possible weapon of bioterrorism. The causative organism is *Yersinia pestis*, a gram-negative rod that is transmitted by fleas from rodents to humans. Infection through the skin disseminates to regional lymph nodes, leading to the clinical syndrome of *bubonic plague.* Infection of the lungs *(pneumonic plague)* can occur either secondary to bacteremic spread from skin or lymph nodes or via airborne transmission of the organism from person to person. Pneumonic plague is highly contagious through aerosolization of the organisms during cough.

Pulmonary involvement is characterized by a widespread bronchopneumonia, which can have regions of homogeneous consolidation. Clinically, patients become acutely ill with high fever, malaise, myalgias, rigors, dyspnea, and cyanosis. Chest radiography shows widespread bronchopneumonia, with a diffuse pattern that can resemble the acute respiratory distress syndrome. Mortality is high unless antibiotic treatment is initiated soon after the onset of symptoms. Streptomycin and doxycycline are the agents of choice.

TULAREMIA

Tularemia is caused by *Francisella tularensis,* a gram-negative coccobacillary organism that infects small mammals and is transmitted to humans by insect vectors (e.g., ticks), exposure to contaminated animals, or inhalation of aerosolized organisms. Although several different forms of clinical presentation may occur with tularemia, depending on the mechanism of transmission and the site of entry, pulmonary tularemia secondary to inhalation of *F. tularensis* is the primary concern for use of this organism as a bioterrorist weapon.

Pulmonary tularemia is characterized by patchy inflammation and consolidation of the lung parenchyma, sometimes with enlargement of hilar lymph nodes and development of pleural effusions. Patients develop fever, chills, malaise, and headache. Chest radiography shows patchy consolidation that may be accompanied by hilar lymphadenopathy and pleural effusions. Treatment consists of streptomycin, and mortality is estimated to be approximately 35% without treatment.

REFERENCES

GENERAL REVIEWS

American Thoracic Society and Infectious Diseases Society of America: Guidelines for the management of adults with hospital-acquired, ventilator-associated, and healthcare-associated pneumonia, *Am J Respir Crit Care Med* 171:388–416, 2005.

Bartlett JG, Dowell SF, Mandell LA, File TM Jr, Musher DM, Fine MJ: Practice guidelines for the management of community-acquired pneumonia in adults, *Clin Infect Dis* 31:347–382, 2000.

Chastre J, Fagon J-Y: Ventilator-associated pneumonia, *Am J Respir Crit Care Med* 165:867–903, 2002.

Ewig S, Bauer T, Torres A: Nosocomial pneumonia, *Thorax* 57:366–371, 2002.

Fine MJ, Smith MA, Carson CA, et al: Prognosis and outcomes of patients with community-acquired pneumonia, *JAMA* 274:134–141, 1996.

Franquet T: Imaging of pneumonia: trends and algorithms, *Eur Respir J* 18:196–208, 2001.

Guthrie R: Community-acquired lower respiratory tract infections. Etiology and treatment, *Chest* 120:2021–2034, 2001.

Halm EA, Teirstein AS: Management of community-acquired pneumonia, *N Engl J Med* 347:2039–2045, 2002.

Hoare Z, Lim WS: Pneumonia: update on diagnosis and management, *BMJ* 332:1077–1079, 2006.

Kollef MH: Prevention of hospital-associated pneumonia and ventilator-associated pneumonia, *Crit Care Med* 32:1396–1405, 2004.

Leong JR, Huang DT: Ventilator-associated pneumonia, *Surg Clin North Am* 86:1409–1429, 2006.

Mandell LA, Wunderink RG, Anzueto A, et al; Infectious Diseases Society of America; American Thoracic Society: Infectious Diseases Society of America/American Thoracic Society consensus guidelines on the management of community-acquired pneumonia in adults, *Clin Infect Dis* 44(suppl 2):S27–S72, 2007.

Niederman MS: Recent advances in community-acquired pneumonia: inpatient and outpatient, *Chest* 131:1205–1215, 2007.

Porzecanski I, Bowton DL: Diagnosis and treatment of ventilator-associated pneumonia, *Chest* 130: 597–604, 2006.

PNEUMONIA CAUSED BY SPECIFIC ORGANISMS

Bartlett JG: Anaerobic bacterial infections of the lung, *Chest* 91:901–909, 1987.

File TM: Streptococcus pneumoniae and community-acquired pneumonia: a cause for concern, *Am J Med* 117(suppl 3A):39S–50S, 2004.

Gupta SK, Sarosi GA: The role of atypical pathogens in community-acquired pneumonia, *Med Clin North Am* 85:1349–1365, 2001.

Hall CB: Respiratory syncytial virus and parainfluenza virus, *N Engl J Med* 344:1917–1928, 2001.

Hammerschlag MR: Chlamydia pneumoniae and the lung, *Eur Respir J* 16:1001–1007, 2000.

Harwell JI, Brown RB: The drug-resistant pneumococcus. Clinical relevance, therapy, and prevention, *Chest* 117:530–541, 2000.

Kaye MG, Fox MJ, Bartlett JG, Braman SS, Glassroth J: The clinical spectrum of Staphylococcus aureus pulmonary infection, *Chest* 97:788–792, 1990.

Lednicky JA: Hantaviruses. A short review, *Arch Pathol Lab Med* 127:30–35, 2003.

Mansel JK, Rosenow EC III, Smith TF, Martin JW Jr: Mycoplasma pneumoniae pneumonia. *Chest* 95: 639–646, 1989.

Marik PE: Aspiration pneumonitis and aspiration pneumonia, *N Engl J Med* 344:665–671, 2001.

Peiris JS, Yuen KY, Osterhaus AD, Stöhr K: The severe acute respiratory syndrome, *N Engl J Med* 349:2431–2441, 2003.

Rose RM, Pinkston P, O'Donnell C, Jensen WA: Viral infection of the lower respiratory tract, *Clin Chest Med* 8:405–418, 1987.

Sanders CV, Kamholz SL, editors: Pneumococcal disease: a symposium in honor of Robert Austrian, MD, *Am J Med* 107(suppl):1S–90S, 1999.

Stout JE, Yu VL: Legionellosis, *N Engl J Med* 337:682–687, 1997.

Tuomanen EI, Austrian R, Masure HR: Pathogenesis of pneumococcal infection, *N Engl J Med* 332:1280–1284, 1995.

Whitney CG, Farley MM, Hadler J, et al; Active Bacterial Core Surveillance Program of the Emerging Infections Program Network: Increasing prevalence of multidrug-resistant Streptococcus pneumoniae in the United States, *N Engl J Med* 343:1917–1924, 2000.

Wilson R, Dowling RB: Pseudomonas aeruginosa and other related species, *Thorax* 53:213–219, 1998.

Writing Committee of the Second World Health Organization Consultation on Clinical Aspects of Human Infection with Avian Influenza A (H5N1) Virus: Update on avian influenza A (H5N1) virus infection in humans, *N Engl J Med* 358: 261–273, 2008.

RESPIRATORY INFECTIONS ASSOCIATED WITH BIOTERRORISM

Bellamy RJ, Freedman AR: Bioterrorism, *QJM* 94:227–234, 2001.

Borio L, Frank D, Mani V, et al: Death due to bioterrorism-related inhalational anthrax. Report of 2 patients, *JAMA* 286:2554–2559, 2001.

Bush LM, Abrams BH, Beall A, Johnson CC: Index case of fatal inhalational anthrax due to bioterrorism in the United States, *N Engl J Med* 345:1607–1610, 2001.

Centers for Disease Control: Recognition of illness associated with the intentional release of a biologic agent, *MMWR* 50:893–897, 2001.

Inglesby TV, O'Toole T, Henderson DA, et al; Working Group on Civilian Biodefense: Anthrax as a biological weapon, 2002. Updated recommendations for management, *JAMA* 287:2236–2252, 2002.

Mayer TA, Bersoff-Matcha S, Murphy C, et al: Clinical presentation of inhalational anthrax following bioterrorism exposure. Report of 2 surviving patients, *JAMA* 286:2549–2553, 2001.

Prentice MB, Rahalison L: Plague, *Lancet* 369:1196–1207, 2007.

Swartz MN: Recognition and management of anthrax—an update, *N Engl J Med* 345:1621–1626, 2001.

24

Tuberculosis and Nontuberculous Mycobacteria

ETIOLOGY AND PATHOGENESIS	**DIAGNOSTIC APPROACH**
DEFINITIONS	**PRINCIPLES OF THERAPY**
PATHOLOGY	**NONTUBERCULOUS**
PATHOPHYSIOLOGY	**MYCOBACTERIA**
CLINICAL MANIFESTATIONS	

Throughout the centuries, few diseases have claimed so many lives, caused so much morbidity, and been so dreaded as tuberculosis. At the turn of the twentieth century, tuberculosis was the single most common cause of death in the United States; more than 80% of the population was infected before the age of 20 years. At the beginning of the twenty-first century, tuberculosis provides a stark example of the disparity in health resources between industrialized nations and the developing world. In the United States and Europe, few diseases have declined so greatly in the frequency of cases and in mortality as has tuberculosis. Two main factors have been responsible: an overall improvement in living conditions and the development of effective chemotherapy, which has made tuberculosis a curable disease. However, in countries with fewer resources, the disease continues to be a health crisis, often striking the young, most productive members of society.

Now more than 125 years since identification of the tubercle bacillus by Robert Koch in 1882, we cannot become complacent about the disease. It has been estimated that approximately one third of the world's population has been infected (i.e., has either latent or active infection) with the tubercle bacillus, with 8 to 10 million new cases of active tuberculosis and approximately 2 to 3 million deaths occurring worldwide each year. The overwhelming majority of cases of active tuberculosis occur in developing countries. Approximately 70 million of the 88 million cases of tuberculosis during the 1990s were from Asia and sub-Saharan Africa, where coinfection with the human immunodeficiency virus (HIV) is a major contributor to the increase in infections. Tuberculosis remains an important public health problem in the United States, particularly in indigent and immigrant populations and in patients with the acquired immunodeficiency syndrome (AIDS; see Chapter 26). Reported cases of tuberculosis in the United States were decreasing until the mid-1980s, at which time the AIDS epidemic and immigration from countries with a high prevalence of tuberculosis combined to result in an increasing frequency of cases. Fortunately, since 1991 the number of cases reported annually in the United States has again begun to decrease. Perhaps most alarming, however, both in the United States and throughout the world, is the relatively recent emergence of drug-resistant strains of the organism, some of which are resistant to multiple antituberculous drugs.

ETIOLOGY AND PATHOGENESIS

The etiologic agent that causes tuberculosis, *Mycobacterium tuberculosis*, is an aerobic, rod-shaped bacterium. An important property of the tubercle bacillus is its ability to retain certain stains even after exposure to acid (discussed in the section on diagnostic approach); thus mycobacteria are said to be *acid-fast*.

Transmission of the disease occurs via small aerosol droplets, generally from 1 to 5 μm in size, that contain the microorganism. The source of these droplets is an individual with tuberculosis who harbors the organism, often excreting tubercle bacilli in the sputum or in small droplets produced during commonplace activities such as speaking, coughing, singing, and laughing. Most commonly, transmission occurs with relatively close contact, often between related individuals or others living in the same household. The disease is not transmitted by fomites (i.e., articles of clothing, eating utensils); direct inhalation of droplets aerosolized by another individual is almost exclusively the mode of spread.

> Transmission of tuberculosis is by inhalation of small aerosol droplets containing the organism.

When droplets containing mycobacteria are inhaled and reach the alveoli, a small focus of *primary* infection develops, consisting of the organisms and an inflammatory process mounted by the host. Alveolar macrophages represent the primary initial defense against organisms reaching the parenchyma, and they are a particularly important component of the resulting inflammatory response. After the initial infection has started, organisms frequently spread via lymphatic vessels to draining hilar lymph nodes as well as via the bloodstream to distant organs and to other regions of lung, particularly the apices. In the majority of cases, even though lymphatic and hematogenous spread may occur, the body's defense mechanisms (in the lung and elsewhere) are capable of controlling and limiting the primary infection. An important component of the body's acquired defense against *M. tuberculosis* is the development of cell-mediated immunity (delayed hypersensitivity) against the mycobacterial organisms. This sensitization and development of a cell-mediated immune response generally occur within several weeks of initial exposure.

The patient usually is unaware of the primary infection. The only tracks left by the organism are those related to the host's response to the bacillus: either the local tissue response or evidence that the host has become sensitized to the tubercle bacillus (i.e., positive delayed hypersensitivity skin test reaction). In a few patients, probably 5% or fewer, the defense mechanisms are unable to control the primary infection, and clinically apparent primary tuberculosis results. This is most common if the host is immunocompromised because of medications, alcoholism, or the presence of HIV/AIDS or malignancy.

Even when the primary infection apparently has been controlled, the tubercle bacillus may not be completely eliminated from the host. A small number of organisms often remain in a dormant or latent state, not killed but also not proliferating or causing any apparent active disease. The majority of patients will never have any further difficulty with development of clinically active tuberculosis. However, in some patients the delicate balance between the organism and host defense mechanisms eventually breaks down, often after many years, and a dormant focus of infection becomes active. These patients with active disease occurring at a time removed from the primary infection "are said to have *reactivation* tuberculosis. For both primary and reactivation disease, the lungs are the most commonly affected site. However, with either type of disease, distant organ systems may be involved as a result of hematogenous spread during the primary phase of the infection. In addition, a disseminated disease, known as *miliary tuberculosis*, may result from hematogenous dissemination of the organisms.

> The majority of active tuberculosis cases involve reactivation of a previously dormant focus within the lungs.

Over the course of a lifetime, it is estimated that approximately 10% of individuals with a normal immune system who have been infected with *M. tuberculosis* (and have not received "preventive" treatment to eradicate dormant organisms) will develop active disease. The risk of developing active tuberculosis is particularly notable within the first 2 years after the initial infection; approximately half of the patients who develop active disease do so within this time frame. The other half of patients who develop active disease do so at some later point in life. These estimates of risk apply to patients with normal host defenses. The risk of developing active tuberculosis is dramatically higher in patients with defective cellular immunity as a consequence of HIV infection and low CD4$^+$ counts.

DEFINITIONS

On the basis of our understanding of disease pathogenesis, a few additional terms are worth defining. First is the distinction between tuberculous infection and tuberculous disease. *Tuberculous infection (or latent tuberculous infection)* is defined by a positive tuberculin skin test or a positive interferon-γ release assay (described in the section on diagnostic approach) but no evidence of active disease. Patients with latent tuberculous infection have been infected by the organism, but the initial infection was controlled by the body's host defense mechanisms and subsequently can be traced only by the positive delayed hypersensitivity skin test response. The small number of remaining organisms are in a dormant or latent state, but they do pose a risk for reactivation at a later time, especially with any impairment in the host's cellular immunity. *Tuberculous disease (or active tuberculosis),* on the other hand, is defined by the presence of clinically active disease in one or more organ systems, ideally with confirmation of the diagnosis by isolation of the organism *M. tuberculosis.*

The other terms worth defining are those that describe different subsets of tuberculous disease. Most common are the terms *primary* and *reactivation tuberculosis,* which refer to disease following the initial exposure and disease that reactivates after a period of latency, respectively. Several other terms are sometimes used to describe clinical disease on the basis of the presumed pathogenesis. The term *progressive primary tuberculosis* reflects primary disease that has not been controlled by host defense mechanisms and has continued to be active beyond the point at which delayed hypersensitivity has developed. As a general rule, cellular immunity develops 2 to 10 weeks after the initial infection, and continuing active disease beyond this time has many of the features of reactivation tuberculosis. The term *postprimary tuberculosis* refers to disease beyond the initial primary infection. Although this term usually refers to reactivation disease, it sometimes includes cases of progressive primary tuberculosis.

The term *reinfection tuberculosis* refers to disease in a previously infected person that results not from reactivation of dormant tubercle bacilli but from new exposure to another source of organisms. This type of infection traditionally has been considered uncommon. It is believed that individuals with prior exposure to tuberculosis who manifest delayed hypersensitivity to the organism are relatively resistant to exogenous reinfection from another source. However, studies using DNA fingerprinting techniques suggest that reinfection with another organism is more common than previously thought, particularly in patients who are infected with HIV.

PATHOLOGY

The pathologic features of pulmonary tuberculosis vary according to the stage of infection. The primary infection in the lung consists of the organisms and a relatively nonspecific inflammatory response in the involved region of parenchyma. Regional lymph nodes often become involved by local spread of the organism, and the combination of the primary area in the lung (the *Ghon lesion)* and involved lymph nodes is termed a *Ranke complex.*

When delayed hypersensitivity is present, either weeks after the primary infection or during a period of reactivation disease, a different pathologic pattern emerges. The hallmarks are the presence of (1) granulomas (collections of activated blood and tissue-derived macrophages termed *epithelioid histiocytes* surrounded by a rim of lymphocytes), and (2) caseous necrosis (foci of necrosis and softening at the center of a granuloma). Within the region of caseous necrosis, the contents can liquefy and slough, leaving behind a cavity, another hallmark of tuberculosis. Other features of the granulomas include multinucleated giant cells and often the presence of tubercle bacilli.

> After development of delayed hypersensitivity, the pathologic hallmarks of tuberculosis are granulomas and caseous necrosis, often with cavity formation.

A process of healing tends to occur at the sites of disease. Fibrosis or scarring ensues, often associated with contraction of the affected area and deposition of calcium. With full-blown tuberculosis, extensive destruction of lung tissue results from large areas of inflammation, granuloma formation, caseous necrosis, and cavitation, along with fibrosis, contraction, and foci of calcification. Interestingly, much of the destruction that occurs during tuberculosis infection requires an intact cellular immune system and appears to be due to the host inflammatory response attempting to contain the infection. As a result, patients with advanced HIV disease often have an atypical presentation in which the organism is widely disseminated but there is little evidence of cavitation and fibrosis.

Tuberculosis is capable of spread, and spread of organisms through the bloodstream at the time of primary infection is probably the rule rather than the exception. When defense mechanisms break down, disease can become apparent at other sites (e.g., liver, kidney, adrenal glands, bones, central nervous system). Spread also occurs to other regions of the lung, either as a result of hematogenous seeding during the primary infection or because of spilling of infected secretions or caseous material into the bronchi and other regions of the lung.

Within the lung, characteristic locations for reactivation tuberculosis are the apical regions of the upper lobes and, to a lesser extent, the superior segment of the lower lobes. It is believed that these are not the sites of the primary infection but rather the favored location for implantation of organisms after hematogenous spread. These regions have a high Po_2 and relatively less perfusion and thus are believed to be particularly suitable for survival of the aerobic tubercle bacilli.

PATHOPHYSIOLOGY

Most of the clinical features of pulmonary tuberculosis can be attributed to one of two aspects of the disease: the presence of a poorly controlled chronic infection or a chronic destructive process within the lung parenchyma. A variety of other manifestations result from extrapulmonary spread of tuberculosis, but these consequences are not considered here.

Why chronic infection within the lung produces systemic manifestations is not entirely clear. However, as implied by the term "consumption," used so frequently in the past, tuberculosis is a disease in which systemic manifestations such as weight loss, wasting, and loss of appetite are prominent features. These and other systemic effects of tuberculosis are discussed in the section on clinical manifestations.

The chronic destructive process involving the pulmonary parenchyma entails progressive scarring and loss of lung tissue. However, respiratory function is generally preserved more than would be expected, perhaps because the disease often is limited to the apical and posterior regions of the upper lobes as well as to the superior segment of the lower lobes. Oxygenation also tends to be surprisingly preserved, presumably because ventilation and perfusion are destroyed simultaneously in the affected lung. Consequently, ventilation-perfusion mismatch is not nearly so great as in many other parenchymal and airway diseases.

CLINICAL MANIFESTATIONS

There is an important distinction—and thus important clinical differences—between tuberculous infection and tuberculous disease (active tuberculosis). Tuberculous infection is the consequence of primary exposure, by which the bacilli have become established in the patient; however, host defense mechanisms have prevented any clinically apparent disease. Specific immunity to the tubercle bacillus can be demonstrated by a positive reaction to a skin test for delayed hypersensitivity or a positive interferon-γ assay; otherwise, there is no evidence for proliferation of bacteria or for tissue involvement by disease. Patients with infection but without disease are not contagious. In contrast, the disease tuberculosis is associated with proliferation of organisms, accompanied by a tissue response and generally (although not always) clinical problems of which the patient is aware.

Patients with pulmonary tuberculosis can manifest (1) systemic symptoms, (2) symptoms referable to the respiratory tract, or (3) an abnormal finding on chest radiograph but no clinical symptoms. When symptoms occur, they generally are insidious rather than acute in onset.

Systemic symptoms often are relatively nonspecific, such as weight loss, anorexia, fatigue, low-grade fever, and night sweats. The most common symptoms resulting from pulmonary involvement are cough, sputum production, and hemoptysis; chest pain occasionally is present. Many patients have neither systemic nor pulmonary symptoms and come to the attention of a physician because of an abnormal finding on chest radiograph, often performed for an unrelated reason.

Patients with extrapulmonary involvement frequently have pulmonary tuberculosis as well, but occasional cases are limited to an extrapulmonary site. The pericardium, pleura, kidney, peritoneum, adrenal glands, and central nervous system each may be involved, with symptoms resulting from the particular organ or region that is affected. With miliary tuberculosis, the disease is disseminated, and patients usually are systemically quite ill.

Physical examination of the patient with pulmonary tuberculosis may show the ravages of a chronic infection, with evidence of wasting and weight loss. This presentation is uncommon in patients with access to health care but is frequently seen in the developing world. Findings on chest examination tend to be relatively insignificant, although sometimes evidence of crackles or rales over affected areas is observed. If a tuberculous pleural effusion is present, the physical findings characteristic of an effusion may be found.

> Common presenting problems with tuberculosis are the following:
> 1. Systemic symptoms: weight loss, fever, night sweats
> 2. Pulmonary symptoms: cough, sputum production, hemoptysis
> 3. Abnormal chest radiographic findings

DIAGNOSTIC APPROACH

One of the most commonly used diagnostic tools, the tuberculin skin test, documents tuberculous infection rather than active disease. A small amount of protein derived from the tubercle bacillus (purified protein derivative [PPD]) is injected intradermally. Individuals who have been exposed to *M. tuberculosis* and have acquired cellular immunity to the organism demonstrate a positive test reaction, seen as induration or swelling at the site of injection after 48 to 72 hours. The criteria for determining a positive skin test reaction vary according to the clinical setting, specifically of the presence or absence of immunosuppression and/or epidemiologic risk factors affecting the likelihood of previous exposure to tuberculosis. Importantly, the test does not distinguish between individuals who have active tuberculosis and those who merely have acquired delayed hypersensitivity from previous infection. However, because reactivation tuberculosis occurs in patients with previous tuberculous infection, a positive skin test reaction does identify individuals at higher risk for subsequent development of active disease.

As for most diagnostic tests, false-negative results can occur with the tuberculin skin test. Faulty administration, an inactive batch of skin-testing material, and underlying diseases that depress cellular immunity, such as HIV, are a few causes of false-negative skin test reactions. On the other hand, not all patients who react to tuberculoprotein have been exposed to *M. tuberculosis*. Infection with nontuberculous mycobacteria, often called *atypical mycobacteria,* is sometimes associated with a positive or a borderline positive skin test reaction to PPD.

Blood tests that detect latent tuberculosis have been developed. The tests involve incubating the patient's T cells with *M. tuberculosis* antigens. Cells from previously sensitized individuals release interferon-γ in response to the antigens, and the interferon-γ is detected by an enzyme-linked assay. Tuberculin skin testing remains more commonly performed than interferon-γ assays. However, blood tests have the advantage of lower labor costs by not requiring patients to return for an office visit for the skin test interpretation. These assays are unaffected by prior bacille Calmette-Guérin (BCG) vaccination (see section on principles of therapy).

For diagnosis of tuberculosis (i.e., actual tuberculous disease), an important initial diagnostic tool is the chest radiograph. In primary disease, the chest radiograph may show a nonspecific infiltrate, often but certainly not exclusively in the lower lobes (in contrast to the upper lobe predominance of reactivation disease). Hilar (and sometimes paratracheal) lymph node enlargement may be seen, reflecting involvement of the draining node by the organism and by the primary infection. Pleural involvement may be seen, with development of a pleural effusion.

> Common features of the chest radiograph in primary tuberculosis are the following:
> 1. Nonspecific infiltrate (often lower lobe)
> 2. Hilar (and paratracheal) node enlargement
> 3. Pleural effusion

When the primary disease heals, the chest radiograph frequently shows some residua of the healing process. Most common are small, calcified lesions within the pulmonary parenchyma, reflecting a collection of calcified granulomas. Calcification within hilar or paratracheal lymph nodes may be seen. The radiographic terminology can be confusing as it is commonly used. The term *granuloma* is actually a pathologic term that describes a microscopic collection of lymphocytes and histiocytes. A calcified nodule on a chest radiograph is frequently called a *calcified granuloma,* but it really represents a small mass of numerous microscopic granulomas.

With reactivation tuberculosis, the most common sites of disease are the apical and posterior segments of the upper lobes and, to a lesser extent, the superior segment of the lower lobes. A variety of patterns can be seen: infiltrates, cavities, nodules, and scarring and contraction (Fig. 24-1). The presence of abnormal findings on a chest radiograph does not necessarily indicate active disease. The disease may be old, stable, and currently inactive, and it is difficult, if not impossible, to gauge activity on the basis of radiographic appearance.

> Radiographic location of reactivation tuberculosis: most commonly apical and posterior segments of upper lobe(s), superior segment of lower lobe(s).

Definitive diagnosis of tuberculosis rests on culturing the organism, either from secretions (e.g., sputum) or from tissue. However, the organisms are slow growing, with possibly 6 weeks required for growth and final identification of the organism. Culture of the organism is important not only for confirmation of the diagnosis but also for testing sensitivity to antituberculous drugs, particularly in light of concerns about resistance to some of the commonly used antituberculous agents.

Another extremely useful procedure for which results are available almost immediately is staining of material obtained from the tracheobronchial tree. The specimens obtained can be sputum, expectorated either spontaneously or following inhalation of

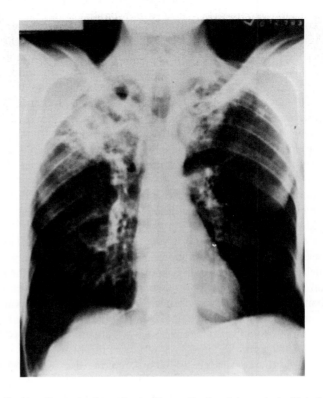

Figure 24-1. Chest radiograph of a patient with reactivation tuberculosis. Note infiltrates with cavitation at both apices, more prominent on the right.

an irritating aerosol (sputum induction), or washings or biopsy samples obtained by fiberoptic bronchoscopy. A hallmark of mycobacterial organisms is their ability to retain certain dyes even after exposure to acid. Their acid-fast property is generally demonstrated with Ziehl-Neelsen or Kinyoun stain or with a fluorescent stain that uses auramine-rhodamine. The finding of a single acid-fast bacillus from sputum or tracheobronchial washings is clinically significant in the majority of cases. One qualification is that nontuberculous mycobacteria, which either cause disease or are present as colonizing organisms or contaminants, have the same staining properties. Therefore, it is critical to determine whether acid-fast bacilli seen on smear represent *M. tuberculosis* or nontuberculous mycobacteria. This distinction can be made either by certain growth characteristics on culture or, more recently, by molecular biologic techniques.

In order for even one tubercle bacillus to be seen on smear, large numbers of organisms must be present in the lungs. Therefore, if few organisms are present, even if they are causing disease, the smear results may be negative, whereas culture findings often will be positive in this setting. In general, the infectiousness of a patient with tuberculosis correlates with the number of organisms the patient is harboring and the presence of organisms on smear. Patients whose sputum is positive by smear tend to be much more infectious than patients whose sputum is positive by culture but negative by smear.

Because of the insensitivity of sputum smears and the time required for *M. tuberculosis* to grow in culture, rapid and more sensitive methods for establishing the diagnosis of tuberculosis have been developed. One technique involves detection of radiolabeled CO_2 after incubation of the specimen with radiolabeled palmitic acid, a metabolic substrate for mycobacteria. Results can be obtained much more quickly with this technique (BACTEC system; Becton, Dickinson, Franklin Lakes, NJ) than with traditional culture techniques. The BACTEC system frequently is combined with very sensitive molecular biologic assays. The BACTEC system indicates when an otherwise undetectable quantity of mycobacteria has grown, thus providing minute quantities of genetic material. The genetic material is processed with molecular biologic techniques, such as amplification of DNA with polymerase chain reaction technology or use of DNA probes to detect ribosomal RNA. These genetic techniques often are applied after identification of acid-fast bacilli on a sputum smear and are used as a rapid method for distinguishing whether the organisms represent *M. tuberculosis* or nontuberculous mycobacteria.

Functional assessment of the patient with tuberculosis often shows surprisingly little impairment of pulmonary function. Such testing is useful primarily for the patient who already has compromised pulmonary function, when there is concern about how much of the patient's reserve has been lost. However, a patient who is potentially contagious should not be evaluated with pulmonary function testing because of the possibility of infecting others during the testing maneuvers. Arterial blood gases often are relatively preserved, with normal or decreased Po_2, depending on the amount of ventilation-perfusion mismatch that has resulted.

PRINCIPLES OF THERAPY

Effective chemotherapy is available for most cases of tuberculosis. Whereas treatment for tuberculosis used to be minimally effective, involving prolonged hospitalization (usually in a sanatorium) or a variety of surgical procedures, the majority of cases now are curable with appropriate drug therapy. Patients are treated for a prolonged period, generally with a minimum of two effective antituberculous agents. Therapy for as few as 6 months with two very effective antituberculous agents, isoniazid and rifampin, supplemented during the first 2 months by a third agent, pyrazinamide, is commonly used in cases of pulmonary tuberculosis, with excellent results in patients with a normal immune system. However, because of concern for organisms resistant to one or more antituberculous agents, a fourth drug (ethambutol) typically is added at the initiation of therapy until drug sensitivity results become available. When resistance to one or more of the usual antituberculous agents is documented, the specific regimen and the duration of therapy must be adjusted accordingly.

Treatment can be administered in an outpatient setting, unless the patient is sufficiently ill to require hospitalization. Patients whose sputum smears initially were positive are generally considered no longer infectious after they have demonstrated a clinical response to antituberculous therapy and after their sputum has become smear-negative on three successive samples. A critical issue determining the success of antituberculous therapy is the patient's compliance with the medical regimen. Erratic or incomplete therapy is associated with a risk of treatment failure and of emergence of resistant organisms, with potentially disastrous consequences. As a result, use of directly observed therapy, in which the drugs are given in a supervised outpatient setting, has become an important component of treatment for many cases of tuberculosis and is essential when there are concerns regarding patient compliance.

Thus, effective therapy for tuberculosis requires long-term chemotherapy for all patients and directly observed therapy for many patients. Treatment is expensive and labor intensive, and is most successful with a well-funded and effective public health system. Even in industrialized nations, this presents difficulties. In many parts of the world, this type of public health system is nonexistent.

In addition to multiple drug therapy administered for active tuberculosis, therapy with isoniazid alone (typically for 9 months) is generally administered to household members of patients with recently diagnosed tuberculosis and to newly infected persons (documented by recent conversion to a positive skin test reaction). Such

A common treatment of pulmonary tuberculosis is isoniazid and rifampin given for 6 months, supplemented by pyrazinamide for the first 2 months and ethambutol until the organism's antimicrobial sensitivity is known.

Isoniazid alone for 9 months is indicated for selected patients with a positive PPD (i.e., tuberculous infection) but no evidence of active disease.

therapy substantially decreases the chances of active tuberculosis developing in these individuals, who are at particularly high risk.

Certain other patients with latent tuberculous infection, documented by a positive tuberculin skin test reaction but no evidence of active disease, are considered candidates for 9 months of treatment with isoniazid alone (or an alternative regimen). Specifically, this category includes patients who satisfy additional criteria (besides a positive PPD reaction) that put them at high risk for reactivation of a dormant infection. Examples include the presence of stable radiographic findings of old active tuberculosis but no prior therapy, or the presence of underlying diseases or treatment that impairs host defense mechanisms. Although this form of single-drug therapy was often called "prophylactic" or "preventive," it actually represents treatment aimed at eradicating a small number of dormant but viable organisms. It has been well demonstrated to be effective in achieving its goal of substantially decreasing the eventual risk for reactivation tuberculosis.

One recent major public health issue has been the development of organisms that are resistant to one or more of the commonly used antituberculous agents. In a survey performed by the Centers for Disease Control and Prevention, approximately 14% of cases of tuberculosis were due to an organism that was resistant to one or more antituberculous agents, and 3.5% of all cases were resistant to both isoniazid and rifampin, the two most effective antituberculous agents. This problem underscores the importance of public health measures to limit person-to-person transmission of tuberculosis as well as efforts to improve patient compliance with antituberculous medication.

The goal of developing an effective vaccine against *M. tuberculosis* remains an important step toward achieving worldwide eradication of tuberculosis. Vaccination with BCG, a live, attenuated strain of *M. bovis,* has been used for many years in various countries around the world, but it has not been recommended for use in the United States except in selected, rare circumstances. Although BCG vaccination appears to decrease the risk of serious and potentially life-threatening forms of tuberculosis in children, its efficacy in preventing pulmonary tuberculosis in adults is questionable. In addition, patients treated with BCG vaccination will, at least initially, have a positive response to a PPD test. Therefore, the PPD test will no longer be useful in detecting actual tuberculosis infection On a public health basis, in areas where TB is uncommon, interference with skin test interpretation is another reason why BCG is not used, although interferon-γ release assays still are accurate in this setting.

NONTUBERCULOUS MYCOBACTERIA

A variety of nontuberculous mycobacteria, sometimes called *atypical mycobacteria,* are potential pulmonary pathogens. They are generally found in water and soil, which appear to be the sources of exposure rather than person-to-person transmission. The most common organisms in this group are classified as belonging to *Mycobacterium avium* complex (MAC), formerly called *Mycobacterium avium-intracellulare.* Other organisms include *M. kansasii, M. xenopi,* and *M. fortuitum.*

The nontuberculous mycobacteria are responsible for disease primarily in two settings: (1) the patient with underlying lung disease, in whom local host defense mechanisms presumably are impaired, and (2) the patient with a defect in systemic immunity, particularly AIDS (see Chapter 26). Nevertheless, disease develops as a result of these organisms in a small number of patients without either of these risk factors. Overall, the recognition of disease from nontuberculous mycobacteria has increased over the past 10 to 20 years, in large part because of its occurrence in patients with AIDS.

Disease caused by nontuberculous mycobacteria can be localized to the lung, where it can mimic tuberculosis, or it can be found after hematogenous dissemination

Atypical mycobacteria are most frequently pathogens in patients with underlying lung disease or AIDS.

throughout the body, particularly in patients with AIDS. Diagnosis of disease caused by these organisms is difficult. The organisms can be found as laboratory contaminants; and, in patients with other underlying lung diseases, the organisms can colonize the respiratory system without being responsible for invasive disease.

When these organisms cause disease, treatment typically involves multiple agents. The organisms frequently are resistant to some of the standard antimycobacterial drugs, so treatment regimens traditionally were complicated and often unsuccessful. Fortunately, the newer macrolide antibiotics, such as clarithromycin and azithromycin, often are effective, and they become particularly useful components of the therapeutic regimen for many of the nontuberculous mycobacteria. A more complete discussion of this topic is beyond the scope of this text, and the reader is referred to the review articles in the references.

REFERENCES

GENERAL REVIEWS

American Thoracic Society: Diagnostic standards and classification of tuberculosis in adults and children, *Am J Respir Crit Care Med* 161:1376–1395, 2000.

Centers for Disease Control and Prevention (CDC): Trends in tuberculosis incidence—United States, 2006, *MMWR Morb Mortal Wkly Rep* 56:245–250, 2007.

Havlir DV, Barnes PF: Current concepts: tuberculosis in patients with human immunodeficiency virus infection, *N Engl J Med* 340:367–373, 1999.

Iseman MD, Huitt GA, editors: Tuberculosis, *Clin Chest Med* 18:1–168, 1997.

Lauzardo M, Ashkin D: Phthisiology at the dawn of the new century, *Chest* 117:1455–1473, 2000.

Yew WW, Leung CC: Update in tuberculosis 2007, *Am J Respir Crit Care Med* 177:479–485, 2008.

PATHOGENESIS

Alland D, Kalkut GE, Moss AR, et al: Transmission of tuberculosis in New York City, *N Engl J Med* 330:1710–1716, 1994.

Barnes PF, Cave MD: Current concepts: molecular epidemiology of tuberculosis, *N Engl J Med* 349:1149–1156, 2003.

Quast TM, Browning RF: Pathogenesis and clinical manifestations of pulmonary tuberculosis, *Dis Mon* 52:413–419, 2006.

Schluger NW: The pathogenesis of tuberculosis: the first one hundred (and twenty-three) years, *Am J Respir Cell Mol Biol* 32:251–256, 2005.

Schluger NW, Rom WN: The host immune response to tuberculosis, *Am J Respir Crit Care Med* 157:679–691, 1998.

Smith I, Nathan C, Peavy HH: Progress and new directions in genetics of tuberculosis: an NHLBI working group report, *Am J Respir Crit Care Med* 172:1491–1496, 2005.

van Crevel R, Ottenhoff TH, van der Meer JW: Innate immunity to Mycobacterium tuberculosis, *Clin Microbiol Rev* 15:294–309, 2002.

CLINICAL MANIFESTATIONS AND DIAGNOSTIC APPROACH

Alvarez S, McCabe WR: Extrapulmonary tuberculosis revisited: a review of experience at Boston City and other hospitals, *Medicine* 63:25–55, 1984.

American Thoracic Society: Diagnostic standards and classification of tuberculosis in adults and children, *Am J Respir Crit Care Med* 161:1376–1395, 2000.

American Thoracic Society: Targeted tuberculin testing and treatment of latent tuberculosis infection, *Am J Respir Crit Care Med* 161:S221–S247, 2000.

Antoniskis D, Amin K, Barnes PF: Pleuritis as a manifestation of reactivation tuberculosis, *Am J Med* 89:447–450, 1990.

Berger HW, Mejia E: Tuberculous pleurisy, *Chest* 63:88–92, 1973.

Sahn SA, Neff TA: Miliary tuberculosis, *Am J Med* 56:495-505, 1974.

Schluger NW: Changing approaches to the diagnosis of tuberculosis, *Am J Respir Crit Care Med* 164:2020–2024, 2001.

Weir MR, Thornton GF: Extrapulmonary tuberculosis, *Am J Med* 79:467–478, 1985.

TREATMENT

American Thoracic Society: Targeted tuberculin testing and treatment of latent tuberculosis infection, *Am J Respir Crit Care Med* 161:S221–S247, 2000.

American Thoracic Society, Centers for Disease Control and Prevention, and Infectious Diseases Society of America: Treatment of tuberculosis, *Am J Respir Crit Care Med* 167:603–662, 2003.

Centers for Disease Control and Prevention (CDC): Emergence of Mycobacterium tuberculosis with extensive resistance to second-line drugs—worldwide, 2000-2004, *MMWR Morb Mortal Wkly Rep* 55:301–305, 2006.

Chaulk CP, Kazandjian VA, Public Health Tuberculosis Guidelines Panel: Directly observed therapy for treatment completion of pulmonary tuberculosis, *JAMA* 279:943–948, 1998.

Cohn DL: Treatment of latent tuberculosis infection, *Semin Respir Infect* 18:249–262, 2003.

European Respiratory Society Task Force: Tuberculosis management in Europe, *Eur Respir J* 14:978-992, 1999.

Horsburgh CR Jr, Feldman S, Ridzon R: Practice guidelines for the treatment of tuberculosis, *Clin Infect Dis* 31:633–639, 2000.

Jasmer RM, Nahid P, Hopewell PC: Latent tuberculosis infection, *N Engl J Med* 347:1860–1866, 2002.

Nahid P, Gonzalez LC, Rudoy I, et al: Treatment outcomes of patients with HIV and tuberculosis, *Am J Respir Crit Care Med* 175:1199–1206, 2007.

Richeldi L: An update on the diagnosis of tuberculosis infection, *Am J Respir Crit Care Med* 174:736–742, 2006.

Small PM, Fujiwara PI: Management of tuberculosis in the United States, *N Engl J Med* 345:189–200, 2001.

NONTUBERCULOUS MYCOBACTERIA

Aksamit TR: Mycobacterium avium complex pulmonary disease in patients with pre-existing lung disease, *Clin Chest Med* 23:643–653, 2002.

American Thoracic Society: Diagnosis and treatment of disease caused by nontuberculous mycobacteria, *Am J Respir Crit Care Med* 156:S1–S25, 1997.

Ellis SM, Hansell DM: Imaging of non-tuberculous (atypical) mycobacterial pulmonary infection, *Clin Radiol* 57:661–669, 2002.

Field SK, Fisher D, Cowie RL: Mycobacterium avium complex pulmonary disease in patients without HIV infection, *Chest* 126:566–581, 2004.

Glassroth J: Pulmonary disease due to nontuberculous mycobacteria, *Chest* 133:243–251, 2008.

Holland SM: Nontuberculous mycobacteria, *Am J Med Sci* 321:49–55, 2001.

Jones D, Havlir DV: Nontuberculous mycobacteria in the HIV infected patient, *Clin Chest Med* 23:665–674, 2002.

Phair JP, Young LS, editors: Clinical challenges of Mycobacterium avium, *Am J Med* 102(suppl):1–55, 1997.

Zumla AI, Grange J: Non-tuberculous mycobacterial pulmonary infections, *Clin Chest Med* 23:369–379, 2002.

25

Miscellaneous Infections Caused by Fungi and *Pneumocystis*

FUNGAL INFECTIONS	Aspergillosis
Histoplasmosis	Other Fungi
Coccidioidomycosis	**PNEUMOCYSTIS INFECTION**
Blastomycosis	

This chapter continues the discussion of infectious diseases involving the lungs and considers miscellaneous infections caused by fungi and *Pneumocystis*. For some of the organisms discussed, infection is clearly a potential problem for the relatively normal host, that is, the individual with intact immunologic defense mechanisms. Histoplasmosis, coccidioidomycosis, and blastomycosis are the major fungal infections in this category; yet even for these diseases, impairment of normal defense mechanisms may substantially alter the presentation, clinical consequences, and natural history of the illness.

For many other fungi and for *Pneumocystis*, the normal host is essentially protected from the organism. Disease occurs almost exclusively as a consequence of an underlying illness or a breakdown of normal defense mechanisms. *Aspergillus* is perhaps the most important fungus of this sort and is the main one considered in this chapter. *Pneumocystis*, which has a debatable taxonomic status, is considered both in this chapter and in the discussion of acquired immunodeficiency syndrome (AIDS) in Chapter 26. The less common fungi (e.g., *Cryptococcus, Mucor,* and *Candida)* and protozoa (e.g., *Toxoplasma)* affecting the immunosuppressed host are not considered in detail here, but further information can be obtained from the references.

FUNGAL INFECTIONS

HISTOPLASMOSIS

Histoplasmosis is caused by the fungus *Histoplasma capsulatum,* found primarily in the soil of river valleys in temperate zones of the world. The central United States, in the Mississippi and Ohio River valleys, is particularly notable as a region in which this organism is endemic. In Canada, the St. Lawrence River valley has a high incidence of the disease. *Histoplasma* is a dimorphic fungus, that is, it exhibits two types of morphology, depending on the conditions for growth. In the soil the organism takes the form of branching hyphae. In the body at 37° C, the organism appears as a round or oval yeast.

Features of *Histoplasma capsulatum* are the following:
1. Common in river valleys of central North America
2. Found in soil contaminated by bird droppings
3. Present in yeast form in tissue
4. Elicits granulomatous response in tissue

Histoplasma organisms flourish best in soil that has been contaminated by bird droppings. When the soil becomes dry or disrupted (e.g., with bulldozing), the infectious spores become airborne, are inhaled by humans, and eventually reach the distal regions of the lung. Contact with chicken houses, bat-infested caves, or starling, blackbird, or pigeon roosts often provides exposure for individuals or groups working in the contaminated area. Riverbanks lined with trees are favorite places for blackbird nesting.

After an individual has been exposed and *H. capsulatum* has entered the lung, the organism (at body temperature) undergoes conversion to the yeast phase. An inflammatory response ensues in the lung parenchyma, with recruitment of phagocytic cells (macrophages). Initially, the yeast may not be killed within the macrophage; therefore, the organism commonly spreads to regional lymph nodes and via the bloodstream to other organs, such as the spleen. Within 3 weeks, lymphocyte-mediated delayed hypersensitivity against *Histoplasma* generally develops, and the pathologic response becomes granulomatous in nature. Central areas of caseation necrosis often occur within the granulomas, making the pathologic response similar to that of tuberculosis.

When the initial or primary lesions heal, residua are absent or take the form of small, fibrotic pulmonary nodules, which may contain areas of calcification. Similarly, small foci of calcification within the spleen may provide evidence of prior infection. However, there are alternatives to this benign pathologic course after exposure. In some cases, particularly in the immunosuppressed host or in the infant or young child, dissemination of the organism to other organs is not controlled by host defense mechanisms, and the patient is said to have *progressive disseminated histoplasmosis*. In other cases, particularly in patients with significant underlying airways disease or emphysema, progressive parenchymal inflammation, destruction, and cavity formation occur in the lung, often called *progressive* or *chronic pulmonary histoplasmosis*.

Types of Infection

Three main clinical syndromes are associated with histoplasmosis, corresponding to the three types of pathologic response just mentioned. In the normal, immunocompetent host a benign, self-limited infection called *acute* or *primary histoplasmosis* generally develops, with relatively few, if any, clinical sequelae. Often the affected person is symptom-free during the acute infection, particularly when the level of exposure has been relatively low. Other individuals have a variety of nonspecific symptoms, ranging from cough, fever, chills, and chest pain to headache, malaise, myalgias, and weight loss. The chest radiograph may reveal several types of patterns, most commonly a pulmonary infiltrate with or without hilar adenopathy. The typical clinical syndrome resolves within a few weeks, even without therapy. The only clues remaining from the acute infection are often one or several pulmonary nodules (which can be calcified) seen on chest radiograph. The nodules represent an encapsulated focus of granulomatous inflammation. Immunologic testing, by means of skin tests or serologic studies, may indicate prior exposure to the organism. Rarely, especially when acute exposure was particularly intense, patients may become quite ill and may die as a result of acute histoplasmosis.

The syndrome of *progressive disseminated histoplasmosis* usually occurs in immunocompromised hosts or in infants or young children. These patients appear to have in common an impairment of cell-mediated immunity that predisposes them to progressive disseminated histoplasmosis. Thus, progressive disseminated histoplasmosis now is seen most commonly in patients treated with corticosteroids or cytotoxic agents or in those who have human immunodeficiency virus (HIV)/AIDS. This potentially life-threatening illness is often associated with widespread pulmonary involvement, accompanied by prominent systemic symptoms and infection of other organ systems.

Chronic pulmonary histoplasmosis is generally seen in individuals with preexisting structural abnormalities of the lung, primarily chronic obstructive lung disease with

Clinical syndromes with histoplasmosis are the following:
1. Acute (primary) histoplasmosis
2. Progressive disseminated histoplasmosis
3. Chronic pulmonary histoplasmosis

emphysema. The clinical and radiographic patterns often resemble those of tuberculosis. Patients may have cough, sputum production, fever, fatigue, and weight loss. The chest radiograph shows disease localized mainly to the upper lobes, with parenchymal infiltrates, often streaky in appearance, and cavity formation.

Diagnosis of histoplasmosis depends on the type of infection: acute, disseminated, or chronic. The options available to the clinician are culture of the organism, identification in tissue, detection of *Histoplasma* antigen in the urine, or documentation of an immunologic response by serologic studies. To identify the organism microscopically, special stains, such as methenamine silver, are required. The specific usefulness and limitations of each of these methods can be found in the references.

Treatment of pulmonary histoplasmosis also depends on the particular type of infection. Acute histoplasmosis generally requires no therapy and is a self-limited illness. Disseminated histoplasmosis requires treatment with a regimen using amphotericin B, typically followed by itraconazole. Chronic pulmonary histoplasmosis is generally treated with itraconazole alone or with amphotericin B followed by itraconazole, depending on the severity of the disease.

COCCIDIOIDOMYCOSIS

Like histoplasmosis, coccidioidomycosis also affects normal hosts, but its clinical consequences may be altered in special categories of patients, especially those with impairment of host defense mechanisms. The causative organism, *Coccidioides immitis,* is a dimorphic fungus. In soil the organisms show mycelia, whereas staining of tissue specimens shows characteristic round, thick-walled structures called *spherules,* which often contain multiple endospores.

Unlike *Histoplasma* organisms, the organisms of *Coccidioides* are limited to the western hemisphere, particularly to the San Joaquin Valley region of California. Other areas in which the organism is endemic include parts of New Mexico, Nevada, Texas, and Arizona, as well as regions of Mexico, Central America, and South America.

After the host inhales contaminated material, some spores may evade the nonspecific host defenses and reach the alveoli, leading to development of primary disease. Pathologically, the inflammatory response to the organism is also a granulomatous one, once delayed hypersensitivity to *Coccidioides* has developed. The normal host generally has a relatively self-limited illness resulting from the primary infection. When dissemination occurs, it usually does so in specific groups of predisposed individuals: immunosuppressed patients, pregnant women, and, for unclear reasons, certain ethnic groups, particularly Filipinos, African-Americans, and Native Americans. Chronic pulmonary coccidioidomycosis is found in some patients as a sequel to primary disease, perhaps related to underlying lung disease or to immune impairment.

Primary infection with *Coccidioides immitis* may be subclinical and unassociated with symptoms, or it may produce respiratory tract symptoms or manifestations of hypersensitivity to the organism. When symptoms occur, they often include fever, cough, headache, and chest pain. Skin manifestations, presumably representing a form of hypersensitivity, are common. One example is erythema nodosum, which consists of tender, red nodules on the anterior surface of the lower legs. Some patients develop polyarthritis, another manifestation of hypersensitivity. The chest radiograph taken during the primary infection frequently shows a pulmonary infiltrate, often with associated hilar adenopathy and sometimes a pleural effusion.

The acute (primary) infection is usually self-limited, resolving within a few weeks. Residual findings on chest radiograph may be absent or may consist of one or more pulmonary nodules or thin-walled cavities. Calcification of the nodules is less common than with histoplasmosis, and the nodules may resemble a primary pulmonary malignancy.

Features of *Coccidioides immitis* are the following:
1. Present in yeast form in tissue
2. Endemic in western and southwestern United States, Mexico, Central and South America
3. Elicits granulomatous response in tissue

Clinical syndromes with coccidioidomycosis are the following:
1. Acute (primary) coccidioidomycosis
2. Disseminated coccidioidomycosis
3. Chronic pulmonary coccidioidomycosis

Disseminated disease, resulting from hematogenous spread of the organism, is often associated with an ominous prognosis. Certain ethnic groups are at high risk for this complication, as are pregnant women and immunosuppressed patients, especially organ transplant recipients and patients with HIV/AIDS.

Chronic pulmonary involvement by coccidioidomycosis can take several forms, including one or more chronic cavities, or upper lobe disease with streaky infiltrates and/or nodules resembling tuberculosis. Patients often have fever, cough (sometimes with hemoptysis), malaise, and weight loss and may appear subacutely or chronically ill.

As with histoplasmosis, diagnosis of coccidioidomycosis depends on the type of clinical presentation and relies on culture, demonstration in tissue (e.g., with methenamine silver staining), and evidence of an immune response to the organism. The specific uses and interpretation of skin testing and serologic techniques for diagnosis are discussed in the various more detailed references. Because of the dangers posed to hospital personnel when culturing the organism, the microbiology laboratory should be notified if there is a high clinical suspicion for coccidioidomycosis in specimens sent for culture.

Treatment considerations are similar to those for histoplasmosis. Primary infections generally do not require therapy, although patients at high risk for dissemination are commonly treated with an oral azole antifungal agent (e.g., fluconazole) or amphotericin B. Chronic pulmonary disease frequently requires therapy with amphotericin B or an oral azole, but occasionally surgery plays a role in specific clinical settings. Disseminated coccidioidomycosis is treated with amphotericin B. Patients who are undergoing prolonged immunosuppressive therapy commonly receive an oral azole.

BLASTOMYCOSIS

Blastomycosis is due to the soil-dwelling fungus *Blastomyces dermatitidis*. It occurs primarily in the midwestern and southeastern United States, often overlapping the areas in which histoplasmosis is seen. Infection is initiated by inhalation of spores that have become airborne. The primary inflammatory response in the lung consists largely of neutrophils; the subsequent response includes macrophages and T lymphocytes. As a result, the findings on histopathology show a combination of granulomas and a pyogenic (neutrophilic) response. If the latter is prominent, the response may mimic a bacterial infection. The organism can disseminate, especially to skin, but the frequency of dissemination is unknown.

Acute infection with
Blastomyces may resemble
a bacterial pneumonia.

Acute pulmonary infection with *Blastomyces* often resembles a bacterial pneumonia. Patients frequently have a relatively abrupt onset of symptoms, including fever, chills, and cough accompanied by purulent sputum production. However, subacute or chronic cases can be seen. Asymptomatic cases of blastomycosis have been reported, but their relative frequency compared with symptomatic cases is unknown. As with the other fungi, patients with impaired cellular immunity are at increased risk for development of more rapidly progressive or severe disease. Skin lesions are common, usually appearing as a characteristic irregular patch with a crusted surface, but nodules and ulcers also may occur.

The chest radiograph of patients with blastomycosis is variable. It may show unilateral or bilateral pulmonary infiltrates, which can resemble bacterial pneumonia, or localized densities, which can resemble carcinoma. Diagnosis often can be confirmed by demonstrating the characteristic yeast forms in sputum or tissue, or by culture of sputum.

Blastomycosis is generally treated with itraconazole (for less severe disease) or amphotericin B (for more severe disease). However, many cases of blastomycosis are self-limited. Whether all cases require treatment, particularly if the diagnosis is made as the disease seems to be resolving clinically, is not clear. However, most authorities agree that a patient with active symptoms when the disease is diagnosed should receive treatment.

ASPERGILLOSIS

Of all the fungi, *Aspergillus* is particularly notable for the variety of clinical presentations seen and the types of individuals predisposed. Unlike *Histoplasma, Coccidioides,* and *Blastomyces, Aspergillus* species are widespread throughout nature and are not limited to particular geographic areas. Unlike these other types of fungi, *Aspergillus* species are not dimorphic in appearance but always occur as mycelia (i.e., branching hyphal forms). Because virtually everyone is exposed to the organism, it is clear that disease must be associated with certain predisposing factors, which now are well defined.

Four major clinical forms of disease caused by *Aspergillus* and the different settings in which these diseases occur are considered here. The first form, *allergic bronchopulmonary aspergillosis,* is a hypersensitivity reaction to airway colonization with *Aspergillus,* seen almost exclusively in patients with underlying asthma or cystic fibrosis. The second form, *aspergilloma,* is a saprophytic colonization of a preexisting cavity in the lung by a mycetoma ("fungus ball") composed of a mass of *Aspergillus* hyphae. The third form, *invasive aspergillosis,* involves tissue invasion by the organism and is seen in patients with significant impairment of their immune defense mechanisms. The fourth and least well-recognized form, *chronic necrotizing pulmonary aspergillosis,* involves a subacute to chronic invasion and destruction of the pulmonary parenchyma by *Aspergillus,* often complicated by cavity formation and secondary development of a mycetoma.

Allergic Bronchopulmonary Aspergillosis

The presence of underlying reactive airways disease—asthma—appears to be the important predisposing factor for development of allergic bronchopulmonary aspergillosis. In this condition the organism resides in the patient's airways, where it appears to be important as an antigen rather than as an infectious, invasive fungus. Both type I (immediate, immunoglobulin E–mediated) and type III (immune complex, immunoglobulin G–mediated) immune reactions to the organism develop in affected persons.

Clinically, patients with allergic bronchopulmonary aspergillosis have manifestations of asthma (wheezing, dyspnea, and cough) and often low-grade fever and production of characteristic brownish plugs of sputum. *Aspergillus* species frequently can be cultured from these plugs of sputum. The chest radiograph may show transient pulmonary infiltrates, which can be a consequence of bronchial obstruction by the plugs or a result of eosinophilic infiltration of lung tissue. Bronchiectasis of proximal airways can be present, and these dilated airways may be filled with mucous plugs.

Diagnosis is made in the proper clinical setting of underlying asthma and is based on culturing the organism, demonstrating the host's immune response to the fungus, or both. For example, skin tests against *Aspergillus* antigen show a positive immediate reaction (reflecting type I immunity), often accompanied by a delayed reaction (called an *Arthus reaction)* after several hours (reflecting type III immunity). Precipitins in the blood and specific immunoglobulin E against the organism frequently can be identified.

Treatment of allergic bronchopulmonary aspergillosis is not aimed at the fungus but at the host's immunologic response to the organism. Therefore, corticosteroids are the mainstay of treatment of this syndrome. However, concomitant therapy with a well-tolerated oral azole agent seems to be associated with better outcomes and now is considered standard treatment.

Features of *Aspergillus* infection are the following:
1. Widespread distribution
2. Present as branching hyphae in tissue

Clinical syndromes with aspergillosis are the following:
1. Allergic bronchopulmonary aspergillosis
2. Aspergilloma
3. Invasive aspergillosis
4. Chronic necrotizing pulmonary aspergillosis

Aspergilloma

The second type of clinical problem resulting from *Aspergillus* is the aspergilloma, or fungus ball. The major predisposing feature for this entity is the presence of a preexisting cavity within the pulmonary parenchyma. Tuberculosis, sarcoidosis, and other fungal infections are a few examples of diseases in which cavities may be seen and therefore in which an aspergilloma may be a complicating problem. In these cases the organism is essentially a saprophyte or colonizer of the cavity, with little tissue invasion. The fungus ball itself represents a mass of fungal mycelia lying within the cavity proper.

Clinically, patients with an aspergilloma present either with hemoptysis or with no symptoms but suggestive findings on chest radiograph. Classically, the radiograph demonstrates an apparent mass in the upper lobes surrounded by a lucent rim, representing air in the cavity around the fungus ball (Fig. 25-1). When the patient changes position, the fungus ball often changes position within the cavity, according to the effects of gravity.

Diagnosis of an aspergilloma is generally strongly suggested by the characteristic radiographic appearance and is confirmed by a culture of the organism or by a demonstration of the presence of precipitins against *Aspergillus* species. Treatment often is unnecessary when the patient has no symptoms from the lesion. In some patients, particularly those with significant amounts of hemoptysis, surgery is performed to remove the diseased area containing the fungus ball. For patients with severe lung disease who are unable to tolerate surgery, bronchial artery embolization can be performed. In this procedure, the bleeding vessel is identified angiographically, and a small piece of synthetic material is released into the vessel to block it and stop the bleeding. Intravenous administration of amphotericin B is not effective treatment of this syndrome, although direct instillation of amphotericin into the cavity has been performed in some cases.

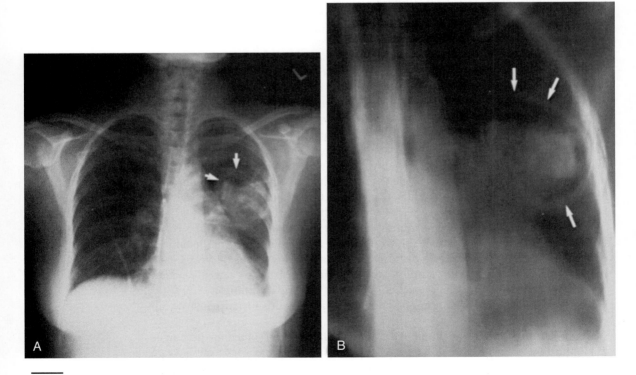

Figure 25-1. Posteroanterior radiograph *(A)* and tomogram *(B)* show aspergilloma in the left lung. Fungus ball appears as a mass sitting within a radiolucent, thin-walled cavity. Arrows outline the cavity wall. (Courtesy Dr. Ferris Hall.)

Invasive Aspergillosis

Invasive aspergillosis is the third clinical presentation of *Aspergillus* infection in the lung. This is the most life-threatening manifestation of *Aspergillus* infection, occurring almost exclusively in patients with marked impairment of host immune defense mechanisms. The most important risk factor is neutropenia (insufficient numbers of polymorphonuclear leukocytes), but patients often also have impairment of cellular immunity as a consequence of treatment with chemotherapeutic agents.

Pathologically, the organism invades and spreads through lung tissue. However, it also tends to invade blood vessels within the lung. As a result of vascular involvement by the fungus, hemoptysis can occur, vessels can become occluded, and areas of pulmonary infarction can develop.

Clinically, patients are extremely ill, with fever, cough, dyspnea, and often pleuritic chest pain. The chest radiograph may show localized or diffuse pulmonary infiltrates, reflecting either tissue invasion and a fungal pneumonia or pulmonary infarction secondary to vascular occlusion.

Diagnosis of invasive aspergillosis generally requires identification of the organism, for example, by methenamine silver staining on a biopsy specimen of lung tissue. Treatment consists of amphotericin B or voriconazole, but the mortality rate is extremely high even with appropriate use of either agent.

Chronic Necrotizing Pulmonary Aspergillosis

The final type of *Aspergillus* infection involving the lung is *chronic necrotizing pulmonary aspergillosis.* In this form, patients frequently have underlying lung disease or some relatively mild impairment of either pulmonary or systemic host defense mechanisms, as occurs with diabetes mellitus or treatment with low-dose corticosteroids. The name of this disorder describes the clinical process, which is characterized by an indolent, localized invasion of pulmonary parenchyma by *Aspergillus* organisms. Necrosis of the involved tissue often results in cavity formation, which may become the site for a mycetoma. Because of tissue invasion, the infection is treated with amphotericin B or an oral azole.

OTHER FUNGI

The remaining fungi are less frequent causes of respiratory infection. *Candida albicans* is an extraordinarily common contaminant of sputum (particularly in patients treated with antibiotics) but is an uncommon cause of pneumonia, even in immunosuppressed patients. *Cryptococcus neoformans* is found primarily in immunosuppressed patients, in whom it causes lung disease and meningitis. Finally, *Mucor* and other zygomycetes are opportunistic fungi that may cause pulmonary infection in the immunocompromised host or in patients with underlying diabetes.

PNEUMOCYSTIS INFECTION

Although *Pneumocystis jiroveci* (formerly called *Pneumocystis carinii)* has been recognized for several decades as a cause of pneumonia in immunocompromised patients, its clinical importance as a major pathogen in AIDS sparked a substantially increased interest in the organism, its treatment, and prevention of infection in high-risk patients. With the current use of highly active antiretroviral therapy for treatment of HIV as well as preventive therapy for *Pneumocystis,* the number of cases of AIDS-related *Pneumocystis* has decreased considerably. Nevertheless, it remains an important pulmonary pathogen, not only in HIV-infected patients but also in a variety of other immunosuppressed patients.

The taxonomy of *Pneumocystis* has changed a number of times since its discovery in 1909. For many years the organism was considered a protozoan; however, techniques involving nucleic acid sequencing of a small ribosomal subunit and study of enzyme structure have shown that the organism is more closely related to fungi than to protozoa. *Pneumocystis* now is classified in a unique category of fungi. There has also been a recent nomenclature change. Previously called *Pneumocystis carinii*, the name has been changed to *Pneumocystis jiroveci,* after the pathologist Jiroveci, who first described the organism in humans.

Pneumocystis appears to be widely distributed in nature. It normally can be found in the lungs of a variety of animals as well as in humans. Yet the organisms do not cause disease in normal hosts, only in individuals with significant impairment in host defenses, specifically cellular immunity. The key cell appears to be the helper T lymphocyte (CD4$^+$), whose numbers, function, or both, can be diminished by specific diseases or by immunosuppressive drugs. Before the recognition of AIDS, *P. jiroveci* pneumonia was seen most commonly in patients with malignancy, organ transplantation, or other diseases requiring treatment with corticosteroids or other immunosuppressive agents. However, after the identification of AIDS and before the introduction of highly active antiretroviral therapy, the majority of cases were seen in patients with AIDS and greatly reduced numbers of CD4$^+$ lymphocytes. The problem of *Pneumocystis* pneumonia as it occurs in AIDS is discussed in more detail in Chapter 26.

Pneumocystis cysts, which are seen in the lung tissue of infected patients, appear on light-microscopic examination as round or cup-shaped structures. They do not stain well with routine hematoxylin and eosin stain; instead they require special stains such as methenamine silver (Fig. 25-2). The tissue response to the organism, seen on microscopic examination of lung tissue, includes infiltration of mononuclear cells within the pulmonary interstitium and exudation of foamy fluid (containing cysts) into alveolar spaces. An exuberant host inflammatory response to the organism contributes to the pulmonary injury. As a result, many patients with *Pneumocystis* pneumonia are treated

Features of *Pneumocystis jiroveci* are the following:
1. Ubiquitous distribution
2. Seen on methenamine silver stain rather than routine tissue stain
3. Tissue response is primarily exudation of foamy fluid into alveoli

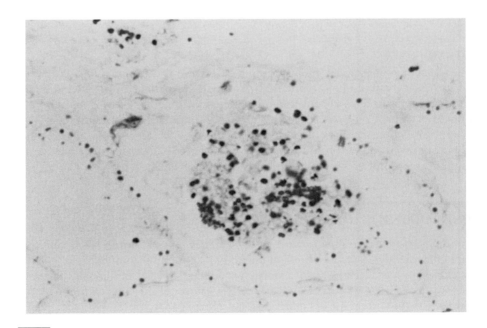

Figure 25-2. High-power photomicrograph of many *Pneumocystis* cysts as seen with methenamine silver staining. Darkly staining cysts are within alveolar lumen. Note foamy exudate in alveolar lumen. (Courtesy Dr. Earl Kasdon.)

with corticosteroids (in addition to antimicrobial therapy against *Pneumocystis*) early in the course of the disease to suppress this response.

Clinically, *Pneumocystis* pneumonia usually manifests in immunocompromised patients with dyspnea and fever. Interestingly, in patients for whom treatment with corticosteroids was the risk factor for developing *Pneumocystis* pneumonia, the symptoms frequently develop and the infection is recognized as the dose of corticosteroids is being tapered. This observation further supports the concept that the host inflammatory reaction to the organism, which is suppressed by corticosteroids and blossoms only as the steroid dose is being tapered, is responsible for much of the clinical presentation. The chest radiograph commonly shows diffuse bilateral infiltrates, which can have the appearance of either an interstitial or an alveolar filling pattern (Fig. 25-3). Due to the alveolar filling and resultant areas of shunting, hypoxemia often is a particularly prominent clinical feature in these patients. Although the disease often is insidious in onset in patients with AIDS, it commonly manifests in other immunocompromised patients as a relatively acute-onset pneumonia that, if untreated, can rapidly progress to respiratory failure and death within days.

Because the organism is extremely difficult to cultivate in the laboratory setting, diagnosis depends on demonstrating the organism on stains of tissue sections, bronchoalveolar lavage fluid, or sputum that has been induced by having the patient inhale a hypertonic saline aerosol. Use of monoclonal antibodies (and, more recently, polymerase chain reaction technology) as a means of detecting the organism in sputum or bronchoalveolar lavage fluid has improved the detection rate compared with use of previous staining methods. No serologic or skin testing methods are available for diagnosis. In

Clinical features of *Pneumocystis* pneumonia are the following:
1. Symptoms: dyspnea, fever
2. Chest radiograph: frequently diffuse interstitial or alveolar infiltrates
3. Hypoxemia

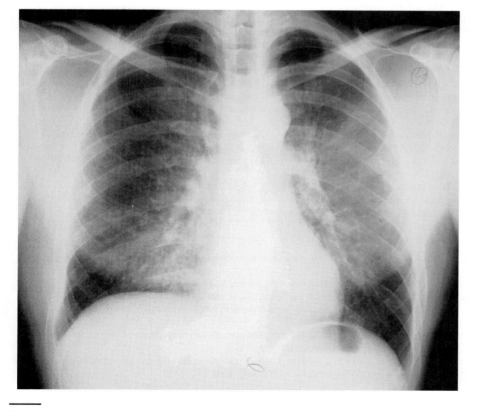

Figure 25-3. Chest radiograph of patient with acquired immunodeficiency syndrome and pneumonia due to *Pneumocystis jiroveci*. Infiltrates representing alveolar filling are most prominent at the right base but also in the left midlung field as diffuse haziness.

non-AIDS patients, the current treatment of choice for *Pneumocystis* infection is a combination of trimethoprim and sulfamethoxazole, which is effective in approximately 80% of patients. In high-risk patients, such as transplant recipients or children receiving chemotherapy for leukemia, low doses of the same agents are used prophylactically to prevent the infection. When patients with *Pneumocystis* pneumonia do not respond or are allergic to the trimethoprim-sulfamethoxazole regimen, alternative drugs, such as atovaquone or pentamidine, are effective. Chapter 26 discusses some of the specific treatment and prophylaxis issues posed by patients with AIDS.

REFERENCES

GENERAL

Baughman RP: The lung in the immunocompromised patient. Infectious complications (part 1), *Respiration* 66:95–109, 1999.

Shelhamer JH, Gill VJ, Quinn TC, et al: Laboratory evaluation of opportunistic pulmonary infections, *Ann Intern Med* 124:585–599, 1996.

Shelhamer JH, Toews GB, Masur H, et al: Respiratory disease in the immunosuppressed patient, *Ann Intern Med* 117:415–431, 1992.

Tamm M: The lung in the immunocompromised patient. Infectious complications (part 2), *Respiration* 66:199–207, 1999.

Wadhwa PD, Morrison VA: Infectious complications of chronic lymphocytic leukemia, *Semin Oncol* 33:240–249, 2006.

FUNGAL INFECTIONS (GENERAL REFERENCES)

Chong S, Lee KS, Yi CA, Chung MJ, Kim TS, Han J: Pulmonary fungal infection: imaging findings in immunocompetent and immunocompromised patients, *Eur J Radiol* 59:371–383, 2006.

Dismukes WE: Introduction to antifungal drugs, *Clin Infect Dis* 30:653–657, 2000.

Goldman M, Johnson PC, Sarosi GA: Fungal pneumonias. The endemic mycoses, *Clin Chest Med* 20: 507–519, 1999.

Pagano L, Caira M, Fianchi L: Pulmonary fungal infections with yeasts and Pneumocystis in patients with hematological malignancy, *Ann Med* 37:259–269, 2005.

Pagano L, Fianchi L, Leone G: Fungal pneumonia due to molds in patients with hematological malignancies, *J Chemother* 18:339–352, 2006.

Patel R: Antifungal agents. Part I. Amphotericin B preparations and flucytosine, *Mayo Clin Proc* 73: 1205–1225, 1998.

Sanchez A, Larsen R: Emerging fungal pathogens in pulmonary disease, *Curr Opin Pulm Med* 13:199–204, 2007.

Saubolle MA: Fungal pneumonias, *Semin Respir Infect* 15:162–177, 2000.

Terrell CL: Antifungal agents. Part II. The azoles, *Mayo Clin Proc* 74:78–100, 1999.

Yao Z, Liao W. Fungal respiratory disease, *Curr Opin Pulm Med* 12:222–227, 2006.

HISTOPLASMOSIS

Buck BE, Malinin TI, Davis JH: Transmission of histoplasmosis by organ transplantation, *N Engl J Med* 344:310, 2001.

Goodwin RA Jr, Des Prez RM: Histoplasmosis, *Am Rev Respir Dis* 117:929–956, 1978.

Goodwin RA, Loyd JE, Des Prez RM: Histoplasmosis in normal hosts, *Medicine* 60:231–266, 1981.

Wheat J: Histoplasmosis. Experience during outbreaks in Indianapolis and review of the literature, *Medicine* 76:339–354, 1997.

Wheat J, Sarosi G, McKinsey D, et al: Practice guidelines for the management of patients with histoplasmosis, *Clin Infect Dis* 30:688–695, 2000.

Wood KL, Hage CA, Knox KS, et al: Histoplasmosis after treatment with anti-tumor necrosis factor-alpha therapy, *Am J Respir Crit Care Med* 167:1279–1282, 2003.

COCCIDIOIDOMYCOSIS

Galgiani JN: Coccidioidomycosis: a regional disease of national importance, *Ann Intern Med* 130:293–300, 1999.

Galgiani JN, Ampel NM, Blair JE, et al: Coccidioidomycosis, *Clin Infect Dis* 41:1217–1223, 2005.

Galgiani JN, Ampel NM, Catanzaro A, et al: Practice guidelines for the treatment of coccidioidomycosis, *Clin Infect Dis* 30:658–661, 2000.

Saubolle MA, McKellar PP, Sussland D: Epidemiologic, clinical and diagnostic aspects of coccidioidomycosis, *J Clin Microbiol* 45:26–30, 2007.

Spinello IM, Johnson RH, Baqu S: Coccidioidomycosis and pregnancy: A review, *Ann NY Acad Sci* 1111:358–364, 2007.

Stevens DA: Coccidioidomycosis, *N Engl J Med* 332:1077–1082, 1995.

BLASTOMYCOSIS

Chapman SW, Bradsher RW Jr, Campbell GD Jr, Pappas PG, Kauffman CA: Practice guidelines for the management of patients with blastomycosis, *Clin Infect Dis* 30:679–683, 2000.

Sarosi GA, Davies SF: Blastomycosis, *Am Rev Respir Dis* 120:911–938, 1979.

ASPERGILLOSIS

Almyroudis NG, Holland SM, Segal BH: Invasive aspergillosis in primary immunodeficiencies, *Med Mycol* 43(suppl 1):S247–S259, 2005.

Binder RE, Faling LJ, Putatch RD, et al: Chronic necrotizing pulmonary aspergillosis: a discrete clinical entity, *Medicine* 60:109–124, 1982.

Cockrill BA, Hales CA: Allergic bronchopulmonary aspergillosis, *Annu Rev Med* 50:303–316, 1999.

Herbert PA, Bayer AS: Fungal pneumonia—IV: invasive pulmonary aspergillosis, *Chest* 80:220–225, 1981.

Herbrecht R, Denning DW, Patterson TF; Invasive Fungal Infections Group of the European Organisation for Research and Treatment of Cancer and the Global Aspergillus Study Group: Voriconazole versus amphotericin B for primary therapy of invasive aspergillosis, *N Engl J Med* 347:408–415, 2002.

Shibuya K, Ando T, Hasegawa C, et al: Pathophysiology of pulmonary aspergillosis, *J Infect Chemother* 10:138–145, 2004.

Paterson DL, Singh N: Invasive aspergillosis in transplant recipients, *Medicine* 78:123–138, 1999.

Reichenberger F, Habicht JM, Gratwohl A, Tamm M: Diagnosis and treatment of invasive pulmonary aspergillosis in neutropenic patients, *Eur Respir J* 19:743–755, 2002.

Ricketti AJ, Greenberger PA, Mintzer RA, Patterson R: Allergic bronchopulmonary aspergillosis, *Chest* 86:773–778, 1984.

Sharma OP, Chwogule R: Many faces of pulmonary aspergillosis, *Eur Respir J* 12:705–715, 1998.

Soubani AO, Chandrasekar PH: The clinical spectrum of pulmonary aspergillosis, *Chest* 121:1988–1999, 2002.

Stevens DA, Kan VL, Judson MA, et al: Practice guidelines for diseases caused by *Aspergillus*, *Clin Infect Dis* 30:696–709, 2000.

PNEUMOCYSTIS INFECTION

Arend SM, Kroon FP, van't Wout JW: *Pneumocystis carinii* pneumonia in patients without AIDS, 1980 through 1993, *Arch Intern Med* 155:2436–2441, 1995.

Hughes WT, Rivera GK, Schell MJ, Thornton D, Lott L: Successful intermittent chemoprophylaxis for *Pneumocystis carinii* pneumonitis, *N Engl J Med* 316:1627–1632, 1987.

Kovacs JA, Gill VJ, Meshnick S, Masur H: New insights into transmission, diagnosis, and drug treatment of *Pneumocystis carinii/jiroveci* pneumonia, *JAMA* 286:2450–2460, 2001.

Masur H, Lane HC, Kovacs JA, Allegra CJ, Edman JC: *Pneumocystis* pneumonia: from bench to clinic, *Ann Intern Med* 111:813–826, 1989.

Peters SG, Prakash UBS: *Pneumocystis carinii* pneumonia, *Ann Intern Med* 82:73–78, 1987.

Pop SM, Kolls JK, Steele C: Pneumocystis: immune recognition and evasion, *Int J Biochem Cell Biol* 38: 17–22, 2006.

Thomas CF, Limper AH: Current insights into the biology and pathogenesis of *Pneumocystis* pneumonia, *Nat Rev Microbiol* 5:298–308, 2007.

Russian DA, Levine SJ: *Pneumocystis carinii* pneumonia in patients without HIV infection, *Am J Med Sci* 321:56–65, 2001.

Yale SH, Limper AH: *Pneumocystis carinii* pneumonia in patients without acquired immunodeficiency syndrome: associated illness and prior corticosteroid therapy, *Mayo Clin Proc* 71:5–13, 1996.

26

Acquired Immunodeficiency Syndrome

ETIOLOGY AND PATHOGENESIS	NONINFECTIOUS
INFECTIOUS COMPLICATIONS	COMPLICATIONS OF AIDS
OF AIDS	Neoplastic Disease
Pneumocystis jiroveci Pneumonia	Inflammatory Disease
Mycobacterial Infection	Pulmonary Vascular Disease
Other Bacterial Infection	DIAGNOSTIC EVALUATION
Viral Infection	OF PULMONARY INFILTRATES
Fungal Infection	IN AIDS

In 1981, a number of cases of immunodeficiency of unknown cause in homosexual males and intravenous drug users were reported. These patients had a variety of unusual infections, including *Pneumocystis jiroveci* pneumonia (then called *Pneumocystis carinii* pneumonia), mucosal candidiasis, and several types of viral infections. In some cases the unusual neoplasm Kaposi's sarcoma also occurred. Evaluation of these patients revealed a marked impairment of cellular immunity, characterized by anergy to skin tests for delayed hypersensitivity and decreased numbers of lymphocytes, specifically with loss of helper-inducer T lymphocytes and a reversal in the normal ratio of helper-to-suppressor T cells. This disease subsequently was given the name *acquired immunodeficiency syndrome* (AIDS).

What initially seemed to be an unusual problem that might be relegated to the realm of medical curiosities has since become one of the major worldwide public health problems confronting the medical profession at the turn of the twenty-first century. Approximately 40 million individuals around the world (including more than 1 million in the United States) currently are infected with human immunodeficiency virus (HIV), with approximately 14,000 new infections occurring worldwide each day. It has been estimated that there are approximately 3 million deaths worldwide per year from HIV/AIDS. In sub-Saharan Africa, HIV/AIDS is the leading cause of death.

During the past 25 years, an enormous amount of research has resulted in identification of the retrovirus responsible for this catastrophic attack on the cellular immune system. At the same time, a wide and unexpected spectrum of clinical problems has been posed by a myriad of opportunistic infections and neoplasms resulting from the profound immunodeficiency in these patients. Fortunately, the development of highly active antiretroviral therapy (HAART) and the development of effective prophylactic regimens against several opportunistic infections have significantly decreased many of the clinical complications of the disease, and the death rate in the United States has declined 80% between 1990 and 2003. Nevertheless, although substantial and rapid progress has been made in the therapy for the disease and in the prevention and treatment of secondary complications, management of patients with AIDS continues to present a major challenge to the medical community. The critical challenge is at the worldwide level, primarily as a result of limited availability of therapeutic and prophylactic agents for the large number of affected individuals in developing nations.

In the United States the largest category of individuals affected by AIDS is men who have sex with men, in whom the responsible virus is transmitted by sexual contact. Persons in the next largest group, intravenous drug users of either sex, introduce the virus into their circulation via infected needles or syringes. Recipients of contaminated blood products, including concentrates of factor VIII used for hemophilia, form another important group at risk for AIDS. Finally, a smaller number of patients contracted AIDS by heterosexual contact, generally with an individual in one of the aforementioned risk groups. In other areas of the world (e.g., sub-Saharan Africa and Asia), AIDS is common in both sexes and is transmitted primarily by heterosexual contact.

Although AIDS potentially leads to complications in almost any organ system, the lungs have been the organ system in which the largest number of complications has occurred. This chapter gives a brief overview of AIDS and focuses on the complications specifically affecting the respiratory system of patients with AIDS.

ETIOLOGY AND PATHOGENESIS

The etiologic agent responsible for AIDS is a retrovirus formerly called human T-cell lymphotropic virus type III (HTLV-III) and now called *human immunodeficiency virus* (HIV). The virus appears to mediate its pathogenic effect by binding to the CD4 receptor on cells that carry this surface receptor. Although the most important cell type affected is the helper-inducer subset of T lymphocytes, cells of the monocyte-macrophage series and certain neural cells also may be infected because they carry the CD4 receptor on their cell surface.

The immunodeficiency occurring with HIV infection results primarily from lysis and depletion of infected CD4$^+$ T lymphocytes. This loss of the helper-inducer cell population may be complicated by altered macrophage function, which probably is secondary to direct effects of the virus and impaired production of cytokines normally affecting macrophage activation and function.

> HIV binds to the CD4 receptor of helper-inducer T lymphocytes.

The major consequence of the immunodeficiency is opportunistic infection with organisms that normally are handled by an adequately functioning cellular immune system. The most common infection involving the lungs in the absence of prophylaxis and HAART is pneumonia caused by *Pneumocystis jiroveci* infection. Pulmonary infection also can result from a wide variety of other respiratory pathogens normally controlled by cell-mediated immune mechanisms, including cytomegalovirus, mycobacteria (*Mycobacterium tuberculosis* and nontuberculous or atypical mycobacteria), and fungi (especially *Cryptococcus, Histoplasma,* and *Coccidioides*). Certain types of bacterial pneumonia, primarily attributable to *Streptococcus pneumoniae* (pneumococcus) and *Haemophilus influenzae,* are also seen with increased frequency in AIDS. Whereas these types of bacterial pneumonia normally might not be predicted to result from the cellular immunodeficiency of AIDS, they probably can be explained by dysregulation of the humoral immune system and impaired antibody production against these organisms.

> Major pulmonary infections with AIDS are the following:
> 1. *Pneumocystis jiroveci (carinii)*
> 2. Cytomegalovirus
> 3. Mycobacteria
> 4. Fungi *(Cryptococcus, Histoplasma, Coccidioides)*
> 5. Bacteria *(Streptococcus pneumoniae, Haemophilus influenzae)*

Even though the majority of pulmonary complications seen in patients with AIDS are infectious, a variety of noninfectious complications also are well recognized. This chapter divides the pulmonary complications of AIDS into these two broad categories—infectious and noninfectious—and concludes with a discussion of the diagnostic evaluation of the patient with AIDS and pulmonary infiltrates.

INFECTIOUS COMPLICATIONS OF AIDS

PNEUMOCYSTIS JIROVECI PNEUMONIA

Since the first identification of cases in 1981, *Pneumocystis* infection has been the most common respiratory complication in patients with AIDS, frequently representing the initial opportunistic infection that establishes the diagnosis of AIDS in the absence of other known causes of immunosuppression. The risk of developing this opportunistic infection is highly dependent on the patient's peripheral blood CD4$^+$ count, with a level less than 200 cells per mm^3 the cutoff below which patients are at high risk for infection. Fortunately, the availability of increasingly effective antiretroviral agents and the more frequent use of prophylaxis against *Pneumocystis* have significantly decreased the likelihood of infection and death resulting from this opportunistic infection.

A general discussion of *Pneumocystis* as a respiratory pathogen was given in Chapter 25. In patients with AIDS, onset of the disease often is more indolent than in immunosuppressed patients without AIDS. Fever, cough, and dyspnea are the usual symptoms bringing the patient to medical attention. The typical chest radiograph shows diffuse interstitial or alveolar infiltrates. Often the lung fields look hazy, a pattern that may be difficult to characterize specifically as either interstitial or alveolar and is commonly described as looking like "ground glass" (see Fig. 25-3). However, atypical radiographic presentations are clearly recognized with documented *Pneumocystis* pneumonia, including even the finding of a normal chest radiograph. High-resolution computed tomographic scanning is particularly sensitive for demonstrating subtle changes associated with *Pneumocystis* pneumonia and generally shows abnormal results even in patients with a normal chest radiograph.

Diagnosis is generally based on finding the organism in respiratory secretions by any number of techniques, especially immunofluorescent staining with a monoclonal antibody. Patients with AIDS often have a surprisingly large burden of organisms, making the organisms easier to obtain than from patients without AIDS. Inducing sputum by having the patient inhale a solution of hypertonic saline frequently is effective and now is used often as the initial diagnostic method when *Pneumocystis* is suspected. Flexible bronchoscopy with bronchoalveolar lavage is another means for recovering the organism, with a positive yield of greater than 85% in patients eventually proven to have *Pneumocystis* pneumonia. Transbronchial biopsy provides a small incremental increase in sensitivity over bronchoalveolar lavage alone.

Treatment of severe pneumonia caused by *Pneumocystis* organisms usually involves one of four regimens: the combination antimicrobial trimethoprim-sulfamethoxazole, the combination of clindamycin and primaquine, or trimetrexate or pentamidine as single agents given intravenously. These four regimens appear to be equally effective; each is successful in approximately 80% of cases. In patients without AIDS treated for *Pneumocystis* pneumonia, the combination trimethoprim-sulfamethoxazole is generally preferred because of fewer side effects. However, patients with AIDS have a peculiar predisposition to allergic reactions to sulfonamides, making the frequency of adverse side effects equivalent to that seen with pentamidine and making necessary a switch to therapy with other drugs in a relatively high proportion of patients. Other agents such as atovaquone or the combination of trimethoprim and dapsone have been used, especially in patients who do not respond to or cannot tolerate one of the more standard agents or who have less severe disease.

In patients with moderate to severe disease caused by *Pneumocystis* pneumonia, adjunctive therapy with corticosteroids often is helpful in averting significant respiratory

Pneumocystis jiroveci pneumonia often has an indolent onset in AIDS.

Diagnosis of Pneumocystis jiroveci is made most commonly on samples obtained by induction of sputum or bronchoalveolar lavage.

Standard therapy for Pneumocystis jiroveci pneumonia is one of four options: trimethoprim-sulfamethoxazole, clindamycin-primaquine, trimetrexate, or pentamidine.

failure. Although steroid therapy would be expected to cause more immunosuppression and make the infection worse, this has not been the case, and the presumed benefit of reducing the inflammatory response in the lung to lysing organisms outweighs any negative effects of the steroids.

In patients with AIDS, oral administration of trimethoprim-sulfamethoxazole (in low doses) or dapsone (either alone or with pyrimethamine) can be used with reasonable effectiveness to prevent *Pneumocystis* pneumonia. Alternatively, patients can receive aerosolized pentamidine once per month by inhalation or oral atovaquone. Such prophylactic therapy is routinely recommended in HIV-infected patients who have a CD4$^+$ count less than 200 cells per mm^3 and in selected other circumstances. Unfortunately, the propensity for development of allergic reactions to trimethoprim-sulfamethoxazole frequently makes this regimen difficult to use in patients with AIDS; therefore, many patients are maintained on one of the other forms of prophylaxis. When *Pneumocystis* pneumonia develops despite use of aerosolized pentamidine prophylaxis, the clinical presentation may be atypical. Unusual radiographic patterns are often seen, especially pulmonary infiltrates limited to the upper lung zones, rather than the more typical pattern of diffuse pulmonary infiltrates.

> Atypical presentations of *Pneumocystis jiroveci* infections commonly are seen in patients receiving aerosolized pentamidine.

MYCOBACTERIAL INFECTION

Mycobacterium tuberculosis has emerged as an important respiratory pathogen in patients with AIDS, not only because it is common but also because it is potentially treatable. Clinical disease may result from primary infection, reactivation of previous infection, or exogenous reinfection. Rather than occurring in all categories of patients with AIDS, disease caused by *M. tuberculosis* is a particular problem in those groups of individuals with a high background prevalence of tuberculosis, for example, intravenous drug users and indigent and immigrant populations.

Because *M. tuberculosis* is a relatively virulent organism that does not require the same degree of immunosuppression to produce disease as do many of the other opportunistic infections, it is often seen early in the course of the disease in patients with AIDS. In this setting, its clinical presentation is similar to that seen in the typical patient with tuberculosis who does not have AIDS. However, it also may occur in AIDS patients who are in a late stage of their disease with more severe immunosuppression, in which case the clinical manifestations often are atypical. In this latter circumstance, upper lobe cavitary disease is less frequent, and disseminated disease is more frequent than is usually seen in patients without AIDS. Interestingly, for patients with AIDS and tuberculosis (or, for that matter, with other opportunistic infections), improvement in the patient's overall immune status, particularly as a result of HAART, can be associated with a paradoxical clinical worsening of the opportunistic infection. In these cases, "reconstitution" of the immune system results in an augmented inflammatory reaction to the opportunistic infection, leading to the apparent clinical worsening.

> Tuberculosis may be an early opportunistic infection in AIDS.

Treatment considerations for tuberculosis in AIDS patients are generally similar to those for patients without AIDS, but with some differences. Because of the risk for disease with nontuberculous mycobacteria, an expanded list of drugs is sometimes given initially to AIDS patients until the organism and its sensitivities are firmly identified. In addition, treatment may be given for a longer duration to AIDS patients, especially if the response to therapy appears slow. Drug interactions with HAART must be carefully considered. Patients with HIV infection who have positive tuberculin skin test reactions (defined as 5 mm or more of induration) but no evidence of active disease should receive 9 months of treatment with isoniazid (or an alternative regimen), similar to the treatment of latent tuberculosis infection in individuals without HIV infection.

The other types of mycobacteria that frequently cause opportunistic infection in AIDS are members of the *Mycobacterium avium* complex (MAC). What is surprising in patients with MAC infection is that the organism is associated primarily with disseminated disease, not with pulmonary disease. Even when disseminated disease is present, pulmonary involvement is not generally a significant part of the clinical picture. Because the risk of MAC infection is associated with extremely low CD4$^+$ counts, prophylactic treatment against MAC, typically with a newer macrolide antibiotic such as azithromycin or clarithromycin, is indicated when the CD4$^+$ count falls below 50 per mm^3.

OTHER BACTERIAL INFECTION

Patients with AIDS appear to have an increased frequency of bacterial pneumonia, primarily attributable to either *S. pneumoniae* or *H. influenzae*. The risk is increased at all levels of CD4$^+$ count and is highest when the count falls below 200 cells per mm^3. Intravenous drug users also appear to be at particularly high risk.

Bacterial pneumonias might not be predicted to be a complication of AIDS because impairment in cellular immunity should not by itself predispose an individual to these infections. However, dysregulation of the humoral immune system accompanies the impairment in cellular immunity. Patients frequently have polyclonal hyperglobulinemia at the same time they demonstrate a poor antibody response after antigen exposure. Presumably, loss of helper-inducer cells results in alteration of the normal interaction between helper-inducer cells and B lymphocytes that regulates antibody production.

VIRAL INFECTION

The most common virus afflicting patients with AIDS is cytomegalovirus (CMV), one of the viruses in the herpesvirus family. The most common sites of clinical involvement are the eye (CMV retinitis) and the gastrointestinal tract. Although CMV frequently can be cultured from lung tissue or bronchoalveolar fluid of patients with AIDS, its role as a clinically important respiratory pathogen is not clear. When patients with CMV in the lungs have clinical respiratory system disease, they almost always have a coexistent organism such as *Pneumocystis* that is thought to be the primary pathogen. Even when typical nuclear and cytoplasmic inclusions are present, the role played by CMV is uncertain in the presence of these other important pathogens, and the usefulness of adding specific treatment for CMV in this setting is unclear.

Other viruses such as herpes simplex, varicella-zoster, and Epstein-Barr virus have been described as potential respiratory pathogens in AIDS, but they are distinctly uncommon and are not considered here.

FUNGAL INFECTION

Several fungi are recognized as causes of respiratory involvement in patients with AIDS, either as isolated respiratory system disease or as part of a disseminated infection. The most common of these fungal infections is due to *Cryptococcus neoformans*, which more commonly causes meningitis than respiratory disease. When respiratory involvement is present, the radiograph may show localized or diffuse disease, and sometimes an associated pleural effusion or intrathoracic lymph node involvement. The lung may be the only organ involved, or involvement may be accompanied by meningitis or disseminated disease. Treatment traditionally has been with amphotericin B, but fluconazole has been used as an alternative agent.

Fungal infections that occur in specific endemic regions—histoplasmosis and coccidioidomycosis—are described in detail in Chapter 25. In patients with AIDS, pulmonary involvement with these organisms is most commonly a manifestation of disseminated disease that resulted either from reactivation of previous disease or from progressive primary infection. Consequently, histoplasmosis and coccidioidomycosis are seen primarily but not exclusively in their respective endemic areas. As is the case in patients without AIDS, amphotericin B (or an oral azole such as itraconazole) is the primary agent used for treatment of either of these infections.

Other fungal infections of the lung are much less common in patients with AIDS. Perhaps surprisingly, even though oral candidiasis (thrush) is extremely common in AIDS, pulmonary infection with *Candida albicans* is extremely uncommon and rarely described except at autopsy. *Aspergillus* infection has been described in AIDS but generally in patients who have other predisposing factors for invasive aspergillosis, especially neutropenia.

NONINFECTIOUS COMPLICATIONS OF AIDS

Although infectious complications affecting the respiratory system are much more common, noninfectious complications are also recognized in patients with AIDS. They fall into the broad categories of neoplastic disease (which includes Kaposi's sarcoma and non-Hodgkin's lymphoma), inflammatory disease (which includes lymphocytic interstitial pneumonitis and nonspecific interstitial pneumonitis), and pulmonary vascular disease (pulmonary hypertension). A brief discussion of each of these potential complications follows.

NEOPLASTIC DISEASE

Kaposi's sarcoma is one of the most common of the neoplastic diseases affecting AIDS patients. In patients with AIDS, it is characterized by slowly progressive cutaneous lesions of the lower extremities in elderly men. It formerly was a rare diagnosis in the United States and was seen in a more aggressive form with frequent visceral involvement in certain parts of Africa. In the early descriptions of AIDS patients in 1981, Kaposi's sarcoma was one of the peculiar clinical manifestations accompanying the profound cellular immunodeficiency. Since then, Kaposi's sarcoma has been recognized as one of the common manifestations, occurring generally with skin involvement but often complicated by dissemination to the lungs and other organ systems. Data from a variety of studies, including the identification of herpesvirus-like DNA sequences in patients with Kaposi's sarcoma (either with or without AIDS) but not in control subjects, indicate that human herpesvirus 8 is the causative agent responsible for Kaposi's sarcoma.

Kaposi's sarcoma is most commonly observed in patients with AIDS as violaceous, vascular-appearing skin lesions. Histologically, these lesions consist of spindle-shaped cells with intervening slitlike vascular spaces. When visceral involvement indicates the presence of dissemination, commonly involved organ systems include the gastrointestinal tract and the lungs. Pulmonary involvement has a variable presentation on chest radiograph. It can appear as diffuse infiltrates, localized disease, or pulmonary nodules. Pleural involvement with resulting pleural effusions can be present and often is a helpful diagnostic point against *Pneumocystis* pneumonia because pleural effusions are uncommon with the latter diagnosis. Involvement of the airways or mediastinal lymph nodes can be seen with intrathoracic Kaposi's sarcoma.

Definitive diagnosis of Kaposi's sarcoma in the lung may be difficult because bronchoalveolar lavage and even transbronchial biopsy infrequently provide sufficient diagnostic material. A more invasive lung biopsy would generally provide diagnostic material but is preferable to avoid because of its invasive nature. When endobronchial involvement is present, the gross appearance of the lesions in the airways may be

Kaposi's sarcoma in the thorax can manifest with parenchymal, airway, lymph node, and pleural involvement.

highly suggestive of the diagnosis. A gallium lung scan may provide another useful clinical clue by demonstrating pulmonary uptake in most opportunistic infections but not in Kaposi's sarcoma.

Therapy for Kaposi's sarcoma involving the lungs is palliative rather than curative, although treatment options have improved greatly in recent years. Patients may have progressive respiratory involvement, often complicated by pulmonary hemorrhage. Although patients may die of disseminated Kaposi's sarcoma, they frequently succumb to coexisting opportunistic infections rather than to the neoplasm.

Another common neoplasm in patients with AIDS is non-Hodgkin's lymphoma. Although extranodal involvement and disseminated disease are common when this malignancy occurs in patients with AIDS, intrathoracic involvement is uncommon. Lung cancer also appears to occur with increased frequency in patients with AIDS. In contrast to Kaposi's sarcoma, HAART does not appear to significantly diminish the incidence of non-Hodgkin's lymphoma or lung cancer.

INFLAMMATORY DISEASE

An occasional patient with AIDS and diffuse pulmonary infiltrates has neither an opportunistic infection nor a neoplasm affecting the lung. Instead, the process is an inflammatory one without any known cause, although viral etiologies (especially Epstein-Barr virus and HIV) have been proposed. In some cases the microscopic appearance is notable for the prominence of lymphocytes and plasma cells infiltrating alveolar septa. In these cases a diagnosis of *lymphocytic interstitial pneumonitis* is made. This particular histologic pattern is a relatively common pulmonary complication seen in children with AIDS but is found infrequently in adults. When treatment is necessary, corticosteroids are used with variable success.

> Lymphocytic interstitial pneumonitis is a common pulmonary complication of AIDS in children.

The other histologic pattern is a nonspecific one with a mixed inflammatory cell infiltrate. Patients with this pattern are diagnosed as having *nonspecific interstitial pneumonitis*. This is an uncommon complication of AIDS about which little is known.

PULMONARY VASCULAR DISEASE

A number of cases of pulmonary arterial hypertension in patients with HIV infection have been reported. Although the association is believed to be a true rather than a coincidental relationship, no clear mechanistic or pathophysiologic explanation is known. The histopathology and clinical features typically are similar to those of idiopathic pulmonary arterial hypertension, but the disease may have a more rapid progression than is generally seen in patients without HIV infection. Treatment is similar to that of idiopathic pulmonary arterial hypertension (see Chapter 14), but use of endothelin-1 receptor antagonists frequently is problematic because of concomitant hepatic disease or concerns about drug interactions. HAART is generally indicated as part of the therapeutic approach.

DIAGNOSTIC EVALUATION OF PULMONARY INFILTRATES IN AIDS

Pulmonary infiltrates, often accompanied by fever, dyspnea, and cough, present a common problem in patients known to have either HIV infection or risk factors for exposure to HIV. Although typical radiographic presentations of some of the afore-mentioned diseases may suggest a particular diagnosis, the findings often are nonspecific. In addition, with the accumulation of experience with AIDS, more atypical presentations of many of these respiratory complications are being recognized. For example, with *Pneumocystis* infection, use of aerosolized pentamidine decreases the likelihood of infection but increases the frequency of atypical radiographic presentations when the infection occurs despite prophylactic therapy.

The initial evaluation of diffuse pulmonary infiltrates frequently focuses on the diagnosis of *Pneumocystis* pneumonia in patients at high risk because they have a CD4 count less than 200/mm³. Induction of sputum accompanied by appropriate staining for *Pneumocystis* often is the first diagnostic procedure because of its noninvasive nature. When sputum induction produces negative findings, flexible bronchoscopy often is the next procedure performed, usually with bronchoalveolar lavage and sometimes with transbronchial biopsy. The diagnosis of Kaposi's sarcoma is strongly suspected if typical lesions are observed in the airways. The yield for *Pneumocystis* is excellent with bronchoalveolar lavage, but making a diagnosis of some of the other infections, neoplasms, and inflammatory processes may require transbronchial biopsy. Surgical lung biopsy is the most invasive of the diagnostic procedures and usually is reserved for situations where a diagnosis is crucial but not forthcoming by less invasive means.

REFERENCES

INFECTIOUS COMPLICATIONS

Baughman RP: Cytomegalovirus: the monster in the closet? *Am J Respir Crit Care Med* 156:1–2, 1997.

Baughman RP, Dohn MN, Frame PT: The continuing utility of bronchoalveolar lavage to diagnose opportunistic infection in AIDS patients, *Am J Med* 97:515–522, 1994.

Beck JM, Rosen MJ, Peavy HH: Pulmonary complications of HIV infection. Report of the fourth NHLBI workshop, *Am J Respir Crit Care Med* 164:2120–2126, 2001.

Boiselle PM, Crans CA, Kaplan MA, Crans CA Jr: The changing face of Pneumocystis carinii pneumonia in AIDS patients, *AJR Am J Roentgenol* 172:1301–1309, 1999.

Bozzette SA, Finkelstein DM, Spector SA, et al: A randomized trial of three antipneumocystis agents in patients with advanced human immunodeficiency virus infection, *N Engl J Med* 332:693–699, 1995.

Burman WJ, Jones BE: Treatment of HIV-related tuberculosis in the era of effective antiretroviral therapy, *Am J Respir Crit Care Med* 164:7–12, 2001.

Girard P-M: Discontinuing Pneumocystis carinii prophylaxis, *N Engl J Med* 344:222–223, 2001.

Hirschtick RE, Glassroth J, Jordan MC, et al: Bacterial pneumonia in persons infected with the human immunodeficiency virus, *N Engl J Med* 333:845–851, 1995.

Johnson MD, Decker CF: Tuberculosis and HIV infection, *Dis Mon* 52:420–427, 2006.

Kovacs JA, Gill VJ, Meshnick S, Masur H: New insights into transmission, diagnosis, and drug treatment of Pneumocystis carinii pneumonia, *JAMA* 286:2450–2460, 2001.

Kovacs JA, Masur H: Prophylaxis against opportunistic infections in patients with human immunodeficiency virus infection, *N Engl J Med* 342:1416–1429, 2000.

Masur H, Kaplan JE, Holmes KK, editors: Guidelines for preventing opportunistic infections among HIV-infected persons—2002, *Ann Intern Med* 137:435–477, 2002.

Meyohas M-C, Roux P, Bollens D, et al: Pulmonary cryptococcosis: localized and disseminated infections in 27 patients with AIDS, *Clin Infect Dis* 21:628–633, 1995.

Minamoto GY, Rosenberg AS: Fungal infections in patients with acquired immunodeficiency syndrome, *Med Clin North Am* 81:381–409, 1997.

National Institutes of Health–University of California Expert Panel for Corticosteroids as Adjunctive Therapy for Pneumocystis Pneumonia: Consensus statement on the use of corticosteroids as adjunctive therapy for Pneumocystis pneumonia in the acquired immunodeficiency syndrome, *N Engl J Med* 323:1500–1504, 1990.

Rigsby MO, Curtis AM: Pulmonary disease from nontuberculous mycobacteria in patients with human immunodeficiency virus, *Chest* 106:913–919, 1994.

Rosen MJ, Narasimhan M: Critical care of immunocompromised patients: human immunodeficiency virus, *Crit Care Med* 34(9 suppl):S245–S250, 2006.

Smego RA, Nagar S, Maloba B, Popara M: A meta-analysis of salvage therapy for Pneumocystis carinii pneumonia, *Arch Intern Med* 161:1529–1533, 2001.

Thomas CF, Limper AH: Pneumocystis pneumonia, *N Engl J Med* 350:2487–2498, 2004.

Wolff AJ, O'Donnell AE: Pulmonary manifestations of HIV infection in the era of highly active antiretroviral therapy, *Chest* 120:1888–1893, 2001.

NEOPLASTIC, INFLAMMATORY, AND PULMONARY VASCULAR COMPLICATIONS

Bazot M, Cadranel J, Benayoun S, Tassart M, Bigot JM, Carette MF: Primary pulmonary AIDS-related lymphoma. Radiographic and CT findings, *Chest* 116:1282–1286, 1999.

Cadranel J, Mayaud C: Intrathoracic Kaposi's sarcoma in patients with AIDS, *Thorax* 50:407–414, 1995.

Mehta NJ, Khan IA, Mehta RN, Sepkowitz DA: HIV-related pulmonary hypertension. Analytic review of 131 cases, *Chest* 118:1133–1141, 2000.

Mesa RA, Edell ES, Dunn WF, Edwards WD: Human immunodeficiency virus infection and pulmonary hypertension: two new cases and a review of 86 reported cases, *Mayo Clin Proc* 73:37–45, 1998.

Stebbing J, Sanitt A, Nelson M, Powles T, Gazzard B, Bower M: A prognostic index for AIDS-associated Kaposi's sarcoma in the era of highly active antiretroviral therapy, *Lancet* 367:1495–1502, 2006.

27

Classification and Pathophysiologic Aspects of Respiratory Failure

Many types of respiratory disease are capable of impairing the normal function of the lung as a gas-exchanging organ. In some cases, the degree of impairment is mild, and the patient suffers relatively few consequences. In other cases, dysfunction is marked, and the patient experiences disabling or life-threatening clinical sequelae. When the respiratory system can no longer function to keep gas exchange at an acceptable level, the patient is said to be in *respiratory failure,* irrespective of the underlying cause.

The tempo for development of respiratory failure varies depending on the nature of the underlying problem. Many of the diseases discussed so far, such as chronic obstructive lung disease and interstitial lung disease, are characterized by a chronic clinical course, accompanied by relatively slow deterioration of pulmonary function and gas exchange. However, because of limited pulmonary reserve, patients with preexisting pulmonary disease also are susceptible to episodes of acute respiratory failure, either from an intercurrent illness or from transient worsening of their underlying disease. On the other hand, respiratory failure, generally acute or subacute in onset, can develop in individuals without preexisting lung disease. The initiating problem in these patients is often a primary respiratory illness or a disorder of another organ system, complicated by major respiratory problems.

This chapter presents an overview of the problem of respiratory failure and discusses the different pathophysiologic types and consequences of respiratory insufficiency. Chapter 28 addresses a specific form of acute respiratory failure known as *acute respiratory distress syndrome,* which does not require the presence of preexisting lung disease. Chapter 29 considers some principles of management of respiratory failure as well as specific modalities of current therapy.

DEFINITION OF RESPIRATORY FAILURE

Respiratory failure probably is best defined as inability of the respiratory system to maintain adequate gas exchange. Exactly where to draw the line for adequate gas exchange is somewhat arbitrary, but in a previously normal individual, arterial Po_2 less than 60 mm Hg or Pco_2 greater than 50 mm Hg generally is considered evidence for acute respiratory failure. In the individual with preexisting lung disease, the situation is even more complicated because the patient chronically has impaired gas exchange and abnormal blood gas values.

For example, it would not be unusual for a patient with significant chronic obstructive lung disease to perform daily activities with Po_2 approximately 60 mm Hg and Pco_2 50 to 55 mm Hg. By the blood gas criteria just mentioned, this patient is always in respiratory failure, but the condition obviously is chronic, not acute. A look at the patient's pH value shows that the kidneys have compensated for the CO_2 retention and that the pH is not far from the normal value of 7.40.

At what point is the condition called acute respiratory failure? Certainly, if an acute respiratory illness such as an acute pneumonia develops, the patient's gas exchange becomes even worse. Po_2 falls further and Pco_2 may rise even higher. In this case, acute respiratory failure is defined as a significant change from the patient's baseline gas-exchange status. If the patient's usual arterial blood gases are known, the task is easier. If the blood gases are not known, the pH value can provide a clue about whether the patient's CO_2 retention is acute or chronic. When a patient is seen initially with Pco_2 70 mm Hg, the implications are quite different if the accompanying pH value is 7.15 as opposed to 7.36.

CLASSIFICATION OF ACUTE RESPIRATORY FAILURE

HYPOXEMIC TYPE

In practice, it is most convenient to classify acute respiratory failure into two major categories, on the basis of the pattern of gas-exchange abnormalities.

In the first category, hypoxemia is the major problem. The patient's Pco_2 is normal or even low. This condition is the hypoxemic variety of acute respiratory failure. For example, localized diseases of the pulmonary parenchyma, such as pneumonia, can result in this type of respiratory failure if the disease is sufficiently severe. However, an even broader group of etiologic factors causes hypoxemic respiratory failure by means of a generalized increase in fluid within the alveolar spaces, often as a result of leakage of fluid from pulmonary capillaries. The latter problem frequently is called *acute respiratory distress syndrome* (ARDS) and can be the consequence of a wide variety of disorders that cause an increase in pulmonary capillary permeability.* Because of the importance of this syndrome as a major form of acute respiratory failure, Chapter 28 focuses entirely on the problem of ARDS.

HYPERCAPNIC/HYPOXEMIC TYPE

In the second category, hypercapnia is present. For the respiratory failure to be considered acute, the pH must show absent or incomplete metabolic compensation for the respiratory acidosis. From the discussion of alveolar gas composition and the alveolar gas equation in Chapter 1, it is apparent that hypercapnia is associated with decreased arterial Po_2 because of altered alveolar Po_2. Therefore, even if ventilation and perfusion are relatively well matched and the fraction of blood shunted across the pulmonary

---

*The abbreviation ARDS was formerly used for *adult respiratory distress syndrome*, but "acute" has now generally replaced "adult" because the entity can occur in children as well.

vasculature is not increased, arterial Po_2 falls in the presence of hypoventilation with consequent hypercapnia. In fact, many cases of hypercapnic respiratory failure have marked ventilation-perfusion mismatch as well, which further accentuates the hypoxemia. With these concepts in mind, it is clear that the hypercapnic form of respiratory failure generally involves not just hypercapnia; rather, it may be more appropriately considered the hypercapnic/hypoxemic form of respiratory failure.

A number of types of respiratory disease are potentially associated with the second form of respiratory failure. How the various disorders result in hypercapnic/hypoxemic respiratory failure is explained in the section on pathogenesis of gas-exchange abnormalities. These disorders primarily include (1) depression of the neurologic system responsible for respiratory control, (2) disease of the respiratory bellows, either the chest wall or the neuromuscular apparatus responsible for thoracic expansion, and (3) chronic obstructive lung disease. More than one of these three problems commonly is present, thus compounding the potential for respiratory insufficiency.

In the hypercapnic/hypoxemic form of respiratory failure, patients often have preexisting disease that is responsible for either chronic respiratory insufficiency or limitations in respiratory reserve sufficient to make patients much more susceptible to decompensation with an acute superimposed problem. This form of respiratory failure is called *acute on chronic respiratory failure,* obviously reflecting the prior problems or limitations with respiratory reserve. This expression has been used especially to describe the patient with chronic obstructive pulmonary disease in whom acute respiratory failure develops at the time of an infection or another acute respiratory insult.

> Causes of hypercapnic/hypoxemic respiratory failure are the following:
> 1. Depression of central nervous system ventilatory control
> 2. Disease of the respiratory bellows
> 3. Chronic obstructive lung disease

PRESENTATION OF GAS-EXCHANGE FAILURE

When acute respiratory failure develops, the patient's symptom complex generally includes the manifestations of hypoxemia, hypercapnia, or both, accompanied by the specific symptoms related to the precipitating disorder. Dyspnea is present in the majority of cases and is the symptom that often suggests to the physician the possibility of respiratory failure.

Impairment of mental abilities is a frequent result of either hypoxemia or hypercapnia. Patients may become disoriented, confused, and unable to conduct their normal level of activity. With profound hypercapnia, patients may become stuporous and eventually lapse into a frank coma. Headache is a common finding in patients with hypercapnia. Dilation of cerebral blood vessels as a consequence of increased Pco_2 probably is an important factor in the pathogenesis of the headache.

Physical findings associated with abnormal gas exchange are relatively few. Patients may be tachypneic, tachycardic, and restless, findings that are relatively nonspecific. Examination of the optic fundus may show papilledema (elevation of the optic disk) resulting from hypercapnia, cerebral vasodilation, and increased pressure at the back of the eye. Findings in the lung are related to the specific form of disease that is present, for example, wheezing and/or rhonchi in chronic obstructive lung disease, or crackles as a result of fluid in the small airways and alveolar spaces. When hypoxemia is severe, patients may become cyanotic, which is apparent as a dusky or bluish hue to the nail beds and the lips.

> Clinical presentation with respiratory failure consists of the following:
> 1. Dyspnea
> 2. Impaired mental status
> 3. Headache
> 4. Tachycardia
> 5. Papilledema (with ↑ Pco_2)
> 6. Variable findings on lung examination
> 7. Cyanosis (with severe hypoxemia)

PATHOGENESIS OF GAS-EXCHANGE ABNORMALITIES

The basic principles of abnormal gas exchange were discussed in Chapter 1. The focus here is on the application of these principles to patients with respiratory failure. A discussion of hypoxemic respiratory failure is followed by a discussion of hypercapnic/hypoxemic failure.

HYPOXEMIC RESPIRATORY FAILURE

In the patient with hypoxemic respiratory failure, two major pathophysiologic factors contribute to lowering of arterial Po_2: ventilation-perfusion mismatch and shunting. In the patient with significant ventilation-perfusion mismatch, regions with a low ventilation-to-perfusion ratio contribute relatively desaturated blood to the systemic circulation. What sorts of problems cause a decrease in ventilation relative to perfusion in a particular region of lung? If an alveolus or a group of alveoli is partially filled with fluid, then a limited amount of ventilation reaches that particular area, whereas perfusion to the region may remain relatively preserved. Similarly, if an airway supplying a region of lung is diseased, either by pathology affecting the airway wall or by secretions occupying the lumen, then ventilation is limited.

When these problems become extreme, ventilation to a region of lung may be totally absent so that a true shunt exists. For example, alveoli may be completely filled with fluid, or an airway may be completely obstructed, preventing any ventilation to the involved area. Although the response of the pulmonary vasculature is to constrict and thereby limit perfusion to an underventilated or a nonventilated portion of the lung, this protective mechanism often cannot compensate fully for the loss of ventilation, and hypoxemia results.

Alveolar filling with fluid and the collapse of small airways and alveoli seem to be the main pathogenetic features leading to ventilation-perfusion mismatch and shunting in ARDS (see Chapter 28). An earlier consideration of the ability of supplemental O_2 to raise the Po_2 in conditions of ventilation-perfusion mismatch versus shunt indicated that O_2 is unable to improve Po_2 significantly for truly shunted blood (see Chapter 1). Therefore, when the shunt fraction of the cardiac output is quite high, oxygenation may be helped surprisingly little by administration of supplemental O_2.

Despite the marked derangement of oxygenation in ARDS, CO_2 elimination typically remains adequate because, at least early in the course of the syndrome, patients are able to maintain alveolar ventilation at an acceptable level. Even when regions of lung have a high ventilation-perfusion ratio and thus effectively act as dead space, patients are generally able to compensate by increasing their overall minute ventilation.

HYPERCAPNIC/HYPOXEMIC RESPIRATORY FAILURE

In the hypercapnic form of respiratory failure, patients are unable to maintain a level of alveolar ventilation sufficient to eliminate CO_2 and to keep arterial Pco_2 within the normal range. Because ventilation is determined by a sequence of events ranging from generation of impulses by the respiratory controller to movement of air through the airways, there are several stages at which problems can adversely affect total minute ventilation. This sequence is shown in Figure 27-1, which also lists some of the disorders that can interfere at each level. Not only is the total ventilation per minute important; the "effectiveness" of the ventilation for CO_2 excretion, that is, the relative amount of alveolar versus dead space ventilation, also is important to ensure proper utilization of inspired gas. If the proportion of each breath going to dead space (i.e., ratio of volume of dead space to tidal volume [V_D/V_T]) increases substantially, then alveolar ventilation may fall to a level sufficient to cause an elevated Pco_2, even if total minute ventilation is preserved.

In the hypercapnic form of respiratory failure, hypoventilation also leads to a decrease in alveolar Po_2. As a result, arterial Po_2 falls even if ventilation-perfusion matching and gas exchange at the alveolar level are well maintained. In practice, however, many of the diseases associated with alveolar hypoventilation, ranging from neuromuscular and chest wall disease to chronic airflow obstruction, are accompanied by significant ventilation-perfusion mismatch. Therefore, patients generally have two major reasons for hypoxemia: hypoventilation and ventilation-perfusion mismatch.

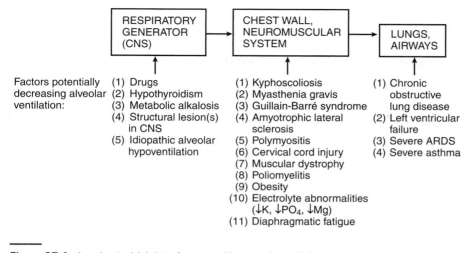

Figure 27-1. Levels at which interference with normal ventilation give rise to alveolar hypoventilation. Factors contributing to decreased ventilation are listed under each level. ARDS = Acute respiratory distress syndrome; CNS = central nervous system.

Interestingly, true shunts usually play a limited role in causing hypoxemia in these disorders, unlike the situation in ARDS.

Given the causes of hypoxemia in the hypercapnic/hypoxemic form of respiratory failure, patients frequently respond to supplemental O_2 with a substantial rise in arterial PO_2. However, most of these patients have at least mild chronic CO_2 retention, with their acute respiratory failure resulting from some precipitating insult or worsening of their underlying disease. Administration of supplemental O_2 to these chronically hypercapnic patients may lead to a further increase in arterial PCO_2 for a number of pathophysiologic reasons (see Chapter 18). With judicious use of supplemental O_2, substantial additional elevation of arterial PCO_2 usually can be avoided.

An elaboration of further features of the hypercapnic/hypoxemic form of respiratory failure follows.

CLINICAL AND THERAPEUTIC ASPECTS OF HYPERCAPNIC/HYPOXEMIC RESPIRATORY FAILURE

Whether the underlying disease is chest wall disease, such as kyphoscoliosis, or chronic obstructive lung disease, this type of respiratory failure often develops in patients who already have some degree of chronic respiratory insufficiency. However, this is not true of all cases. In certain neurologic problems, such as Guillain-Barré syndrome, hypercapnic respiratory failure occurs in a previously healthy individual.

When the patient has chronic disease on which acute respiratory failure is superimposed, the phrase "acute on chronic respiratory failure" is frequently used. In such cases, often a specific, different problem precipitates the acute deterioration, and identification of the problem is important.

What are some of the intercurrent problems or factors that precipitate acute respiratory failure in these patients? Perhaps the most common is an acute respiratory tract infection, such as bronchitis, usually but not always caused by a virus. Bacterial causes must always be investigated, however, because often they are amenable to specific therapy. Use of drugs that suppress the respiratory center, such as sedatives or narcotics, may precipitate hypercapnic respiratory failure by depressing central respiratory drive in a person whose condition already was marginal. Other intercurrent problems

Frequent precipitants of acute on chronic respiratory failure are the following:
1. Respiratory tract infection
2. Drugs (e.g., sedatives, narcotics)
3. Congestive heart failure
4. Less common: pulmonary emboli, exposure to environmental pollutants

include congestive heart failure, pulmonary emboli, and exposure to environmental pollutants, each of which may be sufficient to induce further CO_2 retention in the patient with previously borderline compensation.

The general therapeutic approach to these patients involves three main areas: (1) support of gas exchange, (2) treatment of the acute precipitating event, and (3) treatment of the underlying pulmonary disease. Support of gas exchange involves maintaining adequate oxygenation and elimination of CO_2 (see Chapter 29). Briefly, supplemental O_2, generally in a concentration not much higher than that found in ambient air, is administered to raise Po_2 to an acceptable level (i.e., greater than 60 mm Hg). If CO_2 elimination deteriorates much beyond the usual level of Pco_2, then an acute respiratory acidosis is superimposed on the patient's usual acid–base status. If significant acidemia develops or if the patient's mental status changes significantly as a result of CO_2 retention, then some form of ventilatory assistance, either intubation and mechanical ventilation or noninvasive assisted ventilation with a mask, may be required.

Treating the factor precipitating acute respiratory failure is most successful when bacterial infection or congestive heart failure is responsible for the acute deterioration. Antibiotics for suspected bacterial infection, or diuretics and afterload reduction for congestive heart failure, are appropriate forms of therapy in these circumstances. For patients in whom respiratory secretions seem to be playing a role either chronically or in an acute exacerbation of their disease, attempts to assist in clearance of secretions may be beneficial. In particular, chest physical therapy, in which percussion and vibration of the chest are performed, followed by appropriate positioning to assist gravity in drainage of secretions may be beneficial.

Treatment of the underlying pulmonary disease depends on the nature of the disease. For patients with obstructive lung disease, intensive therapy with bronchodilators and often corticosteroids may be helpful in reversing whatever components of bronchoconstriction and inflammation are present. If neuromuscular or chest wall disease is the underlying problem, then therapy may be available, as is the case with myasthenia gravis. Unfortunately, for many neuromuscular or chest wall diseases, no specific form of therapy exists, and support of gas exchange and treatment of any precipitating factors are the major modes of therapy.

When patients with irreversible chest wall or neuromuscular disease are in frank respiratory failure, they may require some form of ventilatory assistance on a chronic basis (modalities for chronic ventilatory support are discussed in Chapter 29). It is important to emphasize here that the primary decision is whether chronic ventilatory support should be given to a patient with this type of irreversible disease. In many cases the patient, the family, and the physician make the joint decision that life should not be prolonged with chronic ventilator support, given the projected poor quality of life and the irreversible nature of the process.

REFERENCES

GENERAL

Chakrabarti B, Calverley PMA: Management of acute ventilatory failure, *Postgrad Med J* 82:438–445, 2006.

Greene KE, Peters JI: Pathophysiology of acute respiratory failure, *Clin Chest Med* 15:1–12, 1994.

Krachman S, Criner GJ: Hypoventilation syndromes, *Clin Chest Med* 19:139–155, 1998.

Levy MM: Pathophysiology of oxygen delivery in respiratory failure, *Chest* 128(5 suppl 2): 547S–553S, 2005.

Rousso C, Koutsoukou A: Respiratory failure, *Eur Respir J Suppl* 47:3s–14s, 2003.

Weinberger SE, Schwartzstein RM, Weiss JW: Hypercapnia, *N Engl J Med* 321:1223–1231, 1989.

Younes M: Mechanisms of ventilatory failure. In Tierney DF, editor: *Current pulmonology, vol 14*, St. Louis, 1993, Mosby-Year Book, pp. 243–292.

RESPIRATORY FAILURE IN OBSTRUCTIVE LUNG DISEASE

Calverley PM: Respiratory failure in chronic obstructive pulmonary disease, *Eur Respir J Suppl* 47:26s–30s, 2003.

Davidson AC: Critical care management of respiratory failure resulting from COPD, *Thorax* 57: 1079–1084, 2002.

Derenne J-P, Fleury B, Pariente R: Acute respiratory failure of chronic obstructive pulmonary disease, *Am Rev Respir Dis* 138:1006–1033, 1988.

Phipps P, Garrard CS: Acute severe asthma in the intensive care unit, *Thorax* 58:81, 2003.

Plant PK, Elliott MW: Chronic obstructive pulmonary disease. 9: management of ventilatory failure in COPD, *Thorax* 58:537–542, 2003.

Robinson TD, Freiberg DB, Regnis JA, Young IH: The role of hypoventilation and ventilation-perfusion redistribution in oxygen-induced hypercapnia during acute exacerbations of chronic obstructive pulmonary disease, *Am J Respir Crit Care Med* 161:1524–1529, 2000.

RESPIRATORY FAILURE IN NEUROMUSCULAR AND CHEST WALL DISEASE

Bergofsky EH: Respiratory failure in disorders of the thoracic cage, *Am Rev Respir Dis* 119:643–669, 1979.

Gracey DR, Divertie MB, Howard FM Jr: Mechanical ventilation for respiratory failure in myasthenia gravis. *Mayo Clin Proc* 58:597–602, 1983.

Gracey DR, McMichan JC, Divertie MB, Howard FM Jr: Respiratory failure in Guillain-Barré syndrome, *Mayo Clin Proc* 57:742–746, 1982.

Howard RS, Davidson C: Long term ventilation in neurogenic respiratory failure, *J Neurol Neurosurg Psychiatry* 74(suppl 3):iii24–30, 2003.

Mehta S: Neuromuscular disease causing acute respiratory failure, *Respir Care* 51:1016–1021, 2006.

Shneerson JM, Simonds AK: Noninvasive ventilation for chest wall and neuromuscular disorders, *Eur Respir J* 20:480–487, 2002.

Simonds AK: Recent advances in respiratory care for neuromuscular disease, *Chest* 130:1879–1886, 2006.

Acute Respiratory Distress Syndrome

This chapter continues the discussion of respiratory failure with more detailed consideration of one important type of acute respiratory failure: *acute respiratory distress syndrome* (ARDS). Although this entity initially was called the "adult respiratory distress syndrome," it is not limited to adults; therefore "acute" now is considered preferable to "adult" in the naming of this syndrome. ARDS represents a major form of hypoxemic respiratory failure. Its clinical and pathophysiologic features differ considerably from those noted for acute on chronic respiratory failure. ARDS is formally defined by the presence of severe arterial hypoxemia and diffuse, bilateral pulmonary infiltrates that are not due exclusively to cardiogenic or hydrostatic causes. This chapter describes in detail each of these criteria and the associated pathology and pathophysiology.

> ARDS is defined by the presence of severe arterial hypoxemia and bilateral pulmonary infiltrates not attributable exclusively to cardiogenic or hydrostatic causes.

Rather than a specific disease, ARDS truly is a syndrome, resulting from any of a number of etiologic factors. It is perhaps simplest to consider this syndrome as the nonspecific result of acute injury to the lung, characterized by breakdown of the normal barrier that prevents leakage of fluid out of the pulmonary capillaries and into the interstitium and alveolar spaces. Another term, *acute lung injury* (ALI), is formally used to describe a similar process of lung injury in which the disturbance in oxygenation is less severe, whereas ARDS represents the more severe end of the spectrum. A number of other names have been used to describe ARDS, including noncardiogenic pulmonary edema, shock lung, and posttraumatic pulmonary insufficiency.

This chapter first considers the dynamics of fluid transfer between the pulmonary vessels and the alveolar interstitium, because an alteration in this process is important in the pathogenesis of ARDS. Next is an outline of the many types of injury that can result in ARDS and some of the theories proposed to explain how such a diverse group of disorders can produce this syndrome. Following is a discussion of the pathologic, pathophysiologic, and clinical consequences. The chapter concludes with a general approach to treatment. More specific details about support of gas exchange are provided in Chapter 29.

PHYSIOLOGY OF FLUID MOVEMENT IN ALVEOLAR INTERSTITIUM

Despite the diverse group of disorders that can cause ARDS, the net result of the syndrome is the same: a disturbance in the normal barrier that limits leakage of fluid out of the pulmonary capillaries and into the pulmonary parenchyma. Before a discussion of some of the theories explaining how this barrier is damaged, a brief consideration of the determinants of fluid transport among the pulmonary vessels, the interstitial space, and the alveolar lumen may be helpful. The pulmonary parenchyma (Fig. 28-1) consists of (1) small vessels coursing through the alveolar walls, which for simplicity are referred to as the pulmonary capillaries; (2) pulmonary capillary endothelium, the lining cells that normally limit but do not completely prevent fluid movement out of the capillaries; (3) pulmonary interstitium, which is considered here as the alveolar wall exclusive of vessels and the epithelial cells lining the alveolar lumen; (4) lymphatic channels, which are found mainly in perivascular connective tissue in the lung; (5) alveolar epithelial cells, which line the surface of the alveolar lumen; and (6) alveolar lumen or alveolar space.

Movement of fluid out of the pulmonary capillaries and into the interstitial space is determined by a number of factors, including the hydrostatic pressures in the vessels and the pulmonary interstitium, the colloid osmotic pressures in these same two

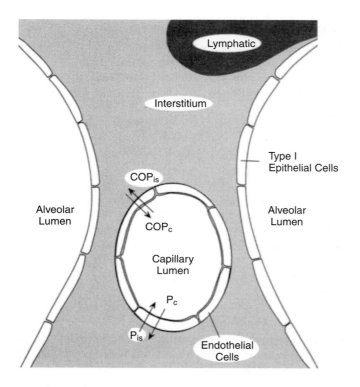

Figure 28-1. Schematic diagram of the lung's gas exchanging region. Forces governing fluid movement between pulmonary capillary lumen and alveolar interstitium are shown. Arrows show direction of fluid movement favored by each of the important forces. Lymphatic vessels are located in perivascular connective tissue rather than within alveolar walls. COP_c = Pulmonary capillary colloid osmotic pressure; COP_{is} = interstitial space colloid osmotic pressure; P_c = pulmonary capillary hydrostatic pressure; P_{is} = interstitial space hydrostatic pressure.

compartments, and the permeability of the endothelium. The effect of these factors in determining fluid transport is summarized in the Starling equation, examined in Chapter 15 with regard to fluid transport across the pleural space. The Starling equation is given as Equation 28-1:

$$F = K[(P_c - P_{is}) - \sigma(COP_c - COP_{is})] \qquad (28\text{-}1)$$

where F = fluid movement; P_c and P_{is} = pulmonary capillary and interstitial hydrostatic pressure, respectively; COP_c and COP_{is} = pulmonary capillary and interstitial colloid osmotic (oncotic) pressure, respectively; K = filtration coefficient; and σ = reflection coefficient (measure of permeability of endothelium for protein).

> Fluid normally moves from the pulmonary capillaries to the interstitial space. Resorption by lymphatics prevents accumulation.

If estimates of the actual numbers are substituted for normal hydrostatic and oncotic pressures in Equation 28-1, F is a positive number, indicating that fluid normally moves out of the pulmonary capillaries and into the interstitial space. Even though the rate of fluid movement out of the pulmonary capillaries is estimated to be approximately 20 mL/hour, this fluid does not accumulate. The lymphatic vessels are quite effective in absorbing both protein and fluid that have left the vasculature and entered the interstitial space. However, if fluid movement into the interstitium increases substantially or if lymphatic drainage is impeded, then fluid accumulates within the interstitial space, resulting in interstitial edema. When sufficient fluid accumulates or the alveolar epithelium is damaged, fluid also moves across the epithelial cell barrier and into the alveolar spaces, resulting in alveolar edema.

TWO MECHANISMS OF FLUID ACCUMULATION

In practice, the forces described in the Starling equation become altered in two main ways, producing interstitial and often alveolar edema (Table 28-1). The first occurs when hydrostatic pressure within the pulmonary capillaries (P_c) is increased, generally as a consequence of elevated left ventricular or left atrial pressure (e.g., in left ventricular failure or mitral stenosis). The resulting pulmonary edema is called *cardiogenic* or *hydrostatic* pulmonary edema, and the cause is essentially an imbalance between the hydrostatic and oncotic forces governing fluid movement. In this form of edema, the permeability barrier that limits movement of protein out of the intravascular space is intact, and the fluid that leaks out has a very low protein content.

In the second mechanism by which fluid accumulates, hydrostatic pressures are normal, but the permeability of the capillary endothelial and alveolar epithelial barriers is increased as a result of damage to one or both of these cell populations. Movement of proteins out of the intravascular space occurs as a consequence of the increase in permeability. The fluid that leaks out has a relatively high protein content, often close to that found in plasma. This second mechanism is the one operative in ARDS. Because an elevation in pulmonary capillary pressure from cardiac disease is not involved, this form of edema is called *noncardiogenic* pulmonary edema.

Table 28-1

CATEGORIES OF PULMONARY EDEMA

Feature	Cardiogenic	Noncardiogenic
Major cause	Left ventricular failure, mitral stenosis	Acute respiratory distress syndrome
Pulmonary capillary pressure	Increased	Normal
Pulmonary capillary permeability	Normal	Increased
Protein content of edema fluid	Low	High

Although cardiogenic and hydrostatic pulmonary edema are mentioned here, subsequent parts of this chapter focus on noncardiogenic edema, that is, ARDS. However, it is important to remember that hydrostatic pressures have an important impact on fluid movement even when the primary problem is a defective permeability barrier. Specifically, higher pulmonary capillary hydrostatic pressures result in more fluid leaking through an abnormally permeable pulmonary capillary endothelium than do lower pressures. At the extreme, some patients with a permeability defect of the pulmonary capillary bed simultaneously have a grossly elevated pulmonary capillary pressure as a result of coincidental left ventricular failure. In these cases, the permeability defect and the elevated hydrostatic pressure work synergistically in contributing to leakage of fluid out of the pulmonary vasculature. Not only is the fluid leak compounded, but when both factors are involved, sorting out the relative importance of each and thus determining the optimal treatment priorities in a given patient can be difficult.

ETIOLOGY

Numerous and varied disorders are associated with the potential to produce ARDS (Table 28-2). What these diverse etiologic factors in ARDS have in common is their ability to cause diffuse injury to the pulmonary parenchyma. Beyond that, defining other features that link the underlying causes is difficult on the basis of our present knowledge. Even the route of injury varies. Some etiologic factors involve inhaled injurious agents; others appear to mediate their effects on the lung via the circulation rather than the airway.

INHALED INJURIOUS AGENTS

Numerous injurious agents that reach the pulmonary parenchyma through the airway have been identified. In some cases, a liquid is responsible; examples include gastric contents, salt or fresh water, and hydrocarbons. With acid gastric contents, especially

Table 28-2	
CAUSES OF DIFFUSE ALVEOLAR DAMAGE AND THE ACUTE RESPIRATORY DISTRESS SYNDROME	
Aspiration	Disseminated intravascular coagulation
Gastric contents	Embolism
Salt/fresh water (near drowning)	Fat embolism
Hydrocarbons	Amniotic fluid embolism
Toxic gas inhalation	Drugs
Nitrogen dioxide (NO_2)	Narcotics
Smoke	Sedatives
Ammonia	Aspirin (rare)
Phosgene	Thiazides (rare)
Bilateral pneumonia	Multiple transfusions
Viral	Pancreatitis
Bacterial	Neurogenic
Pneumocystis jiroveci	Head trauma
Sepsis	Intracranial hemorrhage
Shock (accompanied by other etiologic factors)	Seizures
Trauma	Mechanical ventilation (overdistention and/ or cyclic opening and closing of alveoli)[a]

[a]Generally not a primary cause of acute respiratory distress syndrome but a potential secondary contributor to alveolar damage (see Chapter 29).

when pH is lower than 2.5, patients sustain a "chemical burn" to the pulmonary parenchyma, resulting in damage to the alveolar epithelium. In the case of near drowning, in either fresh or salt water, not only does the inhaled water fill alveolar spaces, but secondary damage to the alveolar-capillary barrier causes fluid to leak from the pulmonary vasculature. Because salt water is hypertonic to plasma, it is capable of drawing fluid from the circulation as a result of an osmotic pressure gradient. Fresh water, on the other hand, is hypotonic to plasma and to cellular contents and thus may enter pulmonary parenchymal cells, with resulting cellular edema. In addition, fresh water appears to inactivate surfactant, a complicating factor that is discussed in more detail in the section on pathophysiology. Finally, aspirated hydrocarbons can be toxic to the distal parenchyma, perhaps in part because they also inactivate surfactant and cause significant changes in surface tension.

A number of inhaled gases have been identified as potential acute toxins and precipitants of ARDS. Nitrogen dioxide is one example, as are some chemical products of combustion inhaled in smoke. High concentrations of oxygen, particularly when given for prolonged periods, have been considered to contribute to alveolar injury. The mechanism of O_2 toxicity is believed to be generation of free radicals and superoxide anions, byproducts of oxidative metabolism that are toxic to pulmonary epithelial and endothelial cells. It is ironic that O_2 can contribute to lung injury given that it is so important in the supportive treatment of ARDS. In patients who require high concentrations of supplemental O_2 to maintain an adequate Po_2, the therapy itself may compound the problem by furthering cellular damage and increasing alveolar-capillary permeability. Chapter 29 discusses an additional way in which treatment of ARDS may worsen alveolar damage through overdistention and/or cyclic opening and closing of alveoli induced by mechanical ventilation.

Infectious agents may produce injury via airway access to the pulmonary parenchyma. Pneumonia is the most common underlying clinical problem associated with development of ARDS. Besides bacterial pneumonia, another important example in recent years was pneumonia resulting from *Pneumocystis jiroveci,* specifically in patients with acquired immunodeficiency syndrome. However, with the common use of highly active antiretroviral therapy as well as the availability of effective prophylactic regimens against *Pneumocystis,* it now is an uncommon cause of ARDS. Another important cause of ARDS is viral pneumonia, which has the capability of damaging parenchymal cells and altering alveolar-capillary permeability.

INJURY VIA THE PULMONARY CIRCULATION

For causes of ARDS that do not involve inhaled agents or toxins, the pulmonary circulation is proposed to initiate the injury in some way. However, in most cases a specific circulating factor has not been identified with certainty, even though several possibilities have been proposed. One of the most common precipitants for ARDS is sepsis, in which microorganisms or their products (especially endotoxin) circulating through the bloodstream initiate a sequence of events resulting in toxicity to parenchymal cells.

Although the term *shock lung* was used many years ago to describe what is now called ARDS, the presence of hypotensive shock alone probably is not sufficient for development of ARDS. Patients in whom ARDS develops seemingly as a result of hypotension usually have complicating potential etiologic factors (e.g., trauma, sepsis) or have received therapy (e.g., blood transfusions) also capable of causing cellular damage.

Patients with the coagulation disorder known as *disseminated intravascular coagulation* (DIC) appear to have the potential for development of ARDS. In DIC, patients have ongoing activation of both the clotting mechanism and the protective fibrinolytic system that prevents clot formation and propagation. Like ARDS, DIC is a syndrome and can occur because of a variety of primary or underlying causes. However, although these two problems frequently are associated, whether and exactly how one causes the other is uncertain.

When fat or amniotic fluid enters the circulation, the material is transported to the lung, resulting in the clinical problems of fat embolism and amniotic fluid embolism, respectively. Presumably these materials are directly toxic to endothelial cells of the pulmonary capillaries, and they certainly have been associated with the development of ARDS.

A variety of drugs, many of which fall into the class of narcotics, are potential causes of ARDS. In most cases an overdose of the drug has been taken, although this is not always the situation. One of the agents most frequently recognized has been heroin, and the name "heroin pulmonary edema" sometimes is used. In addition to heroin and other narcotics, several other drugs have been described as occasionally causing ARDS, including even aspirin and thiazide diuretics. Although the problem of drug-induced pulmonary edema has been well described, the mechanism by which it occurs is not certain.

Some patients with acute pancreatitis develop a clinical picture consistent with noncardiogenic pulmonary edema. In this situation, enzymes released into the circulation from the damaged pancreas have been proposed to directly injure pulmonary parenchymal cells or initiate other indirect pathways, resulting in injury.

Certain disorders of the central nervous system, particularly trauma and intracerebral bleeding associated with increased intracranial pressure, are known to be associated with development of ARDS. Similarly, ARDS occasionally occurs after generalized seizures. An interesting and commonly accepted hypothesis to explain this so-called *neurogenic pulmonary edema* is that intense sympathetic nervous system discharge in response to intracranial hypertension produces extremely high pulmonary capillary pressures, resulting in mechanical damage to the endothelium.

PATHOGENESIS

How do these diverse clinical problems all result in the syndrome of increased pulmonary capillary permeability called ARDS? One important factor appears to be the ability to produce injury to pulmonary capillary endothelial and alveolar epithelial cells (primarily type I epithelial cells, the cytoplasmic processes of which provide most of the surface area lining the alveolar walls). Given the wide variety of insults that can damage these cell types, it seems unlikely that a single common mechanism is operative for all kinds of injury.

In the discussion of some specific causes of ARDS, brief mention was made of a few of the theories of pathogenesis for individual disorders. Here the more generalized cellular and biochemical mechanisms that are operative during the course of injury to the pulmonary epithelial and capillary endothelial cells are considered. A particularly important component of the pathogenesis of acute lung injury and ARDS appears to be the recruitment of inflammatory cells to the lung, especially neutrophils. An early theory explaining recruitment of neutrophils to the lung focused on the complement pathway. When complement is activated by sepsis, C5a is released and is responsible for aggregation of neutrophils within the pulmonary vasculature. These neutrophils may release a variety of substances that are potentially toxic to cellular and noncellular components of the alveolar wall. Superoxide radicals, other byproducts of oxidative metabolism, an array of cytokines, and various proteolytic enzymes all can be released by neutrophils and may be important pathogenetically in producing structural and functional injury to the alveolar wall. Examples of specific mediators include endotoxin, products of arachidonic acid metabolism, and cytokines such as tumor necrosis

The initial injury in ARDS affects alveolar epithelial (type I), capillary endothelial cells, or both.

Proposed important components of the pathogenesis of ARDS include the following:
1. Inflammation in the pulmonary parenchyma, particularly with neutrophils
2. Activation of the vascular endothelium and expression of leukocyte adhesion molecules
3. Release of multiple cytokine mediators, proteases, and oxidants
4. Release of procoagulants and activation of the coagulation system

factor-α, interleukin (IL)-8, endothelin, and transforming growth factor-β. An inflammatory response also can be augmented by a reduction in antiinflammatory mediators, including cytokines such as IL-10 and IL-11.

Activation of complement likely is just one of multiple potential mechanisms for recruiting and sequestering neutrophils in the lungs. Other important factors include cytokines and other mediators that influence neutrophil trafficking in the lungs. Vascular endothelial cells, particularly in the pulmonary vascular system, also become activated, express leukocyte adhesion molecules, and lead to accumulation of neutrophils within the pulmonary vasculature.

Another important process appears to be activation of the coagulation system. Several factors are responsible for what has been called a "procoagulant state," including release of procoagulant tissue factors, a decreased concentration of factors with anticoagulant activity (e.g., protein C and protein S), and increased activity of proteins (e.g., plasminogen activator inhibitor-1) that inhibit fibrinolysis. The result is increased production of thrombin and fibrin as well as evidence of thrombosis within pulmonary capillaries.

Despite extensive research efforts over the past decade to elucidate the mechanisms of acute lung injury, a true understanding of ARDS is still a long way off. Such an understanding will be critical to the development of effective forms of prevention and therapy.

PATHOLOGY

Pathologic features of ARDS are the following:
1. Damage to alveolar type I epithelial cells
2. Interstitial and alveolar fluid
3. Areas of alveolar collapse
4. Inflammatory cell infiltrate
5. Hyperplasia of alveolar type II epithelial cells
6. Hyaline membranes
7. Fibrosis
8. Pulmonary vascular changes

Despite the number of etiologic factors in ARDS, the pathologic findings are relatively similar, regardless of the underlying cause. This pattern of injury accompanying ARDS, as observed by the pathologist, is frequently labeled *diffuse alveolar damage.*

Injury to type I alveolar epithelial cells and pulmonary capillary endothelial cells appears to be the primary factor in pathogenesis. Type I epithelial cells frequently appear necrotic and may slough from the surface of the alveolar wall. Damage to the capillary endothelial cells is generally more difficult, if not impossible, to recognize with light microscopy, and electron microscopy may be necessary to see the subtle ultrastructural changes.

Early in the course of ARDS, often called the *exudative phase,* fluid can be seen in the interstitial space of the alveolar septum as well as in the alveolar lumen. Scattered bleeding and regions of alveolar collapse, which are at least partly related to inactivation of surfactant (by protein-rich alveolar exudates) and to decreased surfactant production resulting from injury to alveolar type II epithelial cells, may be seen. The lung parenchyma shows influx of inflammatory cells, both in the interstitial space and often in the alveolar lumen as well. The cellular response is relatively nonspecific, consisting of neutrophils and macrophages. Fibrin and cellular debris may be seen in or around alveoli.

A characteristic finding in the pathology of ARDS is the presence of *hyaline membranes.* These membranes are believed to represent the protein-rich edema fluid that has filled the alveoli. The membranes are composed of a combination of fibrin, cellular debris, and plasma proteins that are deposited on the alveolar surface. Although they are nonspecific, their presence suggests that alveolar injury and a permeability problem, rather than elevated hydrostatic pressures, are the cause of pulmonary edema.

After approximately 1 to 2 weeks, the exudative phase evolves into a *proliferative phase.* As an important part of the reparative process that occurs during the proliferative phase, alveolar type II epithelial cells replicate in an attempt to replace the damaged type I epithelial cells. These hyperplastic type II epithelial cells often figure quite prominently in the pathologic picture of ARDS.

Another component of the proliferative phase is an accumulation of fibroblasts in the pulmonary parenchyma. In severe and prolonged cases of ARDS, this fibroblastic response becomes particularly important. In some cases, the damaged lung parenchyma is not repaired but goes on to develop significant scar tissue (fibrosis). Often accompanying the fibrosis are changes in the pulmonary vasculature, which include extensive remodeling and compromise of the lumen of small vessels by intimal and medial proliferation and by the formation of in situ thrombosis.

PATHOPHYSIOLOGY

EFFECTS ON GAS EXCHANGE

Most of the clinical consequences of ARDS follow in reasonably logical fashion from the presence of interstitial and alveolar edema. The most striking problem is alveolar flooding, which effectively prevents ventilation of affected alveoli even though perfusion may be relatively preserved. These alveoli, perfused but not ventilated, act as regions in which blood is shunted from the pulmonary arterial to pulmonary venous circulation without ever being oxygenated. This type of shunting is one of the mechanisms of hypoxemia (see Chapter 1), and there is perhaps no better example of shunting than ARDS.

In ARDS there are regions not only of true shunting but also of ventilation-perfusion mismatch. To some extent, this phenomenon results from an uneven distribution of the pathologic process within the lungs. In areas where the interstitium is more edematous or where more fluid is present in the alveoli, ventilation is more impaired (even though some ventilation remains) than in areas that have been relatively spared. Changes in blood flow do not necessarily follow the same distribution as do changes in ventilation, and ventilation-perfusion mismatch results.

In addition to the direct effects of interstitial and alveolar fluid on oxygenation, other changes appear to be secondary to alterations in the production and effectiveness of surfactant. Chapter 8 refers to surfactant as a phospholipid that is responsible for decreasing surface tension and maintaining alveolar patency. When surfactant is absent, as is seen in the respiratory distress syndrome of neonates, there is extensive collapse of alveoli. In ARDS, surfactant production may be adversely affected by injury to alveolar type II epithelial cells. Additionally, evidence suggests that, as a result of extensive fluid within the alveoli, surfactant is inactivated and therefore ineffective in preventing alveolar collapse.

In terms of oxygenation, both ventilation-perfusion mismatch (with regions of low ventilation-perfusion ratio) and true shunting (ventilation-perfusion ratio = 0) are responsible for hypoxemia. Insofar as shunting is responsible for the drop in Po_2, supplemental O_2 alone may not be capable of restoring oxygenation to normal. In practice, Po_2 does rise somewhat with administration of 100% O_2 but not nearly to the level expected after such high concentrations of O_2. Considering the nature of the problem of ARDS, this response to supplemental O_2 should not be surprising. Oxygen improves whatever component of hypoxemia is due to ventilation-perfusion mismatch, but it is ineffective for true shunting.

On the other hand, the absolute level of ventilation in the patient with ARDS remains intact or even increases. As a result, the patient typically does not have difficulty with CO_2 retention, except in terminal stages of the disease or in the presence of another underlying pulmonary process. Even though substantial amounts of what is effectively dead space may be present (as part of the overall ventilation-perfusion mismatch), the patient is able to increase total ventilation to compensate for the regions of maldistribution.

Pathophysiologic features of ARDS are the following:
1. Shunting and $\dot{V}/\dot{Q}$ mismatch
2. Secondary alterations in function of surfactant
3. Increased pulmonary vascular resistance
4. Decreased pulmonary compliance
5. Decreased FRC

CHANGES IN PULMONARY VASCULATURE

The pulmonary vasculature is subject to changes resulting from the overall pathologic process. Pulmonary vascular resistance increases, probably for a variety of reasons. Hypoxemia certainly produces vasoconstriction within the pulmonary arterial system, and fluid in the interstitium may increase interstitial pressure, resulting in a decrease in size and an increase in resistance of the small pulmonary vessels. The lumen of small vessels may be compromised by microthrombi and proliferative changes in vessel walls (discussed earlier in the sections on pathogenesis and pathology).

One consequence of the pulmonary vascular changes is an alteration in the normal distribution of pulmonary blood flow. Naturally, blood flows preferentially to areas with lower resistance, which do not necessarily correspond to the regions receiving the most ventilation. Hence, ventilation-perfusion mismatch again results, with some areas having high and other areas low ventilation-perfusion ratios.

EFFECTS ON MECHANICAL PROPERTIES OF THE LUNGS

When considering the mechanical properties of the lung in ARDS, we must recognize that computed tomographic scanning has demonstrated the distribution of disease to be often more heterogeneous than expected on the basis of the diffuse changes seen on chest radiograph. Whereas some regions have been damaged and are quite abnormal, others appear to have been spared from injury. As a result, the alveoli are not diffusely and relatively homogeneously stiffened. Rather, some regions of the lung have significantly diseased alveoli that ventilate poorly or not at all, whereas other regions have relatively preserved and well-ventilated alveoli. The net result of having fewer effectively "functional" alveoli is that less volume enters the lung for any given inflation pressure; by definition this means that the compliance of the lung is decreased.

> The decreased compliance and low FRC in ARDS are not associated with homogeneously affected alveoli but rather with heterogeneous disease involvement.

The volume of gas contained within the lungs at functional residual capacity (FRC), that is, the resting end-expiratory position of the lungs, also is significantly decreased. Again, on the basis of the heterogeneity of the pathologic process, the decreased FRC is not due to a uniform decrease in volume over all alveoli but rather to a group of alveoli containing little or no gas and another group containing a relatively normal volume of gas. The net result is that patients breathe at a much lower overall lung volume than normal, preferentially ventilating those alveoli that are relatively preserved. The typical breathing pattern resulting from these mechanical changes is characterized by rapid but shallow breaths. This type of breathing pattern is inefficient and demands increased energy expenditure by the patient, which probably contributes to the dyspnea that is so characteristic of patients with ARDS.

CLINICAL FEATURES

Because ARDS is a clinical syndrome with many different causes, the clinical picture reflects not only the presence of noncardiogenic pulmonary edema but also the presence of the underlying disease. Our concern here with the respiratory consequences of ARDS, irrespective of the cause, directs our focus to the clinical effects of the syndrome itself rather than to those of the underlying disorder.

> Clinical features of ARDS are the following:
> 1. Dyspnea, tachypnea
> 2. Rales
> 3. ↓ P_{O_2}, normal or ↓ P_{CO_2}, ↑ AaD_{O_2}
> 4. Radiographic findings of interstitial and alveolar edema

After the initial insult, whatever it may be, there generally is a lag of several hours to 1 day or more before respiratory consequences ensue. In most cases, the first symptom experienced by the patient is dyspnea. At this time, examination often shows the patient to be tachypneic, although the chest radiograph may not reveal significant findings. However, arterial blood gases reflect a disturbance of oxygenation, often with an increase in the alveolar–arterial difference in partial pressure of oxygen (AaD_{O_2}). Alveolar ventilation either is normal or more frequently is increased so that P_{CO_2} is generally below baseline. In the most severe cases, alveolar ventilation cannot be maintained, and P_{CO_2} rises.

As fluid and protein continue to leak from the vasculature into the interstitial and alveolar spaces, the clinical findings become even more florid. Patients may become extremely dyspneic and tachypneic, and chest examination may show the presence of rales. Findings on the chest radiograph become grossly abnormal, revealing interstitial and alveolar edema that can be extensive. The radiographic aspects of ARDS are discussed in the section on diagnostic approach.

As a result of improved ability over the past 40 years to provide respiratory support for these patients, death caused by respiratory failure now is relatively uncommon. Rather, the high mortality seen with ARDS, currently estimated to be approximately 25% to 40%, is related to the underlying cause (particularly sepsis) or to failure of multiple organ systems in these critically ill patients. Patients who are fortunate enough to recover may have surprisingly few respiratory sequelae that are both serious and permanent. Pulmonary function may return essentially to normal, although sophisticated assessment often shows some relatively subtle abnormalities.

DIAGNOSTIC APPROACH

The diagnosis of ARDS is generally based on a combination of clinical and radiographic information (assessment at a macroscopic level) and arterial blood gas values (assessment at a functional level). Although at one time some clinicians and investigators had advocated lung biopsy in patients with presumed ARDS, these procedures were performed primarily for research purposes and never achieved general clinical acceptance.

The chest radiograph in patients with incipient ARDS does not necessarily reveal abnormal findings at the onset of clinical presentation. However, within a short period of time the evidence of interstitial and alveolar edema generally develops, the latter being the most prominent finding on chest radiograph. The edema appears to be diffuse, affecting both lungs relatively symmetrically. As an indication that the fluid is filling alveolar spaces, air bronchograms often appear within the diffuse infiltrates. Unless the patient has prior heart disease and cardiac enlargement unrelated to the present problem, heart size remains normal. A characteristic example of a chest radiograph in a patient with severe ARDS is shown in Figure 3-7.

Arterial blood gas values show hypoxemia and hypocapnia (respiratory alkalosis). Calculation of AaD_{O_2} clearly shows that gas exchange actually is worse than it appears at first glance, with alveolar P_{O_2} elevated as a result of hyperventilation. As the amount of interstitial and alveolar edema increases, oxygenation becomes progressively more abnormal, and severe hypoxemia results. Because true shunting of blood across non-ventilated alveoli is important in the pathogenesis of hypoxemia, P_{O_2} may be relatively unresponsive to administration of supplemental O_2. In order to allow a standardized method for interpreting P_{O_2} in patients receiving different amounts of supplemental oxygen, a ratio of Pa_{O_2} to fractional concentration of inspired oxygen (Pa_{O_2}/F_{IO_2}) less than 200 mm Hg is considered an appropriate gas-exchange criterion for ARDS, whereas ALI is defined by less severe gas-exchange abnormalities and Pa_{O_2}/F_{IO_2} less than 300 mm Hg.

In many cases of ARDS, a direct measurement of pressures within the pulmonary circulation is useful. This measurement is facilitated by use of a catheter inserted into a systemic vein and then passed through the right atrium and right ventricle into the pulmonary artery. The relatively easy passage of this catheter (commonly known as a Swan-Ganz catheter) results from a balloon at the tip, which can be inflated with air and then carried along with blood flow through the tricuspid and pulmonic valves

A pulmonary artery (Swan-Ganz) catheter can measure pulmonary vascular pressures and cardiac output.

into the pulmonary artery. The catheter is positioned at a point in the pulmonary artery where inflation of the balloon occludes the lumen and prevents forward flow. Consequently, if pressure is measured at the tip of the catheter when forward flow has been prevented, the measured pressure theoretically is a reflection of pressure in the left atrium, which corresponds to left ventricular preload. The pressure measured with the balloon inflated is commonly called the *pulmonary artery occlusion pressure* (PAOP) or *pulmonary capillary wedge pressure.*

These measurements can distinguish whether the observed pulmonary edema is cardiogenic or noncardiogenic in origin. In cardiogenic pulmonary edema, the hydrostatic pressure within the pulmonary capillaries is high as a result of "back-pressure" from the pulmonary veins and left atrium. In noncardiogenic pulmonary edema or ARDS, the pressure within the left atrium, measured as the PAOP, is normal, indicating that the interstitial and alveolar fluid results from increased permeability of the pulmonary capillaries and not from high intravascular pressure.

Although use of these catheters for measurement of intravascular pressures is not essential to the diagnosis of ARDS, the information obtained may be useful for determining whether elevated hydrostatic pressures within the capillaries are contributing to the observed pulmonary edema. In addition, the catheters may provide helpful information during the course of the complicated management of these cases, even though their use has not been shown to improve overall patient outcomes.

TREATMENT

Management of ARDS centers on three main issues: (1) treatment of the precipitating disorder; (2) interruption of, or interference with, the pathogenetic sequence of events involved in the development of capillary leak; and (3) support of gas exchange until the pulmonary process improves. Although treatment of the precipitating disorder is not always possible or successful, the principle is relatively simple: As long as the underlying problem persists, the pulmonary capillary leak may remain. In the case of a disorder such as sepsis, management of the infection with appropriate antibiotics (and drainage, if necessary) is crucial to allowing the pulmonary vasculature to regain the normal permeability barrier for protein and fluid.

Approaches aimed at altering the pathogenetic sequence of events in ARDS have focused on developing agents that block the effect of various cytokines or other mediators, such as endotoxin, in patients with septic shock. However, to date, this approach has been unsuccessful, and no agents blocking the effect of a particular mediator have been useful. A more nonspecific approach has been use of corticosteroids in an attempt to block a variety of mediators and to control or reverse the capillary permeability defect allowing fluid and protein to leak into the interstitium and alveolar spaces. This approach is based in part on experimental evidence suggesting that steroids inhibit aggregation of neutrophils induced by activated complement. However, because of disappointing clinical results and the potential for harmful effects, corticosteroids now are generally not considered appropriately indicated for treatment of ARDS, at least early in its course. Preliminary data suggested that steroids may be useful if administered during the later, fibroproliferative phase of ARDS, but a subsequent controlled trial demonstrated no mortality benefit from corticosteroids used in this setting.

Meticulous supportive management, particularly support of gas exchange, is critical for patients with ARDS to survive the acute illness. Given the life-threatening nature of ARDS, patients typically are intubated, ventilated with a mechanical ventilator, and managed in an intensive care unit. Failure of other organ systems besides the respiratory system is common, and patients often present some of the most complex and challenging management problems handled in intensive care units. Because of the importance of mechanical ventilation and ventilatory support in the management of respiratory failure associated with ARDS and with other disorders, Chapter 29 is devoted to a more detailed consideration of mechanical ventilation in the management of respiratory failure.

Because the mortality of ARDS remains considerable, a variety of newer and experimental forms of therapy have been tried. For example, one interesting approach has been the use of inhaled nitric oxide as a selective pulmonary vasodilator. By producing preferential vasodilation in areas of the lung that are well ventilated (because these are the areas to which the gas is delivered), inhaled nitric oxide can facilitate better perfusion of well-ventilated areas, leading to better ventilation-perfusion matching and improved oxygenation. Unfortunately, however, beneficial physiologic effects on gas exchange have not been accompanied by documentation of improved survival in clinical trials conducted to date. In contrast, one large study showed that administration of human recombinant activated protein C, which has both antithrombotic and antiinflammatory effects, improved survival of patients with severe sepsis, one of the common forerunners of ARDS. However, more experience with use of human recombinant activated protein C is needed before its overall role in severe sepsis complicated by ARDS is fully established.

REFERENCES

GENERAL REVIEWS

Arroliga AC, Matthay MA, Weidemann HP, editors: Acute respiratory distress syndrome, *Clin Chest Med* 27:549–754, 2006.

Rubenfeld GD, Herridge MS: Epidemiology and outcomes of acute lung injury, *Chest* 131:554–562, 2007.

Ware LB, Matthay MA: The acute respiratory distress syndrome, *N Engl J Med* 342:1334–1349, 2000.

Wheeler AP, Bernard GR: Acute lung injury and the acute respiratory distress syndrome: a clinical review, *Lancet* 369:1553–1564, 2007.

PATHOGENESIS

Bellingan GJ: The pathogenesis of ALI/ARDS, *Thorax* 57:540–546, 2002.

Matthay MA, Zimmerman GA: Acute lung injury and the acute respiratory distress syndrome. Four decades of inquiry into pathogenesis and rational management, *Am J Respir Cell Mol Biol* 33:319–327, 2005.

Matthay MA, Zimmerman GA, Esmon C, et al: Future research directions in acute lung injury: summary of a National Heart, Lung, and Blood Institute working group, *Am J Respir Crit Care Med* 167:1027–1035, 2003.

Piantadosi CA, Schwartz DA: The acute respiratory distress syndrome, *Ann Intern Med* 141:460–470, 2004.

Suratt BT, Parsons PE: Mechanisms of acute lung injury/acute respiratory distress syndrome, *Clin Chest Med* 27:579–589, 2006.

TREATMENT

Adhibari N, Burns KE, Meade MO: Pharmacologic therapies for adults with acute lung injury and acute respiratory distress syndrome, *Cochrane Database Syst Rev* 4:CD004477, 2004.

Bernard GR, Vincent JL, Laterre PF, et al: Efficacy and safety of recombinant human activated protein C for severe sepsis, *N Engl J Med* 344:699–709, 2001.

Calfee CS, Matthay MA: Nonventilatory treatments for acute lung injury and ARDS, *Chest* 131:913–920, 2007.

Fan E, Needham DM, Stewart TE: Ventilatory management of acute lung injury and acute respiratory distress syndrome, *JAMA* 294:2889–2896, 2005.

Steinberg KP, Hudson LD, Goodman RB, et al: Efficacy and safety of corticosteroids for persistent acute respiratory distress syndrome, *N Engl J Med* 354:1671–1684, 2006.

Management of Respiratory Failure

Supportive therapy aimed at maintaining adequate gas exchange is critical in the management of both acute respiratory failure and chronic respiratory insufficiency. In acute respiratory failure, survival depends on the ability to provide supportive therapy until the patient recovers from the acute illness. In patients with chronic respiratory insufficiency, the goal is to maximize the patient's function and to minimize symptoms and cor pulmonale on a long-term basis. This chapter outlines the goals of supportive therapy and provides a discussion of the ways in which adequate gas exchange can be maintained, focusing on patients with acute respiratory failure. Because the principles for supportive management differ considerably in the two main categories of acute respiratory failure—acute respiratory distress syndrome (ARDS) and acute on chronic respiratory failure—these differences are emphasized in the course of the discussion. The chapter concludes with a consideration of two specific topics applicable to patients with chronic respiratory insufficiency: chronic ventilatory assistance and lung transplantation.

GOALS OF SUPPORTIVE THERAPY FOR GAS EXCHANGE

Adequate uptake of O_2 by the blood, delivery of O_2 to the tissues, and elimination of CO_2 all are parts of normal gas exchange. In terms of O_2 uptake by the blood, almost all the O_2 carried by blood is bound to hemoglobin, and only a small portion is dissolved in plasma. It is apparent from the oxyhemoglobin dissociation curve that elevating Po_2 beyond the point at which hemoglobin is almost completely saturated does not significantly increase the O_2 content of blood. On average, assuming that the dissociation curve is not shifted, hemoglobin is approximately 90% saturated at a Po_2 of 60 mm Hg. Increasing Po_2 to this level is important, but a Po_2 much beyond this level does not provide that much incremental benefit. In practice, patients with respiratory failure often are maintained at a Po_2 slightly higher than 60 mm Hg to allow a "margin of safety" for fluctuations in Po_2.

Oxygen delivery to the tissues, however, depends not only on arterial Po_2 but also on hemoglobin level and cardiac output. In patients who are anemic, O_2 content and thus O_2 transport can be compromised as much by the low hemoglobin level as by hypoxemia (see Equation 1-3). In selected circumstances, blood transfusion may be useful in raising the hemoglobin and O_2 content to more desirable levels.

Similarly, when cardiac output is impaired, tissue O_2 delivery also decreases, and measures to augment cardiac output may improve overall O_2 transport. Unfortunately, some of the measures used to improve arterial Po_2 may have a detrimental effect on cardiac output. As a result, tissue O_2 delivery may not improve (and even may worsen) despite an increase in Po_2. Use of positive-pressure ventilation, particularly with positive end-expiratory pressure, is most important in this regard. This technique is discussed in the section on maintenance of oxygenation.

Elimination of CO_2 by the lungs is important for maintaining adequate acid-base homeostasis. However, achieving an acceptable pH value, not a "normal" Pco_2, is the primary goal in managing respiratory failure and impaired elimination of CO_2. In patients with chronic hypercapnia (and metabolic compensation), abruptly restoring Pco_2 to normal (40 mm Hg) may cause significant alkalosis and thus risk precipitating either arrhythmias or seizures.

> Goals of optimizing O_2 transport to tissues are the following:
> 1. Arterial O_2 saturation >90% (i.e., Po_2 >60 mm Hg)
> 2. Acceptable hemoglobin level (e.g., >10 g/dL, corresponding to hematocrit >30%)
> 3. Normal or near-normal cardiac output

> CO_2 is eliminated to maintain acceptable pH rather than "normal" Pco_2.

MAINTENANCE OF CARBON DIOXIDE ELIMINATION

CO_2 retention is an important aspect of respiratory failure in several types of patients. Most frequently, these patients have some degree of chronic CO_2 retention, and their acute problem is appropriately termed "acute on chronic" respiratory failure. Patients with chronic obstructive lung disease, chest wall disease, and neuromuscular disease all are subject to development of hypercapnia. Hypercapnia may be acute in certain groups of patients—for example, individuals who have suppressed respiratory drive resulting from ingestion of drugs in a suicide attempt and occasional patients with severe asthma and *status asthmaticus*.

If the degree of CO_2 retention is sufficiently great to cause a marked decrease in the patient's pH (<7.25–7.30), ventilatory assistance with a mechanical ventilator often is necessary.* Similarly, if marked CO_2 retention has impaired the patient's mental status, ventilatory assistance is indicated. For the patient who has a good chance of rapid reversal of CO_2 retention with therapy (assuming the level of CO_2 retention is not life threatening), this therapy often is attempted first with the hope of avoiding mechanical ventilation.

Measurements reflecting muscle strength and pulmonary function may be useful for the patient with acute or impending respiratory failure. These measurements serve as an indirect guide to the patient's ability to maintain adequate CO_2 elimination. Hence they also have been used as criteria for instituting ventilatory assistance or, conversely, for deciding when a patient aided by a mechanical ventilator might be weaned from ventilatory support. Although the decision to initiate mechanical ventilation frequently is based on clinical grounds, the objective measurements most commonly used as criteria for mechanical ventilation are (1) vital capacity (<10 mL/kg body weight) and (2) inspiratory force (<25 cm H_2O negative pressure). The latter measurement, which

> Mechanical ventilation often is indicated when arterial Pco_2 has risen sufficiently to cause the following:
> 1. Lowered pH: to 7.25–7.30 or below
> 2. Impaired mental status

---

*To initiate ventilatory support, the patient generally is intubated (i.e., a tube is placed through the nose or mouth, through the vocal cords, and into the trachea), and a mechanical ventilator is connected to the endotracheal tube. An alternative method of assisting ventilation, called *noninvasive positive-pressure ventilation*, is described in the section on chronic ventilatory support.

is also called the *maximal inspiratory pressure,* is performed by having the patient inspire as deeply as possible through tubing connected to a pressure gauge. This technique quantifies the maximal negative pressure that the patient can generate when the airway is occluded. These measurements are most useful in following patients with progressive neuromuscular weakness (e.g., myasthenia gravis) to determine when mechanical ventilation is necessary.

Although these and other specific measurements have been used to determine when a patient requires ventilatory assistance for eliminating CO_2, none of the guidelines is absolute. Some of the many additional factors that enter into such decisions include the nature of the underlying disease, the tempo and direction of change of the patient's illness, and the presence of other medical problems.

MAINTENANCE OF OXYGENATION

Although hypoxemia is a feature of almost all patients with respiratory failure when breathing air (21% O_2), the ease of supporting the patient and restoring adequate Po_2 depends to a great degree on the type of respiratory failure. In most cases of acute on chronic respiratory failure, ventilation-perfusion mismatch and hypoventilation are responsible for hypoxemia. For these mechanisms of hypoxemia, administration of supplemental O_2 is quite effective in improving the Po_2, and particularly high concentrations of inspired O_2 are not necessary. Frequently, O_2 can be administered by face mask or by nasal prongs to provide inhaled concentrations of O_2 not exceeding 40%, and patients are able to achieve a Po_2 greater than 60 mm Hg.

However, patients with chronic hypercapnia may be subject to further increases in Pco_2 when they receive supplemental O_2 (see Chapter 18). If Pco_2 rises to an unacceptably high range, the patient may require intubation and assisted ventilation with a mechanical ventilator to maintain an acceptable Pco_2. Fortunately, this complication is infrequent with judicious use of supplemental O_2.

In the patient with hypoxemic respiratory failure such as ARDS, ventilation-perfusion mismatch and shunting are responsible for hypoxemia. When a large fraction of the cardiac output is being shunted through areas of unventilated lung and, therefore, is not oxygenated during passage through the lungs, supplemental O_2 is relatively ineffective at raising Po_2 to an acceptable level. In these cases, patients may require inspired O_2 concentrations in the range of 60% to 100% and still may have difficulty maintaining Po_2 greater than 60 mm Hg.

Such patients with ARDS also require ventilatory assistance but generally for a different reason than patients with acute on chronic respiratory failure. In the latter patients, an unacceptable degree of CO_2 retention is generally the indication for intubation and mechanical ventilation. In patients with ARDS, oxygenation is extremely difficult to support, CO_2 retention is much less frequent, and hypoxemia rather than hypercapnia is the primary indication for mechanical ventilation.

For patients with hypoxemic respiratory failure, inability to achieve a Po_2 of 60 mm Hg or greater on supplemental O_2 readily administered by face mask (generally in the range of 40%–60%) is often considered reason for intubation and mechanical ventilation. However, such decisions for ventilatory support are not based on just one number. Other factors taken into consideration include the nature of the underlying problem and the likelihood of a rapid response to therapy.

In the setting of ARDS, intubation and mechanical ventilation serve several useful purposes. First, high concentrations of O_2 can be administered much more reliably through a tube inserted into the trachea than through a mask placed over the face. Second, administration of positive pressure by a ventilator relieves the patient of the high work of breathing (see section on reducing work of breathing), allowing the

Mechanical ventilation often is indicated when $Po_2 \geq 60$ mm Hg cannot be achieved with inspired O_2 concentration $\leq 40\%$–60%.

patient to receive more reliable tidal volumes than he or she would spontaneously take, particularly because the poorly compliant lungs of ARDS promote shallow breathing and low tidal volumes. Finally, when a tube is in place in the trachea, positive pressure can be maintained in the airway throughout the respiratory cycle and not just during the inspiratory phase. In common usage, positive airway pressure maintained at the end of expiration in a mechanically ventilated patient is termed *positive end-expiratory pressure* (PEEP).

Why is positive pressure throughout the respiratory cycle beneficial in patients with ARDS? Patients with ARDS often have a great deal of microatelectasis resulting from fluid occupying alveolar spaces, low tidal volumes, and probably both decreased production and inactivation of surfactant. The resting end-expiratory volume of the lung (i.e., functional residual capacity [FRC]) is quite low in these patients but can be increased substantially by administration of PEEP. At the higher FRC, many small airways and alveoli that formerly were closed and received no ventilation are opened and capable of gas exchange. Therefore, blood supplying these regions no longer courses through unventilated alveoli and now can be oxygenated. Measurement of the "shunt fraction" shows that PEEP is quite effective at decreasing the amount of blood that otherwise would not be oxygenated during passage through the lungs.

When the shunt fraction is decreased by PEEP, supplemental O_2 is much more effective at elevating the patient's Po_2 to an acceptable level. The concentration of inspired O_2 then can be lowered, and the patient is less likely to experience O_2 toxicity from extremely high concentrations of O_2.

Beneficial effects of ventilatory assistance in ARDS are the following:
1. More reliable administration of high concentrations of inspired O_2
2. Delivery of more reliable tidal volumes than those achieved spontaneously by the patient
3. Use of PEEP

PEEP is effective in ARDS by increasing FRC and preventing closure of small airways and alveoli.

REDUCING WORK OF BREATHING

One pathophysiologic feature shared by most patients with respiratory failure is an imbalance in the work of breathing relative to the ability of the respiratory muscles to perform that work. In the case of acute on chronic respiratory failure in the patient with chronic obstructive lung disease, the flattened and mechanically disadvantaged diaphragm must cope with an increase in airway resistance. In neuromuscular disease in either the purely acute or the acute on chronic setting, respiratory muscle strength may be insufficient to handle even a relatively normal work of breathing. In the patient with ARDS, the noncompliant (i.e., stiff) lungs require an inordinately high work of breathing even though respiratory muscle strength may be intact.

Consequently, ventilatory assistance in the patient with respiratory failure is important not only for the temporary support of gas exchange but also for the mechanical support of inspiration, allowing the respiratory muscles to rest. Dyspnea often is alleviated when such support is provided and the patient no longer must expend so much energy on the act of breathing. Fatigued respiratory muscles are allowed to recover, and the relatively large amount of blood flow required by overworking respiratory muscles can be shifted to perfusion of other organ systems.

Reducing the work of breathing is a benefit of mechanical ventilation in all forms of acute respiratory failure.

MECHANICAL VENTILATION

Mechanical ventilators are critical to effective management of respiratory failure. By supporting gas exchange and assisting with the work of ventilation for as long a period as necessary, mechanical ventilators can keep a patient alive and as comfortable as possible while the acute process precipitating respiratory failure is treated or allowed to resolve spontaneously. This section briefly describes the operation of mechanical ventilators, the available modes of ventilation, and the complications that can ensue from their use.

Ventilators currently used for management of acute respiratory failure are positive-pressure devices, that is, they deliver gas under positive pressure to the patient during inspiration. Most commonly, the ventilator is used in a *volume-cycled* fashion, meaning that each inspiration is terminated (and passive expiration allowed to occur) after a specified volume has been delivered by the machine. In contrast, in *pressure-limited* ventilation the assistance provided by the ventilator is targeted to a specified level of positive airway pressure. Volume cycling is much more reliable in delivering constant, specifiable tidal volumes than is pressure-limited ventilation. With the latter, changes in lung compliance, airway resistance, and the patient's own inspiratory effort alter the volume of gas delivered as the specified target pressure is reached.

Several ventilatory patterns or modes are available with most mechanical ventilators when used in a volume-cycled fashion (Fig. 29-1). In *controlled ventilation,* ventilation is supplied entirely by the ventilator at a respiratory rate, tidal volume, and inspired O_2 concentration chosen by the physician. If the patient attempts to take a spontaneous breath between the machine-delivered breaths, he or she does not receive any inspired gas. This type of ventilation is uncomfortable for the conscious patient capable of initiating inspiration and therefore can only be used for patients who are comatose, anesthetized, or unable to make any inspiratory effort.

In the *assist-control* mode of ventilation, the ventilator is able to "sense" when the patient initiates inspiration, at which point the machine assists by delivering a specified tidal volume to the patient. Although the tidal volume is set by the machine, the respiratory rate is determined by the number of spontaneous inspiratory efforts made by the patient. However, should the patient's spontaneous respiratory rate fall below a specified level, the machine provides a backup by delivering at least this minimal number of breaths. For example, if the backup rate set on the machine is 10 breaths per minute, the ventilator will automatically deliver a breath if and when 6 seconds have elapsed from the previous breath. Because the respiratory rate with this mode of ventilation is determined by the patient (after the rate is higher than the specified minimal level), fluctuations in minute ventilation can occur if the patient's respiratory rate changes significantly.

A third ventilatory mode is *intermittent mandatory ventilation* (IMV). With IMV, the machine delivers a preset number of breaths per minute at a specified tidal volume and inspired O_2 concentration. Between the machine-delivered breaths, the patient is able to breathe spontaneously from a gas source providing the same inspired O_2 concentration given during the machine-delivered breaths. However, the machine does not assist the spontaneous breaths; therefore, the tidal volume for these breaths is determined by the patient. In a much more commonly used variant of IMV called *synchronized IMV* (SIMV), each of the machine-delivered breaths is timed to coincide with and to assist a patient-initiated breath. If the patient being ventilated by IMV or SIMV modes changes his or her spontaneous respiratory rate significantly, the variation in minute ventilation theoretically is less than in the assist-control mode of ventilation because each breath has not been supplemented by a comparatively large tidal volume delivered by the ventilator. In practice, both assist-control and SIMV are clinically useful and effective modes of ventilation. Little objective information supporting the use of one over the other is available.

Two types of pressure-limited ventilation are used in certain clinical settings. The first is *pressure support ventilation* (PSV). With PSV, the ventilator senses when the patient initiates a breath, at which time the ventilator assists the patient's efforts by providing a specified amount of positive pressure to the airway. This level of pressure support is reached rapidly and is maintained throughout most of inspiration. The ventilator stops providing inspiratory assistance when the patient's inspiratory flow rate falls below a specified target level, such as 25% of the peak inspiratory flow rate. The volume of each breath can be quite variable and is dependent on the preset level

---

With volume-cycled ventilation, inspiration terminates after a specified tidal volume has been delivered by the ventilator. With pressure-limited ventilation, inspiration terminates after the targeted airway pressure has been achieved.

Common modes of mechanical ventilation are assist-control ventilation, synchronized intermittent mandatory ventilation (SIMV), and pressure support ventilation (PSV).

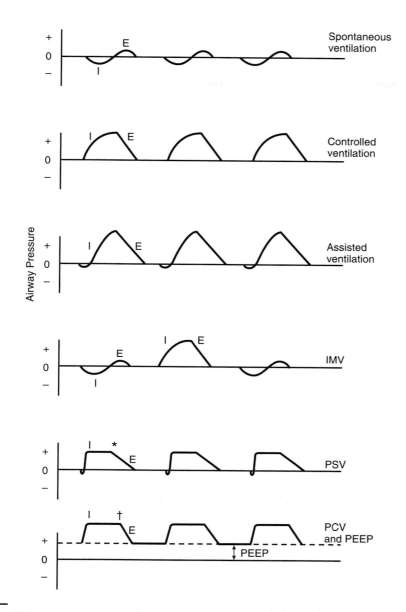

Figure 29-1. Airway pressure during spontaneous ventilation and during mechanical ventilation with several different ventilatory patterns. I = Inspiration; IMV = intermittent mandatory ventilation; E = expiration; PEEP = positive end-expiratory pressure; PCV = pressure-controlled ventilation; PSV = pressure support ventilation. *Inspiratory positive-pressure support ceases when the patient's flow rate falls below a threshold level. †The relative timing of inspiration and expiration is controlled by physician-determined ventilator settings.

of inspiratory pressure support, the patient's pattern of breathing, and the mechanical properties of the lungs. This type of ventilatory support is solely intended to assist a patient's own breathing efforts. If the patient stops making inspiratory efforts, no backup level of support is provided by the ventilator.

In *pressure-controlled ventilation* (PCV), the targeted pressure level is set by the clinician and is achieved rapidly, as is the case with PSV. However, in PSV the patient's spontaneously initiated flow triggers the breath, and a decrease in flow terminates the breath. In contrast, with PCV the initiation of the breath, the duration of inspiration, and the duration of expiration are determined by the clinician and set on the ventilator; the patient's breathing pattern does not influence the timing of the ventilatory assistance. Consequently, as for volume-cycled controlled ventilation, PCV is uncomfortable for the patient, who must be heavily sedated to tolerate the imposed ventilatory pattern. PCV is used primarily in patients with ARDS in whom problems with oxygenation and decreased lung compliance are particularly severe. In these cases, the clinician's control of peak pressure and the relative timing of inspiration and expiration can facilitate improved oxygenation and minimize the risk of complications from high pressure delivered by the ventilator.

An important option available for the intubated patient with hypoxemic respiratory failure (especially when it is due to ARDS) is PEEP. When a patient is assisted by a mechanical ventilator without PEEP, airway (and alveolar) pressure falls during expiration from the positive level achieved at the height of inspiration down to zero. However, if the expiratory portion of the tubing is connected to a valve requiring a pressure of at least 10 cm H_2O, for example, to open it, then the valve closes and expiration ceases when the airway pressure falls to 10 cm H_2O. Consequently, airway pressure at the end of expiration does not fall to zero but remains at the level determined by the specifications of the expiratory valve. On the basis of the pressure required to open the expiratory valve, the level of PEEP can be set as desired.

A variation of PEEP that works on the same principle is *continuous positive airway pressure* (CPAP). The term CPAP is used when the patient is breathing spontaneously (without a mechanical ventilator) and expiratory tubing is connected to a PEEP valve. To use CPAP, the patient can be either intubated or given a tightly fitting face mask. Although no positive pressure is provided by a mechanical ventilator during inspiration, inspired gas is delivered from a reservoir bag under tension or at a sufficiently high flow rate to keep airway pressure positive during inspiration as well as expiration.

With PEEP or CPAP, the benefit comes from the positive pressure within airways and alveoli at the end of expiration. FRC is increased by the positive pressure, and closure of airways and alveoli at the end of expiration is diminished.

In complicated cases of respiratory failure, such as patients with ARDS, a variety of ventilatory strategies are now used. Important goals of these particular strategies are to prevent closure of alveoli during expiration while simultaneously avoiding delivery of excessive volume and pressure to the airways and the alveoli, with the potential for secondary complications (see below). A particularly common strategy is called a *protective, open lung strategy,* in which sufficient PEEP is given to diminish airway closure during expiration, and relatively low tidal volumes (6 mL/kg) are used to protect the lung from inordinately high volumes and pressures delivered during inspiration. In some cases, P_{CO_2} may rise when these relatively low tidal volumes are used, but the elevation in P_{CO_2} above normal levels is considered acceptable according to a strategy of *permissive hypercapnia.* By minimizing the need for high levels of ventilation, this strategy theoretically decreases the risks of developing high alveolar pressures and overdistention and injury of some alveolar units.

> A protective, open lung strategy (using PEEP and avoiding excessive inspiratory inflation pressure and volume) is commonly used in patients with ARDS.

When the underlying problem that precipitated the need for mechanical ventilation has improved, ventilatory support is discontinued, typically after observing the patient during a short (30–120 minute) trial of spontaneous breathing with minimal or no positive pressure delivered by the mechanical ventilator. A useful guideline for assessing the patient's initial response to the spontaneous breathing trial and predicting successful discontinuation of mechanical ventilation is provided by the *rapid shallow breathing index.* This index is the ratio of the patient's respiratory rate divided by the tidal volume (expressed in liters) measured when the patient is not receiving assistance from the ventilator (i.e., during the spontaneous breathing trial). An index less than 105 is predictive of successful weaning, whereas an index greater than 105 is associated with a much higher likelihood of weaning failure.

Although the term "weaning" still is applied to discontinuation of mechanical ventilation, the older technique of slowly decreasing the amount of support provided by the ventilator is generally no longer used. As rational as it seems to wean the patient gradually from ventilatory support, an alternative and superior strategy is to perform a single daily trial of spontaneous breathing. If the patient tolerates the trial, then he or she is extubated; if the trial is unsuccessful, full ventilatory support is resumed for 24 hours until the time of the next daily trial.

Mechanical ventilation can be discontinued after a successful trial of spontaneous breathing.

COMPLICATIONS OF MECHANICAL VENTILATION

Intubation and mechanical ventilation of patients in respiratory failure are not without risks or complications (Table 29-1). The procedure of intubation can be complicated acutely by problems such as arrhythmias, laryngospasm, and malposition of the endotracheal tube (either in the esophagus or in a mainstem bronchus). When a tube remains in the trachea for days to weeks, complications affecting the larynx and trachea can occur. Vocal cord ulcerations and laryngeal stenosis and granulomas may develop. The trachea is subject to ulcerations, stenosis, and tracheomalacia (degeneration of supporting tissues in the tracheal wall) resulting from pressure applied by the inflated balloon at the end of the tube. As a precaution to decrease tracheal complications, tubes are made with cuffs that minimize the pressure exerted on the tracheal wall and the resulting pressure necrosis. For prolonged ventilatory support (weeks to months), a tracheostomy tube, placed directly into the trachea through an incision in the neck, has some advantages over prolonged orotracheal or nasotracheal intubation, including patient comfort and prevention of further vocal cord injury.

The presence of an endotracheal tube puts the patient at significant risk for pneumonia, usually called *ventilator-associated pneumonia*. Several factors appear to contribute to the patient's increased risk for developing pneumonia when intubated and

Table **29-1**
COMPLICATIONS OF INTUBATION AND MECHANICAL VENTILATION

Associated with intubation
  Malposition of tube
    Tube in esophagus
    Tube in mainstem bronchus (usually right)
  Arrhythmias
  Hypoxemia
  Laryngospasm
Associated with endotracheal or tracheostomy tubes
  Vocal cord ulcers
  Laryngeal stenosis/granulomas
  Tracheal stenosis
  Nasal necrosis
  Sinusitis/otitis media (with nasotracheal tubes)
  Occlusion or kinking of tube
  Infection (ventilator-associated pneumonia)
Associated with mechanical ventilation
  Barotrauma (volutrauma)
    Pneumothorax
    Pneumomediastinum
    Subcutaneous emphysema
  Decreased cardiac output (hypotension)
  Alveolar injury (related to overdistention and cytokine release)
  Atelectrauma (associated with cyclic alveolar opening and closing)
  Alveolar hypoventilation or hyperventilation

receiving mechanical ventilation. They include bypassing of the normal anatomic barriers and upper airway clearance mechanisms that prevent organisms from reaching the lower respiratory tract, aspiration of oropharyngeal secretions around the endotracheal tube and into the lower respiratory tract, and bacterial contamination of the endotracheal tube or the ventilator circuitry connected to the endotracheal tube. Organisms causing ventilator-associated pneumonia often are relatively antibiotic-resistant bacteria, including gram-negative bacilli and *Staphylococcus aureus,* leading to significant increases in both duration of hospitalization and mortality.

Administration of positive pressure by a mechanical ventilator has its own attendant problems. Patients receiving positive-pressure ventilation are subject to barotrauma, that is, traumatic changes such as pneumothorax or pneumomediastinum occurring as a result of high alveolar pressures. Because alveolar overdistention with rupture currently is thought to be the cause of these complications, the term *volutrauma* now is used often instead of barotrauma. Development of a pneumothorax in patients receiving mechanical ventilation can have catastrophic consequences if not detected and treated quickly. The ventilator continues to deliver gas under positive pressure to the patient, and the gas enters the pleural space through the rupture. The pressure in the pleural space and thorax increases, and a *tension pneumothorax* results (see Chapter 15), which severely diminishes venous return and cardiac output and causes rapid cardiovascular collapse. In such situations, a tube, catheter, or needle must be immediately inserted to decompress the pleural space, allow resumption of venous return, and enable reexpansion of the lung.

Besides barotrauma, another major adverse effect of positive-pressure ventilation is impairment of cardiovascular function. At least two mechanisms are thought to play a role. The first involves a decrease in venous return to the heart. Whereas the normally negative intrathoracic pressure during inspiration promotes venous return from the periphery, positive inspiratory pressure from a ventilator impedes venous return. The hemodynamic consequences of low cardiac output and blood pressure are even more likely when the patient is also receiving PEEP. In many cases, judicious administration of fluids can restore the effective intravascular volume and reverse the adverse hemodynamic consequences of positive-pressure ventilation.

The second mechanism involves an increase in pulmonary vascular resistance. When alveolar volume is increased with positive-pressure mechanical ventilation, alveolar vessels are compressed, compromising the overall cross-sectional area of the pulmonary vascular bed. As a result, pulmonary vascular resistance and the workload placed on the right ventricle increase. Right ventricular output is potentially compromised, and the right ventricle may dilate. This shifts the interventricular septum toward the left ventricular cavity, also impairing left ventricular filling and stroke volume.

Concern has been raised that the excessive volumes and high levels of pressure provided to the alveoli may be injurious to alveolar structures. Because lung injury in ARDS often is heterogeneously distributed (see Chapter 28), inspired gas is preferentially distributed to the more normal, more compliant alveoli than to the abnormal, less compliant alveoli. This puts the more normal alveoli at particular risk for overdistention. At the same time, more diseased alveoli are subject to collapse (atelectasis) during the expiratory phase of the respiratory cycle because of intraalveolar fluid and/or a disrupted or insufficient surfactant layer. Alveoli that are open during inspiration but collapse during expiration are subject to abnormal shear stresses during the repetitive process of opening and closing, a complication termed *atelectrauma.*

Both alveolar overdistention and atelectrauma may be accompanied by microscopic injury to cells of the alveolar wall and to intercellular attachments, leading to disruption of the normal permeability barrier provided by alveolar epithelial and capillary endothelial cells. In addition, proinflammatory cytokines may be released and perpetuate alveolar injury and inflammation. As a result, positive-pressure ventilation for respiratory failure,

> Barotrauma/volutrauma and impairment of systemic venous return to the heart are important adverse effects of positive-pressure ventilation

especially ARDS, potentially can compound or worsen the process for which it is being used. Therefore, it is currently believed that the pattern of ventilation should avoid both alveolar closure (atelectasis) during expiration and overdistention during inspiration, the former by use of PEEP and the latter by limiting tidal volume to 6 mL/kg and alveolar distending pressure to no more than 30 cm H_2O.

Management of patients receiving positive-pressure ventilation, particularly those with hypoxemic respiratory failure who require PEEP, is complicated. Many factors interact in a complex way, specifically oxygenation, cardiac output, and fluid status. Optimal care requires both sophisticated monitoring of the patient and substantial expertise from the team responsible for patient care. Such care is necessary not only for proper support of vital functions but also for minimizing the complications of therapy.

NONINVASIVE VENTILATORY SUPPORT FOR ACUTE RESPIRATORY FAILURE

When patients with acute respiratory failure require mechanical ventilation, support traditionally has been provided by positive pressure administered through a tube placed into the trachea (i.e., an endotracheal tube). However, use of the tube is associated with risks and complications, such as patient discomfort from the tube itself, injury to the airway mucosa, and development of lower respiratory tract infection (see Table 29-1). An alternative form of support for acute respiratory failure does not require use of an endotracheal tube; rather, positive pressure is provided through a tightly fitting mask placed over the face. This approach has been used for support of patients with a variety of types of acute respiratory failure, including patients with cardiogenic pulmonary edema, those with acute exacerbation of chronic obstructive pulmonary disease, and patients who are not considered suitable candidates for intubation. However, noninvasive ventilatory support is not appropriate if patients are unable to protect their airway; it is most useful when the respiratory failure most likely is readily reversible and therefore of relatively short duration.

SELECTED ASPECTS OF THERAPY FOR CHRONIC RESPIRATORY FAILURE

CHRONIC VENTILATORY SUPPORT

Patients with chronic, irreversible respiratory system disease who require continuous, long-term ventilatory support pose a difficult problem. The first question is whether the patient wishes "to be on a machine" for the rest of his or her life. Some patients clearly wish to prolong life even if it means permanent ventilatory support; others make the decision that life is not worth living if they must be dependent on a ventilator for the remainder of their lives. When the patient chooses to be maintained on a ventilator, support usually is given by positive-pressure ventilation administered through a tracheostomy tube. The care of some patients can be handled at home with the proper support of family and visiting health care personnel. Management of other cases continues in chronic care hospitals or other facilities equipped to care for such patients.

A subgroup of patients with chronic respiratory insufficiency does not require continuous ventilatory support but benefits from nocturnal assistance with ventilation. These patients often have chronic neuromuscular or chest wall disease accompanied by chronic hypercapnia. Although the degree to which respiratory muscle fatigue contributes to the hypercapnia experienced by these patients is not clear, at least part of the rationale for using nocturnal ventilatory support is to afford these patients a number of hours each day when their inspiratory muscles are allowed to rest. After a period of nocturnal rest, the respiratory muscles presumably are better able to handle the work of breathing during the day, and daytime hypercapnia may be improved.

When ventilatory support is needed only during the night, it is generally preferable to avoid a chronic tracheostomy. Several options are available, and the most appropriate depends on the particular patient. Positive pressure can be administered at night through a mouthpiece or a mask (i.e., noninvasive positive-pressure ventilation). Alternatively, inflation of the lungs can be achieved by negative-pressure ventilation, that is, intermittent negative pressure applied outside the chest wall, causing it to expand and the lungs to inflate. The original type of negative-pressure ventilator was the "iron lung," used for ventilatory support from the 1930s through the polio epidemics of the 1950s. Currently, other negative-pressure devices are used more frequently. The two most common types are the "raincoat" (or "poncho") ventilator and the "cuirass" (or "chest shell") ventilator. Unlike the iron lung, which enclosed the entire body below the neck, the raincoat and cuirass ventilators do not enclose or limit movement of the lower half of the body. These negative-pressure ventilatory support devices have been used most frequently for patients with chronic respiratory failure resulting from neuromuscular disease such as muscular dystrophy.

Chronic ventilatory support can be provided by administration of positive pressure to the airway or by a device that produces intermittent negative pressure around the chest wall.

LUNG TRANSPLANTATION

First performed successfully in 1983, lung transplantation is a relatively recent form of therapy for management of severe and disabling chronic pulmonary disease. However, the availability of a lung transplant is limited because only a relatively small number of medical centers have the experience and the capability to perform the procedure and because suitable donor organs are scarce.

Several types of transplantation can be performed, with selection generally based on the underlying clinical problem. Single-lung transplantation has been used effectively in patients with end-stage disease caused by interstitial lung disease, severe emphysema, or pulmonary vascular disease. For patients with cystic fibrosis, in whom chronic bilateral pulmonary infection complicates their lung disease, bilateral lung transplantation has been performed to avoid infection of the new lung by spillover of infected secretions from a remaining diseased lung. When severe cardiac disease accompanies end-stage lung disease, combined heart–lung transplantation may be required. The most recent lung transplantation technique is lobar transplantation from living donors. In this technique, which is used primarily in patients with cystic fibrosis, the recipient is given bilateral implants of a lower lobe from each of two living donors.

In many ways, the lung transplant patient trades the primary lung disease for another disease: that of the transplant recipient. The major potential complications of lung transplantation fall under the general categories of rejection and infection. Because of the risk of rejection, patients are routinely given immunosuppressive drugs, such as prednisone, azathioprine (or mycophenolate mofetil), and cyclosporine (or tacrolimus), as a regimen to prevent rejection. Nevertheless, either acute or chronic rejection can occur despite maintenance immunosuppression. *Acute rejection* often is characterized by fever, impairment of pulmonary function and gas exchange, and pulmonary infiltrates on chest radiograph. Episodes typically occur during the first several months after transplantation and are treated by acute intensification of the immunosuppressive regimen, especially with increased doses of corticosteroids. *Chronic rejection* usually is manifested as bronchiolitis obliterans, which is characterized by progressive inflammation, fibrosis, and obstruction of small airways. The physiologic consequence of this process is progressive airflow obstruction, which typically is unresponsive to augmentation of immunosuppressive therapy. As a result, bronchiolitis obliterans is the major cause of graft failure and death occurring later in

The major complications occurring after lung transplantation are rejection and infection.

Progressive airflow obstruction from bronchiolitis obliterans is thought to represent chronic transplant rejection.

the course after lung transplantation. The main treatment option for posttransplant patients with severe bronchiolitis obliterans is repeat transplantation.

The other major complication of lung transplantation is infection, the risk of which is greatly increased by the need for immunosuppressive therapy. In some cases, organisms (e.g., bacteria, cytomegalovirus) accompanied the donor organ, and development of a complicating infection was precipitated by immunosuppression and impairment of the recipient's defense mechanisms. Patients also are subject to the variety of opportunistic infections that are common to patients with impaired cell-mediated immunity, including other viruses, fungi, and *Pneumocystis*.

Accompanying the growing experience with lung transplantation over the past decade has been a modest improvement in survival. Survival is approximately 75% to 80% at 1 year after transplantation and 60% at 3 years after transplantation. Lung transplantation now is an important but expensive therapeutic option for a highly selected group of patients. As more experience is gained with this form of treatment and as technology and immunosuppressive therapy evolve, we continue to refine our thinking about the role of transplantation in the overall management of patients with severe lung disease.

REFERENCES

MECHANICAL VENTILATION

Antonelli M, Pennisi MA, Conti G: New advances in the use of noninvasive ventilation for acute hypoxaemic respiratory failure, *Eur Respir J* 22(suppl 42):65s–71s, 2003.

Boles J-M, Bion J, Connors A, et al: Weaning from mechanical ventilation, *Eur Respir J* 29:1033–1056, 2007.

Brochard L, Mancebo J, Elliott MW: Noninvasive ventilation for acute respiratory failure, *Eur Respir J* 19:712–721, 2002.

Calfee CS, Matthay MA: Recent advances in mechanical ventilation, *Am J Med* 118:584–591, 2005.

Caples SM, Gay PC: Noninvasive positive pressure ventilation in the intensive care unit: a concise review, *Crit Care Med* 33:2651–2658, 2005.

Chastre J, Fagon JY: Ventilator-associated pneumonia, *Am J Respir Crit Care Med* 165:867–903, 2002.

Fan E, Needham DM, Stewart TE: Ventilatory management of acute lung injury and acute respiratory distress syndrome, *JAMA* 294:2889–2896, 2005.

Girard TD, Bernard GR: Mechanical ventilation in ARDS. A state-of-the-art review, *Chest* 131:921–929, 2007.

Khirani S, Georgopoulos D, Rossi A, Moxham J: Ventilator support in chronic obstructive pulmonary disease: invasive and noninvasive, *Eur Respir Mon* 11(monograph 38):401–429, 2006.

Liesching T, Kwok H, Hill NS: Acute applications of noninvasive positive pressure ventilation, *Chest* 124:699–713, 2003.

MacIntyre NR: Current issues in mechanical ventilation for respiratory failure, *Chest* 128(5 suppl 2):561S–567S, 2005.

MacIntyre NR, Cook DJ, Ely EW Jr, et al: Evidence-based guidelines for weaning and discontinuing ventilatory support: a collective task force facilitated by the American College of Chest Physicians; the American Association for Respiratory Care; and the American College of Critical Care Medicine, *Chest* 120(suppl):375S–395S, 2001.

Malhotra A: Low-tidal-volume ventilation in the acute respiratory distress syndrome, *N Engl J Med* 357:1113–1120, 2007.

Mehta S, Hill NS: Noninvasive ventilation, *Am J Respir Crit Care Med* 163:540–577, 2001.

Pinhu L, Whitehead T, Evans T, Griffiths M: Ventilator-associated lung injury, *Lancet* 361:332–340, 2003.

Rabatin JT, Gay PC: Noninvasive ventilation, *Mayo Clin Proc* 74:817–820, 1999.

Tobin MJ: Advances in mechanical ventilation, *N Engl J Med* 344:1986–1996, 2001.

Vlahakis NE, Hubmayr RD: Cellular stress failure in ventilator-injured lungs, *Am J Respir Crit Care Med* 171:1328–1342, 2005.

CHRONIC VENTILATORY SUPPORT

Consensus Conference Report: clinical indications for noninvasive positive pressure ventilation in chronic respiratory failure due to restrictive lung disease, COPD, and nocturnal hypoventilation, *Chest* 116:521–534, 1999.

Hill NS: Clinical applications of body ventilators, *Chest* 90:897, 1986.

Howard RS, Davidson C: Long term ventilation in neurogenic respiratory failure, *J Neurol Neurosurg Psychiatry* 74(suppl 3):iii24–30, 2003.

MacIntyre NR, Epstein SK, Carson S, et al: Management of patients requiring prolonged mechanical ventilation: report of a NAMDRC consensus conference, *Chest* 128:3937–3954, 2005.

Make BJ, Hill NS, Goldberg AI, et al: Mechanical ventilation beyond the intensive care unit. Report of a consensus conference of the American College of Chest Physicians, *Chest* 113(suppl):289S–344S, 1998.

Peters SG, Viggiano RW: Home mechanical ventilation, *Mayo Clin Proc* 63:1208, 1988.

Simonds AK: Home ventilation, *Eur Respir J Suppl* 47:38s–46s, 2003.

Strumpf DA, Millman RP, Hill NS: The management of chronic hypoventilation, *Chest* 98:474–480, 1990.

LUNG TRANSPLANTATION

Arcasoy SM, Kotloff RM: Lung transplantation, *N Engl J Med* 340:1081–1091, 1999.

Corris PA, Christie JD: Update in transplantation 2006, *Am J Respir Crit Care Med* 175:432–435, 2007.

Nicod LP: Mechanisms of airway obliteration after lung transplantation, *Proc Am Thorac Soc* 3:444–449, 2006.

Orens JB, Estenne M, Arcasoy S, et al; Pulmonary Scientific Council of the International Society for Heart and Lung Transplantation: International guidelines for the selection of lung transplant candidates: 2006 update—a consensus report from the Pulmonary Scientific Council of the International Society for Heart and Lung Transplantation, *J Heart Lung Transplant* 25:745–755, 2006.

Pierson RN III: Lung transplantation: current status and challenges, *Transplantation* 81:1609–1615, 2006.

Trulock EP: Lung transplantation, *Am J Respir Crit Care Med* 155:789–818, 1997.

Sample Problems Using Respiratory Equations

A comatose patient with no spontaneous respiration is placed on mechanical ventilation with the following settings:

Tidal volume (V_T) = 1000 mL

Respiratory frequency (f) = 10 breaths/min

Inspired O_2 concentration = 40% (FI_{O_2} = 0.4)

The following measurements are made:

Arterial P_{CO_2} (Pa_{CO_2}) = 40 mm Hg

Mixed expired P_{CO_2} (PE_{CO_2}) = 30 mm Hg

Arterial P_{O_2} (Pa_{O_2}) = 95 mm Hg

1. Calculate minute ventilation ($\dot{V}_E$), dead space to tidal volume ratio (V_D/V_T), alveolar volume (V_A), and alveolar ventilation ($\dot{V}_A$).
2. If extra tubing with a volume of 250 mL were added to the system in a position such that it provided additional dead space, what would be the new V_D/V_T?
3. With the new system as described in Question 2, what would be the new Pa_{CO_2}?
4. Going back to the original conditions (without added extra tubing), the ventilator settings are changed to new settings:

V_T = 500 mL

f = 20 breaths/min

   a. Calculate the new $\dot{V}_E$, V_A, $\dot{V}_A$, and V_D/V_T.
   b. What would happen to Pa_{CO_2} on the new settings?
   c. What would you expect PE_{CO_2} to be if you now measured it?
5. Using the original ventilator settings and arterial blood gases as given, calculate the alveolar–arterial difference in partial pressure of oxygen (AaD_{O_2}).
6. After the patient is improved, arterial blood gases, measured with the patient breathing room air, are as follows:

P_{O_2} = 75 mm Hg

P_{CO_2} = 40 mm Hg

pH = 7.40

Calculate AaD_{O_2}.
7. The next day, the patient's arterial blood gas values on room air are as follows:

P_{O_2} = 80 mm Hg

P_{CO_2} = 20 mm Hg

pH = 7.55

What is AaD_{O_2}?

Answers

1. $\dot{V}_E$ = 1000 mL/breath × 10 breaths/min = 10,000 mL/min = <u>10 L/min</u>

   V_D/V_T = (40 mm Hg − 30 mm Hg)/40 mm Hg = <u>0.25</u>

   V_A = V_T − V_D = 1000 mL − (0.25 × V_T) = 1000 mL − 250 mL = <u>750 mL</u>

   $\dot{V}_A$ = V_A × f = 750 mL/breath × 10 breaths/min = <u>7.5 L/min</u>

2. New V_D = 250 mL + 250 mL = 500 mL
   New V_D/V_T = 500 mL/1000 mL = <u>0.5</u>

3. Because Pa_{CO_2} is inversely proportional to $\dot{V}_A$, the new Pa_{CO_2} can be calculated from the old and the new $\dot{V}_A$ (assuming $\dot{V}_{CO_2}$ remains constant).
   As per Problem 1, old $\dot{V}_A$ = 7.5 L/min
   New V_A = 1000 mL − new V_D = 1000 mL − 500 mL = 500 mL
   New $\dot{V}_A$ = 500 mL/breath × 10 breaths/min = 5 L/min
   New $\dot{V}_A$ = ⅔ × old $\dot{V}_A$
   New Pa_{CO_2} = ³⁄₂ × old Pa_{CO_2} = ³⁄₂ × 40 mm Hg = <u>60 mm Hg</u>

4. On the basis of the new settings:
   a. $\dot{V}_E$ = 500 mL/breath × 20 breaths/min = <u>10 L/min</u>
      V_A = 500 mL − 250 mL = <u>250 mL</u>
      $\dot{V}_A$ = 250 mL/breath × 20 breaths/min = <u>5 L/min</u>
      V_D/V_T = 250 mL/500 mL = <u>0.5</u>
   b. New Pa_{CO_2} is inversely proportional to the ratio of the new $\dot{V}_A$ to the old $\dot{V}_A$.
      New $\dot{V}_A$/old $\dot{V}_A$ = (5 L/min)/(7.5 L/min) = ⅔
      New Pa_{CO_2} = ³⁄₂ × old Pa_{CO_2} = ³⁄₂ × 40 mm Hg = <u>60 mm Hg</u>
   c. Because V_D/V_T = (Pa_{CO_2} − Pe_{CO_2})/Pa_{CO_2}, substitute the known values and solve the equation for Pe_{CO_2}.
      0.5 = (60 mm Hg − Pe_{CO_2})/60 mm Hg
      Pe_{CO_2} = <u>30 mm Hg</u>

5. Pa_{O_2} = (0.4 × 713 mm Hg) − (40 mm Hg/0.8) = 285 mm Hg − 50 mm Hg = 235 mm Hg
   AaD_{O_2} = Pa_{CO_2} − Pa_{CO_2} = 235 mm Hg − 95 mm Hg = <u>140 mm Hg</u>

6. Pa_{O_2} = 150 mm Hg − (40 mm Hg/0.8) = 100 mm Hg
   AaD_{O_2} = 100 mm Hg − 75 mm Hg = <u>25 mm Hg</u>

7. Pa_{O_2} = 150 mm Hg − (20 mm Hg/0.8) = 125 mm Hg
   AaD_{O_2} = 125 mm Hg − 80 mm Hg = <u>45 mm Hg</u>

Pulmonary Function Tests: Guidelines for Interpretation and Sample Problems

This appendix provides an outline of a simplified approach to the interpretation of pulmonary function tests and gives several examples of test results presented as unknown problems. Because details of the interpretation of these tests may vary among laboratories, the approach here focuses on the general concepts rather than the specific details, providing a step-by-step approach to analyzing pulmonary function tests. The concepts underlying this step-by-step approach are covered in the relevant section on pulmonary function tests in Chapter 3.

ANALYSIS OF PULMONARY FUNCTION TESTS

1. Examination of the lung volumes:
    a. A decrease in total lung capacity (TLC) generally indicates the presence of a restrictive pattern. However, TLC measured by helium dilution may also be artificially depressed when there are poorly communicating or noncommunicating regions within the lung, for example, in bullous lung disease.
    b. Are the lung volumes symmetrically reduced, that is, are TLC, residual volume (RV), functional residual capacity (FRC), and vital capacity (VC) all decreased to approximately the same extent? If so, this suggests interstitial lung disease as the cause of the restrictive pattern. A low diffusing capacity also supports the diagnosis of interstitial lung disease as the cause of the restrictive pattern.
    c. A relatively preserved RV and a normal diffusing capacity suggest another cause of restrictive disease, such as neuromuscular or chest wall disease. Poor effort from the patient also may create this type of pattern.
2. Examination of the mechanics, that is, the flow rates measured from the forced expiratory spirogram:
    a. A decrease in the ratio of forced expiratory volume in 1 second to forced vital capacity (FEV_1/FVC) indicates obstruction. In some cases of airflow obstruction, both FEV_1 and FVC are reduced by approximately the same extent, and FEV_1/FVC may be preserved. Clues to the presence of obstructive disease in this setting are a low forced expiratory flow from 25% to 75% of vital capacity ($FEF_{25\%-75\%}$), a normal to high TLC with a high ratio of RV to TLC, and the configuration of the flow-volume curve.
    b. Interpretation of $FEF_{25\%-75\%}$ (also called *maximal midexpiratory flow* [MMF]):
        (1) $FEF_{25\%-75\%}$ is subject to more variability than most other measurements obtained during a forced expiration, so guidelines for normal values are less well established.

    (2) When lung volumes are low, $FEF_{25\%-75\%}$ also can be decreased without necessarily indicating coexisting airflow obstruction. Therefore, in the presence of decreased lung volumes, a low $FEF_{25\%-75\%}$ indicates obstruction primarily if the decrease in $FEF_{25\%-75\%}$ is out of proportion to the decrease in lung volumes.

    (3) Taking into account the aforementioned qualifications, $FEF_{25\%-75\%}$ may be a relatively sensitive measurement for airway obstruction. An isolated abnormality in $FEF_{25\%-75\%}$ has sometimes been considered a marker for early or very mild airflow obstruction, theoretically reflecting "small airway disease."

3. Interpretation of diffusing capacity of the lung for carbon monoxide ($D_{L}CO$):

  a. Make sure that the value has been corrected for the patient's hemoglobin level. If not, the value will be falsely low if the patient is anemic.

  b. A decrease in the diffusing capacity reflects disease affecting the alveolar-capillary membrane (decreased surface area for gas exchange and/or abnormal thickness of the membrane) or a decrease in pulmonary capillary blood volume.

  c. An increase in the diffusing capacity can reflect increased pulmonary capillary blood volume or erythrocytes within alveolar spaces (pulmonary hemorrhage).

4. Interpretation of the flow-volume curve:

  a. An obstructive pattern is reflected by decreased flow relative to lung volume, generally accompanied by a "scooped out" or "coved" appearance to the descending part of the expiratory curve (see Fig. 3-19).

  b. A restrictive pattern is characterized by decreased volumes, that is, narrowing of the curve along the volume or X-axis, and relatively preserved flow rates. The flow rates often appear increased relative to the small lung volumes, producing a tall, narrow curve.

**Sample Pulmonary Function Test
Results**

1. Female 32 years of age

	Actual	Predicted	% Predicted
Lung Mechanics			
FVC (L)	1.03	3.86	27
FEV_1 (L)	0.97	3.05	32
$FEV_1/FVC \times 100$ (FEV_1 %)	95	79	120
$FEF_{25\%-75\%}$ (L/s)	2.39	3.49	68
Lung Volumes			
VC (L)	1.07	3.86	28
FRC (L)	1.59	2.89	55
TLC (L)	1.99	5.51	36
RV (L)	0.92	1.65	55
RV/TLC $\times$ 100 (%)	46	30	153
D_{LCO} (mL/min/mm Hg)	6.5	11.4	57

Expiratory Flow / Volume

Flow-volume curve

2. Male 60 years of age

	Actual	Predicted	% Predicted
Lung Mechanics			
FVC (L)	2.42	4.62	52
FEV_1 (L)	0.78	3.26	24
$FEV_1/FVC \times 100$ (FEV_1 %)	32	71	45
$FEF_{25\%-75\%}$ (L/s)	0.27	3.10	9
Lung Volumes			
VC (L)	3.23	4.62	70
FRC (L)	5.08	3.94	129
TLC (L)	6.90	7.02	98
RV (L)	3.67	2.40	153
RV/TLC $\times$ 100 (%)	53	34	156
D_{LCO} (mL/min/mm Hg)	6.8	24.5	28

Expiratory Flow / Volume

Flow-volume curve

3. Female 55 years of age

	Actual	Predicted	% Predicted
Lung Mechanics			
FVC (L)	0.93	2.73	34
FEV_1 (L)	0.80	2.03	39
$FEV_1/FVC \times 100$ (FEV_1 %)	86	75	115
$FEF_{25\%-75\%}$ (L/s)	1.60	2.50	64
Lung Volumes			
VC (L)	0.90	2.73	33
FRC (L)	1.50	2.29	66
TLC (L)	2.14	4.18	51
RV (L)	1.24	1.46	85
RV/TLC $\times$ 100 (%)	58	35	166
D_{LCO} (mL/min/mm Hg)	14	12.9	109

Expiratory Flow / Volume

Flow-volume curve

Answers

1. All measurements of lung volume (TLC, VC, FRC, RV) are significantly decreased, indicative of restrictive disease. FEV_1 and FVC are decreased because of the low lung volumes, but FEV_1/FVC is preserved. This finding, along with the fact that $FEF_{25\%-75\%}$ is not decreased out of proportion to the decrease in lung volumes, indicates that there is no obstruction. Diffusing capacity is decreased, suggesting that the restrictive disease is secondary to an abnormality of the pulmonary parenchyma rather than a result of chest wall or neuromuscular disease. The flow-volume curve is tall and narrow, consistent with a restrictive pattern. *Diagnosis:* Interstitial lung disease secondary to pulmonary sarcoidosis.

2. FEV_1 and FVC both are decreased. Because FEV_1 is decreased more than is FVC, FEV_1/FVC is decreased. $FEF_{25\%-75\%}$ also is decreased. These values are indicative of obstructive lung disease. TLC is normal, and RV and FRC are increased. RV/TLC ratio also is increased. Therefore, there is no restriction, but the high RV/TLC ratio indicates there is "air trapping," as is often expected with airflow obstruction. The diffusing capacity is decreased, reflecting loss of alveolar-capillary bed. The flow-volume curve shows an obstructive pattern, characterized by a striking decrease in flow rates, well seen throughout most of the expiratory curve after the initial peak flow rate. This combination of significant airflow obstruction with normal or increased volumes and a low diffusing capacity suggests emphysema.

3. TLC and FRC are reduced, indicating restrictive disease. RV is relatively preserved. FEV_1 and FVC both are decreased, but FEV_1/FVC ratio is preserved. There is no evidence for coexisting obstructive disease. Diffusing capacity is normal, suggesting that the alveolar-capillary bed is preserved. The flow-volume curve is relatively tall and narrow, without any evidence of obstructive disease. *Diagnosis:* Restrictive pattern secondary to chest wall disease (kyphoscoliosis).

Arterial Blood Gases: Guidelines for Interpretation and Sample Problems

The following guidelines are meant to expand on the material presented in Chapter 3 and to simplify the interpretation of arterial blood gas values. Because memorizing a "cookbook" approach can sometimes be counterproductive if the reason why the approach is being used is not clear, these guidelines are meant to supplement a basic understanding of the underlying physiologic principles.

Numerous formulas are used to assess the appropriateness of compensation for a primary acid-base disorder. These formulas are particularly useful for suggesting whether a mixed acid-base disorder is present. Table C-1 lists commonly used formulas that predict the expected degree of respiratory compensation for a primary metabolic problem and metabolic compensation for a primary respiratory problem. These formulas relate arterial PCO_2 and measured HCO_3^-. However, measured values from arterial blood gases include arterial PCO_2 and pH, not serum HCO_3^-. Therefore, to use the formulas in the table, one must either measure serum HCO_3^- (as part of serum electrolyte values) or use a value calculated from PCO_2 and pH according to the Henderson-Hasselbalch equation.

Alternatively, one can use other guidelines relating PCO_2 and pH values. Because these latter guidelines are based on direct measurements obtained with arterial blood gases—and because they are relatively easy to remember—they are used in the method outlined here. However, these easy-to-remember formulas relating PCO_2 and pH become less accurate at the extremes of PCO_2 and pH values. Also, the formulas provide only rough guidelines; the human body does not respond to physiologic disturbances with mathematical precision.

ANALYSIS OF ACID-BASE STATUS

1. Look at the pH value to determine the *net* disturbance in acid-base balance. An alkalotic pH (>7.44) indicates the presence of a primary respiratory alkalosis, a metabolic alkalosis, or both. An acidotic pH (<7.36) indicates the presence of a primary respiratory acidosis, a metabolic acidosis, or both. A normal pH (approximately 7.36–7.44) indicates normal acid-base status or a mixed disturbance (of two balancing problems).

2. Look at PCO_2. A high PCO_2 (>44) indicates that a *respiratory acidosis* is present. A low PCO_2 (<36) indicates that a *respiratory alkalosis* is present. If the pH value moves in the appropriate direction for the PCO_2 change (i.e., $\downarrow$ pH with $\uparrow$ PCO_2; $\uparrow$ pH with $\downarrow$ PCO_2), then the respiratory disorder is the *primary* disturbance. If the pH value does not move in the appropriate direction for the PCO_2 change, then a metabolic disorder is the primary disorder.

Table	C-1

EXPECTED COMPENSATION FOR PRIMARY ACID-BASE DISORDERS

Primary Disorder	Compensatory Response	Expected Magnitude of Response
Metabolic acidosis	↓ Pco_2	$Pco_2 = 1.5 \times (HCO_3^-) + 8 \pm 2$
Metabolic alkalosis	↑ Pco_2	Pco_2 increases 6 mm Hg for each 10 mEq/L increase in HCO_3^-
Respiratory acidosis	↑ HCO_3^-	Acute: HCO_3^- increases 1 mEq/L for each 10 mm Hg increase in Pco_2
		Chronic: HCO_3^- increases 3.5 mEq/L for each 10 mm Hg increase in Pco_2
Respiratory alkalosis	↓ HCO_3^-	Acute: HCO_3^- falls 2 mEq/L for each 10 mm Hg decrease in Pco_2
		Chronic: HCO_3^- falls 5 mEq/L for each 10 mm Hg decrease in Pco_2

Adapted from Narins RG, Emmett M: *Medicine* 59:161–186, 1980. © by Williams & Wilkins, 1980.

3. When a primary respiratory disorder is present, the pH value should change approximately 0.08 units for each 10 mm Hg change in Pco_2 if the process is acute. If the process is chronic, the kidneys compensate (by retaining or losing HCO_3^-) and blunt the pH change in response to any change in Pco_2. The resulting change in pH when the respiratory disorder is chronic is slightly different for acidosis versus alkalosis. With a chronic respiratory acidosis, the expected pH decrease is approximately 0.03 for each 10 mm Hg increase in Pco_2. With a chronic respiratory alkalosis, the expected pH increase is approximately 0.02 for each 10 mm Hg decrease in Pco_2.

4. If a pH change cannot be explained by an alteration in Pco_2, then a primary metabolic disturbance is present. A low pH value with a low Pco_2 indicates a *primary metabolic acidosis* with respiratory compensation. A high pH value with a high Pco_2 can indicate a *primary metabolic alkalosis* with secondary suppression of respiratory drive. However, in many patients the latter pattern of a high pH value with a high Pco_2 often represents a complex acid-base disturbance, such as a chronic compensated respiratory acidosis with a superimposed primary metabolic alkalosis (e.g., as a result of diuretics, vomiting, or nasogastric suction).

5. To determine whether there has been appropriate respiratory compensation for a primary metabolic disorder, a rough guideline is that Pco_2 should approximate the last two digits of the pH value. For example, a Pco_2 of 25 mm Hg accompanying a pH value of 7.25 indicates appropriate respiratory compensation for a primary metabolic acidosis. However, the degree of compensatory hyperventilation (i.e., lowering of Pco_2) for a metabolic acidosis tends to be more predictable than the degree of compensatory hypoventilation (i.e., CO_2 retention) accompanying a metabolic alkalosis.

ANALYSIS OF OXYGENATION

1. When analyzing arterial Po_2, first calculate alveolar Po_2 according to the following equation:

$$P_{AO_2} = (713 \times F_{IO_2}) - \frac{Pco_2}{0.8}$$

For room air, the equation can be simplified as follows: $P_{AO_2} = 150 - (1.25 \times Pco_2)$. Then calculate the alveolar-arterial O_2 gradient ($AaDo_2$), which is the difference between the calculated P_{AO_2} and the measured P_{AO_2}: $AaDo_2 = P_{AO_2} - Pa_{O_2}$.

2. If the patient is hypoxemic, Pco_2 is elevated, and $AaDo_2$ is normal (<15 mm Hg on room air in a young person, although it increases with age), then *hypoventilation* is the cause of the hypoxemia.

3. If the patient is hypoxemic, Pco_2 is normal or low, and $AaDo_2$ is increased, then either $\dot{V}/\dot{Q}$ *mismatch* or *shunting* is present. With $\dot{V}/\dot{Q}$ mismatch, the patient's Pao_2 has a good response to administration of supplemental O_2. With a true shunt, Pao_2 does not rise much with supplemental O_2 (even 100% O_2).

4. If the patient is hypoxemic, Pco_2 is high, and $AaDo_2$ is increased, then the patient has both hypoventilation *and* either $\dot{V}/\dot{Q}$ mismatch or shunt as the cause of the low Pao_2.

SAMPLE PROBLEMS

All blood gases are drawn with the patient breathing room air ($FIo_2 = 0.21$), except as otherwise noted.

1.	Room air	$Po_2 = 45$ mm Hg	$Pco_2 = 30$ mm Hg	pH = 7.47
	(100% O_2)	$Po_2 = 65$ mm Hg	$Pco_2 = 32$ mm Hg	pH = 7.46
2.	Room air	$Po_2 = 45$ mm Hg	$Pco_2 = 30$ mm Hg	pH = 7.47
	(100% O_2)	$Po_2 = 560$ mm Hg	$Pco_2 = 32$ mm Hg	pH = 7.46
3.		$Po_2 = 88$ mm Hg	$Pco_2 = 20$ mm Hg	pH = 7.55
4.		$Po_2 = 65$ mm Hg	$Pco_2 = 60$ mm Hg	pH = 7.35
5.		$Po_2 = 30$ mm Hg	$Pco_2 = 60$ mm Hg	pH = 7.35
6.		$Po_2 = 110$ mm Hg	$Pco_2 = 20$ mm Hg	pH = 7.30
7.		$Po_2 = 55$ mm Hg	$Pco_2 = 48$ mm Hg	pH = 7.49
8.		$Po_2 = 90$ mm Hg	$Pco_2 = 60$ mm Hg	pH = 7.20

Answers

1. Acute respiratory alkalosis. On room air, the patient's $AaDo_2 = 67.5$ mm Hg, which is elevated. The minimal elevation in Po_2 with 100% O_2 indicates that a shunt is the major cause of the hypoxemia.

2. Identical to Problem 1, except that the dramatic increase in Po_2 with 100% O_2 indicates that ventilation-perfusion mismatch is the major cause of the hypoxemia.

3. Acute respiratory alkalosis. Even though Po_2 appears normal, $AaDo_2$ is elevated to 37 mm Hg, indicating the presence of a disorder impairing normal oxygenation of blood.

4. Chronic respiratory acidosis. $AaDo_2 = 10$ mm Hg, indicating that hypoxemia is due to hypoventilation.

5. Chronic respiratory acidosis, as in Problem 4. However, unlike Problem 4, $AaDo_2$ is elevated (to 45 mm Hg), indicating that both hypoventilation and either ventilation-perfusion mismatch or shunting (most likely the former) are responsible for the hypoxemia.

6. Mixed acid-base disorder with a primary metabolic acidosis complicated by a primary respiratory alkalosis. Pco_2 is too low to represent just compensation for the metabolic acidosis, indicating the presence of a respiratory alkalosis as well. $AaDo_2 = 15$ mm Hg, the upper limit of normal for a young adult.

7. The simplest explanation of the acid-base status is a compensated metabolic alkalosis. However, this pattern probably is seen more commonly with a mixed acid-base disorder consisting of a compensated respiratory acidosis complicated by a superimposed primary metabolic alkalosis. $AaDo_2 = 35$ mm Hg. Therefore hypoxemia is due partly to hypoventilation but mostly to ventilation-perfusion mismatch or shunt, probably the former.

8. Something is wrong because $AaDo_2$ is negative (-15 mm Hg). Several possible explanations are as follows: (a) the patient was receiving supplemental O_2; (b) a laboratory error was made; or (c) the blood was not collected or transported properly under anaerobic conditions.

Index

Page numbers followed by *f* refer to figures; *t* refers to tables